Innovative Research in Thermal Imaging for Biology and Medicine

Ricardo Vardasca
University of Porto, Portugal

Joaquim Gabriel Mendes
University of Porto, Portugal

A volume in the Advances in Medical Technologies and Clinical Practice (AMTCP) Book Series

IGI Global
DISSEMINATOR OF KNOWLEDGE

www.igi-global.com

Published in the United States of America by
IGI Global
Medical Information Science Reference (an imprint of IGI Global)
701 E. Chocolate Avenue
Hershey PA, USA 17033
Tel: 717-533-8845
Fax: 717-533-8661
E-mail: cust@igi-global.com
Web site: http://www.igi-global.com

Library of Congress Cataloging-in-Publication Data

Names: Vardasca, Ricardo, 1977- editor. | Gabriel, Joaquim, editor.
Title: Innovative research in thermal imaging for biology and medicine / Ricardo Vardasca and Joaquim Gabriel Mendes, editors.
Description: Hershey, PA : Medical Information Science Reference, [2017] | Includes bibliographical references and index.
Identifiers: LCCN 2016053532| ISBN 9781522520726 (hardcover) | ISBN 9781522520733 (ebook)
Subjects: | MESH: Thermography--methods | Research
Classification: LCC RC78.7.T5 | NLM WN 205 | DDC 616.07/54072--dc23 LC record available at https://lccn.loc.gov/2016053532

This book is published in the IGI Global book series Advances in Medical Technologies and Clinical Practice (AMTCP) (ISSN: 2327-9354; eISSN: 2327-9370)

British Cataloguing in Publication Data
A Cataloguing in Publication record for this book is available from the British Library.

All work contributed to this book is new, previously-unpublished material. The views expressed in this book are those of the authors, but not necessarily of the publisher.

For electronic access to this publication, please contact: eresources@igi-global.com.

Advances in Medical Technologies and Clinical Practice (AMTCP) Book Series

Srikanta Patnaik
SOA University, India
Priti Das
S.C.B. Medical College, India

ISSN:2327-9354
EISSN:2327-9370

Mission

Medical technological innovation continues to provide avenues of research for faster and safer diagnosis and treatments for patients. Practitioners must stay up to date with these latest advancements to provide the best care for nursing and clinical practices.

The **Advances in Medical Technologies and Clinical Practice (AMTCP) Book Series** brings together the most recent research on the latest technology used in areas of nursing informatics, clinical technology, biomedicine, diagnostic technologies, and more. Researchers, students, and practitioners in this field will benefit from this fundamental coverage on the use of technology in clinical practices.

Coverage

- Medical Informatics
- E-Health
- Clinical Studies
- Clinical Data Mining
- Medical Imaging
- Biometrics
- Telemedicine
- Nutrition
- Clinical High-Performance Computing
- Diagnostic Technologies

IGI Global is currently accepting manuscripts for publication within this series. To submit a proposal for a volume in this series, please contact our Acquisition Editors at Acquisitions@igi-global.com or visit: http://www.igi-global.com/publish/.

The Advances in Medical Technologies and Clinical Practice (AMTCP) Book Series (ISSN 2327-9354) is published by IGI Global, 701 E. Chocolate Avenue, Hershey, PA 17033-1240, USA, www.igi-global.com. This series is composed of titles available for purchase individually; each title is edited to be contextually exclusive from any other title within the series. For pricing and ordering information please visit http://www.igi-global.com/book-series/advances-medical-technologies-clinical-practice/73682. Postmaster: Send all address changes to above address.

Titles in this Series

For a list of additional titles in this series, please visit: www.igi-global.com

Internet of Things and Advanced Application in Healthcare
Catarina I. Reis (Polytechnic Institute of Leiria, Portugal) and Marisa da Silva Maximiano (Polytechnic Institute of Leiria, Portugal)
Medical Information Science Reference • copyright 2017 • 349pp • H/C (ISBN: 9781522518204) • US $210.00

Integrating Biologically-Inspired Nanotechnology into Medical Practice
B.K. Nayak (K.M. Centre for Post Graduate Studies, India) Anima Nanda (Sathyabama University, India) and M. Amin Bhat (Sathyabama University, India)
Medical Information Science Reference • copyright 2017 • 394pp • H/C (ISBN: 9781522506102) • US $190.00

Recent Advances in Drug Delivery Technology
Raj K. Keservani (Rajiv Gandhi Proudyogiki Vishwavidyalaya, India) Anil K. Sharma (Delhi Institute of Pharmaceutical Sciences and Research, India) and Rajesh Kumar Kesharwani (National Institute of Technology, Warangal, India)
Medical Information Science Reference • copyright 2017 • 510pp • H/C (ISBN: 9781522507543) • US $215.00

Advancing Medicine through Nanotechnology and Nanomechanics Applications
Keka Talukdar (Nadiha High School, India) Mayank Bhushan (Pondicherry University, India) and Anil Shantappa Malipatil (Guru Nanak Dev Engineering College – Bidar, India)
Medical Information Science Reference • copyright 2017 • 359pp • H/C (ISBN: 9781522510437) • US $195.00

Pattern and Data Analysis in Healthcare Settings
Vivek Tiwari (Maulana Azad National Institute of Technology, India) Basant Tiwari (Devi Ahilya University, India) Ramjeevan Singh Thakur (Maulana Azad National Institute of Technology, India) and Shailendra Gupta (AISECT University, India)
Medical Information Science Reference • copyright 2017 • 358pp • H/C (ISBN: 9781522505365) • US $215.00

Novel Approaches for Drug Delivery
Raj K. Keservani (Rajiv Gandhi Proudyogiki Vishwavidyalaya, India) Anil K. Sharma (Delhi Institute of Pharmaceutical Sciences and Research, India) and Rajesh Kumar Kesharwani (National Institute of Technology, Warangal, India)
Medical Information Science Reference • copyright 2017 • 515pp • H/C (ISBN: 9781522507512) • US $210.00

Emerging Research in the Analysis and Modeling of Gene Regulatory Networks
Ivan V. Ivanov (Texas A&M University, USA) Xiaoning Qian (Texas A&M University, USA) and Ranadip Pal (Texas Tech University, USA)
Medical Information Science Reference • copyright 2016 • 418pp • H/C (ISBN: 9781522503538) • US $195.00

Editorial Advisory Board

Table of Contents

Detailed Table of Contents

imaging and duplex scanning. Such results also suggest that thermovision diagnostics may be useful as a complementary and first of all objective method that can be used in the diagnosis of chronic venous diseases in the lower extremities. It may suggest that thermovision may be used as a screening method or together with an ultrasound diagnosis in different superficial veins disorders.

Enrique Sanchis-Sánchez, University of Valencia, Spain
Rosario Salvador-Palmer, University of Valencia, Spain
Pilar Codoñer-Franch, Hospital Universitario Doctor Peset, Spain
Jose Martín-Guerrero, University of Valencia, Spain
Carlos Vergara-Hernández, CSISP-FISABIO, Spain
Jose María Blasco, University of Valencia, Spain
Esther Ballester, Hospital Universitario Doctor Peset, Spain
Enrique J Sanchis, University of Valencia, Spain
Rolando González-Peña, University of Valencia, Spain
Jose I. Priego-Quesada, University of Valencia, Spain
Rosa M Cibrián, University of Valencia, Spain

The study of the diagnostic accuracy of Infrared Thermal Imaging in the diagnosis of orthopaedic injuries in childhood has been motivated by the high incidence of these injuries throughout the world, being one of the most common reasons for urgent medical consultation. Diagnosis of musculoskeletal injuries usually involves radiography, but this exposes children without fractures to unnecessary ionising radiation. This chapter assesses whether infrared thermography could provide a viable alternative in cases of trauma. To evaluate the accuracy of this technique new thermographic variables have been added to those commonly analysed, such as the extent of the injury and the difference in the size of the area that is at an equal temperature or higher than the maximum temperature of the healthy area. Non-linear cataloguing methods (decision tree models) have also been applied. With the protocol presented, infrared thermal imaging had a sensitivity of 0.91, a specificity of 0.88 and a negative predictive value of 0.95 for diagnosing musculoskeletal injuries.

Francis Ring, University of South Wales, UK
Carl Jones, University of South Wales, UK
Kurt Ammer, University of South Wales, UK
Peter Plassmann, University of South Wales, UK
Ricardo Vardasca, University of Porto, Portugal
Usama I. Bajwa, COMSATS Institute of Information Technology, Pakistan

There are cooling products available for relieving the pain of minor sports injuries, in muscles, tendons, joints, strains, sprains and knocks. These products are based on ice, gel and cold patches. In order to quantify objectively the effect of each type of those products thermal imaging was used. This monitoring method is suitable to quantify quickly large regions of interest in skin areas over time through the thermal radiation perceived by thermal camera sensors. All recorded images were taken in a controlled environment and following a standard capture protocol in terms of subject, equipment and examination room preparation and procedure of conduction the examination. Two experiments were performed. The obtained results demonstrate that quantitative thermal imaging is a simple and objective tool for evaluating topical cooling treatments. However, it is important to assess the emissivity of any applied substance, which could have a significant effect on temperature measurement by remote sensing.

The use of low temperature on the whole human body switched on beneficial physiological reactions. Whole-body cryotherapy is used as a part of rehabilitation. There were reported studies of thermal imaging performed due to whole body cooling in case of patients suffering from different diseases that showed a significant enhancement of the skin temperature gradient observed after cryotherapy. That explains that such therapeutic technique like whole-body cryotherapy can be used as a part of infrared thermography diagnostic procedure.

It is known that the myofascial trigger points (MTP) and myogenous temporomandibular disorders (TMDs) cause regional sympathetic hyperactivity in local temperature due to the cutaneous vasomotor activity and, for detection of functional changes, thermography is used as an complementary diagnostic imaging method. This chapter intends to study two masticatory muscles, masseter and anterior temporalis, in measurement of the cutaneous temperature of volunteers with and without myogenous TMD and MTP. Results: The temperature levels measured at both muscles regions in myogenous TMD volunteers were significantly lower than those measured in controls. Infrared imaging indicated differences between referred and local pain in MTPs of 0.5°C. Conclusions: Infrared imaging measurements seem to indicate that it can be used as an aid in complimentary diagnosing of TMDs and MTPs in masticatory muscles.

The thermoregulation mechanisms during the physical effort can be easily study by using the thermovision. The thermoregulation mechanisms in human body keep the body core temperature on basic level 37 ± 2oC. However, the question is if there are any differences in skin surface temperature distribution between trainee sportsmen and amateur. Is there any possibility to show the sportsman level of practise using the thermal imaging? Would it be possible to evaluate the efficiency of athlete or evaluate the level of sports possibilities in average amateur who just wants to start cycle training. To find how the thermoregulation mechanisms work the different measurements were done i.e. during the cyclist endurance test for group of male cyclist (intermediate level of cycling skill) and during the Aerobic Circuit Training (ACT) for trainee and amateur group of women.

Sports injuries are one of the most important problems in sports. Moreover, professional sports injuries lead to a difficult recovery process for the athletes, reduced athletic performance, and large economic costs. Infrared thermography (IRT) is a safe, non-invasive and low-cost technique that allows for the rapid and non-contact recording of Skin Temperature (Tsk). Recent research results have demonstrated new applications for this technique; among them, the monitoring and prevention of sports injuries appears to be one of the most interesting applications. Although IRT is not as objective as other methods, it may be sufficiently accurate and reliable as a complementary tool considering the theory that musculoskeletal structures should be in thermal equilibrium when in a healthy state. Therefore, the main contribution of IRT is to help identify an injury before it occurs, providing an opportunity for preventative action.

In order to verify whether there is a considerable increase in body skin temperature during different swimming techniques (crawl and backstroke) and identifying the most affected regions. The athlete's thermal symmetry was also analyzed, as well as its modification after the swimming, according to the performed technique. The accuracy of thermography as a method to identify and distinguish these different styles was also evaluated. Ten male swimmers were recruited and two different swimming techniques were assessed, crawl and backstroke. After a 10 minute acclimatization period in the pool, the swimmers were quickly dried with microfiber towels. The thermograms were taken before and after the swimming task, which consisted in a 7x200m protocol in crawl or backstroke. Infrared thermography revealed an increase of temperature after exercise and no significant differences were found between both techniques. Thermal symmetry was not affected by exercise.

This chapter describes an approach to quantifying the local inflammatory response at the injection site after a vaccination by infrared imaging. The aim is to develop a thermographic procedure providing support to evaluate the reactivity of a vaccine. The development of the experimental design had to consider an optimum timeframe for infrared imaging, the variability of the local thermal emission, questions regarding the thermal left-right symmetry and further biometric aspects. To verify this concept, more than 80 participants of the influenza vaccination campaign were involved. Even if this study is based on a well-tolerated seasonal influenza vaccination, nearly 40% of all subjects show a pronounced thermal reaction of approximately 1°C. Apart from this, 25-30% displays no signs of any thermal response. The question of how far thermal imaging will contribute to facilitating the assessment of the reactivity of a vaccine has several aspects which are discussed in this chapter.

Laboratory animals provide important models for studying human diseases, including many types of cancer. Mice are among the most commonly used laboratory animals, allowing for the study of carcinogenic agents, cancer development and for testing innovative preventive and therapeutic strategies. Thus, monitoring angiogenesis in animal models is a major goal for cancer research. Among the currently available imaging techniques, thermography is a useful approach for studying the superficial vascularization of cancer, based on their heat emissions. At this chapter emphasis is placed on thermography and its applications on laboratory animals, in comparison with other available and applicable imaging techniques. In conclusion, thermography may be usefully applied to the study of cancer vascularization in animal models, particularly when using laboratory rodents such as mice. Care is needed in adapting existing approaches to the specificities of each animal species.

Foreword

This book provides a overview of the latest research in biology and medicine which involved infrared thermal imaging. It engaged professionals from different areas of the globe with different expertise, whom had promoted multidisciplinarity and enriched the generated knowledge.

The book is organized in a logical order, it presents ideas in how to conceive a examination laboratory, applications in microvascular and pediatric orthopedics, use of cooling agents and cryotherapy, dentistry, evaluation of physical fitness, prevention of sports injury, monitoring of swimming techniques, assessment of application of vaccines, monitoring of animal models of cancer and ending with assessment of racehorses performance.

It is goal of this publication to contribute for a widespread of infrared imaging knowledge and understanding along with its main applications and future developments.

The editors hope that the reader enjoys reading this publication and it contributes to the endowment of his wisdom in the application of infrared thermal imaging in Biology and Medicine.

Ricardo Vardasca
University of Porto, Portugal

Joaquim Gabriel
University of Porto, Portugal

Preface

INTRODUCTION

The study of temperature in living animals and humans has a long and interesting history. One of the greatest advances in scientific research in this whole area however, has been the ability to harness thermal radiation as a remote sensing technique. Infrared thermal imaging provides an efficient means of recording two-dimensional temperature distributions at the body surface.

The amount of that data now obtainable in fractions of a second is considerable. In the past, individual thermocouples were linked to multichannel recorders in order to monitor temperature over time. A modern day thermogram provides such an increased amount of thermal data, that it seems like comparing the progress of a human on a bicycle with flying in a jet aircraft!

The double technological advantage is of course provided by computing. Digital thermal imaging provides an enormous advantage, in both recording the distribution of temperature and its progress in a dynamic time sequence.

This book brings together a number of studies that reflect the diverse but practical ways in which thermal imaging is contributing to modern physiology of life sciences.

It is now well established that the human skin is an efficient black body radiator. Thermal imaging therefore provides information on skin temperature, and in that sense, should not be confused with many of the medical imaging procedures that are designed to study internal structures or organs.

MODERN RESEARCH STUDIES

It is established from many publications that blood flow and thermoregulation are related, and there are certainly situations where changes in local perfusion can be a major influence on skin temperature distribution. Hence we can see from the first two chapters that thermal imaging has a useful and often complementary role in determining the status of the microcirculation and its clinical relevance.

Another advantage of thermal imaging is that this technique in passive and non-contact, and often proves to be an advantage, especially in diagnostic procedures in children and shown in Chapter 3.

It is understandable that some investigators are cautious of the study of skin temperature that can have many internal and external influences. Research has shown that by careful standardisation of technique, reproducible results can be obtained, making the control of environmental conditions an essential part of any acceptable study of temperature of the skin. However, topically applied medication has become a feature of pharmacology today.

Chapter 4 shows some experiments to document these effects on the skin. In Chapter 5 we also see that cryogenic temperatures, practised in some specialist centres does have a clear influence of body surface temperature, and can influence localised inflammatory disturbances. Thermal imaging is clearly an ideal means of monitoring these effects and the thermal reactions in skin temperature that such therapy can induce.

Chapter 6 presents a methodology for assessing the myogenous temporomandibular disorders and myofascial trigger points in the masticatory muscles, a relevant application in dentistry.

Modern sport scientists have recognised the value of these techniques and have utilised thermal imaging as a means of studying fitness regimes, and elite training effects. Chapter 7 and 8 demonstrate these aspects of sport science. Equally, these procedures are of value in assessing local injuries obtained through sporting activities. Furthermore, of particular interest in this area is the recovery from injury and the search for indicators for the signs of repair or fitness to return to sport, and outlined in Chapter 8 and in Chapter 9 as a means of preventing overstrain or injury as a measure of good and efficient practice.

The sport theme continues through chapter 9 in the study of swimming, where immersion in water, a completely different environment for the human body has measureable effects. Much of the sport science research has much further to go, and without doubt the arrival of cost effective technology for thermal imaging will lead to more research in the months and years ahead.

Chapters 10 and 11 return to the medical theme- in vaccine safety research and in animal models of cancer. These will continue to be of importance in the wider field of disease and pharmacological research.

The final chapter provides some insight into the field of veterinary research. The study of horses in particular has been made over some decades in the past. This is another are where the modern infrared camera technology has been of special value. In earlier years, large and noisy cameras (operating high speed scanning motors) have not been ideally suited to study of the often quite nervous animals. Small portable and silent cameras are now available and are particularly well adaptable for use in veterinary medicine

CONCLUSION

The compilation of research studies embraces a wide biological field, but will provide useful reference data for many researchers entering this area. It is well referenced, and demonstrates that temperature research in medicine now has a further dimension. Non-invasive imaging combined with the wide range of computing and processing make this technology more cost effective than at any time in the last fifty years. The use of careful and critical technique remains essential, but should continue to yield valuable contributions to medical and veterinary science.

Francis J Ring
University of South Wales, UK

Acknowledgment

The editors would like to thank all the authors and reviewers that engaged in the adventure of producing this piece of literature, without their commitment and availability it would be impossible to accomplish.

Most of the studies presented in this research manuscript had involved laboratories, borrowed equipment, anonymous participants and funding, a word of gratitude to those who made this possible.

Chapter 1
Development of a Clinical Microvascular Imaging and Vascular Optics Facility:
The Newcastle Upon Tyne (UK) Experience

John Allen
Freeman Hospital, Newcastle upton Tyne, UK

ABSTRACT

The Newcastle Microvascular Diagnostics Service (MDS) provides a comprehensive array of optical and thermal technologies for assessing micro-circulatory blood flow and function. Thermography is a key modality, although the facility has capability for capillaroscopy, laser Doppler perfusion / speckle contrast imaging, as well as numerous non-imaging techniques. The test portfolio covers four main areas: connective tissue disease and Raynaud's phenomenon, specialist limb studies (i.e. amputation level, muscle compartment perfusion and venous physiology), neurovascular assessment, and burn wound depth assessment. The MDS greatly benefits from a state-of-the-art temperature and humidity-controlled clinical room, enabling thermal physiology investigations to be performed efficiently and with confidence. Extensive research and development (R&D) is also undertaken, with collaborations across a range of academic, clinical and industrial partners. This chapter summarizes the history and development of the MDS, tests performed, R&D undertaken, clinical management, and future service directions.

INTRODUCTION

Background

The microcirculation is the circulation of the blood in the smallest blood vessels in the body, comprising arterioles, capillaries and venules. The main functions of the microcirculation are the delivery of oxygen and nutrients and the removal of carbon dioxide. It also serves to regulate blood flow and tissue perfusion thereby affecting blood pressure and responses to inflammation. Microvascular blood flow and function

DOI: 10.4018/978-1-5225-2072-6.ch001

are therefore very important to study and quantify in health and disease. The microvasculature does, however, present a particular challenge in physiological measurement because the blood vessel structure is spatially inhomogeneous and perfusion can exhibit high variability over time (Allen & Howell, 2014).

Often optical-based techniques are used for the microvascular assessment and the Newcastle upon Tyne Microvascular Diagnostics Service (MDS) in the UK provides a comprehensive array of optical and thermal non-invasive technologies for this purpose. The author's main roles are the development and management of a state-of-the-art clinical microvascular, thermal imaging assessment facilities, and associated patient clinical measurement services. Measurement technologies are mostly imaging-based and currently include thermal imaging, capillaroscopy, laser Doppler perfusion imaging and flowmetry, photoplethysmography, tissue oxygen spectroscopy, fluorescence spectroscopy, venous physiology, invasive muscle tissue perfusion, autonomic function assessment, skin heating and iontophoresis vasodilatation, and tissue objective colour spectrophotometry. Many patient groups can potentially benefit, including those with Raynaud's phenomenon, connective tissue disease, diabetes, chronic exertional muscle compartment syndrome, inflammation, chronic fatigue, burn wounds, and patients with endothelial and/or autonomic dysfunction. The measurement facility gives capability for both routine clinical measurements and provides an excellent resource for undertaking collaborative and clinically focused research and development work. The author is founder of the measurement facility and has worked with national experts to develop business plans, to procure the specialist measurement room, to introduce microvascular technologies, and also to introduce local associated measurement protocols in the form of standard operating procedures (SOP) (Allen, 2012).

This chapter summarizes the history and development of the MDS, the routine clinical services offered, and also the research and development currently undertaken. The aim of this chapter is also to emphasize the many potential opportunities for collaboration and innovation in this specialist field.

CLINICAL VASCULAR OPTICS MEASUREMENT SERVICE

History and Development: The Clinical Need

The Microvascular Diagnostics Service was founded by the author *circa* 2000 with its main imaging focus of thermography. Prior to this there were minimal resources secured for measurement equipment, staffing or room infrastructure. The patient workload was small (typically 50 patient tests per year) and with no formal service income generated from the patient work. Staffing for service delivery was also limited. The Freeman Hospital, which is part of the Newcastle upon Tyne Hospital NHS Foundation Trust (NuTH), is a centre of excellence in cardiovascular, cancer, transplantation and musculoskeletal / rheumatology and offers increasing support for developing innovative clinical measurement services for its clinical specialists and patients.

Circa 2000, there was already an established vascular ultrasound ('large blood vessel') assessment service within NuTH, but this at the time gave only limited information about patients with conditions such as Raynaud's and connective tissue diseases (e.g. systemic sclerosis). The first formal business plan was thus made in 2000/1 with Freeman Hospital colleagues in Vascular Surgery (Mr Timothy Lees), Anaesthesia (Dr Angus Pridie) and Rheumatology (Dr Ian Griffiths) to secure the purchase of a thermal imaging system (SC300 by FLIR Systems) and a capillaroscopy imaging system (KK Technology) for microvascular assessments of patients with suspected Raynaud's and connective tissue disease.

In the early years all microvascular measurements were performed in a converted clinical room that had basic temperature control but was however shared with a multitude of other staff working in research and device development. Service capacity was therefore limited because of related room access issues. The opportunity then arose *circa* 2004 to plan for a purpose built microvascular measurement facility within the new Northern Centre for Cancer Care (NCCC) building development at Freeman Hospital which was being designed to accommodate cancer services and the then Regional Medical Physics Department (RMPD) (in 2016 became Northern Medical Physics and Clinical Engineering). A business plan was written with Professor Brian Diffey, the then Clinical Director of the department. The microvascular room was designed for versatility – future proofing for new imaging modalities and research and development (R&D) opportunities. It was then in late 2008 that the new building was complete, then ready for occupying by early 2009. There was significant work involved in the commissioning and acceptance testing against specification of the microvascular room and its facilities (environmental control specification defined below). Following commissioning the facility was available full-time for patient testing from around mid-2009 leading to the current workload of approximately 500 patients studied per year (i.e. ~1000 tests). The facility has expansion capacity for clinical work and associated service R&D.

As well as the room and the imaging systems there were other very important developments for the service. In 2009 a bespoke patient database was introduced, essential for tracking patient appointments and activity and meeting the UK 6 week diagnostic waiting time limit. From 2010 a clinical technologist (Steve Burnett) was assigned to the service, followed by research scientists Costanzo Di Maria (from 2011), Audrey Macdonald (from 2014), and Dr Sam Urwin (from 2015). The move to the new facility, the introduction of the bespoke Information Technology database resource, and having dedicated staff resources were key turning points for the MDS. The training of service staff and allocated students is also very important with the aim to have continuity of provision and succession in case of staff leaving / retiring. Having scientific researchers aligned to the service also supports significant development work, also vital for future proofing of the facility. The service now has referrals from across the North East of England, and for 2013-4 financial year was from approximately 75 consultants in more than 20 hospitals. There are formal Service Level Agreements (SLAs), i.e. contracts, set up with several hospital Trusts in the region to provide an efficient way of securing block income for services delivered to an agreed quality.

Several peer-review papers are published each year from MDS research work undertaken. Furthermore, in the last few years significant grant funding in vascular optics research has been secured – opening up many further collaborative opportunities. It has taken more than 15 years (part-time) to get to its current operational capability. The successful industrial collaborations with National Physical Laboratory (NPL), Moor Instruments and Philips Research are considered success indicators, and underlining the developing clinical specialism of Microvascular / Vascular Optics in the UK. There also have been awards associated with the MDS: for innovation in public services and also innovation in vascular optics device development work including novel vascular disease detection using optical pulse methods.

Clinical Measurement Facility

Skin blood flow can be strongly influenced by environmental temperature, humidity, or even ambient noise. Consequently, measurements need to be performed in a stable controlled environment facility otherwise confidence in the diagnostic result can be compromised. MDS greatly benefits from a state-of-the-art purpose-built temperature and humidity-controlled room, enabling investigations to be performed efficiently and with confidence (Figure 1).

Figure 1. Vascular optics measurement facility - set up for a research assessment using a combination of tissue oxygenation spectrophotometry, tissue fluorescence, tissue objective colour spectrophotometry and capillaroscopy
Source: Photograph: Juliet Chenery-Robson. Reproduced with permission

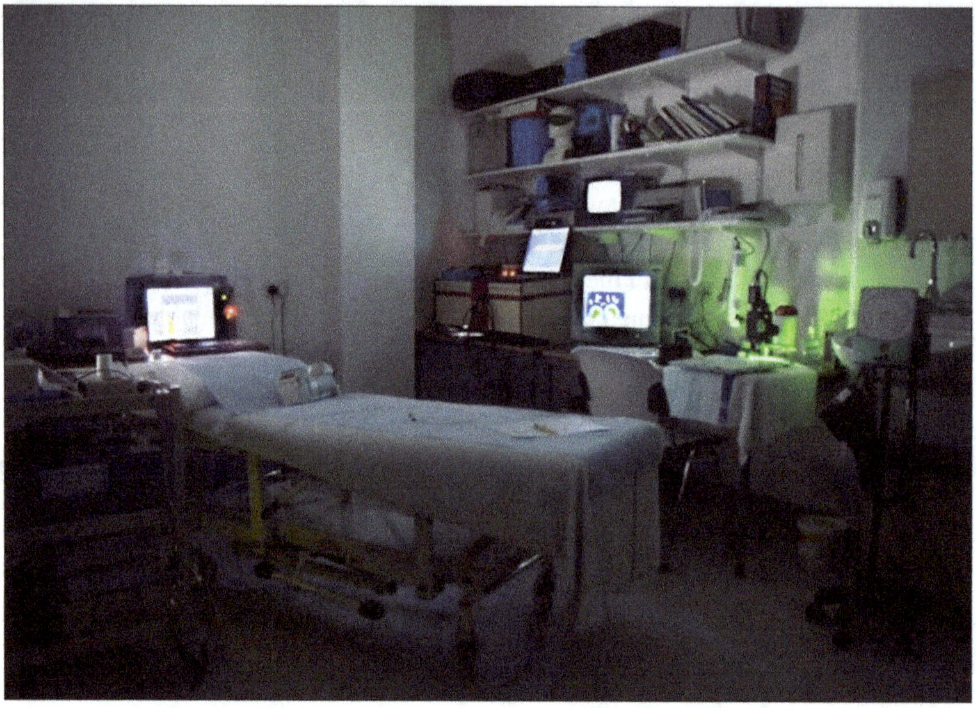

vascular optics measurement facility

The main design operating temperature is "normothermic" at 23.5 °C and 40-50% RH. The room's special air conditioning system can also be programmed to shift operating conditions between "cold" (e.g. 15 °C) and "hot" (30 °C) ambient temperatures for whole body thermal physiology assessment (with peak rate of change between hot and cold settings at close to 0.5 °C per minute). The room heating protocol can be used for specialist tests that need to induce whole body peripheral vasodilatation and the room cooling protocol used for inducing vasoconstriction. The cool room protocol at 18 °C is also used in the protocols for selected tissue inflammation studies.

The Microvascular room has been specifically designed for medical thermal imaging and microvascular measurements. It is close to square in shape and with a floor area of 20 m^2 (wall height 2.7 m). The room has minimal circulating draughts enabled by using special ceiling manifolds with swirl design. There are no windows or external building walls. All surfaces are clinical grade and wall matt paint (emulsion paint, HTM56 Cat 6) used to help reduce optical and heat reflections. Lighting is controllable by dimmer and on-off switch. A wall control enables the clinician to set the room temperature and relative humidity setpoints. At the room entrance there are shielding doors, sufficient to allow a standard hospital bed to pass through. The doors also act as a thermal buffer to help maintain tight room temperature control when staff and / or patients come and go from the adjacent waiting area and reception. The doors have vision panels with privacy blind.

The essential requirements for the controlled environmental controlled facility (adapted from original room specification):

1. The standard operating temperature range of room is 20 to 25 °C and must be held to better than 1 °C of a particular setting within this range for up to 1 hour, i.e. with the doors remaining closed throughout. However, if tighter control can be achieved without significant increases in cost and / or engineering then this must be considered. The 'normothermic' temperature of 23.5 °C will be the most frequently used setting for microvascular measurements. Local i.e. wall-mounted control of required room temperature is needed.
2. Lower and upper limits of operating temperature of at least 18 and 30 °C, respectively.
3. The standard operating relative humidity of the room is 45 ±5% at 23.5 °C. With the latest version of the room environmental control system the relative humidity setpoint can also be adjusted at the normothermic temperature setting.
4. Overall air speed should be kept as low as possible and any forced draughts must not to be directed at a patient who will normally be positioned about the centre of the room during their measurement.
5. The normothermic temperature and relative humidity specifications given above should be attainable when the room has at least 3 adult occupants with thermal imager and associated computer hardware running.
6. A target peak rate of change of room temperature of 0.5 °C per minute is required when moving from one control setpoint temperature setting to another.

Figure 2 shows the room temperature changes against set point for a 6 hour setpoint test cycle. Good stability and control is achieved at 18, 23.5 and 25 °C setpoints. This room test cycle is now performed regularly as part of service quality assurance (QA).

Microvascular Test Portfolio

The test portfolio covers four main areas: connective tissue disease and Raynaud's phenomenon assessments, specialist limb studies (i.e. amputation level, muscle compartment perfusion and venous physiology), neurovascular assessment and burn wound depth assessment. Figure 3 shows the standard issue microvascular test card used for patient referrals by the clinician.

The established measurement portfolio is provided for patient assessments from across the different clinical directorates within the hospital Trust, including rheumatology, paediatrics, vascular surgery, immunology, dermatology, neurology, respiratory medicine, regional burns centre, care of the elderly, and falls and syncope assessment. Such testing includes the investigation of peripheral skin blood flow and temperature in patients with connective tissue disease, Raynaud's phenomenon, diabetes, complex regional pain syndrome, renal fistula, inflammation, and peripheral vascular disease.

Typically, a microvascular assessment on a single patient would take approximately 1 hour to perform and 30 minutes to report. Each patient would tend to have more than 1 test performed as well as an appropriate clinical history taken. To date, the majority of patients attending the MDS will have thermography and this illustrates the great utility of this imaging technology. At current workload, approximately 500 patients are seen per year (i.e. 1000+ tests). The general increase in workload since the service was introduced some 15 years ago can be seen in Figure 4. Year on year since imaging was introduced at the

Figure 2. Example of the room temperature controlled over 6 hours from 9 am i.e. over a working day. The room temperature setpoint is switched to 18 °C (at 11 am), to 23.5 °C (12-30 pm), and then to 25 °C (1-30 pm). At steady state the variability in the measured room temperature is well within specification. The speed of room warming and cooling to setpoint demand can also be estimated. The room temperature control between these operating ranges is checked at regular intervals as part of the service quality assurance (QA)

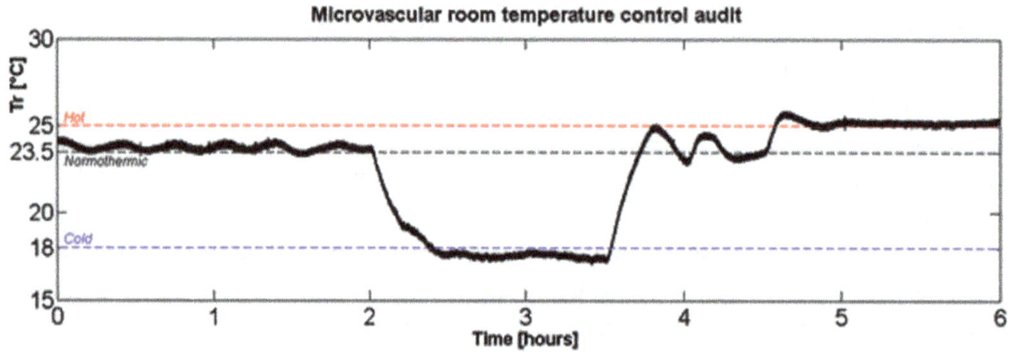

Figure 3. Microvascular test request card as used for patient referrals to the service. The portfolio test options are on the main left hand column, patient details to upper part, plus internal appointment booking notes to the right hand side. A clinical extract is also requested from the referring clinician to aid appropriate booking for the test and also for the subsequent reporting of the measurements

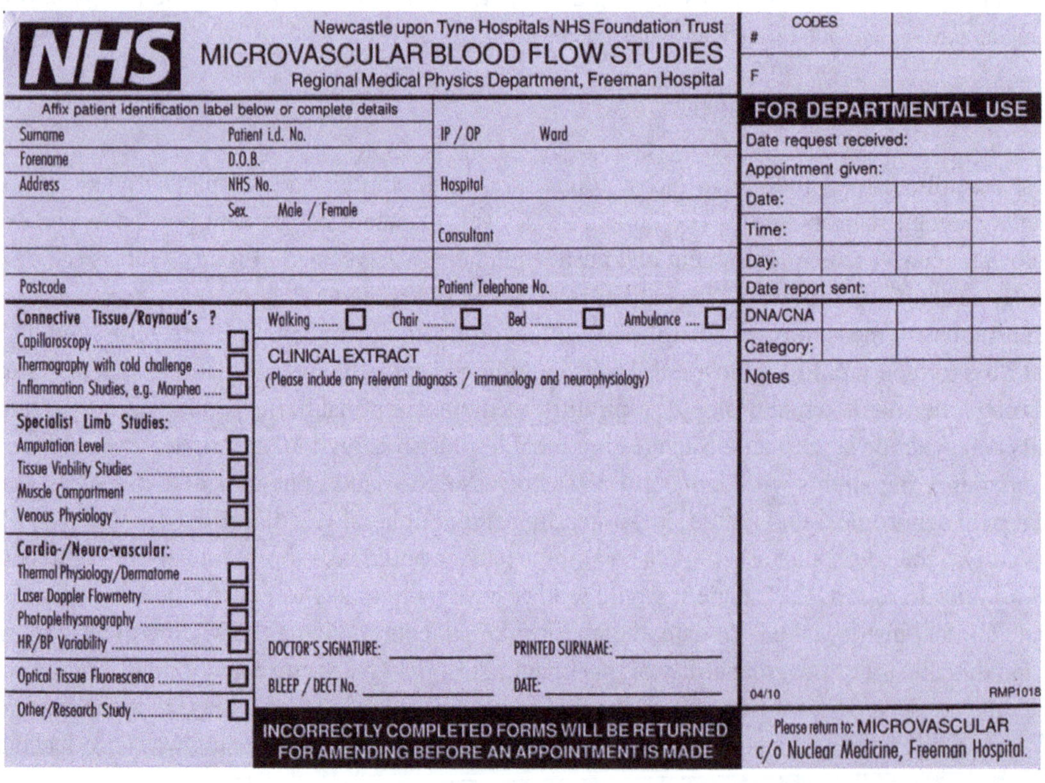

NHS
Newcastle upon Tyne Hospitals NHS Foundation Trust
MICROVASCULAR BLOOD FLOW STUDIES
Regional Medical Physics Department, Freeman Hospital

CODES
#
F

Affix patient identification label below or complete details

Surname — Patient i.d. No. — IP / OP — Ward
Forename — D.O.B.
Address — NHS No. — Hospital
Sex. Male / Female
Consultant
Postcode — Patient Telephone No.

FOR DEPARTMENTAL USE
Date request received:
Appointment given:
Date:
Time:
Day:
Date report sent:
DNA/CNA
Category:
Notes

Connective Tissue/Raynaud's ?
Capillaroscopy ☐
Thermography with cold challenge ☐
Inflammation Studies, e.g. Morphea ☐

Specialist Limb Studies:
Amputation Level ☐
Tissue Viability Studies ☐
Muscle Compartment ☐
Venous Physiology ☐

Cardio-/Neuro-vascular:
Thermal Physiology/Dermatome ☐
Laser Doppler Flowmetry ☐
Photoplethysmography ☐
HR/BP Variability ☐

Optical Tissue Fluorescence ☐

Other/Research Study ☐

Walking ☐ Chair ☐ Bed ☐ Ambulance ☐

CLINICAL EXTRACT
(Please include any relevant diagnosis / immunology and neurophysiology)

DOCTOR'S SIGNATURE: ________ PRINTED SURNAME: ________
BLEEP / DECT No. ________ DATE: ________

INCORRECTLY COMPLETED FORMS WILL BE RETURNED FOR AMENDING BEFORE AN APPOINTMENT IS MADE

04/10 RMP1018

Please return to: MICROVASCULAR c/o Nuclear Medicine, Freeman Hospital.

Figure 4. General increases in workload for the MDS. Most patients have thermography tests during their visit to the facility. Time points of note are that in 2009 the high-specification measurement room was introduced as well as the addition of the patient database. Up until 2010 the service was managed and operated solely by the Lead Clinical Scientist (JA) and with minimal infrastructure support. Service Level Agreements were established in 2011, to help provide a longer-term stable financial platform for a clinical technologist and a research scientist to join the service

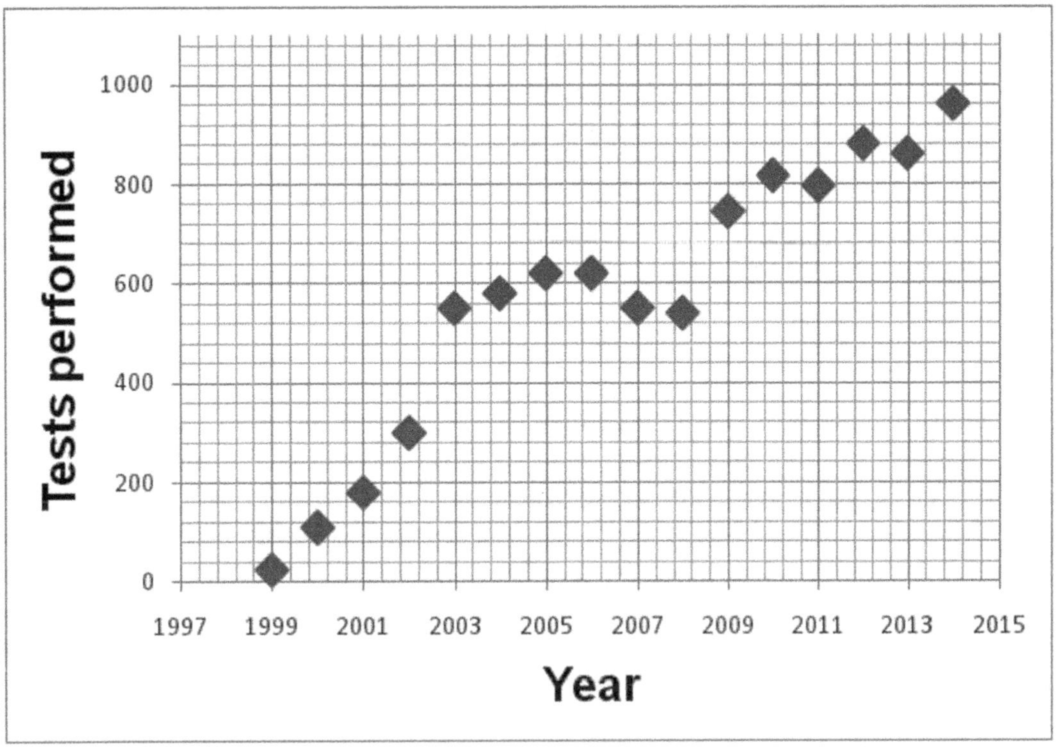

MDS the majority (at least 90%) of routine clinical tests performed have been diagnostics in Raynaud's and connective tissue disease.

Microvascular and Vascular Optic Measurement Modalities

There is a range of measurement technologies available – generally classed as either imaging or non-imaging. This range is highlighted briefly in this section but it is the medical thermal imaging which is the focus of this chapter for the book.

Imaging Modalities

The imaging modalities include thermal imaging (far infrared, camera models FLIR Systems type A40 and type SC300) (Ring & Ammer, 2012), capillaroscopy (Bollinger & Fagrell, 1990; Cutolo, 2010), and laser Doppler perfusion imaging (LDPI) (Fullerton *et al.*, 2002). In recent years other imaging technologies have been loaned and evaluated with a view to opportunity for patient service enhancement, i.e. subject to resources becoming available, and these include optical coherence tomography (OCT), hyperspectral imaging, laser speckle contrast imaging (Briers, 2001; Cheng *et al.*, 2004), and short wave infrared imaging (SWIR).

Non-Imaging Modalities

The non-imaging techniques include photoplethysmography (Allen, 2007; McKay *et al.*, 2014), laser Doppler flowmetry (iontophoresis and thermal hyperaemia challenge capability) (Anderson *et al.*, 2004; Agarwal *et al.*, 2012), tissue colour and fluorescence (i.e. UV) spectroscopy, arterial stiffness tonometry, invasive tissue pressure and volume measurements for muscle and venous physiology assessments, autonomic function (i.e. BP and heart rate variability) assessment and with tilt table capability (Allen *et al.*, 2012), plus the visible and near infrared spectroscopy of tissue oxygen.

Medical Thermal Imaging

Pre-Test Protocol for Thermal Imaging

A very important and sometimes overlooked part of the measurement procedure is the pre-test protocol that should consider both acclimatization time and also patient preparation (Ammer, 2008). In the MDS an acclimatization period of 30 minutes is used to cover both cardiovascular and thermal settling. Our protocol development experiments have shown that even healthy controls can take 30 minutes for their extremities (i.e. the hands) to thermally stabilize to be ready for imaging (Allen *et al.*, 2014).

As well as the acclimatization period it is important to ask the patient to consider diet, medicine, exercise, skin preparation, dress and turning up for their appointment in good time and not to be rushed or stressed. These pre-test guidance notes are added to our standard appointment letter that goes out to each patient. Compliance with these notes should help reduce the measurement uncertainty and aid confidence in interpretation. The patient letter guidance notes the following type of guidance and language.

To improve the diagnostic accuracy and reliability of your study you are requested to read and follow the pre-test guidance given below:

- **Diet:** In the 2 hours before your study is due to start please refrain from chocolate, tea, coffee, caffeinated soft drinks (e.g. cola), alcoholic beverages, smoking cigarettes, and taking non-prescribed stimulating drugs or substances. If not prescribed also avoid decongestant remedies. You may of course eat a light meal and drink water or juice prior to coming to the hospital.
- **Medication:** Continue taking any prescribed medicine as usual.
- **Exercise:** Avoid physical exercise or exertion in the 2 hours before your study.
- **Skin Preparation:** Avoid hand and foot skin moisturizer (or other cream), talcum powder or nail varnish.
- **Dress:** Do dress appropriately for the weather conditions. If you are sensitive to the cold then please wrap up well to keep warm and in the colder months remember to wear gloves on your way to the hospital. When in the measurement room you will need to wear suitable clothing that allows us to study the temperature of the skin surface from just above the elbows down to the hands. The clothing around the upper arms should also be loose fitting (not restrictive). If it is acceptable and possible to do so then please remove hand jewellery (e.g. rings) before coming to the hospital.

- **Relaxed:** Do arrive for your appointment in good time so you are not unduly stressed when you arrive.

On the day of the test the patient is also asked to complete a brief health questionnaire – this information will be used in the subsequent interpretation and reporting of the images (see Appendices).

Vasospastic Conditions: Raynaud's Phenomenon

One of the main applications of thermal imaging in the MDS is for the assessment of patients with vasospastic conditions. The main condition studied is Raynaud's phenomenon (RP). RP is skin vasospasm on exposure to even just mild cold or emotional stress. It has a female predilection (female to male) of 4:1. The main sites affected are the fingers and toes with distinct colour changes with the classic reported episodic phases of white (pallor), blue (cyanosis) and red (rubor), and in addition there can be numbness and paraesthesia. These classically described phases however are not present in all patients with RP and not always in RP patients with a high degree of skin pigmentation. The incidence of primary RP is in the range 3-10%. Approximately 10% of apparent RP patients who seek medical help eventually develop a secondary disorder (Spencer-Green, 1998). See Figure 5.

There are many conditions that RP can be secondary to but autoimmune connective tissue disease (CTD) is a main area of study. One CTD, known as systemic sclerosis (SSc) is associated with significant changes in the microcirculation. SSc has a varied presentation with fibrosis of the skin and internal

Figure 5. (a) Example visible image from a patient with Raynaud's. The white (pallor) phase is clearly seen in at least 3 fingers. The blue (cyanosis) and red (rubor) phases often follow this in a sequence. It is important to note that the classic three episodic colour phases ascribed to Raynaud are not always seen. Furthermore, in a patient with a high degree of skin melanin they can have grey, yellow or orange skin colour changes. Thermal imaging can give a representation of skin blood flow irrespective of skin colour. (b) shows the hands of a patient with the connective tissue disease systemic sclerosis (SSc). The image is an exaggerated case but the skin tightening and scarring on the fingers can be seen leading to flexing of the digits. SSc is of varied presentation and as well as thickening, hardening and tightening of the skin can have internal organ involvement. The majority of patients with SSc tend to also have Raynaud's

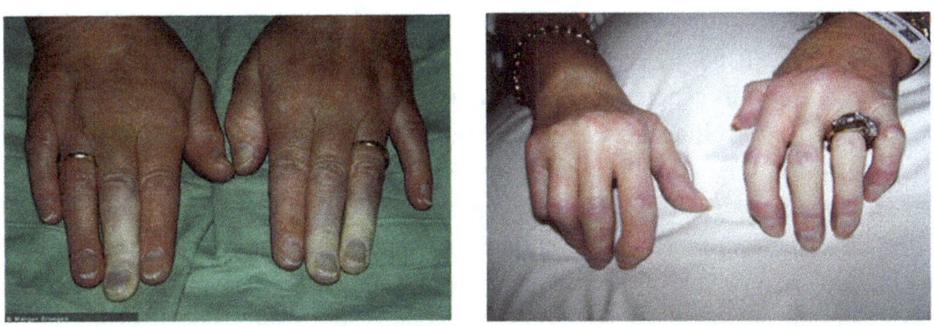

(a) Classic blanching of fingers in a patient with Raynaud's

(b) Systemic sclerosis (SSc)

organs, thickening, hardening and tightening of the skin and patients usually have RP also (Herrick 2008). SSc can be hard to diagnose early since the standard blood tests i.e. immunological screening tests are not always reliable. Microvascular imaging can aid in the diagnosis of SSc and other connective tissue diseases in association with RP. Thermal imaging can help assess the thermoregulatory microcirculation whereas other imaging techniques such as capillaroscopy (Cutolo, 2010; Cutolo *et al.,* 2010) assess the nutritional arm of the microcirculation. Patients referred to MDS for Raynaud's assessment nearly always have both of these microvascular imaging tests (Allen *et al.,* 2015a).

Since RP is not an uncommon condition it is important to note that with limited resources it is appropriate to target the test to specific patient groups. It is considered appropriate in our centre to refer patients who have the following; long-standing Raynaud's with their symptoms worsening recently; adult 30 years+ with recent onset RP (i.e. <1 year); RP and abnormal immunology (e.g. anti-nuclear antibody positive, ANA+); recent tissue viability problems at the finger and/or toe pads leading to digital ulceration; other clinical indicators (including asymmetric Raynaud's and frequent swelling of the fingers).

The standard protocol used in our centre for RP testing is 30 minutes of acclimatization in the waiting area and then 10 minutes in the microvascular measurement room with their hands resting gently on a thermally insulated measurement table - palms down. A mild cold challenge provocation to the hands is performed for 1 minute (lightly gloved and water temperature 20 °C) and an imaging follow-up time to allow for re-warming of at least 10 minutes. In the Newcastle protocol thermal images of the hands are collected at 1 minute intervals (Kumar *et al.,* 2006). The test assesses the degree of vasospasm in the peripheral circulation to cold, and post-challenge it is expected that healthy subjects to have rapid symmetrical re-warming from the fingertips, but for RP patients their response is usually clearly delayed. In RP secondary to SSc the presentation may appear thermally patchy, and in systemic lupus erythematosus (SLE, "lupus") the presentation may be thermally challenging to explain. Care needs to be taken in the image interpretation for the report, and should be made focussed and reported in clinical context by using information from the health questionnaire completed by the patient. Knowing the relevant medical history is particularly useful if there are multiple conditions and/or injuries contributing to some degree to the thermal presentations seen. See Figure 6.

A lot of emphasis is placed on the hands for microvascular assessment in RP. However it can be that patients have more problems with their feet. In the MDS we do not regularly assess the feet using cold challenge testing but instead focus on just their baseline resting state. By imaging the feet at rest the coldness of the toes, the degree of thermal asymmetry (i.e. right – left temperature difference for a region of interest which could be a localised spot or the whole hand, foot or limb) and also clear joint inflammation may be localised.

The main emphasis of this chapter is on medical thermography but the technique of capillaroscopy does need to be mentioned (Bollinger & Fagrell, 1990; Cutolo, 2010; Cutolo *et al.,* 2010). Capillaroscopy is the systematic examination of the nailfold regions of the fingers to assess the architectural structure of the capillary network, their density and distribution, shape and size (Figure 7). Nailfold capillaroscopy (NFC) can provide evidence of microvascular damage (microangiopathy) which when present can also be problematic in internal organs of the body. In primary RP patients the capillaries may exhibit only minor changes from the normal range but in SSc they can be strikingly abnormal. In other connective tissue diseases such as lupus and diabetes there can also be microangiopathy, but not usually to the degree seen in patients with SSc.

Figure 6. Example thermal images post-cold challenge from patients with Raynaud's. In image (a) the left the thumbs are thermally spared and there is general bilateral similarity. In image (b) on the right there is clear thermal asymmetry and with the left hand showing a much greater delay in warming. It is challenging to explain the presentation on the right by peripheral nerve injury alone. These images show the power of thermal imaging as a non-contact technique to provide evidence for Raynaud's and also for helping to point to whether it may be of primary form or secondary to a disease such as a connective tissue disease

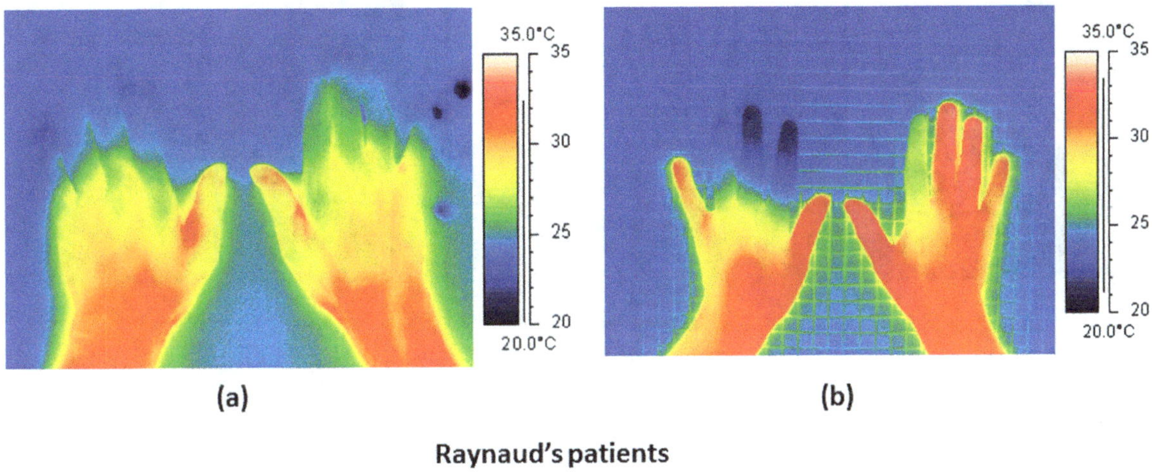

Nailfold capillaroscopy technology uses a green or blue light source to illuminate the skin at the nailfold area and with a drop of contact oil (e.g. liquid paraffin) it allows the red blood cell columns within capillaries to be imaged with good contrast to surrounding non-vascular tissues. In the MDS all fingers studied are imaged and graded, and an overall interpretation made by the capillaroscopist. Care is taken to note potential artefact relating to damaged cuticles and micro-trauma. NFC is relatively easy to perform but the interpretation of the images requires significant training and experience. Capillaroscopy is performed on all patients referred to the MDS for thermography to assess Raynaud's.

Patients with suspected Raynaud's can have a third test when they come to the MDS and this is an assessment of the tissue viability at the finger and toe pads in those deemed at risk of developing digital ulcers. A tissue oxygenation spectrophotometer is a vascular optics technique that can measure tissue oxygen saturation (SO2) values to very low levels (Figure 8) (Abel *et al.*, 2014).

Other Vasospastic Conditions

There are other types of vasospastic conditions that are occasionally referred to the facility for microvascular assessment. These include erythromelalgia (EM) and complex regional pain syndrome (CRPS) (Gorodkin *et al.*, 2004). Both of the these conditions may initially present on thermal imaging similar to Raynaud's patients and so careful clinical history taking and subsequent image interpretation and reporting are needed. EM can affect both the upper and lower limbs and can demonstrate a range of thermal characteristics, presenting with very hot feet and sometimes paradoxically with a cold sensitivity at the hands (Figure 9). EM patients can also experience burning hot lower limb sensations at night even though the feet are extremely cold to the touch. In CRPS the patient can be very sensitive to light

Figure 7. One finger is studied at a time in the region of interest shown in the figure. The finger nail fold site is chosen as the capillaries usually lay parallel to the skin surface rather than be perpendicular as is the case with most other skin sites. The upper two images show example capillary morphologies from healthy subjects and the lower two images show example capillary morphologies from patients with systemic sclerosis (SSc). In SSc there is often clear microangiopathy which includes dilated loops to the grade of giant / mega, avascular fields, marked extravasation, and / or angiogenesis

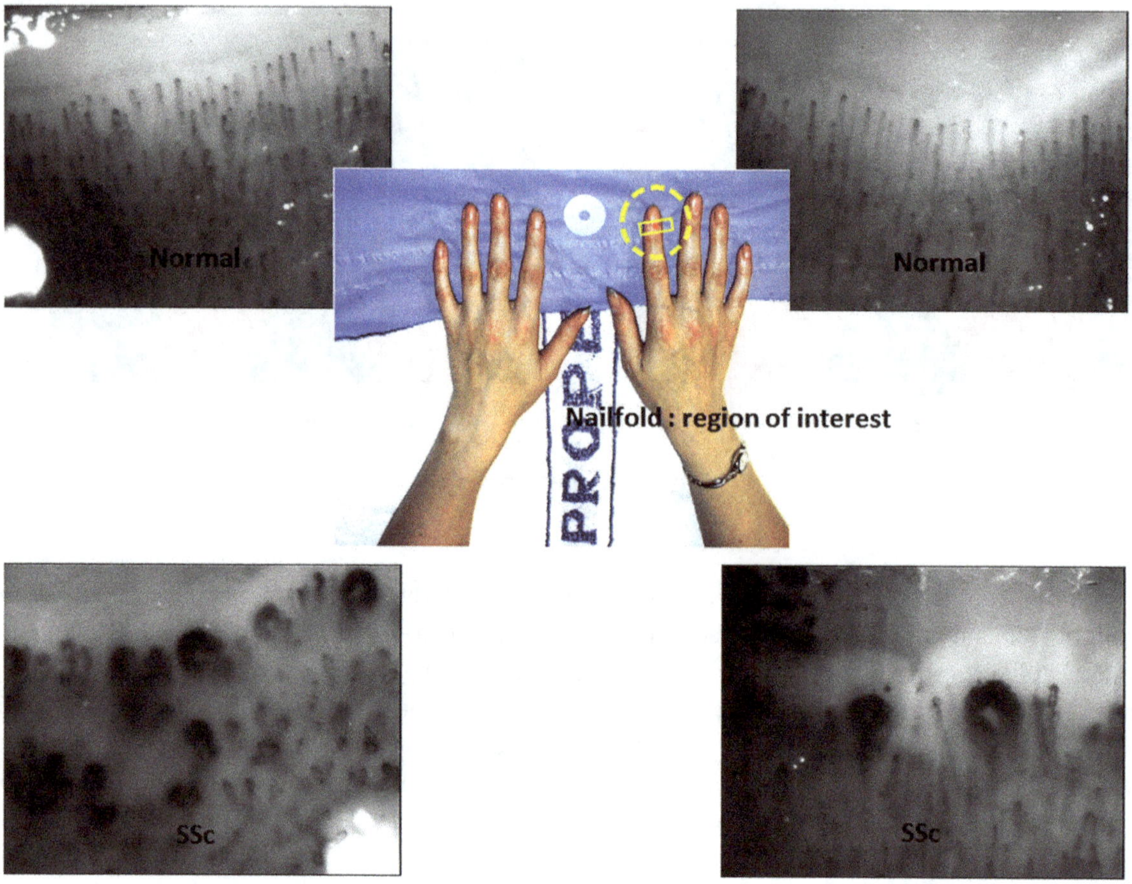

touch on the skin (Figure 10) and also have abnormalities in nail growth and sweating. It is considered within the MDS that further R&D work is needed to better formalise vascular optics tests for EM and CRPS patients.

Tissue Inflammation

Thermal imaging can be used to detect local areas of raised heat related to tissue inflammation (Figures 11 to 13). Generally, inflammation studies can be carried out using a cooled room protocol (18 °C). Thermography has value in assessing patients with morphea (localised scleroderma) to detect the presence of active inflammation where significant local warming and / or thermal asymmetry can be seen at sites of active lesion (Howell *et al.*, 2009). Incidental observations of likely inflammation can be seen on thermography in patients referred with other conditions, e.g. arthritis, diabetes mellitus, and deep vein

Figure 8. A clinical scientist (JA) using a tissue oxygenation spectrophotometry system (O2C "Oxygen to See" device, LEA Medizintechnik GmbH). The technology can be used to assess tissue oxygen saturation in Raynaud's patients deemed at risk of tissue viability problems at the fingers and toes. The spectrophotometry device shines white light onto the skin and quickly determines the absorption characteristics in the green part of the spectrum, with a pulsatile biphasic characteristic obtained for tissue oxygen saturation levels approaching 100% and a damped monophasic characteristic for poor tissue oxygenation levels. Unlike pulse oximetry the technique of tissue oxygen spectrophotometry does not need a pulse to work – it can make measurements from a wide range of tissue sites. The spectrophotometry technique is also routinely used MDS for assessing lower limb amputation level in end-stage vascular disease patients, with leg measurements points shown in the figure

Source: Allen & Howell 2014 © IOP Publishing. Reproduced with permission. All rights reserved

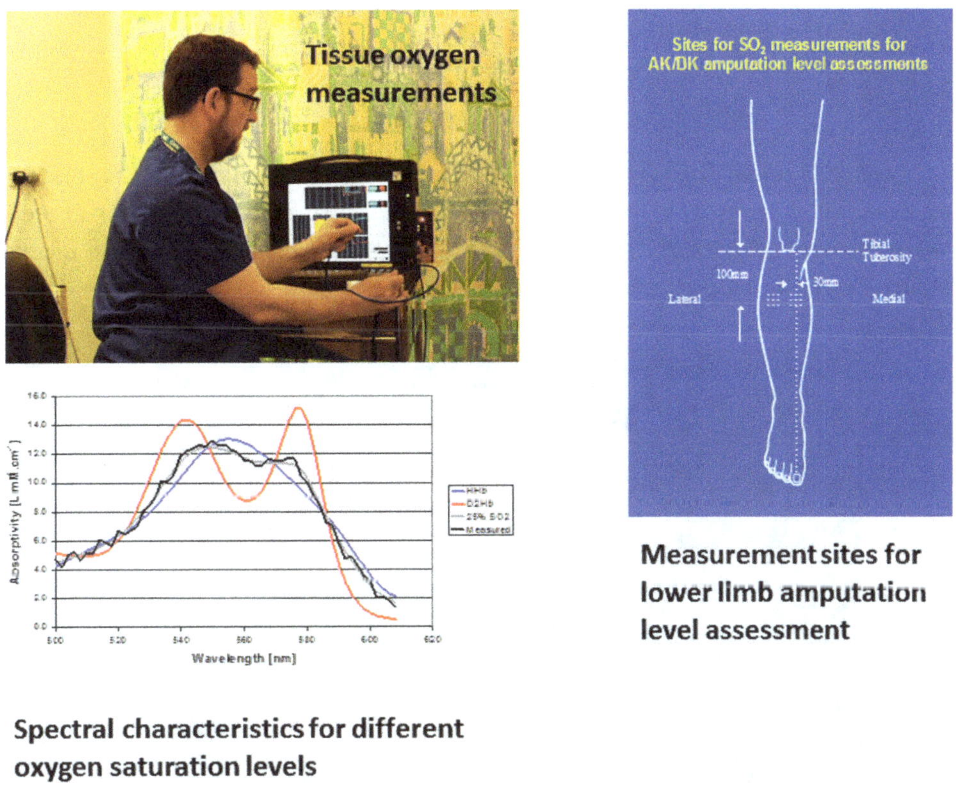

thrombosis (DVT) (Allen *et al.,* 2015b). Research is underway by the microvascular team in conjunction with endocrinology and ophthalmology to evaluate thermography for assessing patients with thyroid eye disease to determine if their disease is likely to be in an active disease state (Allen *et al.,* 2011; Perros *et al.,* 2012; Di Maria *et al.,* 2014; Di Maria *et al.,* 2015).

Autonomic Function

Autonomic function assessments have been undertaken using thermal imaging in patients with restless legs syndrome (RLS). The microvascular team developed a measurement protocol utilising the MDS controlled environment room to explore thermoregulation between normothermic, cold (e.g. 18 °C, for

Figure 9. A patient diagnosed with erythromelalgia showing the markedly hot feet at rest. This is in contrast to the hands for which the mild cold challenge response suggests a tendency to cold sensitivity

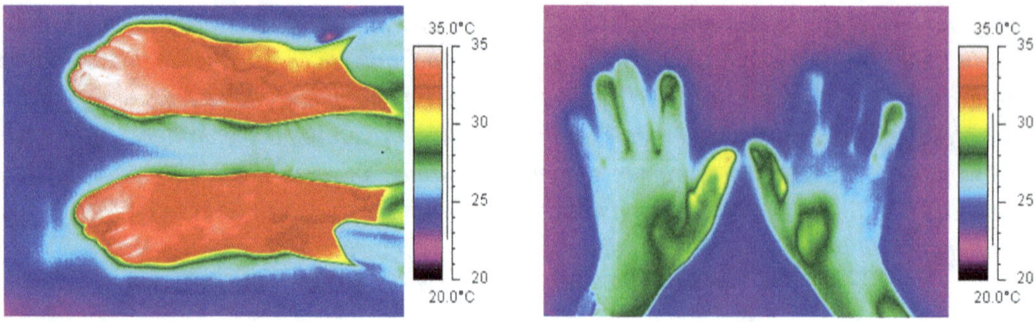

erythromelalgia

Figure 10. Complex Regional Pain Syndrome (CRPS) with its onset in this patient suggested as following just routine minor surgery at the left great toe. There is extensive vasoconstriction to the left foot as shown by the clear marked thermal asymmetry. CRPS, however, is considered to have a central origin rather than just localised to the affected digit or extremity

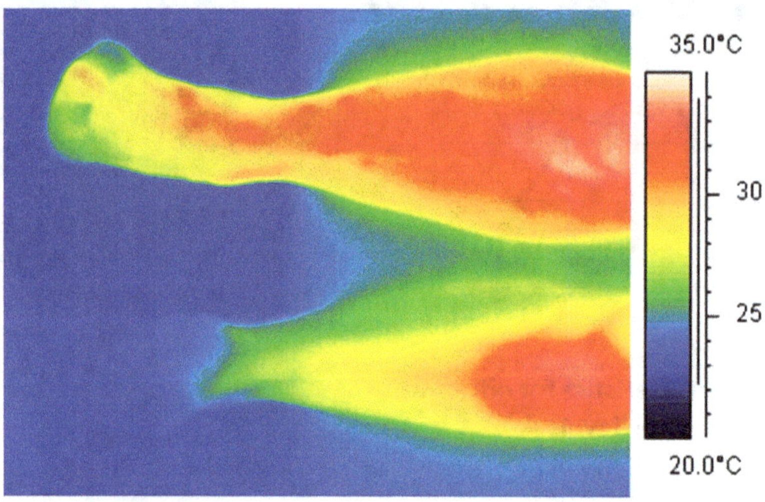

Complex regional pain syndrome

peripheral vasoconstriction) and hot (e.g. 30 °C, for peripheral vasodilatation) states. In a recent study of 12 patients with RLS compared to 12 controls thermal imaging an exploratory analysis found significant differences between foot temperatures in patients with restless legs syndrome compared with controls during the hot room phase ($p<0.05$). Notably, patients with restless legs syndrome had more uniform foot temperatures, whereas controls had a wider variability in surface temperature across the feet (Anderson *et al.*, 2013).

Figure 11. Example of morphea with a strip of raised skin temperature to the distal right calf segment. This clear thermal asymmetry would be consistent with active inflammation

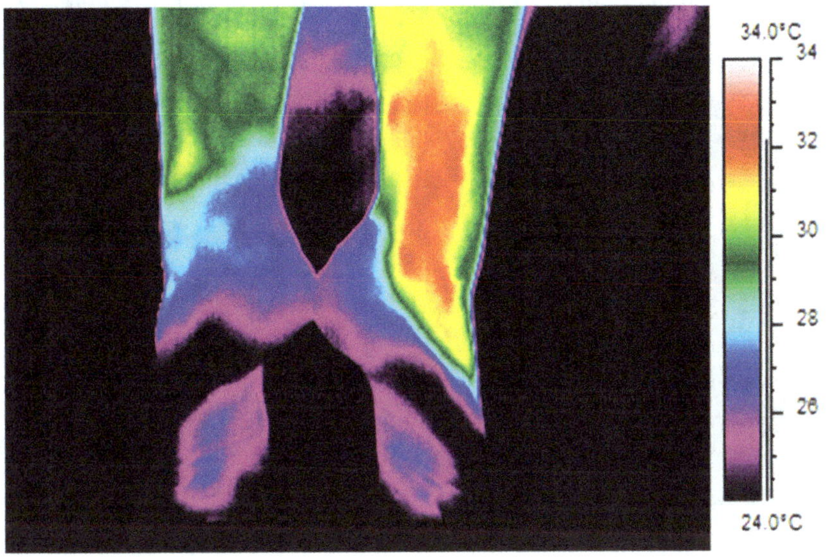

morphea

Figure 12. (a) Locally elevated temperatures at knuckle joints of the right hand, consistent with inflammation. (b) Charcot joint inflammation at the ankle of a patient with diabetes. (c) lower limb deep vein thrombosis (DVT) with elevated temperatures to the right leg, and clear thermal asymmetry between legs

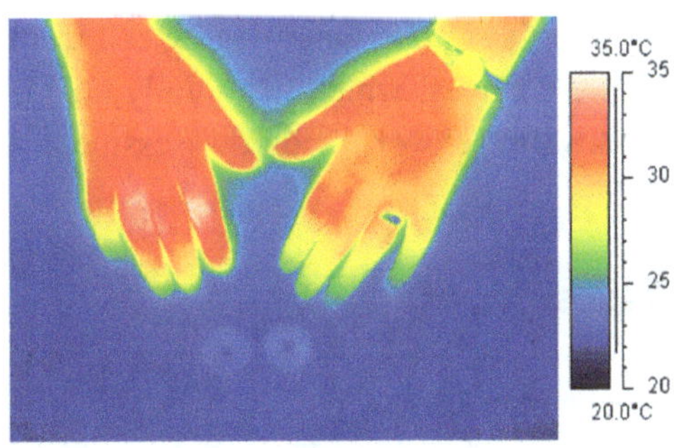

(a) joint inflammation

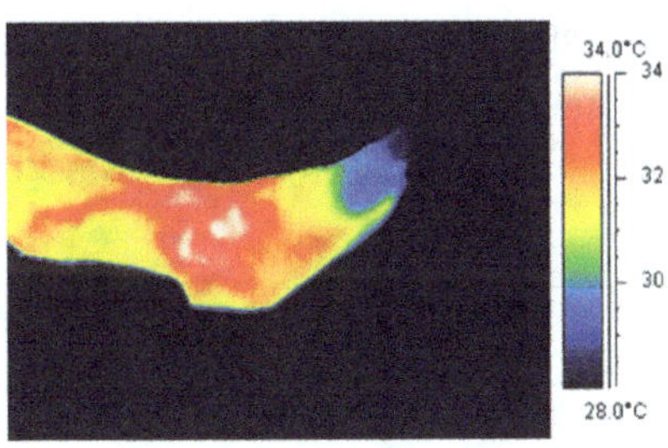

(b) Charcot joint

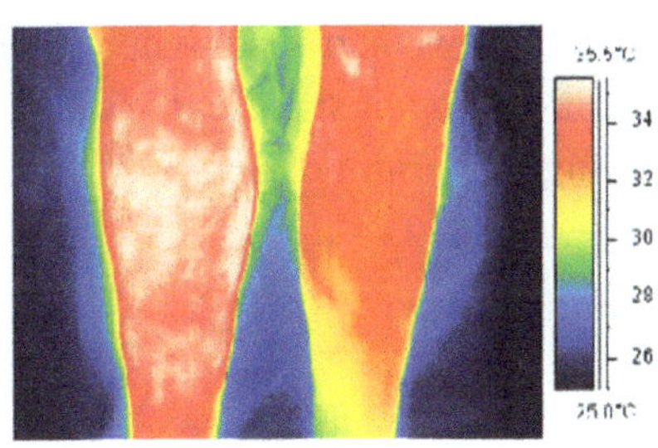

(c) DVT

Figure 13. Thyroid eye disease (TED) is an autoimmune thyroid condition but also involves inflammation at the tissues surrounding the eyes. There are surgical and pharmacological treatments available but it is important for the clinician to know if the disease is active or not. Example "close-up" images from patients with (a) active and (b) inactive disease states

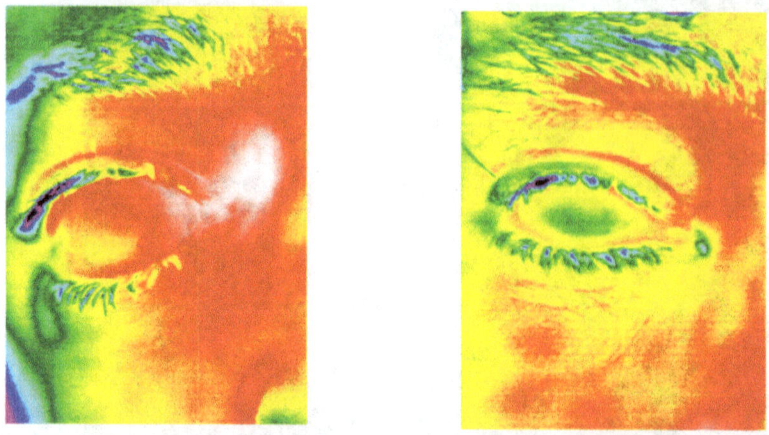

(a) active thyroid eye disease **(b) inactive disease**

Thermography may also have a role in the treatment with botulinum toxin A and facial sweating in Frey syndrome. Frey syndrome classically causes gustatory sweating and facial flushing. In the study by Green *et al* 2014 images were taken after patients chewed a sialagogue and 2 weeks later they were given injections of botulinum toxin A. Images taken 4 weeks after treatment showed a considerable reduction in sweating and facial flushing, which was supported by the results of quality of life questionnaires completed before and after treatment. Thermal imaging can identify areas of gustatory sweating, associated vascular and temperature changes, which potentially enable treatment to be targeted accurately. Thermography also has an advantage over standard assessment, i.e. it is cleaner than the Minor's starch iodine test.

Renal Fistula Vascular Assessment

Vascular access on the arms is needed for haemodialysis, to enable blood to be extracted at high flows but lower than arterial pressures. A shunt is surgically added between a vein and artery and often at a site on the arm (Figure 14). Thermal imaging has been shown to be potentially useful for the following; localising the area of the fistula, since there appears to be a linear relationship between degree of thermal asymmetry at the arms then it is possible for the level of shunt blood flow to be estimated clinically and remotely, identification of significant vascular steal from the hand from a shunt that is too efficient, and also identifying the failure of a shunt due to coagulation (Figure 15) (Allen *et al.,* 2006; Allen *et al.,* 2015c).

Figure 14. Thermal images of the arms where the brachial shunt can clearly be located. The hot arterialized blood from the brachial artery flows into the more superficial venous blood vessels directly. The hands are warm and show thermal symmetry, i.e. no evidence of vascular steal

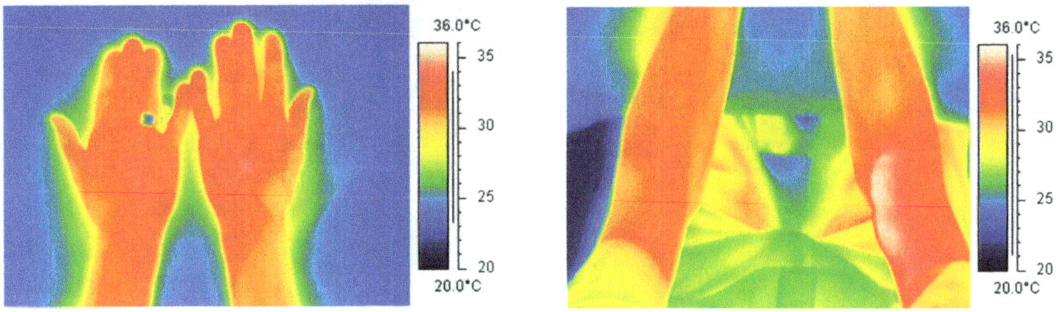

healthy brachial fistula

Figure 15. Thermography has potential to detect potential problems with a fistula, with (a) thermal steal from the left hand i.e. the side of the shunt, and (b) shunt occlusion where no clear thermal lines on the shunt side and no clear thermal asymmetry seen

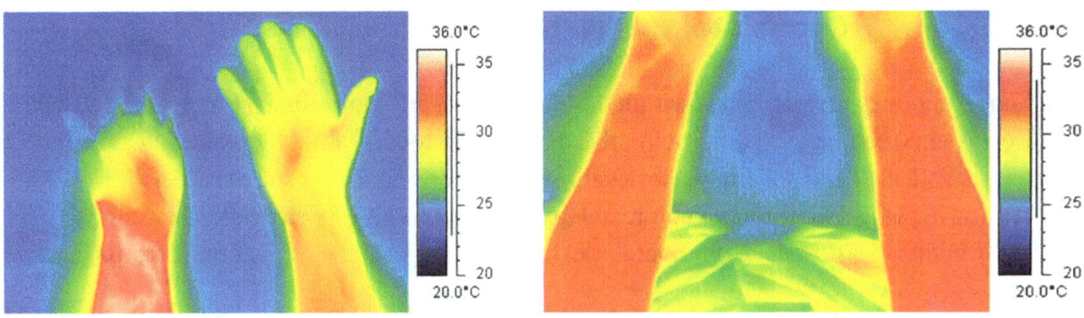

(a) vascular steal, left hand **(b) occluded fistula?**

Cancer

Increased heat can be linked to tumours and angiogenesis. Superficial fatty tumours i.e. lipomas can sometimes be seen in patients with the rare mitochondrial disease myoclonic epilepsy with ragged red-fibers (MERRF) Figure 16). MERRF is a muscle disease that has a wide spectrum of disease and disability, and currently no treatment exists.

Figure 16. Example image from a patient with MERRF. The areas associated with lipomas can be seen on the posterior view example
Source: Allen and Gorman, 2015d. © IOP Publishing. Reproduced with permission. All rights reserved

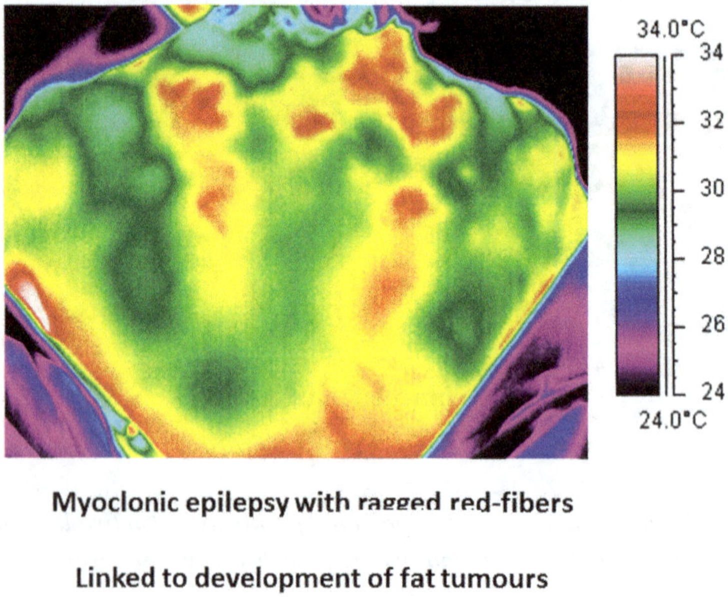

Colorectal Cancer: Gastrointestinal (GI) Perfusion

Most measurements are currently made within the environmentally controlled facility although the FLIR A40 (FLIR Systems) can be used as a roving thermal camera for research in other clinical settings and environments. Work has been undertaken to develop the protocols for operating theatre use for measuring bowel perfusion in patients undergoing colorectal resection, including considerations of safety, infection control, fitting within measurement time boundaries of procedure and imaging internal organs (Figure 17).

Management of the Clinical Measurement Service: The Wider Picture

As well as the measurement facility, portfolio of tests, and measurement technologies it is important to mention the key management aspects relating to the clinical measurement service. The wider aspect of management is seldom addressed in texts on thermography and clinical microvascular measurement - an overview is provided below as an outline example. The management infrastructure is an evolving process and the systems in place should hold the service in a good place to develop and expand, meeting the needs of patients by providing needed and clinically relevant diagnostics.

Clinical Governance and Audit

MDS falls under the department's Clinical Governance framework and the lead scientist attends monthly meetings where audit, risk, health and safety, near misses, bench marking, QIPP (Quality, Innovation, Productivity and Prevention), targets and protocols are discussed. This provides a forum to share ideas,

Figure 17. A tract of bowel exposed during colorectal resection surgery imaged using thermal imaging technology (FLIR Systems A40). The normal tract (i.e. ROI boundary labeled as normal) is visibly hotter than the tract which was de-vascularised (i.e. boundary labeled as de-vascularised), reflecting blood perfusion
Source: Image courtesy of Costanzo Di Maria, Northern Medical Physics and Clinical Engineering

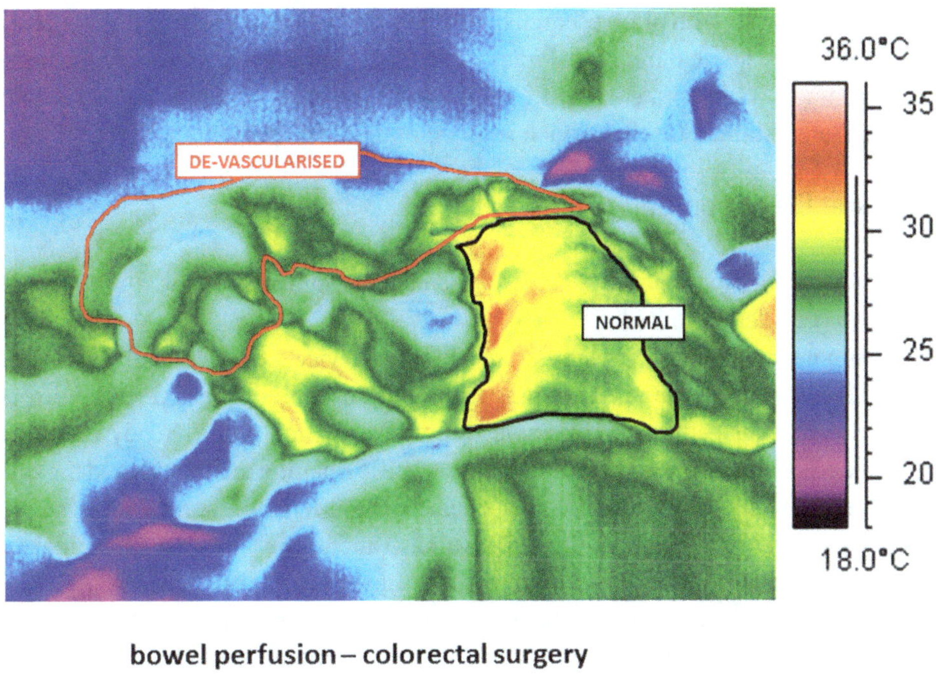

improve methods of working, and helps the team to realize the wider picture and goals of the department and hospital.

Audit is a very important part of the clinical measurement service management process. Activities are performed annually and formerly registered with the hospital Clinical Risk department. The process of service peer review is also covered here. The named external auditor for the Newcastle service (Dr Kevin Howell, Clinical Scientist, Royal Free Hospital, London) and formal registered activities are carried out and documented at least 1-2 times per year. The peer review often includes inspecting a series of sample reports and a log of the more complex case histories discussed. Audit can also be undertaken for research and development work undertaken within the service. Other activities that could come under audit include a patient satisfaction survey, test effectiveness from medical records and outcomes, and accuracy checks of data held on the MDS patient database.

Financial Opportunities

There are usually many financial considerations in establishing and running a clinical measurement service. Forming business plans takes significant effort and justifying the significant outlay for equipment procurement and replacement, staff, measurement rooms and support infrastructure is a challenge. Formal costs do exist for routine NHS patients and also for private patients for the main scans provided i.e. thermography and capillaroscopy. An overall package is provided rather than trying to price individual specialized tests that can be performed but not routinely requested. The Newcastle service has a number of formal Service Level Agreements established with regional hospital Trusts and each commits the service to deliver a diagnostic, to a certain quality, and within a certain timeframe. Other sources of funding include research grants and historically this has been one of the main positive actions for MDS development in its early years, with pilot research funds kick-starting new tests and collaborations within the hospital. A decade ago the field of clinical microvascular technology was in a relative infancy but to many clinicians starting to collaborate in the field the innovative pilot research was notably fruitful. A list of the main funding obtained for the service is given in the R&D section that follows later.

Staff Training and Development

Currently, there are few training courses for microvascular measurement in the UK. The literature on such training is also considered limited.

Appendix A summarizes a training plan devised by the service Lead Clinical Scientist for future trainee clinical scientists to learn the main imaging techniques used in connective tissue disease assessment, MDS operational management, and be able to produce outline reports ready for finalizing and signing off by the service lead. There is a reading list on specific imaging techniques and the training plan draws these together, and building on excellent materials from a) Medical Thermal Imaging provided by University of South Wales (formerly Glamorgan University) and b) the Genova based Eular Capillaroscopy course for which the author has been a member of teaching faculty on the technique. There is also specialist imaging training from some manufacturers, including Burn wound depth assessments using Laser Doppler Perfusion Imaging (i.e. Moor Instruments) with competencies tested for image collection and interpretation. For general medical laser use there is the Laser Core of Knowledge certification.

General professional training also includes hospital mandatory training including; fire safety, infection control, information governance, manual handling and lifting, cardiopulmonary resuscitation, and child protection (to Level 2). Other NHS training can include laser safety and prevention of falls. Continuing Professional Development (CPD) is mandatory with qualifying CPD activities logged and an annual return made to the national body (Institute of Physics and Engineering in Medicine, IPEM). CPD comprises work-based learning and self-directed learning. Research and development training includes Good Clinical Practice (GCP) training and update, and Informed Consent and Ethics training. There are also opportunities for Public and Patient Involvement (PPI) and Project Management training from the National Institute of Health Research (NIHR) if a member of NIHR Faculty.

As well as the abovementioned training and CPD each staff member has an annual appraisal, with main focus in our hospital on professional leadership behaviors.

Quality Assurance

There are several aspects to quality assurance (QA). One can be with equipment, including the measurement environment and the thermal imaging system (Plassmann et al., 2006; Howell & Smith, 2009), but can also relate to staff training and standards of test reporting.

A range of thermal imaging performance characteristics can be obtained using a black body reference that can be adjusted to provide a traceable reference source that includes a physiological test range (e.g. 15 to 40 °C). Various tests can be performed to include camera linearity and offset across the temperature range (could be within 1 to 2 °C, depending on camera purchased), settling time of camera from first switch on (can be more than 1 hour in some of the older cameras), spatial resolution and consistency across image quadrants, and accuracy for when using non-standard use lenses e.g. close-up lens (Richards *et al.,* 2013). Black body QA measurements can be tested at the normothermic temperature setting but also drift and offset characteristics need to be known across a range of room operating settings (e.g. at the cool room protocol temperature of 18 °C, and at the warm room protocol temperature of 25 °C). It is likely cameras can have offset errors and so it is important to know their performance under the range of ambient conditions that the device will be used clinically. Figure 18 shows the black body test configuration used to assess the performance of the FLIR SC300 and A40 thermal cameras used in the microvascular service. Figure 19 gives an example Bland Altman type test result quantifying the level of agreement between the SC300 thermal camera across a range of black body reference temperatures in the physiological range, for a cooled room setting.

As well as good measurement technique it is vital that the measurements are interpreted correctly and reported clearly and accurately. For example, with thermal imaging the technique can be sensitive to detecting clinical abnormalities but is not always specific as to saying what those abnormalities relate to. The microvascular specialist therefore needs to have an appropriate level of knowledge, including neurophysiology and immunology, to make a reliable interpretation. It is recommended good technique to ask a patient to complete a health questionnaire (an example of one used in Newcastle centre for Raynaud's assessments is given in Appendix B), and to go through this with the patient, seeking clari-

Figure 18. Example set-up for test equipment for black body reference checks in the target range of 20 to 40 °C: for FLIR SC300 and FLIR A40 cameras. A Land P80P blackbody thermal reference system has a PRT reference source traceable to national standards. The blackbody cavity emissivity is >0.995 (noting also that human skin emissivity is close to 0.98)

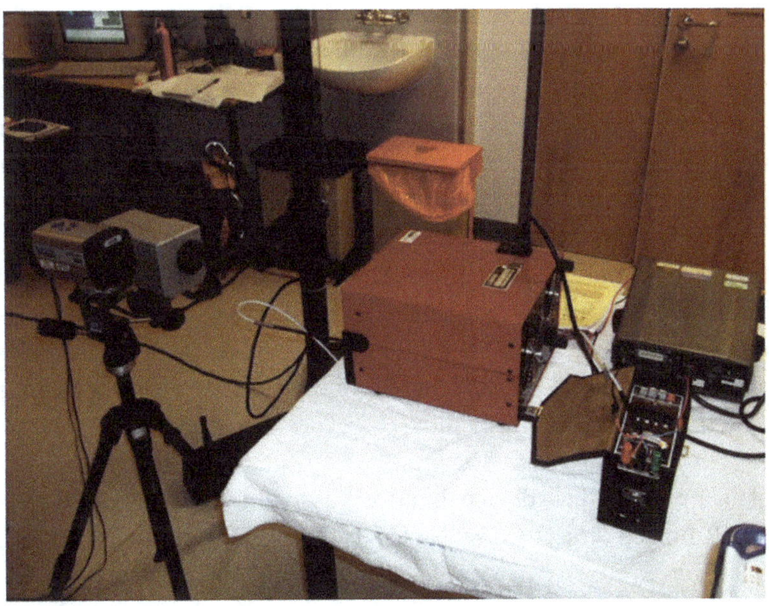

set-up : black body calibration checks of service thermal cameras

Figure 19. Example Bland Altman plot for an FLIR SC300 thermal imager showing the relationship between measurement error (SC300 measured - black body [BB] reference) and the mean of BB and SC300 temperatures. This test example was performed at a cooled room setting

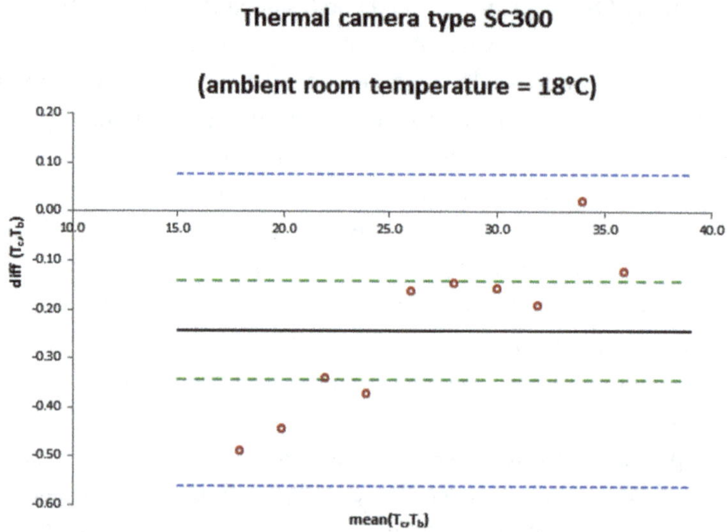

fication where needed. This information can help distinguish between different causes for the thermal presentations seen. The test report also needs to be accurate, non-speculative, defensible, and traceable.

Research and Development

Capital funding has been secured with clinical colleagues for specialist measurement facilities, totaling approximately one quarter of a million pounds. In addition to this the service Lead Clinical Scientist has been a collaborator on a wide range of medical physics research and development projects with clinical specialists in Rheumatology, Paediatric and Adult Cardiology, Vascular Surgery, Hepatology, Chronic Fatigue Syndrome, Diabetic Medicine, Endocrinology and Neurology. Grant funding has also been secured with industrial partners to international level. The vascular optics field is growing and has capability to be awarded significant grant funding - there are currently 3 UKCRN Portfolio projects underway within the service amounting to significant involvement in projects with total partner linked funding of £2.7M. One of the projects – developing a novel vascular assessment device is being led by the MDS lead and with grant funding at £1.3M for this R&D (Wilkes et al., 2015).

The current research projects associated with the service are listed below, highlighting the diversity of work undertaken and the partnerships formed:

1. Development of an optical medical device for novel vascular assessment in a Primary Care setting: optical pulse. NIHR funded project led by NuTH (NIHR Reference II-C1-0412-20003). UKCRN Portfolio.
2. Novel thermal imaging measurement and analysis techniques for detecting inflammation in thyroid eye disease.

3. A pilot study of new spectrophotometry device developed by NMPCE to measure tissue oxygen saturation.
4. Novel photoplethysmography cardiovascular assessments in patients with Raynaud's phenomenon and systemic sclerosis: a pilot study.
5. Role of medical thermography in treatment of Frey's syndrome with botulinum toxin A.
6. Finger optical pulse microvascular responses to deep inspiratory gasp using wavelet analysis.
7. Novel assessment of microvascular changes in idiopathic restless legs syndrome (Willis-Ekbom disease): thermal imaging and laser Doppler flowmetry.
8. Gastro-intestinal (GI) microvascular assessments to reduce colorectal leak: thermal imaging and laser speckle contrast imaging. Novel intra-operative imaging.
9. Laser Doppler assessments of dermal circulatory changes in people with coronary artery disease.
10. Chronic fatigue syndrome and impaired peripheral optical pulse characteristics on orthostasis.
11. Novel optical assessment of tissue composition and viability using fluorescence spectroscopy and tissue oxygenation spectrophotometry in patients with systemic sclerosis.
12. The effect of a low-cost vibrating cushion on tissue oxygen saturation at the ischial tuberosity compared to standard tilt-in-space wheelchair responses.
13. An innovative optical imaging system for the early identification, monitoring, evaluation and diagnosis of foot ulcers. NIHR funded project led by National Physical Laboratory, Teddington, UK (NIHR Reference II-LA-0813-20007). A multi-centred study with Newcastle upon Tyne forming one of the 3 clinical assessment sites for the device development. UKCRN Portfolio. (Petrova et al 2016).
14. Validation of laser Speckle imaging and thermography in patients with Raynaud's phenomenon secondary to systemic sclerosis. Arthritis Research funded project led by Manchester University. A multi-centred study with Newcastle upon Tyne forming one of the 7 clinical assessment sites. UKCRN Portfolio.
15. Reliability of nailfold capillary density measurement as a possible outcome measure for systemic sclerosis-related microangiopathy. Led by Manchester University. A multi-centred study with Newcastle upon Tyne forming one of at least 7 European clinical capillary grading sites.
16. Novel vascular optics wearable sensor technologies for cardiovascular assessment. A collaborative pilot study with a leading US industrial partner.

Dissemination

Findings from the majority of the projects undertaken have been presented at national / international level. There is great scope for wider dissemination; including peer review publication and targeted impact. Targeted dissemination of specific projects in the list could have far reaching impact in relation to NHS commissioning of services and clinical care pathways.

Partners and Outreach

Outreach work is very important for a variety of reasons. Microvascular is a relatively new area of medical diagnostics and as thus is not often known about by the public. Outreach and partnerships help communicate the work done and tests available for a variety of patient groups. Good public relations have existed with the University of the Third Age (U3A, Wearside Branch), northern IET retired members group, the Workers' Educational Association (WEA), and the Reyrolle Heritage Trust. The service lead is a STEM Ambassador and has promoted Medical Physics at more than 20 schools across the North East region to hundreds of students, with thermal imaging a key technology demonstrated. The service lead has also given formal presentations at Westminster (Benson & Allen, 2015) and at the Bradford Science Festival (2015). There are also links internationally with academic establishments in the US, India, Holland, China, Cuba and Russia, and also with UK universities i.e. Nottingham and Loughborough Universities, and Glamorgan University (now University of South Wales) for which the service lead has acted as external PhD examiner.

Future Directions in Terms of Developments and Research in the MDS

The clinical direction of the MDS facility will be to continue supporting the clinical measurement needs of the regional hospital specialists and their patients. Capillaroscopy and thermal imaging will therefore remain, for the foreseeable future, key measurements to be provided at expert level in the field of connective tissue disease. Strategically, the lead clinical scientist is also looking at opportunities in optical cancer diagnostics and thermal physiology. The measurement facility, its clinical infrastructure and clinical expertise are considered future proofed for many years to come. Staff resourcing for the service will need to expand to give resilience. A Clinical Scientist grade staff formal training programme has been established by the service lead. The service lead is now looking for PhD students to cover some areas of the R&D projects highlighted previously. Clinical technologist support will also be expanded in the coming years.

There is great scope to advance the knowledge in the field of vascular optics and also to develop novel medical devices. Examples have been given for devices that can be used in primary care as well as in hospitals, helping to drive care closer to home for the patient. Medical device work also opens up further opportunities to collaborate with leading industrial partners.

Experience has shown that R&D work needs to be focused and prioritized so that chosen research projects have a realistic chance of turning into the real tests that are needed by the clinicians for their patients, and be diagnostic / screening tests that are funded and clinically supported.

CONCLUSION

This chapter has summarized the history and development of the Newcastle upon Tyne Microvascular Diagnostics Service, its portfolio of tests available, the clinically focused research and development, and also key aspects of operational and scientific management. The utility of thermal imaging has been highlighted, and when combined with other modalities, including capillaroscopy, laser Doppler perfusion imaging and laser speckle contrast imaging, it enables an extensive array of tests to be covered across many different medical specialties. This chapter has also given an introduction to service management aspects, a topic seldom covered in the formal clinical measurement literature. Good operational and business management are very important for patient safety and quality as well as future proofing a measurement service.

The MDS is a powerhouse. It can be considered highly successful in terms of growth in patient referrals, income secured through focused business planning, significant research and development funding awarded, publications, and the comprehensive range of academic, clinical, and industrial partnerships formed to date. All these aspects are important pieces of the service development and delivery jigsaw. MDS has come a long way on its fifteen year plus journey and it is exciting to consider where microvascular diagnostics will be in the next decade or two. There are many great opportunities for the specialism of vascular optics.

REFERENCES

Abel, G., Allen, J., & Drinnan, M. (2014). A pilot study of a new spectrophotometry device to measure tissue oxygen saturation. *Physiological Measurement*, *35*(9), 1769–1780. doi:10.1088/0967-3334/35/9/1769 PMID:25119876

Agarwal, S. C., Allen, J., Murray, J., & Purcell, I. F. (2012). Laser Doppler assessment of dermal circulatory changes in people with coronary artery disease. *Microvascular Research*, *84*(1), 55–59. doi:10.1016/j.mvr.2012.02.002 PMID:22366028

Allen, J. (2007). Topical Review: Photoplethysmography and its application in clinical physiological measurement. *Physiological Measurement*, *28*(3), R1–R39. doi:10.1088/0967-3334/28/3/R01 PMID:17322588

Allen, J. (2012). *Development of a clinical vascular optics measurement facility – the Newcastle upon Tyne experience.XII European Congress of Thermology*, Porto, Portugal.

Allen, J., Di Maria, C., Burnett, S., Forrest, I., & Griffiths, B. (2015a). *Imaging assessments of patients with suspected systemic sclerosis and associated inflammatory lung disease. In Infrared imaging: A casebook in clinical medicine*. Institute of Physics Publishing.

Allen, J., & Gorman, G. (2015d). *Thermographic assessment of the presence of fatty tumours in myoclonic epilepsy with ragged red fibres. In Infrared imaging: A casebook in clinical medicine*. Institute of Physics Publishing.

Allen, J., & Howell, K. J. (2014). Topical Review: Clinical Microvascular Imaging: Techniques and opportunities for clinical physiological measurements. *Physiological Measurement*, *35*(7), R91–R141. doi:10.1088/0967-3334/35/7/R91 PMID:24910968

Allen, J., Murray, A., Di Maria, C., & Newton, J. L. (2012). Chronic fatigue syndrome and impaired peripheral pulse characteristics on orthostasis - a new potential diagnostic biomarker. *Physiological Measurement*, *33*(2), 231–241. doi:10.1088/0967-3334/33/2/231 PMID:22273713

Allen, J., Oates, C., & Talbot, D. (2015c). *Thermal imaging and its potential for arterio-venous fistula function assessment. In Infrared imaging: A casebook in clinical medicine*. Institute of Physics Publishing.

Allen, J., Oates, C. P., Chishti, A. D., Ahmed, I. A. M., Talbot, D., & Murray, A. (2006). Thermography and colour duplex ultrasound assessments of arterio-venous fistula function in renal patients. *Physiological Measurement*, *27*(1), 51–60. doi:10.1088/0967-3334/27/1/005 PMID:16365510

Allen, J., Perros, P., Dickinson, J., & Murray, A. (2011). An exploratory look at the thermal characteristics of the eyes in patients with thyroid eye disease. International Consensus Guidelines on Medical Thermography. Iguazu Falls, Brazil 23-26 Nov 2011. *Thermology International*, *21*, 148.

Allen, J., Robertshaw, D., & Leech, N. (2015b). *Thermal imaging potential for assessing diabetic Charcot foot syndrome. In Infrared imaging: A casebook in clinical medicine*. Institute of Physics Publishing.

Allen, J., Young, A. L., & Griffiths, B. (2014). Subject preparation and thermal acclimatization prior to mild cold challenge testing using dynamic thermal imaging. *Pan American Journal of Medical Thermology*, *1*(1), 51–54. doi:10.18073/2358-4696/pajmt.v1n1p51-54

Ammer K. (2008). The Glamorgan Protocol for recording and evaluation of thermal images of the human body. *Thermology International, 18*, 125–44.

Anderson, K., Di Maria, C., & Allen, J. (2013). Novel assessment of microvascular changes in idiopathic restless legs syndrome (Willis-Ekbom disease). *Journal of Sleep Research*, *22*(3), 315–321. doi:10.1111/jsr.12025 PMID:23397977

Anderson, M. E., Moore, T. L., Lunt, M., & Herrick, A. L. (2004). Digital iontophoresis of vasoactive substances as measured by laser Doppler imaging - a non-invasive technique by which to measure microvascular dysfunction in Raynauds phenomenon. *Rheumatology (Oxford, England)*, *43*(8), 986–991. doi:10.1093/rheumatology/keh244 PMID:15199217

Benson, E., & Allen, J. (2015). *Illuminating light in medical diagnostics and treatment*. British Science Week seminar on light. Portcullis House.

Bollinger, A., & Fagrell, B. (1990). *Clinical capillaroscopy: a guide to its use in clinical research and practice*. Toronto: Hogrefe & Huber Publishers.

Briers, J. D. (2001). Laser Doppler, speckle and related techniques for blood perfusion mapping and imaging. *Physiological Measurement*, *22*(4), R35–R66. doi:10.1088/0967-3334/22/4/201 PMID:11761081

Cheng, H., Luo, Q., Liu, Q., Lu, Q., Gong, H., & Zeng, S. (2004). Laser speckle imaging of blood flow in microcirculation. *Physics in Medicine and Biology*, *49*(7), 1347–1357. doi:10.1088/0031-9155/49/7/020 PMID:15128210

Cutolo, M. (2010). *Atlas of capillaroscopy in rheumatic diseases*. Milan: Elsevier.

Cutolo, M., Sulli, A., & Smith, V. (2010). Assessing microvascular changes in systemic sclerosis diagnosis and management. *Nature Reviews. Rheumatology*, *6*(10), 578–587. doi:10.1038/nrrheum.2010.104 PMID:20703220

Di Maria, C., Allen, J., Dickinson, J., Neoh, C., & Perros, P. (2014). 2014 Novel thermal imaging analysis technique for detecting inflammation in thyroid eye disease. *The Journal of Clinical Endocrinology*, *99*(12), 4600–4606. doi:10.1210/jc.2014-1957 PMID:25238202

Di Maria, C., Perros, P., Dickinson, J., & Allen, J. (2015). *Exploratory thermal and laser speckle contrast imaging measurements of eye inflammation in a case of thyroid eye disease. In Infrared imaging: A casebook in clinical medicine*. Institute of Physics Publishing.

Fullerton, A., Stücker, M., Wilhelm, K. P., Wårdell, K., Anderson, C., Fischer, T., & Serup, J. et al. (2002). Guidelines for visualization of cutaneous blood flow by laser Doppler perfusion imaging. A report from the Standardization Group of the European Society of Contact Dermatitis based upon the HIRELADO European community project. *Contact Dermatitis*, *46*(3), 129–140. doi:10.1034/j.1600-0536.2002.460301.x PMID:12000320

Gorodkin, R., Moore, T., & Herrick, A. (2004). Assessment of endothelial function in complex regional pain syndrome type I using iontophoresis and laser Doppler imaging. *Rheumatology (Oxford, England)*, *43*(6), 727–730. doi:10.1093/rheumatology/keh158 PMID:15026582

Green, R. J., Endersby, S., Allen, J., & Adams, J. (2014). Role of medical thermography in treatment of Freys syndrome with botulinum toxin A. Short Communication. *The British Journal of Oral & Maxillofacial Surgery*, *52*(1), 90–92. doi:10.1016/j.bjoms.2013.09.013 PMID:24238875

Herrick, A. (2008). Diagnosis and management of scleroderma peripheral vascular disease. *Rheumatic Disease Clinics of North America, 34*, 89-114.

Herrick, A. L., & Clark, S. (1998). Quantifying digital vascular disease in patients with primary Raynauds phenomenon and systemic sclerosis. *Annals of the Rheumatic Diseases*, *57*(2), 70–78. doi:10.1136/ard.57.2.70 PMID:9613334

Howell, K. J., Lavorato, A., Visentin, M. T., Smith, R. E., Schaefer, G., Jones, C. D., & Woo, P. et al. (2009). Validation of a protocol for the assessment of skin temperature and blood flow in childhood localised scleroderma. *Skin Research and Technology*, *15*(3), 346–356. doi:10.1111/j.1600-0846.2009.00371.x PMID:19624432

Howell, K. J., & Smith, R. E. (2009). Guidelines for specifying and testing a thermal camera for medical applications. *Thermology International, 19*, 5-12.

Kumar, N., Allen, J., Murray, A., & Griffiths, B. (2006). The assessment of single dose Sildenafil Citrate (Viagra) in the treatment of Raynaud's phenomenon in patients with systemic sclerosis. *The Journal of Rheumatology*, *33*, 1918–1919. PMID:16960964

McKay, N., Griffiths, B., di Maria, C., Hedley, S., Murray, A., & Allen, J. (2014). Novel photoplethysmography cardiovascular assessments in patients with Raynauds phenomenon and systemic sclerosis: A pilot study. *Rheumatology*, *53*(10), 1855–1863. doi:10.1093/rheumatology/keu196 PMID:24850874

Perros, P., Di Maria, C., Dickinson, J., & Allen, J. (2012). Thermal imaging and characteristics in Graves' Orbitopathy. European Thyroid Journal, 1(S1), 123-65.

Petrova, N., MacDonald, A., Ainarkar, S., Plassmann, P., Ring, F., Simpson, R., & Edmonds, M. et al. (2016). Infrared thermometry reveals no differences of the skin temperatures at the plantar, dorsal, medial and lateral sites between the right foot and left foot in healthy volunteers. *Diabetic Medicine*, *33*(Suppl. 1), 35–196.

Plassmann, P., Ring, E. F. J., & Jones, C. D. (2006). Quality assurance of thermal imaging systems in medicine. *Thermology International, 16*, 10-5.

Richards, R. E., Allen, J., Burnett, S., Howell, K. J., & Smith, R. E. (2013). Evaluation of three thermal imagers for skin temperature measurement using a blackbody source and a spatial resolution test object. *Thermology International*, *23*, 17–23.

Ring, E. F. J., & Ammer, K. (2012). Infrared thermal imaging in medicine. *Physiological Measurement*, *33*(3), R33–R46. doi:10.1088/0967-3334/33/3/R33 PMID:22370242

Spencer-Green, G. (1998). Outcomes in primary Raynaud phenomenon: A meta-analysis of the frequency, rates, and predictors of transition to secondary diseases. *Archives of Internal Medicine*, *158*(6), 595–600. doi:10.1001/archinte.158.6.595 PMID:9521223

Wilkes, S., Stansby, G., Sims, A. J., Haining, S., & Allen, J. (2015). Peripheral arterial disease: Diagnostic challenges and how photoplethysmography may help. *The British Journal of General Practice*, *65*(635), 323–324. doi:10.3399/bjgp15X685489 PMID:26009528

APPENDIX A

Clinical Scientist Outline Training Plan for Microvascular Imaging in the Assessment of Connective Tissue Disease / Raynaud's Phenomenon (CTD/RP)

Scientist Trainee: Dr Jigsaw

Commitment: 1 clinic day per week. It is expected that training in the CTD/RP specialism should be completed within a period equivalent to 6 months full-time.

Start Date / Period: To plan in the 6 levels / overall duration dependent on staff availability and commitments. An important time planning factor will also be the trainee's levels of patient and NHS clinical service experience to date. Furthermore, scanning exposure to sufficient SSc patient numbers is very important – the extent of patient availability depending on the clinical centre and specialist consultants based there.

Supervisor: e.g. Dr John Allen. Can delegate team member(s), as appropriate.

Stage A. Level I – Clinical Service Overview and Familiarization

Know the microvascular measurement portfolio for both clinical service and also R&D – including (Freeman Hospital based) CTD/RP studies, tissue inflammation assessment, muscle and venous physiology, amputation service, autonomic function, and R&D. Burn wound depth assessment service.

Observe selected microvascular studies across the service portfolio (selected sessions). Support service / associated documentation.

Assessment: End of Level I interview (supervisor/trainee).

Stage A. Level II – Infrastructure / Service Management

Know service R&D activities and plans: short, medium and long-term. Microvascular appointments – diary, key secretarial and clerical staff, nurse support, and chaperoning. Communications relating to appointments – voicemail / mobile DECT phone / email etc. Patient / care-relative handling skills. Infection control – monthly audit, Health and safety, Service audit activities. Microvascular database, Patient workload "Activity" software and monthly reporting. Service documentation – request cards, SLAs and invoicing. Calibration of specific equipment. Equipment management, MDS room – temperature and humidity controls, clinical stocks, Estates – fault reporting, etc. Data – imaging archive, systems of work. Patient confidentiality. Hospital complaints procedures. Security. Service SOPs.

Continue to observe selected microvascular studies across the service portfolio (selected sessions). Also, an overview visit to the Newcastle burn wound depth assessment facility.

Assessment: End of Level II interview (supervisor/trainee, and 1 member of the clinical measurement group).

Stage B. Level I – Connective Tissue Microvascular Specialism

Understand clinical problems and key diagnostic questions – in rheumatology i.e. connective tissue disease and Raynaud's. Understand thermal imaging and capillaroscopy optical imaging and tissue oxygen saturation (SO2) measurement technologies. Observe measurements in weekly clinics – expecting ~2 patients per week to have a likely CTD (1 SSc) – to give patient examples to consider as well as an array of healthy and patient control subjects. Understand the importance of the supporting MV clinical questionnaire and clinical hand / foot examinations.

Assessment: Critical appraisal of thermal imaging and capillaroscopy methods in context of assessing patients with CTD (Aim to keep within a 1000 word limit). Needs to know important literature.

Stage B. Level II – Supervised Microvascular Imaging Measurements

Undertake supervised imaging: thermal imaging (i.e. mild cold provocation to hands, resting foot measurements) and also capillaroscopy on an agreed number of healthy staff volunteers from the service and allied areas. Know pre-test protocol letter details. Understand main pitfalls, artifacts and limitations. Know service SOPs.

Undertake supervised measurements – with patients pre-selected by supervisor to try and maximize scleroderma pattern patients in sample. Continue observation of measurements in weekly clinics.

Build on patient / care-relative handling skills – specifics for CTD / RP patients. Learn about specifics of clinical questionnaire and hand / foot examination. Know about nails in health and disease. Know about key immunology. Learn other key documentation needed for measurements. It is vital the trainee has sufficient exposure to the range of SSc patients that might be expected for such a service. Regular attendance and flexibility are very important because of the nature of clinical work. Regular attendance is also paramount to keep abreast of changes and updates on management infrastructure, work by others in the service to maximize synergy and output from the team.

Assessments

1. Undertake full microvascular imaging studies on an agreed number of CTD / RP patients – observed with competency assessed by the supervisor. There must be a minimum number of scleroderma spectrum patterns studied for this set.
2. Write a specific new SOP for an aspect of the service and its enhancement – with topic agreed with supervisor.
3. Write a systematic review for an aspect of the service and its enhancement – with topic agreed by supervisor.

Stage B. Level III – Reporting of CTD/RP Microvascular Imaging Studies

"Mechanics" of reporting – methods for producing key documents needed for thermography and capillaroscopy, and interpretation / recommendation summary. Data – imaging archive, systems of work.

Depending on staff availability and session workload aim to spend up to 1 session per week observing reporting, viewing example historical image sets and reports and also some from supervised measurements. Continue imaging measurements aspect for other session times per week. Use the Newcastle atlas examples for capillary grading – study and learn. This level will aim to include the trainee joining the supervisor in his annual audit / peer review with the external auditor – with additional aims to see how another UK measurement centre undertakes microvascular studies and to appreciate their specific clinical setting.

Assessments: Performing imaging set, clinical interview and produce full patient reporting on an agreed number of patients, as learning examples. Each report will be discussed in detail with the supervisor. End of stage B meeting with supervisor/trainee, and 1 member of the clinical measurement group.

Stage C. Level I - Trainee Delegated to Cover at Least 1 Fixed Measurement Session Per Week

Continued observation of microvascular clinics - 1 or 2 sessions per week as agreed with supervisor and linked to needs of service. Also, aiming for trainee to be at demonstrated competency level to cover up to 1 day per week of clinics, specifically doing CTD / RP measurements and producing patient reports. This role will involve working in parallel with the service technologist or other clinical scientist staff as per the needs of the service. Patient reports can be issued by the trainee after verification and counter-signing by the service clinical scientist. The trainee is expected to be at a level that they have a full awareness of the service, can perform all aspects of the work area if clinical needs require it, and have the experience to take delegated responsibility in supervising other service staff as appropriate. The trainee should be able to make appropriate resource decisions and also demonstrate a level of initiative. They must also know their professional limitations and to seek advice from senior staff and/or clinicians when appropriate.

Assessments: Supervisor audit of a minimum of an agreed number of microvascular imaging tests and subsequent reports. End of stage C meeting with supervisor/trainee, and 1 member of the clinical measurement group, and the service technologist.

APPENDIX B

Clinical Questionnaire for CTD/RP Imaging and Reporting: Wider Context

1. Do your FINGERS clearly change colour when exposed to just *mild* cold? If so then please note below what is the general colour pattern sequence:

WHITE (sometimes called pallor) ?
BLUE / PURPLE (cyanosis) ?
RED (rubor) ?
OTHER (e.g. yellow or grey)?

2. If the fingers do change colour then does this last a long time, i.e. is it EPISODIC lasting say up to an hour or more PERSISTENT lasting over many hours / days? (EPISODIC / PERSISTENT)?

3. Are the FINGERS affected much more than the THUMBS, or about the same?

4. Summarize OTHER SYMPTOMS you might get in the cold with the hands (pain / numbness etc)?

5. Is one hand affected with the colour changes much more than the other side? If so then which HAND is worse the RIGHT or the LEFT one?

6. Are the FEET affected by cold? If so do the toes also change colour?

7. Which are worse – the HANDS or the FEET, or are they about the same?

8. What generally triggers an event: COLD / EMOTION / LIMB POSITION?

9. Are the Raynaud's symptoms worse in WINTER than in SUMMER?

10. Are the overall Raynaud's symptoms of RECENT onset in the last year? If not recent then approximately how many years have you experienced these?

11. Have the Raynaud's symptoms generally worsened in recent months?

12. Do you or have you taken medicines to help treat the Raynaud's symptoms (Y / N)?

13. Summarize any significant INJURIES, falls and / or hobbies with risk of personal injury:

General Information

1. Are you RIGHT handed or LEFT handed (RH / LH, please circle)?
2. Do you SMOKE (Y / N / EX-SMOKER)?
3. Are you a DIABETIC patient (Y / N)?
4. Do you have an underactive THYROID (Y / N)?
5. Are you currently seeing any other medical specialists (Y / N), if so which?
6. Summarize your current and past WORK HISTORY:

Specific Symptoms

1. Do your fingers swell up with the heat (Y / N)?
2. Noticed permanent changes to the skin on the hands: becoming shiny, leathery or scar like? (Y / N)?
3. Ulcers to your fingertips (Y / N)? At the toes recently (Y / N)?
4. Is there a tendency to sweating at the palms, even if the hands are cold (Y / N)?
5. Is your skin very sensitive to sunlight – enough to cause a rash for example (Y / N)?
6. Do you get a lot of bother and discomfort with your neck, back and/or shoulders (Y/N)?
7. Symptoms of "pins and needles" sensations in the arms / legs at night time, if so which side(s) (Y/N)?
8. Do you tend to get very achy and stiff joints, especially in the morning on waking (Y / N)?
9. Do you get restless legs (Y / N)? Sensations of "burning hot" feet at night (Y / N)?
10. Do you often get the following: Very dry mouth (Y / N)? Very dry eyes (Y / N)?
11. Noticed bother recently with swallowing food / choking on food (Y / N)?
12. Noticed recent bother with gastric acid reflux coming up (Y / N)?
13. Noticed recently getting breathless easily, i.e. just by "walking and talking" (Y / N)?
14. Do suffer from bad fatigue (Y / N)? If so is there any "dizziness" on standing up (Y / N)?
15. Please summarize any other diagnostic tests carried out recently (e.g. nerve / lung studies / bloods etc.)

APPENDIX C

Acronyms and Terms

ANA anti-nuclear antibody
BB black body
CPD continuing professional development
CRPS complex regional pain syndrome
CTD connective tissue disease
DVT deep vein thrombosis
EM erythromelalgia
GCP good clinical practice
GI gastrointestinal
IET Institution of Engineering and Technology
IPEM Institute of Physics and Engineering in Medicine
LDPI laser Doppler perfusion imaging
MDS Microvascular Diagnostics Service
MERRF myoclonic epilepsy with ragged red-fibers
NuTH The Newcastle upon Tyne Hospitals NHS Foundation Trust
NFC nailfold capillaroscopy
NIHR National Institute of Health Research
NMPCE Northern Medical Physics and Clinical Engineering
PPI Public and Patient Involvement
QA Quality Assurance
QIPP Quality, Innovation, Productivity and Prevention
RLS restless legs syndrome
ROI Region of Interest
RP Raynaud's phenomenon
SLE systemic lupus erythematosus
SO2 tissue oxygen saturation
SOP standard operating procedure
SSc systemic sclerosis
STEM Science, Technology, Engineering and Mathematics
SWIR short wave infrared
TED thyroid eye disease
U3A University of the Third Age
UKCRN United Kingdom Clinical Research Network
UV ultraviolet
WEA Workers' Educational Association

Chapter 2
Thermal Diagnostics in Chronic Venous Disease

Armand Cholewka
University of Silesia, Poland

Agnieszka Cholewka
Institute of Oncology, Poland

Karolina Sieroń-Stołtny
Medical University of Silesia, Poland

Zofia Drzazga
University of Silesia, Poland

Joanna Kajewska
University of Silesia, Poland

Agata Stanek
Medical University of Silesia, Poland

ABSTRACT

The aim of the study was to determine the diagnostic usefulness of thermal imaging as tool to find quantitative parameters in lower-limb primary chronic venous diseases and insufficiency of superficial veins. There were significant differences obtained in thermal maps of lower extremities between patients and healthy. The correlations were obtained between temperature parameters counted from thermal imaging and duplex scanning. Such results also suggest that thermovision diagnostics may be useful as a complementary and first of all objective method that can be used in the diagnosis of chronic venous diseases in the lower extremities. It may suggest that thermovision may be used as a screening method or together with an ultrasound diagnosis in different superficial veins disorders.

INTRODUCTION

There are many different diseases that physicians may called civilization's problems. One of them is undoubtedly chronic venous disease. There are factors that can cause serious vein diseases i.e. obesity, diabetes, lack of exercises and hypertension. When patients with chronic venous disease are considered it is often observed that few of these factors appear together. Risk factors of chronic venous disease include inheritance (genetic predisposition), age, sex, obesity (mainly in women), pregnancy, long-time standing or sitting, smoking and insufficient movement. The other important factors that can contribute to chronic venous disease (CVD) are the lack of fibre in food, congestion, peroral contraception or hormonal substitution treatment, wearing high heels, garters and higher body height. The occurrence of

DOI: 10.4018/978-1-5225-2072-6.ch002

chronic venous disease in the population is connected with the lifestyle of modern society. The etiology of CVD still remains unclear. The cause of chronic venous disease is multifactorial and represents a combination of internal and external influences (Švestková & Pospíšilová, 2008).

Some commonly mentioned conditions associated with venous ulcers include older age, obesity, hypertension, heart failure, diabetes, rheumatoid arthritis, nephrosis, and a history of venous thrombosis (Nelzen, Bergqvist, & Lindhagen, 1991; Scott, LaMorte, Gorin, & Menzoian, 1995).

Subjective symptoms on lower limbs are connected with chronic venous disease include pain in the limbs, feeling of heavy legs, feelings of intumescences, pressure or burning of the skin (Švestková & Pospíšilová, 2008).

CHRONIC VENOUS DIESEASE (CVD)

Chronic venous disease ranks among civilization diseases and its occurrence increases in both sexes nearly linearly with age. However the probability of venous insufficiency occurring increases with number of pregnancies. The probability of lower-limb venous disease appearing is estimated at 40-50% for men and 50-55% for women, whereas visible varicose veins and chronic venous insufficiency are, respectively, present in 10-15% and 2-7% of the male population and 20-25% and 3-7% of the female population. Moreover it usually is observed for people beyond 50 years old however it can be seen also in younger people (Švestková & Pospíšilová, 2008; Chiesa, Marone, Limoni, Volonte, Schaefer, & Petrini, 2005). For example in the United States, an estimated 23% of adults have varicose veins, and 6% have more advanced chronic venous disease (CVD), including skin changes and venous ulcers (Sieroń, Cierpka, Rybak, & Stanek, 2009; Kaplan, Criqui, Denenberg, Bergan, & Fronek, 2003). Such symptoms may cause pain and discomfort, what lead to absence or disability of work, and a deterioration of a healthy quality of life (Van den Oever, Hepp, Debbaut & Simon, 1998; Kaplan, Criqui, Denenberg, Bergan, & Fronek, 2003). It is also observed that it usually afflicts industrial countries. Therefore chronic venous disease is considered as civilization problem (Van den Oever, Hepp, Debbaut, & Simon, 1998; Kaplan, Criqui, Denenberg, Bergan, & Fronek, 2003).

That is why the chronic venous disease (CVD) of the lower extremities is one of the most widespread diseases in the populations of Western European countries and the USA (Milic, 2011).

The most frequent symptoms of chronic venous disease are dilated cutaneous veins, such as telangiectases and reticular veins, or varicose veins. That is why it is also used the term chronic venous insufficiency (CVI) which describes more advanced problems of the venous system of the lower extremities including edema, skin changes, and even ulcerations. In turn, the term chronic venous disease (CVD) is used to represent the full spectrum of manifestations of chronic venous disease. Veins diseases have a significant meaning on healthcare resources. There was reported that millions of people seek medical help for their health as well as cosmetic appearance annually. However it should be noted that cosmetic consequences may adversely affect an individual's quality of life and are associated with other symptoms. It should be underlined that serious consequences of chronic venous insufficiency i.e. venous ulcers have an estimated prevalence of about 0.3%, although active or healed ulcers occurred in 1% of the adult population. It has been reported that in United States about 2.5 million people have chronic venous insufficiency and 20% of that number develops in venous ulcers. The healing process of venous ulcers is different and can last long time – even few years is common for more than 50% of venous ulcers. Delayed healing and recurrent ulceration is common in patients with ulcers on lower extremities. Moreover the socioeconomic impact of venous ulceration is very serious, resulting frequently in absence to engage in social and occupational activities, what significantly reduce the quality of life. Venous ulcers influence on loss of productive work hours, what was estimated at 2 million workdays/year, and may cause early retirement, which is found in up to 12.5% of workers with venous ulcers (Robert, Eberhardt, Joseph, & Raffetto, 2014; International Angiology, 2014). The important thing in understanding this problem is that the cost of CVD includes not only its investigation, its treatment, and also the loss of working days of the afflicted patients (Kurz et al., 1999). A very interesting fact is that in 1991 in France the cost of CVI treatment represented 2.6% of the total healthcare budget for that year (Lafuma, Fagnani, Peltier-Pujol, & Rauss, 1994). On the other hand in Sweden, the average weekly cost of treating venous leg ulcers in 2002 was 101 Euros, with an estimated annual cost of 73 million Euros (Tennvall, Andersson, Bjellerup, Hjelmgren, & Oien, 2004). The veins of the lower extremity are divided into the superficial and deep venous system connected by a series of perforator veins. The superficial venous system is located above the muscular fascial layer. The deep venous system is located below the muscular fascial and serves as collecting veins and the outflow from the extremity (Eberhardt & Rafeto, 2005; Caggiati, Bergan, Gloviczki, Jantet, Wendell-Smith, & Partsch, 2002).

CURRENT DIAGNOSIS OF CVD

The diagnosis of CVI is made via patient history and physical examination with the assistance of non-invasive testing. Invasive testing also may be used to establish the diagnosis, but it is typically reserved for assessing disease severity or when surgical intervention is being contemplated (Eberhardt & Rafeto, 2005). The physical examination plays an important role in guiding therapy in chronic venous insufficiency. Typical examination and palpation may reveal visual evidences for chronic venous disease. Physician examines the skin surface and looking for irregularities or bulges to suggest the presence of varicose veins. There might be also seen hyperpigmentation, stasis dermatitis, atrophic blanche (white scarring at the site of previous ulcerations with a paucity of capillaries), or lipodermatosclerosis. These mentioned symptoms are very useful in making a diagnosis. It can be seen varicose veins track follow the course of the affected superficial vein, such as the great or short saphenous veins. For better see such symptoms of CVD examination should be done on the patient in the upright posture to allow maximal distention of the veins and from multiple directions. The presence of edema and its severity are assessed. The early evidence of chronic veins disorders may be calf fullness or increased limb girth, so the calf muscle consistency should be assessed. Additionally measurement of the limb girth should be performed. There was also reported that long-standing edema may become more springy to palpation. Palpation is also helpful in diagnosis of dilated veins due to revealing tenderness of those ones. Ulcers are seen with more advanced level of disease. The venous ulcers usually occur in the medial supramalleolar area at the site of major perforating veins and the greatest hydrostatic pressure what suggest the Trendelenberg test to be performed. During this test patient is lying down to empty the lower extremity veins. The upright posture is resumed after applying a test or it can be also used manual compression at various levels of the low extremities. When authors consider varicose of superficial veins they will remain collapsed if compression is more proximal or cephalic to the point of reflux. With deep (or combined) venous insufficiency, the varicose veins will appear despite the use of the test or manual compression (Eberhardt & Rafeto, 2005).

The other diagnostic technique in chronic venous disorder or chronic venous insufficiency is using of continuous wave Doppler typical assist in the bedside evaluation. The presence and direction of flow in the veins may be determined after Valsalva test or the sudden release of thigh or calf compression. In these movement the minimal signal should be detected toward the feet. This technique may be used to assess the great and short saphenous veins. The problem is that the lack of direct visualization of the vessels leaves uncertainty about the precise site of reflux. There are also another diagnostics technique used in CVD. The most known and common used is venous duplex imaging. This technique as a non invasive technique is also is used to confirm the presence and evaluation of CVI as well as to assess its etiology and severity. Duplex ultrasound imaging is very useful in evaluation of disease, especially pulsed Doppler bring information about the anatomic extent of disease involving the deep and superficial blood supply systems problems, as well as it can give us also very important information about perforations of veins. The duplex examination is standard used to exclude the exclude DVT (Deep Vein Thrombosis) or venous obstruction. There are also used the compressibility tests complimented by flow characteristics what can exclude the thrombosis. Due to Trendelenberg tests the direction of flow may be assessed even in 30° reverse position during provocative maneuvers like Valsalva maneuver, or after augmenting flow with limb compression. Moreover use of a cuff inflation-deflation method with rapid cuff deflation in the standing position is preferred to induce reflux (Robert, Eberhardt, Joseph & Raffetto,2014; Markel, Meissner, Manzo, Bergelin, & Strandness, 1994). In evaluation of reflux the most important thing is the direction of flow due to any significant flow toward the feet is suggestive as a reflux. The duration of reflux is known as the reflux time. The reflux is connected with wrong direction of blood flow and reverse through the valves in veins. A reflux time in the range above of 0.5 second is connected with wrong their functioning and diagnosis as the presence of reflux, although a more refined definition with a variable "cutoff" based on location has been suggested (Robert, Eberhardt, Joseph & Raffetto, 2014; Markel, Meissner, Manzo, Bergelin, & Strandness, 1994). The definition of venous reflux is retrograde flow greater than 500 ms (0.5 sec) in the superficial system, and greater than 1000 ms (1.0 sec) in the femoral or popliteal segment (Labropoulos, Tiongson, Pryor, Tassiopoulos, Kang, Ashraf Mansour, & Baker, 2003). This is very good moment to underline the possibility of use the thermal imaging to diagnosis a reflux due to increase of temperature in vicinity of veins region where the valves malfunction occurred. It lead to increase the temperature of skin surface especially when the superficial veins are considered – in thermovision is very important that the best temperature gradient changes can be observed only for superficial veins diseases. On the other hand it should be realized that the longer the duration of reflux or the greater the reflux time implies more severe disease which also may be seen in thermovision (Labropolous et al., 2003). It was also try to correlate other parameters such as the reflux velocity and even the calculated reflux volume with temperature gradient changes or some temperature parameters derived from thermograms however the correlation coefficients were found poor. But all these parameters are commonly used to assess the severity of reflux and can be used as the parameters to assess of the severity of disease (Cholewka, Stanek, Klimas, Sieroń, & Drzazga, 2014; Neglen, Egger, Olivier, & Raju, 2004). It should be underlined that there was also weak correlation obtained of the severity of disease by duplex imaging with both plethysmographic techniques and clinical manifestations what put the investigators to find other non-invasive techniques which might be used as quantitative diagnostics techniques in assess of severity of the veins disease. Maybe it will be possible to do it with modern thermal imaging. However, nowadays, the venous duplex reflux evaluation, it is considered the most common, non-invasive technique used in diagnostics of chronic venous insufficiency. It is known that Dupplex ultrasound imaging may give information about local valve function and its disorders however combine of body cooling and thermal imaging can also bring interesting and useful information about valves health state what was reported in the literature (Labropolous et al., 2003; Cholewka et al., 2010). Such information may be important when the proper therapy is considered, however if the contribution of the reflux to global hemodynamics is required, the deeper diagnosis is needed (Robert, Eberhardt, Joseph, & Raffetto, 2014). One of the technique that is necessary in chronic venous disease is photopletysmography. It relies on measuring the backscatter of light emitted from a diode with a photosensor what can give information about relative changes in blood volume in the dermis of the limb. The probe of photopletysmograph is placed to the foot and make moves to empty the foot with calf muscle contraction. Then return of blood is observed by increased backscatter of light detected in probe. That gives possibilities to calculate the refill time. Such measurement is not quantitative. However it may be used as a parameter to correlate with other techniques towards diagnosis CVI (Robert, Eberhardt, Joseph, & Raffetto,2014; Abramowitz, Queral, Finn, Nora, Peterson, Bergan & Yao, 1979). It was found that venous refill time between 18 to 20 seconds, depending on the patient's position during the study, may indicate the chronic venous insufficiency but bigger values of refill time may prove normal flow (Robert, Eberhardt, Joseph, & Raffetto, 2014; Abramowitz, Queral, Finn, Nora, Peterson, Bergan, & Yao, 1979; Nicolaides & Miles, 1987). It seems that it will be possible to correlate the time of refill with some temperature parameters derived from thermograms in similar tests due to temperature gradient changes during filling and flowing of blood in big superficial venous. There is also air plethysmography (APG) which gives possibility to measure reflux, obstruction, and muscle pump dysfunction (Christopoulos, Nicoliades, & Szendro, 1988; Criado, Farber, Marston, Daniel, Burnham, & Keagy, 1998). Cuff surrounding the calf and changes of the air volume in it gives information about changes in limb volume. Such measurement is done during maneuvers to empty and fill the venous system in the lower extremities. Venous outflow is evaluate during rapid cuff deflation on an elevated limb that has a proximal venous occlusion cuff applied. The outflow fraction at defined value is the primary parameter used to evaluate the adequacy of outflow. Then the limb position is changed to evaluate the venous filling. The rate of refill is used to determine the presence and severity of reflux. The most important parameter is the venous filling index which values for normal flow and insufficiency that point to chronic venous insufficiency has been defined (Criado, Farber, Marston, Daniel, Burnham, & Keagy, 1998; Harada, Katz, & Comerota, 1995). The ability of the calf muscle pump to eject blood is determined in test similar to that used in the liquid crystal thermography, which relies on few exercises - single and 10 repetitive contractions of calf muscle during toe raises. It changes the blood supply what lead to change the temperature inside examinated veins as well as on the skin surface what gives the possibility to use also in the other chronic venous insufficiency diagnosis tests like thermal imaging. Evaluation of some temperature parameters changes may give some possibility to derive some quantitative parameters in diagnosis of chronic venous insufficiency. However it seems that it rather should be treated as a additional technique and very individual one. It should be also known that there are also invasive techniques that could be used in chronic venous insufficiency like ascending or descending phlebography or venography (Criado, Daniel, Marston, Mansfield, & Keagy, 1995). Ascending phlebography requires the injection of contrast in the dorsum of the foot with its visualization while traveling up the lower extremity in the deep venous system. The ascending phlebography is considered as a gold standard to determine the patency of veins. However nowadays modern medicine is looking for noninvasive and less risk diagnosis techniques so ascending phlebography is very rarely used despite it could give many details of venous anatomy what may be helpful in planning of surgical interventions and bring information useful to distinguish primary from secondary stage of the disease. On the other hand there is descending phlebography which involves proximal injection of contrast in a semivertical posture on a tilt table with the use of the Valsalva maneuver (Robert, Eberhardt, Joseph, & Raffetto, 2014; Kamida, Kistner, Eklof, & Masuda, 2001; Masuda, Arfvidsson, Eklof, & Kistner, 2001; Nicolaides & Zukowski, 1986). The descending phlebography is also very useful to identify reflux in the common femoral vein and at the saphenofemoral junction. The other invasive diagnostics technique used in chronic venous insufficiency is ambulatory venous pressure (AVP) which is called the hemodynamic gold standard in assessing chronic venous insufficiency (Masuda, Arfvidsson, Eklof, & Kistner, 2001; Nicolaides & Zukowski, 1986). The difficulty and risk in this method relies on necessarily of insertion a needle into the pedal vein with connection to a pressure transducer. Test is performed at rest and after exercise, usually in the form of toe raises. Moreover in this technique pressure also is monitored before and after the placement of an ankle cuff to help distinguish between deep and superficial veins system reflux (Neglen & Raju, 2000).

The last mentioned techniques are invasive and bring the risk for the patients during examination so they are very seldom used in clinical practice (Eberhardt & Rafeto, 2005).

PATOPHYSIOLOGY OF THE VENOUS SYSTEM OF THE LOWER LIMB

One way or another chronic venous disorders or its more advanced form chronic venous insufficiency are the diseases for which symptoms and health complications have a huge impact on patients' quality of life so it seems that the fast, non-invasive and early screening diagnosis is needed. It should be also underlined that modern medicine requires fast, sensitive and non-invasive diagnosis techniques. So angiology needs easy to use, noninvasive techniques for the early diagnosis veins problem. There is another problem of chronic venous disease – it can lead to very serious health complications as ulceration or even to lameness due to amputation of lower limb. However such serious effects needs time to make disease advancement. It usually occur when few other civilization diseases appear together at the same time i.e. obesity, diabetes, and hypertension (Sieroń, Cierpka, Rybak, & Stanek, 2009; Wilkinson, Bunker, Edwards, Scurr, & Smith, 1993; Hess, 2005). Chronic venous disease is usually connected with abnormal function of the vein's valves and a narrowing its diameter. Such elements cause the blood stasis and a filling up of a part of the blood circulation system what leads to leukocyte entrapment and an inflammatory state surrounding the run of vein (Cholewka, Stanek, Klimas, Sieroń, & Drzazga, 2014). When the blood pressure is too high it becomes too sticky and coagulates fast one must be concerned about the dangerous condition of vein thrombosis. Moreover capillaries become more pervious for blood cells and swelling occurs. In some cases, it is possible to see a widening of superficial veins that protrude along the skin. This is the result of varicose veins which are occur two times more often in women than men as well mostly for people in their sixties or older, obese, and those who are disabled and unable to move as a result of certain diseases. The long - lasting standstill of the patient implicates muscles disorders and as a result problems with muscle pump as well as in the circulation of blood (Sieroń, Cierpka, Rybak, & Stanek, 2009; Wilkinson, Bunker, Edwards, Scurr, & Smith, 1993; Sukovatykh & Kniazev, 2007). The mentioned above disorders are connected with metabolism changes what lead to skin temperature changes especially when the diseases are connected with superficial veins which are close to skin surface. The skin temperature gradient can be easily seen in thermal imaging. This is the reason why it could be possible to use thermal imaging in such diseases. It should be also emphasized that finding new, cheap and fast diagnostics techniques complementary to standard techniques used nowadays i.e. duplex in veins disorders, is important especially that thermal imaging can show the temperature changes as a first symptom before tissue changes has become visible for ultrasound and big vessel blood circulation problems occur (Cholewka, Stanek, Klimas, Sieroń, & Drzazga, 2014; Cholewka et al,2010); Cholewka, Stanek, Kwiatek, Sieroń & Drzazga, 2013; Mercer & Ring, 2009).

Yet, the increased temperature manifested in the superficial vein track may be associated with some functional problems of venous valves caused by, for example, blood stasis. It may lead to other pathological vein changes like vein deformation which can be seen on the skin surface as areas with higher temperature, unlike the healthy lower limb, discussed in the previous work (Laurikka, Sisto, Tarkka, Auvinen, & Hakama, 2002). There are some processes that play a main role in venous insufficiency such as leukocyte entrapment, hyperviscosity of blood and fibrin cuff. These processes may have influence on soft tissue metabolism and the skin temperature gradient. The number of morphotic elements in blood influences blood flow in capillaries due to their influence on viscosity. The interaction of morphotic blood elements with endothelium cells is also very important. The friction has an influence on the temperature inside the vessels as well as on surrounding soft tissues as a result of leukocytosis influence which leads to an increase in resistance and blood pressure. The erythrocytes are smaller than white blood cells and flow faster and can lead to an aggregation of erythrocytes, and force white blood cells to the vessel walls. This is called the leucocytes-erythrocytes train. It leads to process of leucocytes rolling, and an adhesis to endothelium cells causes the leucocytes entrapment. Such processes lead to damage in endothelium and to a migration of leucocytes through the blood vessel walls (Laurikka, Sisto, Tarkka, Auvinen, & Hakama, 2002; Švestková & Pospíšilová, 2008; Milic, 2011). Resultingly it can lead

Figure 1. The thermal images of representative patient's limbs in anterior and posterior position

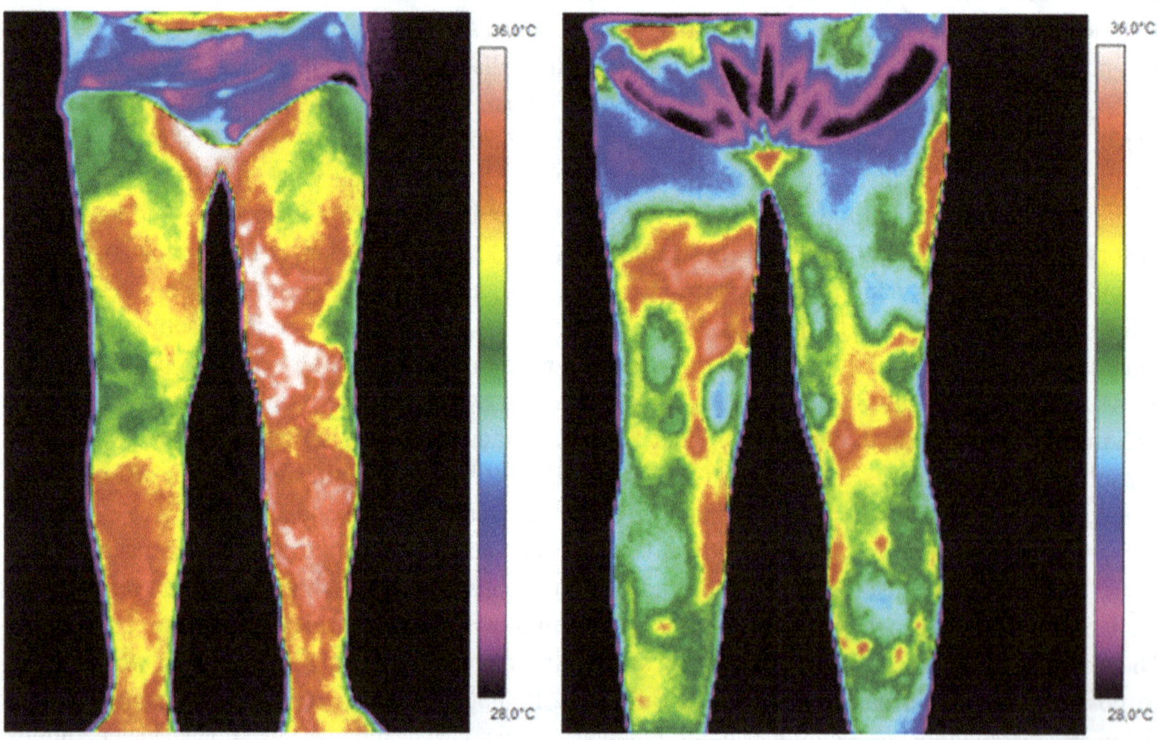

to a release of cytotoxic substances and changes to blood cells; the vessel walls can be damaged which enables the increase of permeability and start of an inflammatory state. The results are easy to derive in thermal imaging because they lead to gradient temperature changes, mostly in the path of the afflicted vein. The very critical aspect is that these processes take place in small vessels so they are strictly connected with microcirculation and cannot be visible in duplex *ultrasonography*.

However it should be noted that blood flow is defined by the volume of blood that is moving through a volume of tissue per unit of time and flow velocity is inversely related to the vascular cross-sectional area. In venous congestion the blood flow is high, but the flow velocity is low. Increase of blood viscosity and thrombus formation reduce the blood flow velocity in front of stenotic or partially obstructed venous vessels and this process may result in venous stasis. Thermal imaging used to the extended varicose veins when they are located in the superficial skin layers, cannot provide information on the direction of blood flow inside of veins but it is not the point of this technique. It is not necessary to measure the velocity and direction of blood flow by using the thermovision. It can be obtained by Duplex sonography which based on the velocity of blood cells, and is appropriate for measuring velocity and its direction. Temperature gradients define the direction of heat flow and are equal to the temperature differences between any sites in a 3-dimensional body. Changes in microcirculation contribute to skin temperature and seemingly the differences in the temperature gradient are easily correlated with the medical diagnosis and for that reason it was interesting to check the correlation between the temperature and area parameters with the duplex *ultrasonography* parameters.

CLASSIFICATION OF CVD

There is normally used by physicians CEAP scale which contain describing the clinical class, etiology, anatomy, and pathophysiology and the ultrasound parameters derived from Dupplex scanning in diagnosis of venous disorders. The term - *chronic venous disorder (CVD)* describes the full spectrum of venous abnormalities. The Guideline Committee recommends using the *Classification of chronic venous disorders* the CEAP scale for CVD. The classification is based on clinical signs of venous disease (C), etiology (E), anatomy (A), and the underlying pathophysiology (P). Clinical class includes the full spectrum of venous disorders, from no signs of visible venous disease (C0) to telangiectasia or reticular veins (C1), varicose veins (C2), edema (C3), skin changes, such as pigmentation or eczema (C4a) or lipodermatosclerosis or atrophie blanche (C4b), and healed (C5) or active (C6) ulcer. Etiology can be congenital (Ec), primary (Ep), or secondary (Es). The CEAP classification in CVD is used to distinguish venous disease from congenital varicosity and post - thrombotic venous insufficiency due to differences in evaluation and treatment of such three diseases (Sieroń, Cierpka, Rybak & Stanek, 2009; Gloviczki et all, 2011).

However, there are some limitations to the CEAP clinical classification, which is arbitrary and subjective with inadequate delineation of the categories. Therefore a venous severity score was developed to complement the CEAP classification and further define the severity of chronic venous insufficiency. It been shown to be useful to evaluate the response to treatment. The venous severity scoring provides a numeric score based on 3 components:

1. The venous clinical severity score,
2. The anatomic segment disease score, and
3. The disability score.

The venous clinical severity score consists of 10 attributes (pain, varicose veins, venous edema, skin pigmentation, inflammation, induration, number of ulcers, duration of ulcers, size of ulcers, and compressive therapy) with 4 grades (absent, mild, moderate, severe). The venous anatomic segmental score assigns a numerical value to segments of the venous system in the lower extremity that account for both reflux and obstruction. On the other hand the venous disability score comes from the ability to perform normal activities of daily living with or without compressive stockings (Eberhardt & Raffetto, 2005; Rutherford, Padberg, Comerota, Kistner, Meissner, & Moneta, 2000).

THERMAL IMAGING AS A NEW DIAGNOSTIC METHOD FOR CVD

The main diagnosis techniques that can give not only qualitative but much more important quantitative parameters used in chronic venous diseases diagnostics procedures are: ultrasound - Duplex scanning, which allows the evaluation of visibility, compressibility, and venous flow, including, the measurement of the duration of reflux, and augmentation, plethysmography - used for evaluation of calf muscle pump function, global venous reflux, and venous outflow obstruction and also used liquid crystal thermography (Sieroń, Cierpka, Rybak, & Stanek, 2009; Nicolaides, 2000; Gloviczki et al., 2011). The first two techniques and theirs application in medicine are very wide described in the literature were shortly described earlier in this chapter (Sieroń, Cierpka, Rybak, & Stanek, 2009). They are not the aim of this chapter. But very interested fast, quite cheap and can give some additional diagnostic information for physician is liquid crystal thermography as well as much more sensitive and accuracy is thermal imaging – thermovision which gives information about temperature gradient so the metabolism not only connected with superficial veins but also describes metabolism of soft tissues in the very superficial skin layer. Such temperature gradient changes and the thermal map of the whole lower extremities may give important and useful information about health state of the blood supply system in the lower extremities. Analyzing the useful of the first one method which is liquid crystal thermography it should be pointed that such imaging technique can be used as a screening test to localize incompetent perforators what was reported in the literature (Ammer, 2004). Liquid crystal thermography diagnosis technique requires to stick the liquid

Figure 2. Thermal image of inside limb parts representative for healthy group

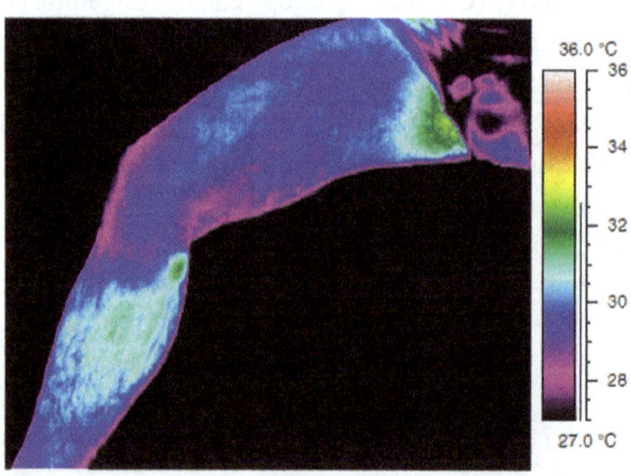

Area	Temperature °C
Right lower limb : T_{mean}	29.8

crystal thermographic plates to the thigh or leg usually after 20 tiptoe rises. Thermography is performed immediately after a tiptoe exercise what demonstrates incompetent perforating veins as "hot spots" after short time nedeed to thermodynamic equilibrium between liquid crystals and the body (Maksymowicz, Dudek, Bauer, Jurek, & Drozd, 2007; Mercer & Ring, 2009). Liquid crystal thermography diagnosis qualitative parameters compared with duplex scanning, showed the positive predictive value of this test of about 91% (Ammer, 2004; Thomas, Cobby, Davies, Jeans, & Whicher, 1989).

However it should be noted that liquid crystal thermography is not popular technique used in chronic venous disease because sometimes it requires doing exercises by patient what may be problematic - standing up the toes and back on the heels even 20 times and physician hast o stick the liquid crystal plate to the tibia. Then the time is needed to obtain thermodynamic equilibrium between liquid crystal plates and the body and after that it is possible to see the inefficient lancination veins as hot-spots (Beesley & Fegan, 1970; Patil, Williams, & Williams, 1970). Also developing is diagnosis is breast cancer studied by liquid crystal thermography. Such examination can show hot spots connected with tumor tissues (Kalodiki et al., 1995). It was also reported that liquid crystals are used in chronic back pain as well as in cosmetology and in diabetes in developing of feet ulceration (Rosenberg & Marchese, 1963; Beesley & Fegan, 1970). However it should be noted that it can be treated only as a qualitative tool with average temperature sensitivity.

It seems that there should be possibilities to use the other diagnostic technique – thermovision which is still developing through the years and nowadays the newest thermal cameras have sensitivity even less than 25 mK (Patil, Williams, & Williams, 1970). This is very important information because thermal imaging may give not only visible pathological changes but possibly also these ones which are not visible in other diagnostic techniques but connected with some malfunction in capillaries due to inflammatory state and thermoregulation problems (Harding, 1995; Sayre, Kelechi, & Neal, 2007). Such problems occurred in soft tissues result from blood supply changes undoubtedly influence on metabolism which changes manifest in body surface temperature gradient (Labropoulos, Tiongson, Pryor, Tassiopoulos, Kang, Mansour, & Baker, 2003; Bradbury, Murie, & Ruckley, 1993; Einspahr et al., 2007; Ammer, 2004; Ring, 2001).

Changes in blood supply especially in big veins or in capillaries that run in superficial skin layer are very good aims for thermovision. That is why it is used in i.e. vascular diseases, dermatological diseases, breast cancer, dermatological diseases, Raynaud phenomenon, foot ulceration among patients with diabetes mellitus, and lower back pain. There are many other medical specialities where thermal imaging gives important information about health state and therapy effects. It has been also reported that thermovision was used in physiological measurements with radiographic investigations. It was found that thermal imaging can show three to five times bigger areas characterized with a changed temperature gradient than a physician could see (Labropoulos, Tiongson, Pryor, Tassiopoulos, Kang, Mansour, & Baker, 2003; Bradbury, Murie, & Ruckley, 1993; Bauer, Hurnik, Zdziarski, Mielczarek, & Podbielska, 1997; Nicolaides, 2000; Herrick & Clark, 1998; Rok, 2012). It is due the high sensitivity of modern thermovision cameras, tissue metabolism, as well as circulation changes in capillaries. A Very important influence on skin temperature has activity of the endothelium cells that excrete active substances which are responsible for the vasoconstriction and vasodilatation of the vessels what play the main role in microcirculation (Sieroń, Cierpka, Rybak, & Stanek, 2009; Cholewka, Stanek, Klimas, Sieroń, & Drzazga, 2004). All advantages of thermal imaging mentioned above suggest thermovision as a very good and promising diagnostic technique that can be used in many diseases. However there are also some disadvantages of thermal imaging like its poor specificity which may be important in study of venous disorders. Thermal images can't identify the increased cutaneous perfusion. The presence of inflammatory effects in both deep and superficial vessels can be misleading when thermovision is used only. However thermal imaging is easy to perform and can give some important information connected to blood supply and metabolism changes on chosen skin areas. The technique may be effective not only in tracing the run of the superficial vessels but it gives opportunities to find some quantitative parameters useful in evaluation of health state of the patient especially when modern thermal cameras and support with computer programming is considered.

Therefore the purpose of this chapter was to present and discuss the usefulness of thermovision in chronic primary venous disease as well as show some relations between the known diagnostics parameters used as a gold standard like ones taken from duplex ultrasonography with temperature parameters obtained from thermograms.

The thermal imaging of the lower extremities skin surface should be performed by using a high sensivity Thermovision Camera. The emissivity should set in the range of 0.97 to 0.98. The patients before the examination should not exercise, eat hot meals or use of stimulants such as alcohol or drugs. Patients should stand in stable temperature and should wear cotton clothes that does not oppress their bodies approximately 20 minutes before the infrared examination. Patients should be instructed that before and during the examination should not touch the lower limbs. Examination should be performed in a air-conditioned room where the temperature is stable (23±1 °C). The distance between the camera and the patient's body should be about 1.0 – 1.5m (depending on the size of the limb). It is necessary to follow the standard protocol of infrared imaging in medicine.

CVD AND THERMOVISION: CARRIED OUT RESEARCH

In the literature can by presented some attempts to show usefulness of thermal imaging in venous disorders (Herrick & Clark, 1998; Bagavathiappan et al., 2009). For example thermography was used to measure blood flow indirectly, by measuring skin surface temperature. There were also tries to combining thermography with the structural detail of other imaging modalities what gave good synergy of anatomic and physiologic predictors of plaque vulnerability. Moreover there were trials performed for patients with suspected deep venous thrombosis who had thermography performed prior to ascending phlebography. It was obtained high agreement (79%). However it was not possible to diagnose consistently limited or early thrombosis, especially in the calf muscle veins. It was concluded that venous insufficiency produced the majority of false positives. However there is lack of papers tried to find out some correlation between parameters normally used in CVD diagnosis as: mean venous reflux duration and range of vein insufficiency, which are counted by duplex scan with thermal parameters derived from thermograms. There can be found paper in which the Authors tried to correlate mentioned above parameters with temperature and areas counted from thermograms. The parameters were:

- Mean temperature derived from isotherm area. Isotherm areas were marked using the mean temperature of the whole lower limb. The temperature higher than the mean limb temperature was taken as a temperature threshold used for the isotherm area in lower limb thermal images,
- Mean temperature of lower extremity, counted from limb area in thermograms,
- Range of isotherm area (Thermal range), that describes the range of area characterized by higher temperature seen along the venous run,

- Temperature difference described as difference between mean temperature of isotherm and mean temperature of lower limb surface,
- And ratio of whole lower extremity area and chosen isotherm area (Cholewka, Stanek, Klimas, Sieroń, & Drzazga, 2014).

The problem in using thermal imaging in diagnostics of CVD in not the possibility of visualization superficial veins as a hot spots but the set of procedures of imaging of lower extremities and show the results of the imaging as a complementary to duplex parameters. The important is to show in quantitative parameters what can't be shown and calculated by using ultrasound.

It is known that skin temperature is an indicator of the metabolism inside the organism especially when it is located in superficial tissues like it is in CVD so it seem to be a very interesting and pertinent issue for thermal imaging what was presented in Figure 3. One can see the areas characterized with higher temperature which are result of inflammatory states connected with venous disorders. It can be easily traced run of veins what was presented in literature area (Cholewka, Stanek, Klimas, Sieroń, & Drzazga, 2014; Cholewka et al., 2010; Bagavathiappan et al., 2009). However the question is if it is possible to obtain from such images important quantitative information that can agree or even close to those ones obtained from duplex scanning. That is why the thermograms from Figure 3 were presented in other way what can give us more possibilities in diagnostics – see Figure 4.

The thermograms in Figure 3a and 3c show elongated areas close to tracks of the vessels with a higher temperature than in healthy extremity. Such increased temperature seems to be associated with blood stasis due to a malfunction in the vein's valves and point to areas connected with vein deformation and inflammatory states. These processes manifest on the skin surface as areas with a higher temperature what is not seen on the thermogram of healthy lower limb (Figure 3a - right limb and Figure 3b). The differences in the temperature gradient can be easy correlated with the medical report (Cholewka, Stanek, Klimas, Sieroń, & Drzazga, 2014; Cholewka et al., 2010; Cholewka et al., 2012; Bauer, Hurnik, Zdziarski, Mielczarek, & Podbielska, 1997).

Why it is possible to see such thermal map in CVD? The answer is in the processes taking place inside and outside vessels as well as in blood cells.

The leukocyte entrapment, hyperviscosity of blood, and fibrin cuff are processes that influence blood flow but the interaction with endothelium cells is very important in developing of the disease because also the leukocytosis can lead to increase in of blood pressure. Moreover erythrocytes are smaller than white blood cells so they move faster and it can lead to a phenomenon called a leucocytes-erythrocytes train which causes an aggregation of erythrocytes that push the white blood cells to the vessel walls. Then the leucocytes entrapment may occur what is the process of its adhesion and accumulation to endothelium cells. All these processes can lead to migration of cells through the blood vessel walls (Sieroń, Cierpka, Rybak, & Stanek, 2009; Bradbury, Murie & Ruckley, 1993; Shor, 2007; Beesley & Fegan, 1970). Notably, described processes take place in small vessels and capillaries so they can be not visible during duplex scanning. That is why the thermovision can show temperature gradient changes due to decreased of blood flow, an increase of friction inside vessels because of their influence on heat production. Other process that can be observed during the development of vein insufficiency is the migration of leucocytes towards the main skin and lead to dysfunction of fibrinolysis, embolism inside the capillaries, hypoxia and trophic ulceration, what was reported in literature (Cholewka, Stanek, Klimas, Sieroń, & Drzazga, 2014; Cholewka et al., 2010; Cholewka et al., 2012). There were not visible such thermal effect in healthy limbs. Thermograms did not show such big temperature gradient changes along

Figure 3. The thermal images of the inside limb parts suffering from CVD. 3a presents a patient back view and 3b and 3c present thermograms for two lower extremities showed separately. Temperature parameters collected in the table show differences in mean temperatures between the left and right lower extremity

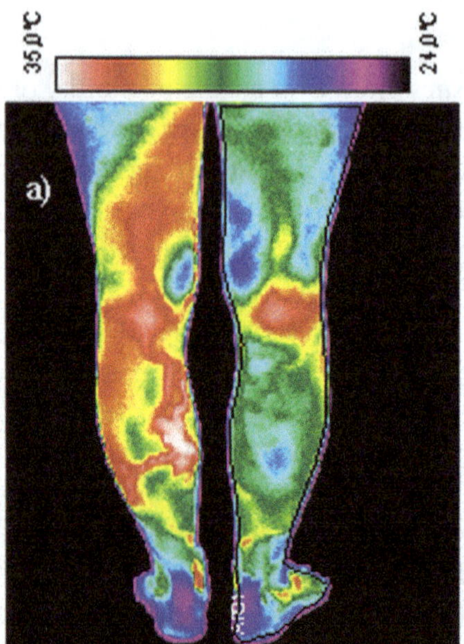

Area	Temperature °C
Left thigh: T mean	31,0
Right thigh: T mean	30,1

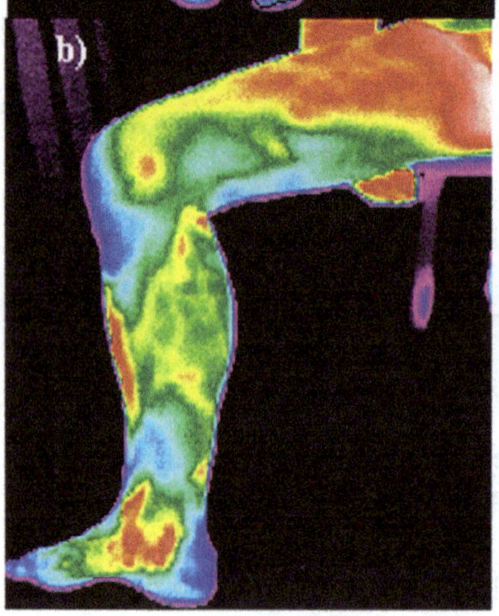

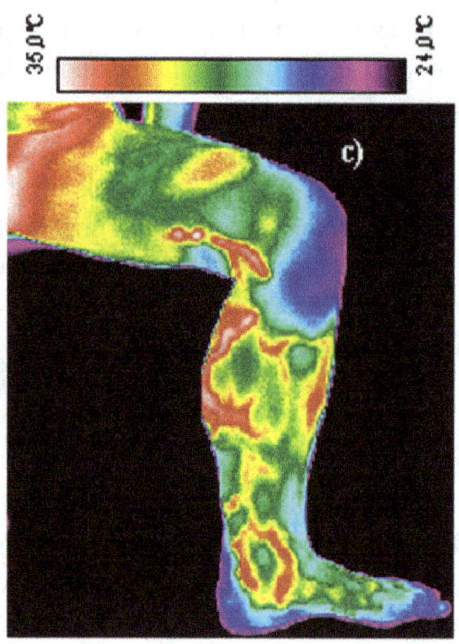

the run of the superficial veins and the skin temperature was much lower than for the patients with CVD. It was presented in earlier work (Cholewka, Stanek, Klimas, Sieroń, & Drzazga, 2014).

The other way to analyze thermograms of lower extremities of patients suffering from chronic venous disease is presented in Figure 4. The thermograms has marked isotherm areas that were done by using the temperature threshold set above the mean (in this case it was 31,0° C) limb temperature. The respective classic thermograms of presented patient are presented in Figure 3. The idea of such way to thermal diagnosis of chronic venous disease was presented in the literature (Cholewka, Stanek, Klimas, Sieroń, & Drzazga, 2014).

Figure 4. Thermal images of representative patient suffering from CVD and respective images, with marked isotherm areas. The temperature above the mean (in this case it was 31,0° C) limb temperature was taken as a temperature threshold used for obtain the isotherm areas

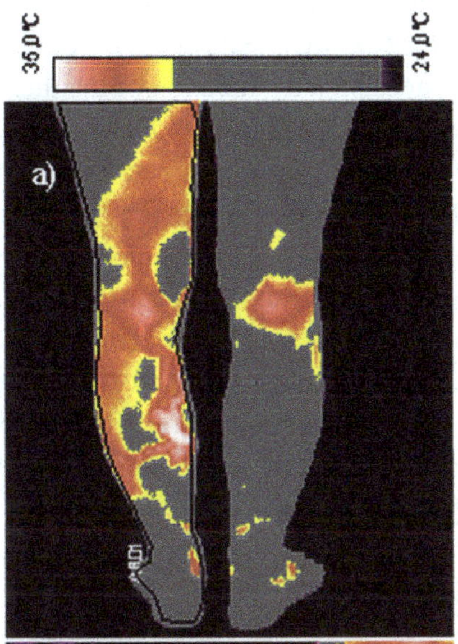

Area	Temperature °C
Left thigh: T mean	31,0
Right thigh: T mean	30,1

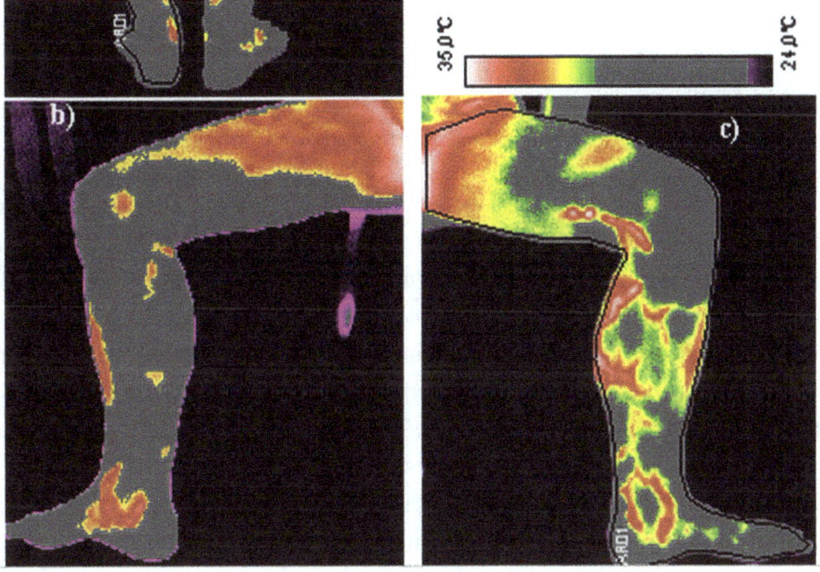

One can see the much bigger isotherm area on the left limb than on the right and the mean temperature of the left limb surface is higher than the right (in this case it was 0,9° C). Such designation seems to give some new information. It should be realized that most of the processes connected with venous disease are also relate to capillaries and microcirculation in the superficial tissues. That is why it may cause the temperature gradient changes on skin. Such presentation of this problem point out to probability of correlation between the temperature parameters counted from the thermograms and parameters from the ultrasound examination i.e. mean reflux duration and the range of vein insufficiency. That is why it has to be checked and there were some statistical analysis performed. The Authors focused on the duplex parameters (mean venous reflux duration and range of vein insufficiency) and the temperature parameters (mean temperature derived from isotherm area, mean temperature of lower extremity, range of isotherm area (counted along the limb), temperature difference described as difference between mean temperature of isotherm and mean temperature of lower limb surface, ratio of whole lower extremity area and isotherm area). Performed analysis showed medium negative correlation between the mean Venous Reflux Diuration and the Lower Limb mean temperature as well as the mean Venous Reflux Diuration and the mean temperature of the isotherm area. It should be considered that high value of mean venous reflux duration is connected with a low blood circulation what influences on a dysfunction of the thermoregulation in the soft tissues. That explains why reflux is higher in the inflammatory state around the vessel and it is seen on the thermograms as a bigger areas characterized by increased temperature. Moreover excluded parts of microcirculation system due to low or even lack of blood flow causes ischemia and anoxia of soft tissues and bigger venous stasis which may lead to colder lower extremities. The developing of the disease leads to structural and functional changes in the endothelium what causes a migration of leucocytes through the blood vessel walls. It is usually seen as a bigger skin temperature gradient as well as ramification of the vessels what also can be easily seen on thermograms. Performed other analysis tried to find out possibility of finding some dependences between the range of vein insufficiency counted by duplex scanning and the range of isotherm area marked on thermograms. Such study showed medium positive correlation what may suggest the thermal imaging as a helpful modality to evaluate the range of great saphenous vein insufficiency (Cholewka, Stanek, Klimas, Sieroń, & Drzazga, 2014).

CONCLUSION

Thermal imaging as a completely non-invasive technique can be helpful in the diagnosis of superficial vein insufficiency and promising diagnostics technique of lower extremities veins dysfunctions. It may be possible to optimise this thermal method of diagnosis in chronic venous disease but the study should involve a bigger group of patients and automatic algorithm of thermograms analysis which should be close to standard protocol of medical thermovision imaging (Ring & Ammer, 2000). Changes of the limb temperature gradient during the development of disease stays in good correlation with the physiological processes occurring in soft tissues and capillaries. In addition, many details can be seen which could not be seen in duplex scanning. Thermal imaging is used as a technique that can show the metabolism and functional changes manifested as changes in skin temperature.

It seems that thermal imaging in cooperation with duplex scanning may provide some early symptoms of blood circulation disorders which may be useful in prophylaxis and prognosis of veins or microcirculation problems in lower extremities because of possibility to show on thermograms things that cannot be seen in ultrasound diagnostics as the metabolism and functional changes manifested in skin temperature gradient. However, every patient should be taken into consideration individually. The innovative is using the thermal imaging in screening on venous diseases especially that Authors showed some correlation between standard parameters of Duplex USG and thermal parameters. Obtained results may provide to use thermal imaging as a standard used by family medicine physicians. It is very important to evaluate the standard protocol for using thermovision for chronic vein diseases insufficiency (Cholewka, Stanek, Klimas, Sieroń, & Drzazga, 2014).

REFERENCES

Abramowit, Queral, Finn, Nora, & Peterson, Bergan, & Yao. (1979). The use of photoplethsmography in the assessment of venous insufficiency: A comparison to venous pressure measurements. *Surgery*, *86*, 434–441. PMID:473029

Ammer. (2004). Temperature effects of thermotherapy determined by infrared measurements. *Phys Med, 20*(S1), 64-66.

Bagavathiappan, S., Philip, J., Raj, K., & Panicker, K. (2009). Infrared thermal imaging for detection of peripheral vascular disorders. *Journal of Medical Physics*, *34*(1), 43–47. doi:10.4103/0971-6203.48720 PMID:20126565

Bauer, Hurnik, & Zdziarski, Mielczarek, & Podbielska. (1997). Thermovision and its applications in medicine. *Acta Bio-Optica et Informatica Medica*, *3*(2-4), 121–131.

Bauer, Hurnik, Zdziarski, Mielczarek, & Skrzek, Podbielska, & Zagrobelny. (1997). Thermovison evaluation of cryotherapy effects. *Acta Bio-Optica et Informatica Medica*, *3*(2-4), 133–140.

Belcaro, Dugall, Luzzi, Ippolito, & Cesarone. (2014). Postpartum Varicose Veins: Supplementation with Pycnogenol or Elastic Compression—A 12-Month Follow-Up. *International Journal of Angiology*. Available at http://santurel.net/_library/_files/Pycnogenol-studie-spataders.pdf

Benbow, C., & Bowsher, W. (1994). The prediction of diabetic neuropathic plantar foot ulceration by liquid-crystal contact thermography. *Diabetes Care*, *17*(8), 835–839. doi:10.2337/diacare.17.8.835 PMID:7956627

Bollinger, Isenring, & Franzeck. (1982). U.K.: Lymphatic microangiopathy: a complication of severe chronic venous incompetence (CVI). *Lymphology*, *15*(2), 60–65. PMID:7109680

Bollinger, L., Leu, A. J., Hoffmann, U., & Franzeck, U. K. (1997). Microvascular changes in venous disease: An update. *Angiology*, *48*(1), 27–32. doi:10.1177/000331979704800105 PMID:8995340

Bradbury, M., Murie, J. A., & Ruckley, C. V. (1993). Role of leucocyte in the pathogenesis of vascular disease. *British Journal of Surgery*, *80*(12), 1503–1512. doi:10.1002/bjs.1800801204 PMID:8298912

Briain, L., & Takano, F. (2003). Intravascular Modalities for Detection of Vulnerable Plaque. *Arteriosclerosis, Thrombosis, and Vascular Biology*, *23*(8), 1333–1342. doi:10.1161/01.ATV.0000080948.08888.BF PMID:12805071

Browne, S., Sivananthan, U. M., Sabroe, I., & Rees, M. R. (1992). Use of thermal imaging to monitor crural thrombolysis. *Blood Coagulation & Fibrinolysis*, *3*(4), 489–492. doi:10.1097/00001721-199208000-00019 PMID:1420827

Caggiati, B., & Gloviczki, J. (2002). International Interdisciplinary Consensus Committee on Venous Anatomical Terminology. Nomenclature of the veins of the lower limbs: An international interdisciplinary consensus statement. *Journal of Vascular Surgery*, *36*(2), 416–422. doi:10.1067/mva.2002.125847 PMID:12170230

Cameron, S., Sachdev, D., Gishen, P., & Martin, J. F. (1991). Liquid crystal thermography as a screening test for deep vein thrombosis in patients with cerebral infarction. *European Journal of Clinical Investigation*, *21*(5), 548–550. doi:10.1111/j.1365-2362.1991.tb01408.x PMID:1752294

Chiesa, M., & Limoni, V. (2005). Demographic factors and their relationship with the presence of CVI signs in Italy: The 24-cities cohort study. *European Journal of Vascular and Endovascular Surgery*, *30*(6), 674–680. doi:10.1016/j.ejvs.2005.06.016 PMID:16055355

Cholewka, K., & Stanek, K. (2012). Thermal imaging and TC oximetry measurements of hyperbaric oxygen therapy (HBO) effects on trophic ulceration of the crura. *Journal of Thermal Analysis and Calorimetry*, *108*(1), 25–31. doi:10.1007/s10973-011-1934-6

Cholewka, Stanek, & Klimas, Sieroń, & Drzazga. (2014). Thermal Imaging Application In Chronic Venous Disease. *Pilot Study*, *115*, 1609–1618.

Cholewka, Stanek, & Kwiatek, Sieroń, & Drzazga. (2013). Does the temperature gradient correlate with photodynamic diagnosis parameter NCV? *Photodiagnosis and Photodynamic Therapy*, *10*, 33–38. doi:10.1016/j.pdpdt.2012.07.001 PMID:23465370

Christopoulos, N., Nicolaides, A. N., & Szendro, G. (1988). Venous reflux: Quantification and correlation with clinical severity. *British Journal of Surgery*, *75*(4), 352–356. doi:10.1002/bjs.1800750419 PMID:3359149

Criado, D., & Marston, M. (1995). Physiologic variation in lower extremity venous valvular function. *Annals of Vascular Surgery*, *9*(1), 102–108. doi:10.1007/BF02015323 PMID:7703053

Criado, F., & Marston, D. (1998). The role of air plethysmography in the diagnosis of chronic venous insufficiency. *Journal of Vascular Surgery*, *27*(4), 660–670. doi:10.1016/S0741-5214(98)70231-9 PMID:9576079

Da Silva, Navarro, & Batalheiro. (1992). The importance of chronic venous insufficiency: Various preliminary data on its medico-social consequences. *Phlebologie*, *45*, 439–443. PMID:1302319

Davison, Ewing, & Fergason. (1972). Detection of breast cancer by liquid crystal thermography: A preliminary report. *Cancer, 29*, 1123-1132.

Dragan & MILIC. (2011). Prevalence and socioeconomic data in chronic venous disease: How useful are they in planning appropriate management? *Medicographia*, *33*, 253.

Eberhardt, R. T. (2005). Chronic Venous Insufficiency. *Circulation*, *111*(18), 2398–2409. doi:10.1161/01.CIR.0000164199.72440.08 PMID:15883226

Einspahr, T., & Saboda, N. (2007). Expression of vascular endothelial growth factor in early cutaneous melanocytic lesion progression. *Cancer*, *110*(11), 2519–2527. doi:10.1002/cncr.23076 PMID:17932890

Fegan, W. G., & Beesley, W. H. (1970). An investigation into the localisation of incompetent perforating veins. *British Journal of Surgery*, *57*(1), 30–32. doi:10.1002/bjs.1800570106 PMID:5411584

Fowkes, L., & Evans, A. (2001). Lifestyle risk factors for lower limb venous reflux in the general population: Edinburgh Vein Study. *International Journal of Epidemiology*, *30*(4), 846–852. doi:10.1093/ije/30.4.846 PMID:11511615

Gloviczki, Comerota, Dalsing, Eklof, & Gillespie. (2011). The care of patients with varicose veins and associated chronic venous diseases: Clinical practice guidelines of the Society for Vascular Surgery and the American Venous Forum. *J Vasc Surg, 5*, 1S-48S.

Guex, Myon, & Didier, Nguyen Le, & Taieb. (2005). Chronic venous disease: Health status of a population and care impact on this health status through quality of life questionnaires. *International Angiology*, *24*, 258–264. PMID:16158036

Guex, Z., & Boussetta, N. L. (2007). Construction and validation of a patient reported outcome dedicated to chronic venous disorder: SQOR-V (Specific Quality of Life and Outcome Response-Venous). *Journal des Maladies Vasculaires*, *32*(3), 135–137. doi:10.1016/j.jmv.2007.05.004 PMID:17616292

Harada, K., Katz, M. L., & Comerota, A. (1995). A non-invasive screening test to detect critical deep venous reflux. *Journal of Vascular Surgery*, *22*(5), 532–537. doi:10.1016/S0741-5214(95)70033-1 PMID:7494351

Harding. (1995). Liquid crystal thermography in the investigation of deep venous thrombosis: A prospective study of 800 patients. In *The Thermal Image in Medicine and Biology*. Uhlen Verlag.

Harding. (1995). Thermal imaging in the investigation of deep venous thrombosis. *Proceedings of the 1995 IEEE Engineering in Medicine and Biology conference and 21st Canadian Medica/and Biological Engineering Conference.*

Herrick, A. L., & Clark, S. (1998). Quantifying digital vascular disease in patients with primary Raynauds phenomenon and systemic sclerosis. *Annals of the Rheumatic Diseases*, *57*(2), 70–78. doi:10.1136/ard.57.2.70 PMID:9613334

Hess. (2005). Identifying and managing venous dermatitis. *Adv Skin Wound Care., 18*(5), 42-3.

Jung, Z., & Kalicki, M. (2015). Thermal imaging in the screening diagnosis of crural varices in adolescents. In F. Ring, A. Jung, & J. Zuber (Eds.), Infrared Imaging. A casebook in clinical medicine. IOP Publishing.

Kalodiki, Calahoras, & Geroulakos. (1995). Liquid crystal thermography and duplex in the preoperative marking of varicose veins. *Phlebology*, *10*, 110–114.

Kamida, Eklof, & Masuda. (2001). Lower extremity ascending and descending venography. In Handbook of Venous Disorders (2nd ed.). New York, NY: Arnold.

Kaplan, C., & Denenberg, B. (2003). Quality of life in patients with chronic venous disease: San Diego population study. *Journal of Vascular Surgery*, *37*(5), 1047–1053. doi:10.1067/mva.2003.168 PMID:12756353

Kurz, Kahn, & Abenhaim. (1999). Chronic venous disorders of the leg: epidemiology, outcomes, diagnosis and management: summary of an evidence-based report of the VEINES task force. *International Angiology*, *18*, 83–102. PMID:10424364

Labropolous, T. (2003). Definition of venous reflux in lower extremity veins. *Journal of Vascular Surgery, 38*(4), 793–798. doi:10.1016/S0741-5214(03)00424-5 PMID:14560232

Labropoulos, T., Pryor, T., & Kang, A. M. (2003). Definition of venous reflux in the lowerextremity veins. *Journal of Vascular Surgery, 38*(4), 793–798. doi:10.1016/S0741-5214(03)00424-5 PMID:14560232

Lafuma, Fagnani, Peltier-Pujol, & Rauss. (1994). Venous disease in France: An unrecognized public health problem[in French]. *Journal des Maladies Vasculaires, 19*, 185–189. PMID:7798803

Laurikka, S., & Tarkka, A. (2002). Risk indicators for varicose veins in forty to sixty-year-olds in the Tampere varicose vein study. *World Journal of Surgery, 26*(6), 648–651. doi:10.1007/s00268-001-0283-1 PMID:12053212

Maksymowicz, Dudek, & Bauer, Jurek, & Drozd. (2007). Assessment of the possibilities of applications of the thermovision technique in medico-legal diagnosis. *Annales Academiae Medicae Stetinensis, 53*(suppl. 2), 102–106. PMID:20143690

Markel, M., & Manzo, B. (1994). A comparison of the cuff deflation method with Valsavas maneuver and limb compression in detecting venous valvular reflux. *Archives of Surgery (Chicago, Ill.), 129*(7), 701–705. doi:10.1001/archsurg.1994.01420310033005 PMID:8024449

Martins, Ribeiro, & Cury. (2012). Diagnostic Evaluation of Chronic Venous Insufficiency Cases Using Thermal Imaging. *Thermology International, 22*(3), 169-176.

Masuda, Eklof, & Kistner. (2001). Direct venous pressure: Role in the assessment of venous disease. In Handbook of Venous Disorders (2nd ed.). New York, NY: Arnold.

Mercer, Nielsen, & Hoffmann. (2008). Improvement of wound healing by water-filtered infrared-A (wIRA) in patients with chronic venous stasis ulcers of the lower legs including evaluation using infrared thermography. *GMS German Medical Science, 6*, 1-26.

Mercer & Ring. (2009). Fever screening and infrared thermal imaging: Concerns and guidelines. *Thermology International, 19*, 67–69.

Milic. (2011). Prevalence and socioeconomic data in chronic venous disease: How useful are they in planning appropriate management? *Medicographia, 33*, 253-258.

Neglen, E., Egger, J. F. III, Olivier, J., & Raju, S. (2004). Hemodynamic and clinical impact of ultrasound-derived venous reflux parameters. *Journal of Vascular Surgery, 40*(2), 303–310. doi:10.1016/j.jvs.2004.05.009 PMID:15297826

Neglen, P., & Raju, S. (2000). Ambulatory venous pressure revisited. *Journal of Vascular Surgery, 31*(6), 1206–1213. doi:10.1067/mva.2000.105669 PMID:10842158

Nelzen, B., Bergqvist, D., & Lindhagen, A. (1991). Leg ulcer etiology–a cross-sectional population study. *Journal of Vascular Surgery, 14*(4), 557–564. doi:10.1016/0741-5214(91)90251-O PMID:1920653

Nicolaides, A. N., & Miles, C. (1987). Photoplethysmography in the assessment of venous insufficiency. *Journal of Vascular Surgery, 5*(3), 405–412. doi:10.1016/0741-5214(87)90047-4 PMID:3334678

Nicolaides, A. N., & Zukowski, A. J. (1986). The value of dynamic venous pressure measurements. *World Journal of Surgery*, *10*(6), 919–924. doi:10.1007/BF01658640 PMID:3798938

Nicolaides. (2000). Investigation of chronic venous insufficiency: A consensus statement. *Circulation, 102*, e126-e163.

Patil, W., Williams, L., & Williams, K. L. (1970). Thermographic localisation of incompetent perforating veins in the leg. *British Medical Journal*, *1*(5690), 195–197. doi:10.1136/bmj.1.5690.195 PMID:4904934

Raffetto, J. D., & Khalil, R. A. (2008). Mechanisms of varicose vein formation: Valve dysfunction and wall dilation. *Phlebology*, *23*(2), 85–98. doi:10.1258/phleb.2007.007027 PMID:18453484

Ring & Ammer. (2000). The technique of infrared imaging in medicine. *Thermol Intern*, *10*, 7–14.

Ring. (2001). Provocation tests in thermal imaging. *Abs. Thermology Int., 11*, 2.

Ritchie, S., Soulen, R. L., & Lapayowker, M. S. (1979). Thermographic diagnosis of deep venous thrombosis. *Radiology*, *131*(2), 341–344. doi:10.1148/131.2.341 PMID:441316

Rok. (2012). *The use of thermovision in diagnostics and therapy* (Doctoral Thesis). Jagiellonian Univeristy, Kraków, Poland.

Rosenberg & Marchese. (1963). Perforator vein localisation by heat emission detection. *Surgery*, *53*, 575–578. PMID:13974907

Rutherford, P., & Comerota, K. (2000). Venous severity scoring: An adjunct to venous outcome assessment. *Journal of Vascular Surgery*, *31*(6), 1307–1312. doi:10.1067/mva.2000.107094 PMID:10842165

Sayre, K., Kelechi, T. J., & Neal, D. (2007). Sudden increase in skin temperature predicts venous ulcers: A case study. *Journal of Vascular Nursing*, *25*(3), 46–50. doi:10.1016/j.jvn.2007.06.002 PMID:17723909

Scott, LaMorte, Gorin, & Menzoian. (1995). Risk factors for chronic venous insufficiency: A Dual case-control study. *J Vasc Surg., 22*(5), 622-628.

Shor & Pronin. (2006). Local signs of the reperfusion syndrome in obliterating atherosclerosis of the lower extremity arteries and their treatment. *Klin Khir*, *1*, 34–37. PMID:16719070

Stess, S., & Moss, G. (1986). Use of liquid crystal thermography in the evaluation of the diabetic foot. *Diabetes Care*, *9*(3), 267–272. doi:10.2337/diacare.9.3.267 PMID:3731992

Sukovatykh & Kniazev. (2007). The mechanisms of critical impairments of microcirculation in patients with chronic ischemia of lower extremities. *Vestnik Khirurgii Imeni I. I. Grekova*, *166*(4), 20–24. PMID:17966649

Švestková & Pospíšilová. (1991). Risk Factors Of Chronic Venous Disease Inception. *Current Problems in Surgery*, *28*, 339–400.

Švestková & Pospíšilová. (2008). Risk Factors Of Chronic Venous Disease Inception. *Scripta Medica*, *81*(2), 117–128.

Tennvall, Andersso, & Bjellerup, Hjelmgren, & Oien. (2004). Treatment of venous leg ulcers can be better and cheaper. Annual costs calculation based on an inquiry study. *Lakartidningen*, *101*, 1506–1510, 1512–1513. PMID:15150953

Thomas, C., & Davies, J. (1989). Liquid crystal thermography and C reactive protein in the detection of deep venous thrombosis. *BMJ (Clinical Research Ed.)*, *299*(6705), 951–952. doi:10.1136/bmj.299.6705.951 PMID:2508949

Van den Oever, Hepp, Debbaut, & Simon. (1998). Socio-economic impact of chronic venous insufficiency. An underestimated public health problem. *International Angiology*, *17*, 161–167. PMID:9821029

Wilkinson, B., & Edwards, S. (1993). Leukocytes: Their role in the etiopathogenesis of skin damage in venous disease. *Journal of Vascular Surgery*, *17*(4), 669–675. doi:10.1016/0741-5214(93)90109-Y PMID:8464084

Chapter 3
Clinical Applications:
Infrared Thermal Diagnosis of Orthopaedic Injuries in Childhood

Enrique Sanchis-Sánchez
University of Valencia, Spain

Jose María Blasco
University of Valencia, Spain

Rosario Salvador-Palmer
University of Valencia, Spain

Esther Ballester
Hospital Universitario Doctor Peset, Spain

Pilar Codoñer-Franch
Hospital Universitario Doctor Peset, Spain

Enrique J Sanchis
University of Valencia, Spain

Jose Martín-Guerrero
University of Valencia, Spain

Rolando González-Peña
University of Valencia, Spain

Carlos Vergara-Hernández
CSISP-FISABIO, Spain

Jose I. Priego-Quesada
University of Valencia, Spain

Rosa M Cibrián
University of Valencia, Spain

ABSTRACT

The study of the diagnostic accuracy of Infrared Thermal Imaging in the diagnosis of orthopaedic injuries in childhood has been motivated by the high incidence of these injuries throughout the world, being one of the most common reasons for urgent medical consultation. Diagnosis of musculoskeletal injuries usually involves radiography, but this exposes children without fractures to unnecessary ionising radiation. This chapter assesses whether infrared thermography could provide a viable alternative in cases of trauma. To evaluate the accuracy of this technique new thermographic variables have been added to those commonly analysed, such as the extent of the injury and the difference in the size of the area that is at an equal temperature or higher than the maximum temperature of the healthy area. Non-linear cataloguing methods (decision tree models) have also been applied. With the protocol presented, infrared thermal imaging had a sensitivity of 0.91, a specificity of 0.88 and a negative predictive value of 0.95 for diagnosing musculoskeletal injuries.

DOI: 10.4018/978-1-5225-2072-6.ch003

INTRODUCTION

Musculoskeletal injuries (fractures, sprains, dislocations, contusions and compartment syndrome) are a leading cause of paediatric injuries in western countries (Collard, Verhagen, Van Mechelen, Heymans, & Chinapaw, 2011) and one of the main reasons why children visit paediatric emergency departments. At the hospital where the study was carried out, 65% of paediatric emergencies involved traumatological injuries. The diagnostic reaction towards these injuries is varied: while the case history and physical exploration constitute the first step in the clinical process, the interpretation of the diagnostic studies through imaging is essential, X-rays being the most commonly used means. Most paediatric fractures occur in the limbs and, although the effective radiation dose is very small, this procedure can be unnecessary for children without a bone fracture at the same time as exposing them to ionizing radiation (Schulze-Rath, Hammer, & Blettner, 2008; Mettler et al., 2009).

Moreover, the X-ray does not allow one to directly detect a relatively common type of traumatological injury such as epiphysiolysis type 1 (Salter-Harris fractures), as they involve fissures of the ligament and, therefore, require a complementary study.

Bone fractures usually trigger a local inflammatory response, evident through a set of signs and symptoms amongst which is a notable increase in skin temperature in the affected area. Infrared Thermal Imaging (ITI) is a useful addition to the diagnostic tools available to clinicians, as it can detect localized variations in temperature, such as those that occur when there is a fracture (Head & Elliott 2002; Pascoe, Mercer, & De Weerd, 2006; Arthur, Khan, & Barclay, 2011), as well as having the advantages of being easy to use and harmless (Awerbuch, 1991).The authors have, therefore, undertaken a systematic review looking into the diagnostic possibilities of infrared thermal imaging for musculoskeletal injuries (Sanchis-Sánchez et al., 2014), as very few studies on the use of infrared thermal imaging in children's limb injuries (Saxena & Willital, 2008; Silva et al., 2012) have been published.

The review found only three studies from the 1980s whose aim was to evaluate the diagnostic potential of infrared thermal imaging in stress fractures. Results from this systematic review showed high heterogeneity for sensitivity, negative likelihood ratio and diagnostic odds ratio, together with moderate combined values for specificity (0.69; 95% CI: 0.49–0.85) and low values for positive likelihood ratio (2.31; 95% CI: 0.63–8.47). These values limit the clinical use of thermal imaging.

However, in the studies consulted it was observed that, on the one hand, they did not consider several variables that could be of interest, such as the size of the injury, and, on the other hand, that the statistical treatment of the data provided by the thermographic images had been undertaken using conventional statistical tests such as Logistic Regressions, even though the type of variables considered would allow them to be analysed using other statistical tests, namely non-linear cataloguing, which would be more appropriate for dealing with complex clinical issues.

This chapter, therefore, presents a protocol for evaluating the thermographic images of traumatological injuries. A greater number of study variables and non-linear cataloguing methods are employed in the form of decision trees to discriminate between fractures and other musculoskeletal injuries (Breiman, Friedman, Olshen, & Stone, 1984). Using this protocol infrared thermal imaging had a sensitivity of 0.91, a specificity of 0.88 and a negative predictive value of 0.95 for diagnosing musculoskeletal injuries.

BACKGROUND: APPLICATIONS OF THERMAL IMAGING IN THE FIELD OF MEDICINE

Health Applications

Over the last five decades there has been a steady increase in the use of infrared thermal imaging cameras in order to obtain correlations between thermal physiology and skin temperature. Thermal imaging has been mainly used to investigate diseases in which skin temperature may reflect the presence of inflammation in the underlying tissues, or where blood flow is either increased or reduced due to a clinical abnormality. In principle, thermal imaging can be applied in medicine, either as a diagnostic test or as an outcome measurement in clinical trials (Ring & Ammer, 2012).

ITI has been successfully used in the diagnosis of breast cancer, diabetic neuropathy and peripheral vascular disorders. It has also been used to diagnose musculoskeletal injuries, detect neurological problems and rheumatic diseases, also in gynaecology, dermatology, ophthalmology, kidney transplants, cardiology, surgery, thermoregulation control and fever screening (Jones, 1998; Lahiri, Bagavathiappan, Jayakumar, & Philip, 2012).

New generation infrared detectors provide thermal images that are now becoming a diagnostic tool and an increasingly accepted medical alternative for carrying out measurements of abnormal temperature patterns. The interpretation of the encoded ITIs with a colour and temperature scale is a quicker and comparatively easy process.

Currently, research into this field is centred on the automatic analysis of temperature distribution in the region of interest (ROI) and their statistical analysis for detecting abnormalities. Moreover, thermal images can be stored digitally and, following the use of different software packages for processing, can be compared with a thermal pattern. In this way, and due to the clinical nature of diseases, abnormal thermal patterns on the surface of the skin can be monitored.

In 1964 Barnes showed that ITI can provide information on physical anomalies and, therefore, can be useful in diagnosing physical disease (Barnes, 1964). Since then a large number of authors have conducted research in the field of medicine. Thus, Jiang et al. (Jiang et al., 2005) undertook a review of the outlook for ITI in medical thermal imaging and E. F. J. Ring, Jung, and Zuber (Ring, Jung, & Zuber, 2009), suggested several opportunities for using ITI in the medical field.

At present, ITI is of general use in research into breast cancer (Arora, 2008; Ng, 2009; Kontos, Wilson, & Fentiman, 2011) where tumours are characterized by an increase in angiogenesis and, therefore, an increase in metabolic activity leading to higher temperature gradients in comparison with adjoining tissues. It is also well established in surgery such as in in coronary artery bypass operations, as it allows one to supervise the resumption of blood flow through the coronary blood vessels (Wild, Schütte, Pau, Kramp, & Just, 2003). In plastic surgery it is used to assess the reperfusion of skin flaps (de Weerd, Mercer, & Setså, 2006).

In addition, Hildebrandt et al. (Hildebrandt, Raschner, & Ammer, 2010; Hildebrandt, Zeilberger, Ring, & Raschner, 2012) included more recent and important uses classified into three fields of research; injuries to soft tissues, vascular disorders and vasomotor disorders and affirmed that it is used in a variety of medical applications in the fields of neurology, oncology, traumatology and dermatology.

In the review undertaken by Lahiri et al. (Lahiri et al., 2012) it was said that so far ITI had successfully been used in fields such as: the study of thermoregulation, the detection of breast cancer, the diagnosis of diabetic neuropathy and vascular disorders, detecting fever, diagnostics in odontology; applications in dermatology; control of blood pressure; diagnosing rheumatic diseases, diagnosing dry-eye syndrome and other ocular diseases; diagnosing hepatic diseases; renal diseases, heart surgery operations, and gynaecology.

The latest update on the advances of ITI in medicine (Diakides, Diakides, Lupo, Paul, & Balcerak, 2013) provided the following list of ITI applications in medicine:

- Oncology,
- Treatment and control of pain,
- Vascular disorders,
- Rheumatic diseases/arthritis,
- Neurology,
- Surgery (heart, transplants, etc.),
- Ophthalmology,
- Dermatology,
- Burns,
- Ulcers,
- Monitoring the efficacy of pharmacological treatments and other therapies,
- Thyroids,
- Odontology,
- Respiratory disorders,
- Sport and
- Physical rehabilitation.

There are institutions dedicated to the research and practical applications of ITI throughout the world and this has led to a growing number of publications in scientific journals (Diakides et al., 2013).

This chapter deals with the study of musculoskeletal injuries through thermal imaging, which is less commonly analysed in scientific bibliography. However, for all the areas of medicine, it should be pointed out that, even ITI offers a visual and quantitative map of the distribution of skin temperature, a clinical evaluation for interpreting the thermal images is required. 2 In this chapter the possibilities of a protocol will be discussed so that, from the quantification of variables in thermal imaging and the use of decision trees for their analysis, it may be able to discriminate between fractures and non-fractures in a parallel study to the clinical assessment.

Application for the Study of Musculoskeletal Injuries

Epidemiological studies show that 80% of fractures happen to children over the age of 6, 70% of them in the upper limb, the most frequent causes being a casual fall at an early age and sports injuries (Collard et al., 2011). The possibility that a child suffers a fracture during their growth period is greater in boys (42%) than in girls (27%) (Landin, 1997).

Of fractures to the upper limbs, 45.1% are to the radius (mostly to its metaphysis and distal physis); 18.4% in the humerus (metaphysis and distal physis); 15.1% to the tibia; 13.8% to the clavicle and 7.6% to the femur. Fissure fractures represent 21.7% of injuries. Ligament injuries and dislocations, as well as fractures of the hip and spine, are less frequent, as the physis absorbs the forces and cedes earlier. Special mention, owing to their complications, should be made of epiphysiolysis, fractures that affect the physis or growth plate that represent between 15% and 20% of all fractures, being most frequent during the latter stages of adolescence and predominantly in the upper limb (Gascó-Gómez de Membrillera, Gascó-Adrien, & Barra-Pla, 2002). These fractures can be classified according to the Salter and Harris classification in different degrees. Those of type I affect only the area of cartilage growth, with separation between the metaphysis and the epiphysis, but with displacement of the fragments and, hence, do not appear in an X-ray image.

It is, therefore, of interest to be able to discriminate, from the thermal imaging point of view, cases of fracture as opposed to other types of traumatological injuries such as contusions or sprains that do not require the undertaking of an X-ray for their treatment and to see whether thermal imaging can identify epiphysiolysis type 1, which does not appear in X-rays.

A wide-ranging systematic review on the use of thermal imaging for studying musculoskeletal injuries (Saxena et al., 2008) concluded that the establishment of a rigorous protocol and an adequate analysis of the data for improving the results obtained to date would be desirable.

MAIN FOCUS OF THE CHAPTER

The study design is based on the evaluation of the diagnostic accuracy of thermal imaging for diagnosing traumatological injuries (fracture, non-fracture) to individuals of a paediatric age. The aim of this type of study design consisted of estimating the measuring capacity (diagnostic test) for discriminating between individuals who suffer an illness and those who do not, but who present a similar symptomology. It set off from the hypothesis that the injury can be measured validly and reliably through a "*gold standard*", i.e., a reference procedure.

The determination of the sample and its characteristics was based on the results obtained in the previously undertaken systematic review [8], establishing, on the one hand, that to be able to successfully estimate a sensitivity of 0.8 and a specificity of 0.6, with α=0.05 and an accuracy in the estimate of 0.1, a sample of 155 individuals attending the paediatric emergency service was required (62 injured -fractures- and 93 non-injured -contusions and sprains-). Inclusion and exclusion criteria in the study were then defined. The population sample with traumatisms was obtained from cases attending the paediatric emergencies service of the Hospital Universitario Dr. Peset of Valencia, with suspected bone fractures. The harmlessness of the test and what it consisted of was explained to all study subjects and to their parents or legal guardians and the consent of the parents or guardians was requested, as all subjects were minors. Without this requirement they could not be included in the study. The study was approved by the Ethics Committee of the Hospital in which the study was carried out.

The inclusion criteria for the study were as follows:

- Between 1 and 14 years of age
- Informed consent of the legal guardian
- Diagnosis of suspected bone fracture in limbs

- X-ray available for confirming the diagnosis

And as exclusion criteria:

- Time elapsed since the origin of the injury greater than 72 hours
- The consumption of anti-inflammatory drugs in the 3 hours prior to the test
- Wearing a plastercast or other type of fixed ferule
- Non-fulfilment of one or more requirements of the measuring protocol that will be detailed further on: impossible rest, contact with the region of interest during the waiting period, shower or bath in the previous 2 hours, fever (≥ 38 ºC), use of creams, lotions or local application of ice on the regions of interest within the 3 hours prior to the test.

Applying these criteria, 145 of the 208 patients evaluated were eligible for inclusion.

Image-Capture Protocol

Table 1 shows the criteria used in the image-capture protocol.

The image-capture room, therefore, was acclimatized to 24 ºC. There was no source of direct air that could have an effect on the exploration zone and there was a relative humidity of 40%. Here the study participants uncovered the affected zone and its contralateral zone, remaining at rest in the ward for 10 minutes without having any contact with the ROI, as established in the thermal imaging measuring protocol for acclimatization.

The position of the children for capturing the image depended on their clinical state and the region of interest (ROI), which could be undertaken in standing, lying or sitting position. Depending on the injured area between 2 and 4 images were taken (anterior, posterior, lateral and medial).

Without having the definitive diagnosis available, thermal images were taken on the ROI of the injured and uninjured zones and with the following values of reference (Ring et al., 2000; Hassan et al., 2007; Practice guidelines, 2012a; Practice guidelines, 2012b; Vardasca & Simoes, 2013):

- Emissivity (ε) of 0.98,
- Distance camera-patient of 0.8 m,
- Projection angle of 0º.

During the image-capture process, expanded polystyrene sheets, placed behind the ROI, were used to prevent possible thermal contamination of the area. Information was also gathered on the atmospheric temperature and the relative humidity of the image-capture room, so that they could be introduced as correction parameters in the image analyses and into the thermal imaging camera itself (Ring et al., 2000).

Furthermore, information on the definitive diagnosis of the pathologies of interest was gathered once issued by the traumatology team. The diagnosis was based on a combination of clinical criteria and a radiological study (simple X-ray) carried out by the radiology team. The traumatology and radiology teams of the hospital did not have any knowledge at any time of the results of the ITI.

Figure 1 presents the ITI images corresponding to some of the patients analyzed. These images were processed following the protocol indicated below.

Table 1. Criteria used in the image-capture protocol

Aspects to Consider	Recommendations	Criteria Used in the Protocol
Room characteristics	Sufficient space so that the patients can remain at rest with the aim of establishing their temperature.	Room with sufficient area for patient rest.
Room temperature control between 18 °C and 26 °C (Ring & Ammer, 2000)	Use of temperature indicator.	According with the protocol, the image-capture room was acclimatized to 24 ºC and with a relative humidity of 40%.
	The flow of air-conditioning must be low and not directly aimed at the patient.	No source of direct air that could affect the zone of exploration.
Background or atmospheric radiation	Take measures to reduce the radiation of the surroundings: Reduce the distance between the patient and the camera.	Distance of 0.8 m, angle of 0º.
	Isolate the object or zone of interest from possible thermal sources nearby. Avoid as much as possible reflection that can be produced on the walls around the patient during the taking of the thermogram in the nearby area.	Use of expanded polystyrene sheets placed behind the ROI and under the lights.
Image-capture system	Mounting the camera. Operating the camera.	20 minutes before carrying out the technique, switch on the camera.
The patient	Norms prior to undertaking the test (Usuki, Kanekura, Aradono, & Kanzaki, 1998): Use of cosmetics in the 12 previous hours. Pharmacological treatment. Stabilization stage of the temperature 10-15 minutes (Ring et al., 2000). Avoid contact with the zones to be explored Positioning for capturing the image Standardize the distance camera-patient for each region of the body.	Exclusion criteria: consumption of anti-inflammatory drugs and/or use of creams, lotions or local application of ice on the ROI within the 3 hours prior to the test. Zone affected and its contralateral zone uncovered, remaining in the room for 10 minutes without making any contact with the ROI.

Processing the Images and Study Variables

Although thermal imaging already provides a map of temperatures that allow one to see evidence of asymmetries between the healthy and pathological zones, a protocol was established for obtaining quantifying variables of the injury that may later allow a statistical study to be undertaken to assess the diagnostic capability of this technique.

In order to carry out the analysis, differences between the ROI in the injured and the healthy area were analysed, given that thermal symmetry of the upper and lower limbs exists in healthy subjects (Vardasca, Ring, Plassmann, & Jones, 2012). ROIs were determined using an adapted version of the Glamorgan Standard Capture Protocol (Ammer & Ring, 2007; Ammer, 2008), which selects the limits of the ROI based on anatomical markers. The variables analysed were:

- The difference between the mean temperatures of the injured and healthy ROI (ΔTmean),
- The difference between the maximum temperatures of both the injured and healthy ROI (ΔTmax) and

Figure 1. Thermographic images of some of the patients analysed. a) Fractures. b) Sprains. c) Contusions

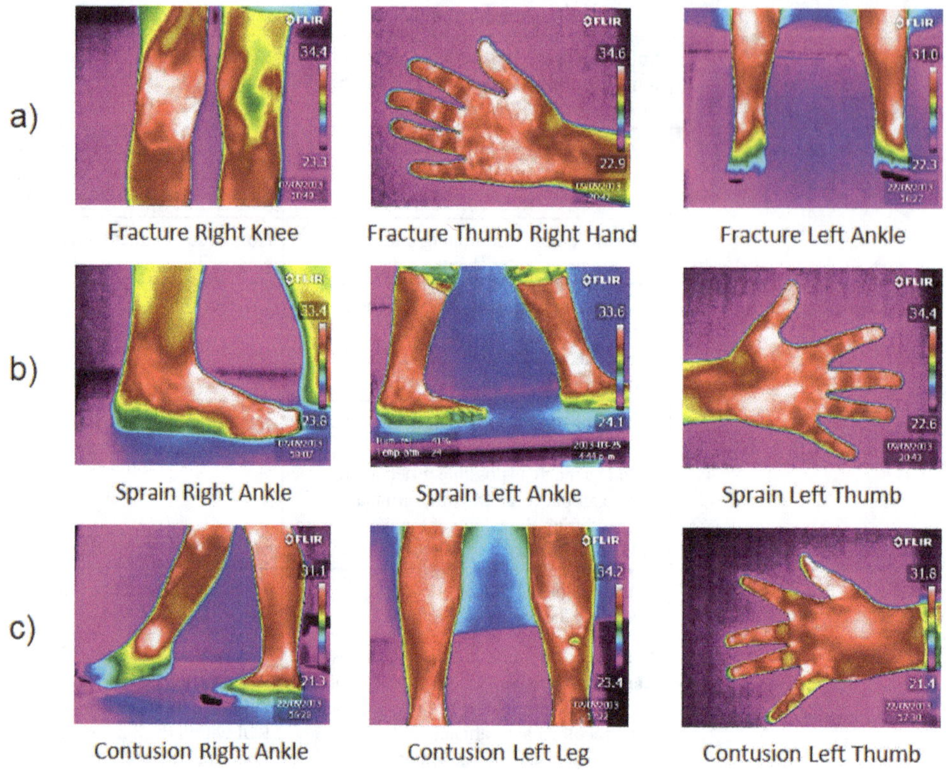

- The difference between the area covered by each ROI at the same isotherm, which is the number of pixels at maximum temperature in the ROI of the healthy area, compared to the number in the injured area that were equal to, or greater than the said temperature in the healthy area (Δpix) (Sanchis-Sánchez et al., 2014) (Figure 2).

Although other authors have reported on the first two variables, the third proposed variable (Δpix) was innovative.

The images were initially processed using FLIR® Tools Plus 3.1.13080.1002 (FLIR® Systems, Wilsonville, OR) software to obtain the mean and maximum temperatures of the ROI. They were then processed by an application from Matlab®[1] (v.R2011b, MathWorks, Natick, MA, US) (Figure 3), which was carried out ad hoc for the Δpix analysis.

For determining the ROIs, an adaptation of the Glamorgan Standard Capture Protocol (Ammer et al., 2007) was used, which consisted of selecting the limits of the same based on anatomical references. This adaptation involved:

1. The selection of an anatomical reference (for example: tibial malleolus, kneecap, styloid process, olecranon…).
2. The drawing of a line to determine the width of the ROI (Figure 2).

Figure 2. Determining the height and width of the ROI

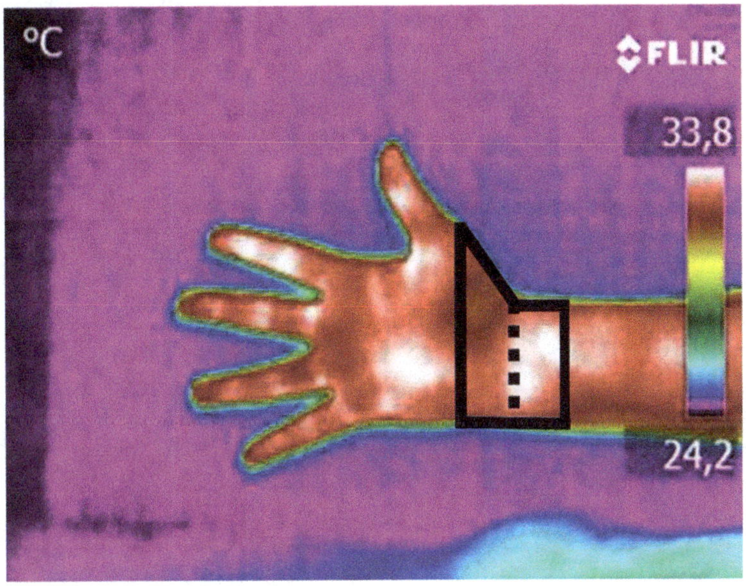

3. For calculating the height measurement of the ROI, based on the anatomical reference, proportions were established with respect to the width of the ROI. Thus, in lower limbs a proportion of 2/3 of the width value of the ROI was used, and for upper limbs, a proportion of 1/3 of the width value was established (Figure 2).

Once the ROI was established, the mean temperatures and absolute maximums of the ROI were calculated together with the differences of mean temperatures (ΔTmean) and the difference of maximum temperatures (ΔTmax) of the injured and healthy ROIs.

For obtaining the new variable, Δpix, the colour images were transformed to the grey scale with the same FLIR software in order to use them in specifically designed software and to determine the differences of area (in the form of number of pixels) between the ROIs of the healthy and injured limbs. Specific software was programmed using a Matlab® tool.

The aim of the program was to determine the temperatures measured on the images of each projection and to undertake a comparison between the healthy and injured limbs of each participant in the study. By doing this it could be established whether differences existed between the injured and the healthy limbs in the ROIs in terms of the number of pixels.

The program, moreover, provides both the maximum temperature that has been measured in the image of the healthy limb (taken as the temperature of reference) and its position and the area that that zone, considered as reference on the image itself, occupies. In the image of the injured limb, it establishes the area occupied by those temperature measurements that have turned out to be equal or greater than the reference. Using this information, the thermometric parameters, their distribution and their size could be obtained for the later statistical analysis of the results.

For these new ROIs, obtained in the healthy and injured zones, the mean and maximum temperatures were determined and the differences of those mean temperatures (ΔTmean), maximum temperatures (ΔTmax) were established as variables of interest. Likewise the size of the area composed by the same

Figure 3. This figure is a plot of the Matlab user interface where, A: is the select analysis area; B: establishes the part of the body or joint to be analysed; C: is the application console, and informs about possible errors, but also about how to use the software; D: select ROI analysis button; E: representation of thermographic pictures, where the ROI has to be selected and where the difference of temperature of the injured area will be shown in blue (healthy) and red (injured) after the diagnosis; F: diagnosis, probability of fracture, in this case P = 1 (100%); G: Print diagnosis report button; H: reset button

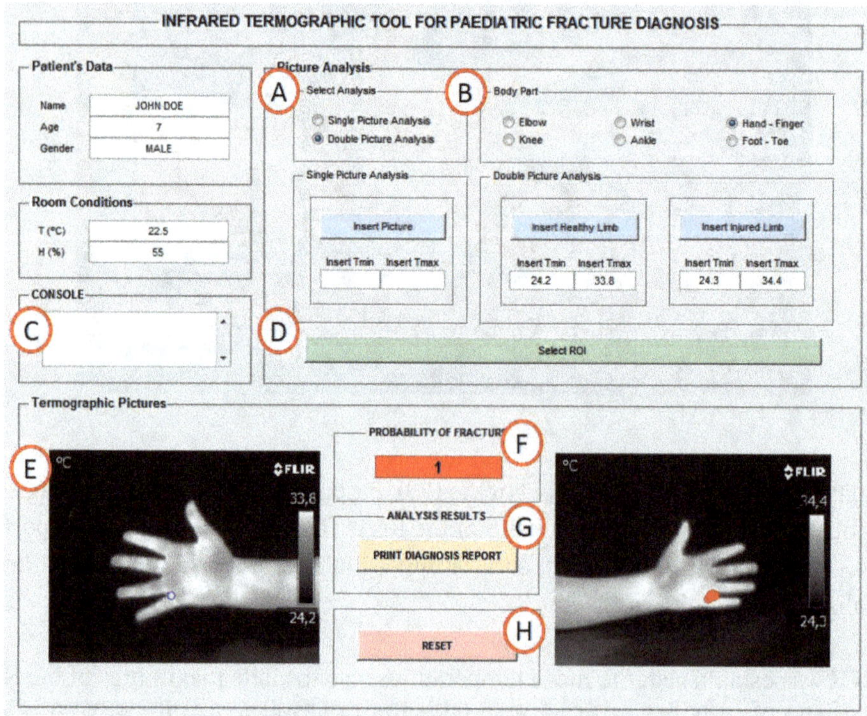

isotherm in each ROI (number of pixels at maximum temperature in the ROIs of the injured zones that are equal to or greater than that threshold, Δpix) was determined.

Interactive software was developed in which commands were introduced by keyboard and the results and images were shown on the screen.

Figure 4 shows the program flow chart that begins with a reading of the image of the healthy limb, calculating the maximum and minimum temperatures.

The functioning of the program is sequential, undertaking the following operations:

1. First of all, the analysis of the image (or figure in the context of the program) of the healthy limb is undertaken. The program undertakes a binary reading of 8 bits of the image, creating a matrix of dimensions $M_{158x256}$. This size corresponds to the resolution of the thermal imaging camera. In this way the thermometric data measured of each pixel in the corresponding space of the matrix are stored.
2. Later, the same program shows the image on the screen and asks the user to introduce the maximum and minimum temperatures measured. These are already known, as they were obtained by the software associated with the camera (FLIR). The introduced data are necessary, as they correspond

Figure 4. Program flow chart

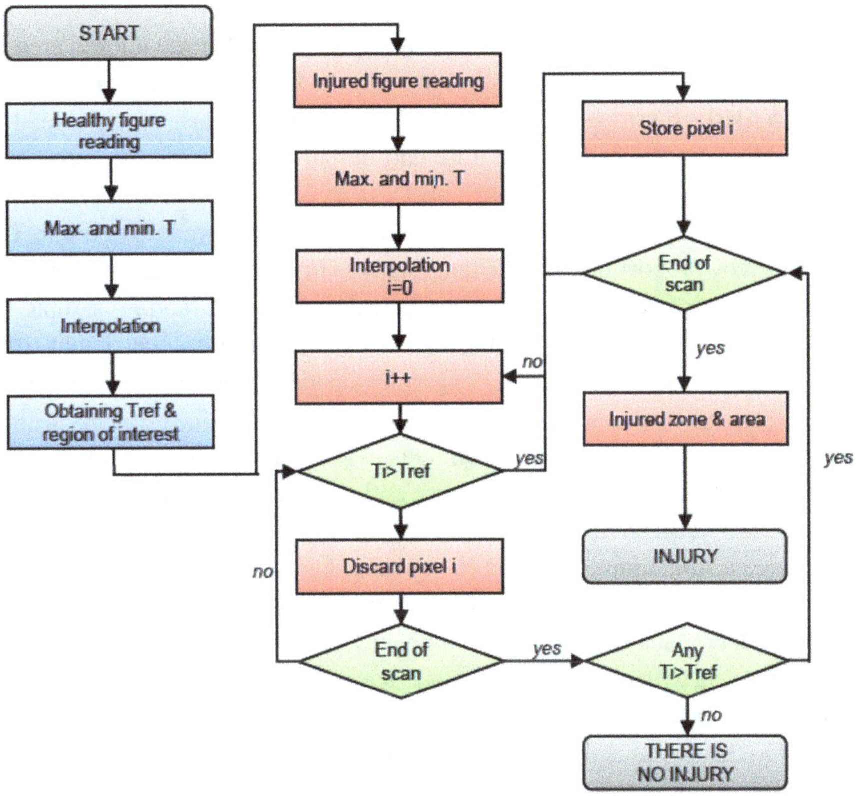

to the maximum and minimum values (0 and 255) of the stored binary reading. By undertaking an interpolation, the different temperatures measured in each pixel are obtained according to their measured binary value.

3. The next step is to select which area of the figure is to be analysed. Logically, this area corresponds to the same part of the locomotor system under study as in the injured area. Having done that, the program shows the image of the healthy limb, but on this occasion indicates the position and size of area occupied by that maximum temperature. It is that which will later be taken as the reference for analysing the image of the injured limb, as pixels with greater temperatures will indicate an injury.
4. Having analysed the image of the healthy limb, the same operation is undertaken for the injured limb, i.e. reading of image, establishment of maximum and minimum temperatures, interpolation and selection of the ROI. Having taken these steps, the program finally shows the image of the injured limb, indicating on the image itself all those points of the ROI with a temperature higher than that of the reference. It, therefore, shows the area and quantifies its size.
5. To calculate the ΔTmean, ΔTmax and Δpix, a protocol was drawn up for the analysis process: in the case of the participants with traumatism, the interpretation was undertaken without having any diagnosis of the injury and by means of a dual analysis independently of the ITIs.

Statistical Analysis

The following variables were analysed: patient's age and gender; whether the injured area was in the upper or lower body; whether the lesion extension was minor (e.g., finger), moderate (e.g., wrist, elbow), or major (e.g., forearm, leg); the thermographic variables of temperature variation referred to as ΔTmean, ΔTmax and Δpix and the atmospheric temperature and humidity in the room where the imaging was undertaken.

A descriptive analysis of the demographic variables of the samples was carried out. The qualitative variables were described by proportions and the quantitative variables by mean and standard deviations.

Interobserver and intraobserver reliabilities were calculated using a random sample of 33 patients to analyse the ΔTmean, ΔTmax and Δpix, with the intraclass correlation coefficient (ICC). The time between the two measures of the same thermal imaging of a patient, made by the same observer, ranged from 10 to 15 days.

Non-linear cataloguing, in the form of decision trees, was used to address the prognostic model and classify patients with trauma injury into patients with and without bone fractures. Those systems classify an input vector into predefined classes by using the answers from a series of sequential questions, which referred always to a single input variable (Breiman et al., 1984).

Decision trees are produced using the so-called entropy of the information, which intuitively provides information of the disorder or lack of regularity of a given variable (i.e. a low entropy level of a variable indicates that it is regular and with ordered values, and vice versa). Different indices are widely accepted for performing the entropy measurement, the so-called Gini's Index (I_G) being the most common choice, and also the one used in this work. A detailed description of the calculation of this index can consulted in Gelfand, Ravishankar, and Delp, (Gelfand, Ravishankar, & Delp, 1991).

Similar to the concept of probability and conditional probability, entropy also has conditional entropy; it means that entropy decreases in relation to the information given by a given measurement. Within this framework, once the result of an event is known, the information gain is related to the entropy decrease. Indeed, decision trees are based on the calculation of the conditional entropies weighted to the proportion of examples that fits a given attribute. Taking into account the structure of the trees, the variables in the first hierarchical levels are the most relevant ones for the model. This allows not only to develop a classification, but also a deeper knowledge of the problem in an intuitive way, since the outcome of the model can be obtained by means of rules, and the most relevant rules for the model are those that appear in the first hierarchy levels.

Two of the most widely accepted models have been used in this work, namely, CART (Classification and Regression Trees) (Kass, 1980) and CHAID trees (Chi-square Automatic Interaction Detection) (Kass, 1908). On the one hand, CART tends to generate non-homogenous datasets on the objective variable, always producing child nodes from a parent node, this also being its primary limitation. On the other hand, CHAID splits the information into two or more child nodes from the beginning of the tree construction. After testing both approaches, and taking into account the better performance of CART in presence of categorical features, CART was finally selected as it usually produces more meaningful rules, with higher values of sensitivity and specificity. It should also be emphasized that a 10-fold validation process was carried out to guarantee the application of the model to new data.

The diagnostic accuracy of thermal imaging was evaluated by means of sensitivity, specificity, positive predictive value, negative predictive value, positive likelihood ratio, negative likelihood ratio and diagnostic odds ratio. Sensitivity and specificity are statistical measures of the performance of a binary classification test or classification function. They quantify the diagnostic ability of the test. In clinical practice they allow to establish how good the test is at predicting abnormality, for instance the proportion of patients with abnormal test results (Altman, & Bland, 1994). Positive and negative predictive values are useful when considering the value of a test. The sensitivity and specificity of a quantitative test are dependent on the cut-off value above or below which the test is positive. In general, the higher the sensitivity, the lower the specificity, and vice versa. To better understand those concepts, some definitions are needed:

1. True positive, when the patient has the disease and the test is positive (correctly identified);
2. False positive, when the patient does not have the disease but the test is positive (incorrectly identified);
3. True negative, when the patient does not have the disease and the test is negative (correctly identified) and
4. False negative, when the patient has the disease but the test is negative (incorrectly identified).

Afterwards, likelihood ratios are used for assessing the value of the diagnostic tests performance, while the diagnostic odds ratio provides the measure of effectiveness of a diagnostic test.

This is followed by the graphic parameterization of the efficiency of the model on the diagnostic variables, using the area under the Receiver Operating Characteristic (ROC) (Fawcett, 2006).

Figures 5 and 6 show considerable mean and maximum temperature differences. Likewise differences of area (number of pixels) between the healthy and the injured limb can be observed, at the same time as allowing to clearly view the zone where the traumatism has been received.

These images show considerable differences of mean and maximum temperatures between the same healthy and injured zones. You can also see the differences of area (number of pixels) between the healthy and the injured limb. Furthermore, the thermal imaging technique, although not being quantifiable data, allows seeing the zone where the traumatism has been received.

Interobserver reliability provided ICC values of 0.95 (95%CI: 0.9-0.97) and intraobserver reliability was always higher than 0.92 (95% CI: 0.83-0.96).

When the thermographic images of the 145 study subjects were analysed, 12 outliers had decreased temperature in the injured area, which may correspond to different physiological responses to trauma. These cases should be analysed independently to establish a thermographic pattern that explains such behaviour but, due to their small numbers, they were not considered in the current study. Therefore, the final sample was 133 patients.

Results

Descriptive data are shown in Table 2. The patients' ages ranged from one to 14 years and the patients who had sustained a fracture were aged from two to 14 years old. The ratio of males and females with fractures was 1.3:1 - 57% of males and 43% of females – which corresponded to the prospective and consecutive study carried out, where all cases that came to the hospital during the three-month study who met the inclusion criteria were included. Based on their pathologies, 65% of the subjects did not have a fracture whilst 35% (46 children) did. Salter-Harris fractures accounted for 46% of them. Of these, two were forearms, six were fingers, two were metacarpal bones, six were wrists and five were ankles. With regard to the rest of fractures (54%), four were forearms, two were elbows, nine were fingers, seven were

Figure 5. Healthy right knee (Tmean=30.8 ºC) and injured left knee (Tmean=31.8 ºC)

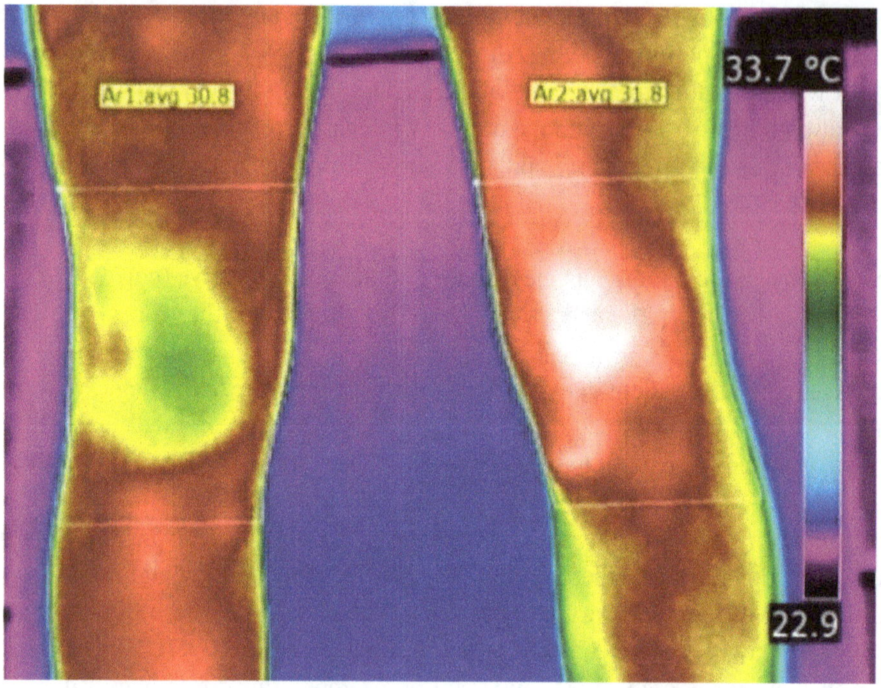

Figure 6. Healthy right knee (Nº pixels=3) and injured left knee (Nº pixels=1 906)

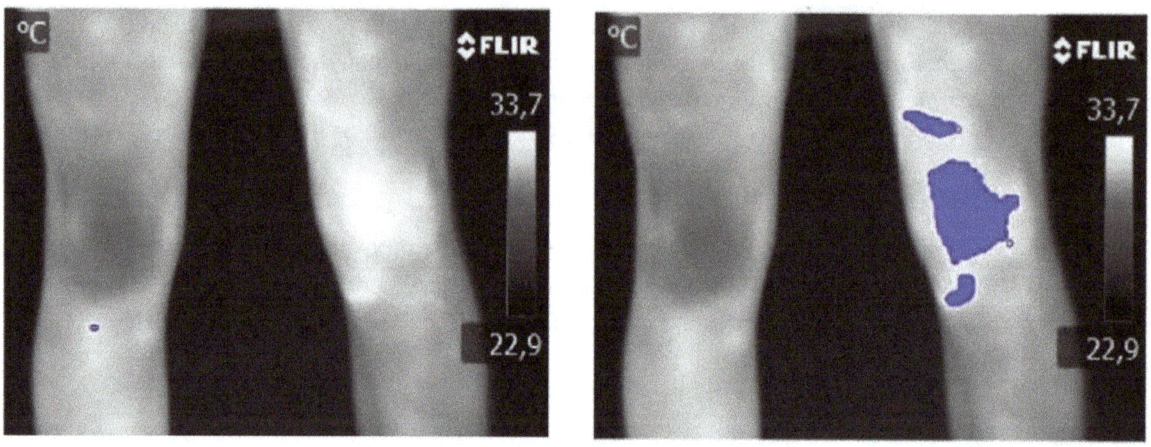

wrists, one was metatarsal bones and two were ankles. The majority of the fractures (80%) were in the upper body. Table 2 shows the mean values of the ΔTmean, ΔTmax y and Δpix, variables measured on the thermographic images.

The Classification and Regression Trees (CART), to discriminate between patients with and without fracture incorporated all the variables analysed, except the patient's gender (see decision tree in ADDITIONAL MATERIAL).

Table 2. Descriptive data (n = 133 subjects)

Variable	Fracture (n=46)	Contusion (n=53)	Sprain (n=34)	Total non-fracture (n=87)	*P* Value [a]
Gender [b]	26/20	25/28	13/21	38/49	0.27
Age, mean (SD), years	9.9 (2.8)	10.3 (3.1)	10.6 (2.1)	10.4 (2.8)	0.52
Zone [c]	37/9	36/17	9/25	45/42	< 0.001
ΔTmean, mean (SD), ºC	0.44 (0.88)	0.16 (0.58)	-0.39 (0.75)	-0.06 (0.7)	< 0.001
ΔTmax, mean (SD), ºC	0.47 (0.81)	0.17 (0.64)	-0.26 (0.74)	0 (0.71)	0.001
Δpix, mean (SD), No.pixels	562.4 (1020)	248.5 (395)	213.1 (441.2)	234.6 (406.3)	0.008

Abbreviations: ΔTmean, difference of average temperatures (injured-healthy ROI); ΔTmax, difference of maximum temperatures (injured-healthy ROI); Δpix, difference of areas (pixels). SD, standard deviation.

[a]Differences between fracture, contusion and sprain groups (Chi-square test for proportions & Kruskal-Wallis test for means).

[b]Gender: Male/Female.

[c]Zone: Upper body/Lower body.

The decision tree model incorporated ΔTmean as a first order variable and Δpix as a second order variable, reducing the ΔTmax to the fourth level of the tree. Therefore, if ΔTmean is equal to, or greater than, 1.525ºC, the model shows the injury probability of being a bone fracture as one (100%). For smaller values of this variable, the tree includes the values of the other variables in the study: the Δpix in the second level, the injury location (lower or upper limbs) and injury extension (minor, moderate or major extension) in the third level, the ΔTmax and humidity in the fourth level and the variables of age and atmospheric temperature in the lower levels.

Depending on the values considered, it is possible to work out the probability of whether the bone is fractured. The decision tree offered 22 possible outcomes and in 15 of them the diagnosis of fracture or non-fracture was definitive, with a score of one or zero. In the remaining seven outputs, the probability of a fracture was not definitive. One output indicated a 75% probability of a fracture, three outputs indicated a probability of 50% and three indicated a probability of less than 22% (22%, 14% and 10%).

The diagnostic accuracy values obtained for this prognostic method, taking into account all the tree outputs, can be illustrated using a receiver operating characteristic (ROC) curve (Figure 7). The diagnostic capacity of the method is given by the area under the curve (AUC), which in our case was 0.97, very close to one. The diagnostic values with clinical interest are shown in Table 3, with a high predictive negative value of 0.95. This implies that four of the 46 fractures were not properly classified by the decision tree. Of these, three were Salter-Harris type 1 fractures and one was a fracture of the first finger of the right hand caused by hitting a ball.

The results obtained here differ from those presented in a recent systematic review, which looked at the diagnostic possibilities of infrared thermal imaging in musculoskeletal lesions (Sanchis-Sánchez et al., 2014). The review found three studies from the 1980s that aimed to evaluate the diagnostic potential of infrared thermal imaging in stress fractures. Results from this systematic review showed high heterogeneity for sensitivity, negative likelihood ratio and diagnostic odds ratio, together with moderate combined values for specificity (0.69; 95% CI: 0.49–0.85) and low values for positive likelihood ratio (2.31; 95% CI: 0.63–8.47).

Figure 7. ROC curve for this diagnostic method based on CART. Delong's test for ROC curve offers a p-value < 0.001. AUC - area under the curve

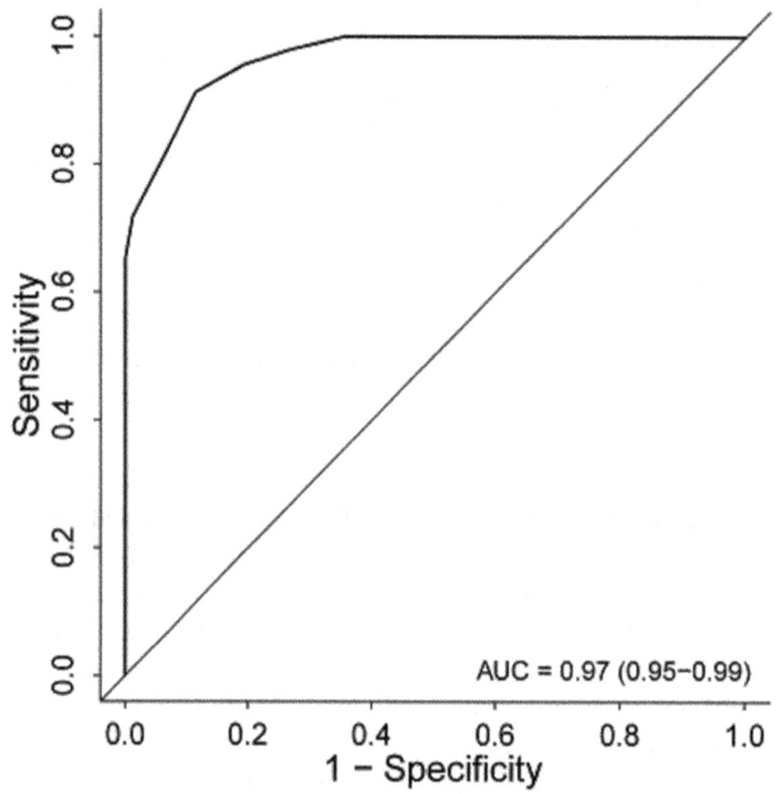

Table 3. Diagnostic performance of method, using decision tree model (CART)

	Se	Sp	PPV	NPV	PLR	NLR	DOR	AUC
Value	0.91 (42/46)	0.89 (77/87)	0.81 (42/52)	0.95 (77/81)	7.94	0.1	80.85	0.97
95% CI	[0.79-0.98]	[0.8-0.94]	[0.67-0.90]	[0.88-0.99]	[4.4-14.33]	[0.04-0.25]	[24-274]	[0.95-0.99]

Abbreviations: Se, sensitivity; Sp, specificity; PPV, positive predictive value; NPV, negative predictive value; PLR, positive likelihood ratio; NLR, negative likelihood ratio, DOR, diagnostic odds ratio; AUC, area under the curve. CI, confidence interval.

Our results show that implementing the non-linear cataloguing method and incorporating a new variable measured on the thermal image, the area of injury (Δpix), makes infrared thermal imaging more effective when predicting bone fractures in children than previous studies. It showed high discriminatory power, with a sensitivity of 0.91 and a specificity of 0.88. In addition, the 10-fold analysis suggests that these indices really are indicative of the ability of the model to solve the problem. The results obtained here provide a more accurate approximation of the real diagnostic potential of infrared thermal imaging.

The decision tree modelling incorporated Δpix as a second order variable. With regard to the scientific literature on infrared thermal imaging, it has not been identified any research that quantifies the injured area using Δpix. Therefore, this variable can be assumed to be important for distinguishing bone fractures.

The strengths of this study are that the protocol presented allowed to use thermal imaging to aid the diagnosis of limb fractures, with high values of diagnostic ability - sensitivity, specificity, and positive and negative predictive values. This is also a non-invasive and low-cost method that could provide fast screening at the patient's bedside. Three of the four fracture cases not detected by thermal imaging were Salter-Harris type 1 fractures and they were not detected by radiography either. Only the fracture of the first finger of the right hand could actually be considered a false negative as far as the X-ray is concerned.

Therefore, the routine diagnostic criterion for Salter-Harris type 1 fractures is clinical judgement, based on the swelling and localized pain on palpation of the physis.

An expected limitation of infrared thermal imaging was the time needed for acclimatization, especially by the youngest children, who needed to be distracted so that the technique could be executed correctly and ensure that no contact was made with the skin in the ROI. It was challenging to overcome this issue, even with the help of family members.

On the other hand, 12 patients were excluded of the analysis because it was noted that they had abnormal temperature values in the injured areas. It could reflect a hidden pattern in the classification of subjects. A larger number of cases would improve the resolution of the decision tree and would allow to carry out a specific study in order to consider these outliers and improve the clinical suitability of the method.

The results obtained by our study are a significant improvement on the diagnostic values reported by other authors. They show how useful and practical thermal imaging is for physical examinations, due to its low cost and safety. It could provide fast screening at the bedside.

The good negative predictive value achieved using this technique (0.95; 95% CI: 0.88-0.99) shows that it is a promising method.

SOLUTIONS AND RECOMMENDATIONS

Thermal imaging is a very attractive technique for the study of paediatric pathologies that are accompanied by variations of body temperature as it is a harmless technique (non-invasive and non-ionizing); it allows to locate of the injured zone; it requires no contact with the child; it is quick, direct without great technical complications and is of a relatively moderate cost.

As recent studies have shown, in order to ensure a correct application of thermal imaging in the field of health, it is necessary to incorporate standardization through the definition and use of normalization protocols for image capturing, for selecting ROIs, and for processing images (Jones & Plassmann, 2002; Ring et al., 2003; Ring et al., 2012).

A protocol was designed in this study for capturing images, based on the criteria that other authors had used and incorporating others such as the use of expanded polystyrene sheets to prevent contamination or noise that light sources produce in the measuring room. Likewise a protocol was drawn up for analysing the images.

The choice of the quantifying variables was of great importance for undertaking this study. The variables ΔTmean and ΔTmax have been used by different authors (Goodman, Heaslet, Pagliano, & Rubin, 1985; Katz et al., 2008; Kolosovas-Machuca, & González, 2011; Diakides et al., 2013) reflecting satisfactory results. However, two variables have been incorporated into this study that to date had not been taken into account in other studies. These variables are as follows:

1. Δpix, which corresponds to the difference in the size of the area found at the same temperature (isotherm) or higher to the temperature of reference in the healthy zone.
2. Extension, that corresponds to the size of the anatomical segment analysed.

The intra-observer and inter-observer reliability of the variables measured on the thermal image present some very high values in all cases, close to 1, so ensuring the reproducibility of this protocol in analysing images for the variables ΔTmean, ΔTmax and Δpix. Moreover, the use of anatomical references and proportions to define the ROIs allows health professionals to make use of this technique without the need for exhaustive training or prior knowledge.

The greater sensitivity and specificity using data mining through decision trees, as opposed to traditional statistical treatment (logistic regression), may be due to the fact that many real problems and especially those related with human beings, are intrinsically non-linear and, therefore, only a non-linear model can provide sufficiently satisfactory results.

In the decision tree model, the ΔTmean variable and the Δpix variable were incorporated as first and second order respectively, so reducing the hierarchical level of ΔTmax to the fourth level of the tree. Although, in the scientific literature on ITI, no investigation was identified that employed a quantification of the injured area, in this study the Δpix measurement proposed is postulated as of great importance for distinguishing between fractures and non-fractures and is perhaps of interest for the study of other pathologies.

The sensibility and specificity results obtained in our study differ from those revealed in a systematic review that involved three studies from the 1980s, the aim of which was to evaluate the diagnosis potential of ITI in stress fractures (Sanchis-Sánchez et al., 2014), although it must be considered that the characteristics of our sample are different from those papers, because our sample had a larger number of patients and a lower prevalence of fractures. The papers analized in the cited systematic review showed some poor results that varied between large heterogeneity for Sensitivity, negative likelihood ratio and diagnostic odds ratio; some moderate combined values for Specificity (0.69; 95% CI: 0.49-0.85) and low positive likelihood ratio (2.31; 95% CI: 0.63-8.47). However, on considering those studies individually (Meurman, Somer, & Sjovall, 1980; Devereaux, Parr, Lachmann, Page-Thomas, & Hazleman, 1984; Goodman et al., 1985), it can be appreciated how diverse factors converge that could have skewed their results. In particular can be observed obsolescence due to the use of low precision equipment; samples with high prevalence of fractures; absence of screening between the ITI and the standard of reference; control over the measuring environment and confounding variables; absence of an objective criterion to define the diagnostic threshold and linear and univariate analysis. Given that those factors were tackled in the present study, we consider that the results obtained here provide a more reliable assessment of the real diagnosis potential of ITI.

One limitation to this investigation, as has already been mentioned, is the 12 outlier values obtained (9% of the sample), that could reflect a hidden pattern in the classification of the subjects. A possible way of tackling this limitation would be to choose, as the ROI of reference, a zone of the same limb (even though the temperature variations found do not recommend its use, which was why this study did not focus on one single body zone) or undertaking the study with a much wider sample that would make the presence of this above-mentioned hidden pattern visible. A greater percentage of the sample would require it to be analysed in greater depth, as a group of specific characteristics.

This study offers new contributions to the use of ITI in the health field as a result of its rigorousness in the careful gathering of the sample; in the methodology used in data gathering, in the application of an image-capturing protocol; in the adaptation of the Glamorgan protocol; in the incorporation of the extension variable on the third level of hierarchy and the area variable with the analysis of the difference between pixels of the areas, as well as through the design and development of an interactive software using MATLAB.

It is also important to stress the finding that the use of decision tree is especially appropriate in analysing variables such as those used in this study. The authors stress the fact no study has been found in the literature consulted that makes mention of this issue.

FUTURE RESEARCH DIRECTIONS

This technique should be used with a larger cohort of patients in order to develop a diagnostic method to rule out fractures.

In this study the injured area with a healthy area in the other limb is compared. However, this was not possible if the patient attended the emergency unit wearing a bandage or fixed cast, or had used ice to reduce the inflammation, as the ROI would no longer be comparable to the healthy limb. To overcome this problem, the authors propose to use a healthy area of the injured limb for comparison purposes.

New future lines of work will have to check the existence of a hidden pattern in a certain group of children, as to consider only the injuries produced in lower limbs (in the three groups studied, fracture, sprains and contusions), negative average values were found for ΔTmax and ΔTmean, which does not tally with the inflammatory process that justifies the use of ITI as a diagnostic tool in musculoskeletal injuries. However, two hypotheses have been found in the literature that could explain this phenomenon (Awerbuch, 1991; Di Benedetto, Huston, Sharp, & Jones, 1996):

1. The increase and reduction in muscle tone or muscle "pump" (in healthy and injured zones, respectively) would produce an anomalous reading of the temperature increase.
2. The activation of oxidative mechanisms with the involvement of small nervous fibres (causing vasoconstriction) could reduce the temperature of the injured zone.

In addition to these hypotheses there are others related with the information provided by the patients on the application of ice or the consumption of anti-inflammatory drugs or other aspects of the acclimatization process. With more cases collected, it may be possible to establish a diagnostic rule for this behaviour pattern.

It would, therefore, be useful to replicate this study in different populations (adults, the elderly…) in order to discover if the results could be extrapolated to other ages.

CONCLUSION

Thermal imaging is a very attractive technique for the study of paediatric pathologies that are accompanied by variations in body temperature, given that it is a harmless technique (non-invasive and non-ionizing); it allows to locate the injured zone; it does not require contact with the child; it is fast, direct, without excessive technical complications and involves a relatively moderate cost.

The incorporation of certain new variables on the thermal image, such as Δpix, corresponding to the difference in the size of area that is found to be at a temperature equal to (isotherm) or greater than the temperature of reference in the healthy area, and Extension, corresponding to the size of the anatomical segment analysed, together with the use of non-linear cataloguing methods could provide thermal imaging with greater possibilities of use in the clinic.

REFERENCES

Altman, D. G., & Bland, J. M. (1994). Diagnostic tests. 1: Sensitivity and specificity. *British Medical Journal, 308*(6943), 1552. doi:10.1136/bmj.308.6943.1552 PMID:8019315

Ammer, K. (2008). The Glamorgan Protocol for recording and evaluation of thermal images of the human body. *Thermology International, 18*(4), 125–129.

Ammer, K., & Ring, F. E. (2007). Standard procedures for infrared imaging in medicine. In N. A. Diakides & J. D. Bronzino (Eds.), *Medical infrared imaging. Principles and Practice* (pp. 32.1–32.14). Boca Raton, FL: Taylor & Francis. doi:10.1201/9781420008340.ch22

Arora, N., Martins, D., Ruggerio, D., Tousimis, E., Swistel, A. J., Osborne, M. P., & Simmons, R. M. (2008). Effectiveness of a noninvasive digital infrared thermal imaging system in the detection of breast cancer. *American Journal of Surgery, 196*(4), 523–526. doi:10.1016/j.amjsurg.2008.06.015 PMID:18809055

Arthur, D. T., Khan, M. M., & Barclay, L. C. (2011). Thermographic investigation of osseous stress pathology. In *Engineering in Medicine and Biology Society, EMBC, 2011 Annual International Conference of the IEEE* (pp. 6250 - 6253). doi:10.1109/IEMBS.2011.6091543

Awerbuch, M. S. (1991). Thermography--its current diagnostic status in musculoskeletal medicine. *The Medical Journal of Australia, 154*(7), 441–444. PMID:2005838

Barnes, R. B. (1964). Thermography. (Thermography & its clinical applications). *Annals of the New York Academy of Sciences, 121*(1), 34–48. doi:10.1111/j.1749-6632.1964.tb13683.x PMID:14237524

Breiman, L., Friedman, J. H., Olshen, R., & Stone, C. J. (1984). *Classification and regression trees.* Monterey, CA: Wadsworth.

Collard, D. C., Verhagen, E. A., Van Mechelen, W., Heymans, M. W., & Chinapaw, M. J. (2011). Economic burden of physical activity–related injuries in Dutch children aged 10–12. *British Journal of Sports Medicine, 45*(13), 1058–1063. doi:10.1136/bjsm.2010.082545 PMID:21685503 de Weerd, L., Mercer, J. B., & Setså, L. B. (2006). Intraoperative dynamic infrared thermography and free-flap surgery. *Annals of Plastic Surgery*, *57*(3), 279–284. doi:10.1097/01.sap.0000218579.17185.c9 PMID:16929195

Devereaux, M. D., Parr, G. R., Lachmann, S. M., Page-Thomas, P., & Hazleman, B. L. (1984). The diagnosis of stress fractures in athletes. *Journal of the American Medical Association*, *252*(4), 531–533. doi:10.1001/jama.1984.03350040061027 PMID:6737649

Di Benedetto, M., Huston, C. W., Sharp, M. W., & Jones, B. (1996). Regional Hypothermia in Response to Minor Injury1. *American Journal of Physical Medicine & Rehabilitation*, *75*(4), 270–277. doi:10.1097/00002060-199607000-00006 PMID:8777022

Diakides, N. A., Diakides, M., Lupo, I., Paul, J., & Balcerak, R. (2013). Advances in Medical Infrared Imaging: An Update. In N. A. Diakides, M. Diakides, & J. D. Bronzino (Eds.), *Medical Infrared Imaging. Principles and practice. Boca Ratón* (pp. 1.1–1.14). CRC Press.

Fawcett, T. (2006). An introduction to ROC analysis. *Pattern Recognition Letters*, *27*(8), 861–874. doi:10.1016/j.patrec.2005.10.010

Gascó-Gómez de Membrillera, J., Gascó-Adrien, J., & Barra-Pla, A. (2002). Conceptos básicos en Traumatología infantil. Epidemiología. Tratamiento cerrado de las fracturas. Tratamiento abierto de las fracturas. Remodelamiento de fracturas mal consolidadas. *Pediatría Integral*, *6*(6), 535–546.

Gelfand, S. B., Ravishankar, C. S., & Delp, E. J. (1991). An Iterative Growing and Pruning Algorithm for Classification Tree Design. *IEEE Transactions on Pattern Analysis and Machine Intelligence*, *13*(2), 163–174. doi:10.1109/34.67645

Goodman, P. H., Heaslet, M. W., Pagliano, J. W., & Rubin, B. D. (1985). Stress-fracture diagnosis by computer-assisted thermography. *The Physician and Sportsmedicine*, *13*(4), 114–132. doi:10.1080/00913847.1985.11708772 PMID:27421377

Hassan, M., Chernomordik, V., Vogel, A., Hattery, D., Gannot, I., Little, R., & Yarchoan, R. (2007). Infrared imaging for functional monitoring of disease processes. In N. A. Diakides & J. D. Bronzino (Eds.), *Medical Infrared Imaging. Principles and practice* (pp. 14.11–14.28). Taylor & Francis.

Head, J. F., & Elliott, R. L. (2002). Infrared imaging: Making progress in fulfilling its medical promise. *Engineering in Medicine and Biology Magazine, IEEE*, *21*(6), 80–85. doi:10.1109/MEMB.2002.1175142 PMID:12613215

Hildebrandt, C., Raschner, C., & Ammer, K. (2010). An overview of recent application of medical infrared thermography in sports medicine in Austria. *Sensors (Basel, Switzerland)*, *10*(5), 4700–4715. doi:10.3390/s100504700 PMID:22399901

Hildebrandt, C., Zeilberger, K., Ring, E. F. J., & Raschner, C. (2012). The Application of Medical Infrared Thermography in Sports Medicine. In An International Perspective on Topics in Sports Medicine and Sports Injury. doi:10.5772/28383

Jiang, L. J., Ng, E. Y. K., Yeo, A. C. B., Wu, S., Pan, F., Yau, W. Y., & Yang, Y. et al. (2005). A perspective on medical infrared imaging. *Journal of Medical Engineering & Technology*, *29*(6), 257–267. doi: 10.1080/03091900512331333158 PMID:16287675

Jones, B. F. (1998). A reappraisal of the use of infrared thermal image analysis in medicine. *Medical Imaging. IEEE Transactions on*, *17*(6), 1019–1027. doi:10.1109/42.746635

Jones, B. F., & Plassmann, P. (2002). Digital infrared thermal imaging of human skin. *IEEE Engineering in Medicine and Biology Magazine*, *21*(6), 41–48. doi:10.1109/MEMB.2002.1175137 PMID:12613210

Kass, G. V. (1980). An Exploratory Technique for Investigating Large Quantities of Categorical Data. *Journal of Applied Statistics*, *29*(2), 119–127. doi:10.2307/2986296

Katz, L. M., Nauriyal, V., Nagaraj, S., Finch, A., Pearlstein, K., Szymanowski, A., & Pearlstein, R. D. et al. (2008). Infrared imaging of trauma patients for detection of acute compartment syndrome of the leg. *Critical Care Medicine*, *36*(6), 1756–1761. doi:10.1097/CCM.0b013e318174d800 PMID:18496371

Kolosovas-Machuca, E. S., & González, F. J. (2011). Distribution of skin temperature in Mexican children. *Skin Research and Technology*, *17*(3), 326–331. doi:10.1111/j.1600-0846.2011.00501.x PMID:21338404

Kontos, M., Wilson, R., & Fentiman, I. (2011). Digital infrared thermal imaging (DITI) of breast lesions: Sensitivity and specificity of detection of primary breast cancers. *Clinical Radiology*, *66*(6), 536–539. doi:10.1016/j.crad.2011.01.009 PMID:21377664

Lahiri, B. B., Bagavathiappan, S., Jayakumar, T., & Philip, J. (2012). Medical applications of infrared thermography: A review. *Infrared Physics & Technology*, *55*(4), 221–235. doi:10.1016/j.infrared.2012.03.007

Landin, L. A. (1997). Epidemiology of childrens fractures. *Journal of Pediatric Orthopaedics. Part B*, *6*(2), 79–83. doi:10.1097/01202412-199704000-00002 PMID:9165435

Mettler, F. A. Jr, Bhargavan, M., Faulkner, K., Gilley, D. B., Gray, J. E., Ibbott, G. S., & Yoshizumi, T. T. et al. (2009). Radiologic and Nuclear Medicine Studies in the United States and Worldwide: Frequency, Radiation Dose, and Comparison with Other Radiation Sources—1950–2007 1. *Radiology*, *253*(2), 520–531. doi:10.1148/radiol.2532082010 PMID:19789227

Meurman, K., Somer, K., & Sjovall, J. (1980). Thermography of stress fractures in military personnel. *Acta Thermographica*, *5*, 132–136.

Ng, E. Y.-K. (2009). A review of thermography as promising noninvasive detection modality for breast tumor. *International Journal of Thermal Sciences*, *48*(5), 849–859. doi:10.1016/j.ijthermalsci.2008.06.015

Pascoe, D. D., Mercer, J. B., & De Weerd, L. (2006). Physiology of thermal signals. In J. D. Bronzino (Ed.), *Medical devices and systems* (pp. 21.1–21.20). doi:10.1201/9781420003864.ch21

Practice Guidelines Committee of the American Academy of Thermology. (2012a). *Guidelines for Breast Thermography*. Retrieved from http://www.aathermology.org/

Practice Guidelines Committee of the American Academy of Thermology. (2012b). *Guidelines for Neuromusculoskeletical Infrared Thermography Sympathetic Skin Response (SSR) Studies*. Retrieved from http://www.aathermology.org/

Ring, E. F. J., & Ammer, K. (2000). The technique of infrared imaging in medicine. *Thermology International, 10*(1), 7-14.

Ring, E. F. J., & Ammer, K. (2012). Infrared thermal imaging in medicine. *Physiological Measurement, 33*(3), R33-46. doi: 10.1088/0967-3334/33/3/R33

Ring, E. F. J., Ammer, K., Jung, A., Murawski, P., Wiecek, B., Zuber, J., & Jones, B. F. et al. (2003, December). Standardization of infrared imaging. *Conference Proceedings; ... Annual International Conference of the IEEE Engineering in Medicine and Biology Society. IEEE Engineering in Medicine and Biology Society. Conference, 2,* 1183–1185. PMID:17271897

Ring, F., Jung, A., & Zuber, J. (2009). New opportunities for infrared thermography in medicine. *Acta Bio-Optika et Informatica Medica, 15,* 28–30.

Sanchis-Sánchez, E., Salvador-Palmer, R., Codoñer-Franch, P., Martín, J., Vergara-Hernández, C., Blasco, J., & Cibrián, R. et al. (2014). Infrared thermography is useful for ruling out fractures in paediatric emergencies. *European Journal of Pediatrics,* 1–7. doi:10.1007/s00431-014-2425-0 PMID:25241828

Sanchis-Sánchez, E., Vergara-Hernández, C., Cibrián, R. M., Salvador, R., Sanchis, E., & Codoñer-Franch, P. (2014). Infrared thermal imaging in the diagnosis of musculoskeletal injuries: A systematic review and meta-analysis. *AJR. American Journal of Roentgenology, 203*(4), 875–882. doi:10.2214/AJR.13.11716 PMID:25247955

Saxena, A. K., & Willital, G. H. (2008). Infrared thermography: Experience from a decade of pediatric imaging. *European Journal of Pediatrics, 167*(7), 757–764. doi:10.1007/s00431-007-0583-z PMID:17762940

Schulze-Rath, R., Hammer, G. P., & Blettner, M. (2008). Are pre-or postnatal diagnostic X-rays a risk factor for childhood cancer? A systematic review. *Radiation and Environmental Biophysics, 47*(3), 301–312. doi:10.1007/s00411-008-0171-2 PMID:18528700

Silva, C. T., Naveed, N., Bokhari, S., Baker, K. E., Staib, L. H., Ibrahim, S. M., & Goodman, T. R. et al. (2012). Early assessment of the efficacy of digital infrared thermal imaging in pediatric extremity trauma. *Emergency Radiology, 19*(3), 203–209. doi:10.1007/s10140-012-1027-2 PMID:22362422

Usuki, K., Kanekura, T., Aradono, K., & Kanzaki, T. (1998). Effects of nicotine on peripheral cutaneous blood flow and skin temperature. *Journal of Dermatological Science, 16*(3), 173–181. doi:10.1016/S0923-1811(97)00049-2 PMID:9651814

Vardasca, R., Ring, E. F. J., Plassmann, P., & Jones, C. D. (2012). Thermal symmetry of the upper and lower extremities in healthy subjects. *Thermology International, 22*(2), 53-60.

Vardasca, R., & Simoes, R. (2013). Current Issues in Medical Thermography. In *Topics in Medical Image Processing and Computational Vision* (pp. 223–237). Springer Netherlands. doi:10.1007/978-94-007-0726-9_12

Wild, W., Schütte, S. R., Pau, H. W., Kramp, B., & Just, T. (2003). Infrared thermography as a non-invasive application for medical diagnostic. In *Proceedings XVII IMEKO World Congress* (pp. 22-27).

APPENDIX

List of Abbreviations

ΔTmax: Differences of maximum temperatures.
ΔTmean: Differences of average temperatures.
Δpix: Differences of areas.
AUC: Area under the curve.
CART: Classification and regression trees.
CHAID: Chi-square automatic interaction detection.
CI: Confidence interval.
DOR: Diagnostic odds ratio.
ICC: Intraclass correlation coefficient.
I_G: Gini's index.
ITI: Infrared thermal imaging.
NLR: Negative likelihood ratio.
NPV: Negative predictive value.
PLR: Positive likelihood ratio.
PPV: Positive predictive value.
ROC: Receiver operating characteristic.
ROI: Region of interest.
SD: Standard deviation.
Se: Sensitivity.
Sp: Specificity.

Chapter 4
Cooling Agents' Effect Monitoring When Applied to Skin of Healthy Human Subjects

Francis Ring
University of South Wales, UK

Peter Plassmann
University of South Wales, UK

Carl Jones
University of South Wales, UK

Ricardo Vardasca
University of Porto, Portugal

Kurt Ammer
University of South Wales, UK

Usama I. Bajwa
COMSATS Institute of Information Technology, Pakistan

ABSTRACT

There are cooling products available for relieving the pain of minor sports injuries, in muscles, tendons, joints, strains, sprains and knocks. These products are based on ice, gel and cold patches. In order to quantify objectively the effect of each type of those products thermal imaging was used. This monitoring method is suitable to quantify quickly large regions of interest in skin areas over time through the thermal radiation perceived by thermal camera sensors. All recorded images were taken in a controlled environment and following a standard capture protocol in terms of subject, equipment and examination room preparation and procedure of conduction the examination. Two experiments were performed. The obtained results demonstrate that quantitative thermal imaging is a simple and objective tool for evaluating topical cooling treatments. However, it is important to assess the emissivity of any applied substance, which could have a significant effect on temperature measurement by remote sensing.

INTRODUCTION

The temperature effects of cryotherapy were monitored by means of infrared technology in the past (Ammer, 2014) and the temperature course of knee joint after treatment with cold packs was shown with thermal imaging (Schmidt, Mäurer & Rusch, 1979).

DOI: 10.4018/978-1-5225-2072-6.ch004

A study (Hug et al., 2012) assessed the hydration and cooling effect of an anti-inflammatory gel and concluded that there was a statistically significant increase in skin hydration as well as a rapid cooling effect lasting approximately 30 min, after application of the gel. The small relative increase in water loss may be associated with an additional skin surface water loss secondary to the increased water content brought into the skin by the gel. The use of the gel did not induce any skin irritation and was found acceptable to use by the majority of participants in the trial.

A more recent research (Lasanen, 2016) on the effect of cooling of concentrated menthol demonstrated that menthol concentration was not connected to skin cooling, while moderate menthol concentration of 4.6% may induce stronger cooling sensation compared to low (0.5%) or high (10.0%) menthol concentration gels.

In a pilot study, it has been shown that the cooling effect of gel applied to the forearm of volunteers, could be successfully monitored by infrared thermal imaging (Ammer, 2014 & Airaksinen, 2003). The gel was applied for 2, 4, and 8 minutes, and the thermal recovery recorded by thermal imaging. In the following study the objective and subjective cooling effect of Deep Freeze Cold Gel by applying with and without rubbing into the skin. The temperature decrease from both methods did not reach statistical difference, although the treated area remained cold for longer using the layering application.

It was also shown that the emissivity of the gel was high and close to that of the human skin surface. As a result of this finding it was deemed to be permissible to measure the temperature of the gel with the imaging technique while it was in contact with the skin, and over longer periods of time.

The area of skin chosen for this study was over the lumbar spine. A region of 10x10 cm was used to make a comparison between the cooling effect of a block of ice of that size and the same area coated with the deep freeze gel. The gel was layered on the skin, as evenly as possible according to the protocol, and this was left for 50 minutes, after which it was removed by wiping clear with paper tissues.

The ice was prepared in a thin plastic box measuring 10x10 centimeter and 2.5 centimeter deep. This was wrapped in a plastic sheeting to prevent water from melting ice reaching the skin while in contact. The ice was strapped to the back to maintain firm contact with the skin for 10 minutes. The time of contact chosen for the ice was taken as that used by an average application in domestic use. Physiotherapists may use up to 20 minutes contact but with crushed ice contained in several layers of cotton toweling. To obtain useful results of the re-warming of the skin within one hour, the shorter time of 10 minutes was found to be ideal for the purposes of this study.

Deep Freeze Cold Patch (Mentholatum Co Ltd, UK) is a product designed to produce a cooling effect when applied to the skin. This study has objectively investigated the extent of cooling and the effect of time of application of the Deep Freeze Cold Patch to the skin of healthy volunteers.

AIM

The aim of this study was to compare the objective and subjective cooling effects of Deep Freeze gel with that of a standard ice pack applied to the skin of human volunteers and to investigate the cooling effect of the new product designed to provide a sustained topical cooling effect when applied to the skin. This study reports the thermal effects from the application of the product Deep Freeze Cold Patch to the forearm and the anterior thigh of human healthy volunteers using infrared thermal imaging.

SKIN THERMOREGULATION

The thermoregulation (Guyton, 2006) is a set of mechanisms that keep the body temperature within certain limits, despite fluctuations in temperature of the external environment. The skin is the largest and heaviest organ of the human body and makes the interface with the external environment, having a very important role in thermoregulation of the human body. Skin temperature is highly influenced by cutaneous blood flow.

The skin and extremities, contrary to what happens at the level of the deep body regions (central body region), have greater variation of temperature range. Adipose tissue has natural insulating function (low heat conduction), and separates the skin (most sensitive region to external temperature changes) of the central body region (stable temperature). Cutaneous blood flow connects between the skin and core body region.

Cutaneous irrigation consists of a complex system of vascular branches, which are part of venous plexus, arterioles and arteriovenous anastomoses (essentially present at the level of exposed areas such as the feet, hands and nose). The subcutaneous venous plexus is supplied by arterioles and arteriovenous anastomoses, so that the subcutaneous blood flow will vary depending on the greater or lesser degree of vasoconstriction latter. The modulation of arterial tone depends primarily the sympathetic nervous system.

Thus, higher or lower blood supply mediates internal heat flow to the skin, from which the heat can then be dissipated to the environment. The heat conduction passing a total vasoconstriction for full vasodilation increases by about 8 times. It can then be said that the skin acts as a controlled heat radiation system, which can be monitored through infrared thermal imaging.

There are two types of cutaneous thermal sensors that influence the local skin thermoregulation: cold sensitive (in larger numbers) and heat sensitive. The information transmitted by these receptors is enriched by information from pain receptors specifically stimulated by extreme temperature variations, which explains that they can be perceived as pain.

The degree of stimulation (pulses per second) of the different thermal receptors allows humans gradations of thermal sensations. The rate of temperature installation also modulates the degree of stimulation, verifying that the persistence of exposure to a certain temperature gradually in a lower thermal stimulation of receptors (the phenomenon of adaptation).

Thermal receptors are located immediately below the skin and distributed in different percentages depending on body area (e.g., in the case of cold receptors - the lips 15-25/cm^2, the fingers 3-5/cm^2, chest and back <1/cm2). The cold receptors are consistently more numerous, but the relationship between the cold receptors/heat receptors can range from 3:1 to 10:1. The existence of a greater number of receptors sensitive to cold due to the fact that in the middle neutral environment, the metabolic rate of the human being consistently produce more heat than is required to maintain the core body temperature at 37 °C.

The information of the thermal receptors progresses along with the information of skin painful receptors within C fibers unmyelinated (transmission speed 0.4-2m/s), and fiber A small myelinated delta (transmission speed 20m/s) to the blade superficial dorsal horn of the spinal cord.

By these means cold provocation is much more effective than heat provocation in assessing the possible effect of topical solutions for inflammation and pain relief, which cause local vasodilatation.

METHODOLOGY

This research has 2 separated studies, one comparing Deep Freeze gel with ice packs (Experiment 1) and other evaluating the effect of Deep Freeze Patch in the arm and thigh of volunteers (Experiment 2).

Experiment 1

Six healthy volunteers were recruited, two female and four male for the study. The males had a mean age of 26.5 years (24-30 years) and the females were aged 32 and 26 years. All were asked to read the prepared information sheet about the study and signed the consent form in the presence of a witness.

All measurements were made in a stable air-conditioned laboratory at 22°C, with diffuse airflow to avoid draughts. The subjects were positioned on an examination couch in the prone position. Clothing was removed from the waist to shoulders. Female subjects did not need to remove underwear, but the lumbar and thoracic spine area was exposed for 10-15 minutes until stable temperature reading were obtained.

A FLIR SC500 Thermacam infrared imager was positioned over the subject to image the lumbar spine region. The distance between the camera and the skin area under test varied a little depending on body size, the usual distance used in the study was approximately 70 centimeters.

The thermal image was continually monitored on an image processing system running special software CTHERM. Baseline images were recorded when spot temperatures monitored from four points in the required area of the lumbar region were unchanged for 5 minutes.

After the baseline image, the treatment was applied as described above. Gel was layered on a marked area of skin 10x10 centimeters, and ice was applied with a plastic covered container of the same dimensions. Automatic frame grabbing was started at 3 minutes intervals for 1 hour. The ice packs were removed at 10 minutes into the experiment.

Throughout the whole experiment the subjects remained on the couch beneath the camera to allow continuous visual monitoring, and regular frame grabbing as described.

The images (approx. 250 in number) were analyzed by locating a region of interest ROI over the treated area. To take account of any effects from the lateral diffusion of cooling or temperature change at the perimeter of the treated area, the ROI was made slightly larger than the 10x10 cm target area of skin. The total area of the ROI was between 10 and 15% larger than the cooled area.

The subjects were asked to respond to four questions indicating their assessment of sensation for each treatment.

The questions supplied were:

- **Question:** How would you describe the sensation from the patch? Or how did the patch feel when first placed on the skin?
- **Answers:** Cool 3, Cold 9
- **Question:** Did you feel this was too cold? Not cold enough? About right?
- **Answers:** Too cold: 1, Not cold enough: 0, about right: 11
- **Question:** Overall impression of the patch?
- **Answers:** Very Good: 9, acceptable: 2, Cold: 1.
- **Question:** What would you use this cooling patch for? Injury, swelling, arthritis
- **Answers:** Injury: 12, Swelling: 4, Arthritis: 1

The temperature changes was indicated at the start of treatment and 10 minutes later. Comfort was indicated at 20 minutes and 60 minutes of the procedure by a line analogue scale.

Experiment 2

Twelve healthy volunteers were recruited to the study. 10 males and two females were tested under identical conditions. The ages ranged from 19-30 years, the mean of 10 males was 23 years, and two females 19, and 21 years were included. The mean age of the whole group was 22.5 years. Each volunteer attended on two occasions, with each visit lasting for three hours 30 minutes including acclimatization to achieve a stable baseline temperature. The test laboratory was air-conditioned at 23ºC ± 1.0ºC, and relative humidity was inferior to 50%. No direct draughts on the subject were allowed throughout the study. After acclimatization for 15 minutes, with both arms and legs exposed.

Basic demographic data, name, age, and gender were recorded. In the reported data, personal identification has been replaced by an index code to preserve confidentiality. Each volunteer used a questionnaire to assess the subjective effects of the Patch application during and after the test.

Non-contact thermal imaging was performed with an FLIR A40 digital infrared camera calibrated at 30ºC for quantitative temperature measurements was linked to an image processing station was mounted vertically over the seated subjects, who had either their arms resting on a table, or their thighs positioned from the sitting position, parallel to the floor. Accurate focusing was ensured prior to each captured image. The subject was positioned with both arms placed forwards on a flat surface. The IR focal plane array camera was positioned at 90° from the dorsal surface of the arms and hands. Automatic sequence grabbing of the images was achieved with the special infrared imaging software CTHERM.

One limb is cooled with the patch and the other left exposed to the ambient to act as a control. The patch, measuring 10x15 centimeters, was applied to the mid anterior forearm on the first test, and to the mid anterior thigh on the second test. The tests on each subject were conducted on different days to avoid any persistent effects from skin cooling that might influence the response. The time duration for application of the patch (tested by a pilot study) was maintained in position for three hours at each site.

The process was repeated on a separate day for application to the legs. For this test the subject was seated on a chair, with the camera set vertically above to image both legs simultaneously, both feet on the floor. The patch was applied to one mid thigh, the choice of left or right for the patch application was randomized.

During the study, temperature sampling of the area of skin covered by the patch was performed by peeling the patch and applying it back (approximately 95%) for infrared imaging measurements and then carefully replaced on exactly the same area of skin.

To perform the infrared image during the application period of the patch, the dressing was peeled back from the skin to 5 mm, to expose the treated area. Immediately after the image was recorded, the patch was replaced in the same position. The time delay for this process was less than 10 seconds. A pilot test was performed and the results showed that this was the most effective method to use.

Infrared thermal images (Thermograms) were recorded as follows: Baseline before application, then at the following time intervals: 15,30, 45, 60, 90, 120, 150, and 180 minutes.

RESULTS

The results are divided by experience for a better understanding of each one.

Experiment 1

The mean of median temperature plots for each subject is shown in Figure 1. In addition, the graphic plot for maximum – minimum temperature and standard deviation were calculated to assess the evenness of cooling and or re-warming of the skin. All the graphs show the measurements made from the selected regions of interest.

The subjects when treated with the gel showed that temperature of the gel surface remained reasonably stable throughout the treatment period. Some slight variation was found in the first 10 minutes, probably indicating the effect of the body temperature on the gel itself. There was a slight upward trend in temperature towards the end of the test period. This may indicate a slowing down of the cooling action of the gel on the skin below.

From these data, the dramatic change caused by the application of ice, and the re-warming of the skin after removal is shown. In the case of gel application, it is clear that the changes in max-min. temperature occur in the first 3 minutes of application, as the gel stabilizes, and becomes more even in temperature recorded by the imaging system. The downward trend in temperature difference occurs around 50-55 minutes as shown in the median temperature measurements that increased at this time.

Figure 1. Mean of median temperature in °C resulting from gel and ice application, bars do indicate the standard deviation, T-Student test p = 0.056

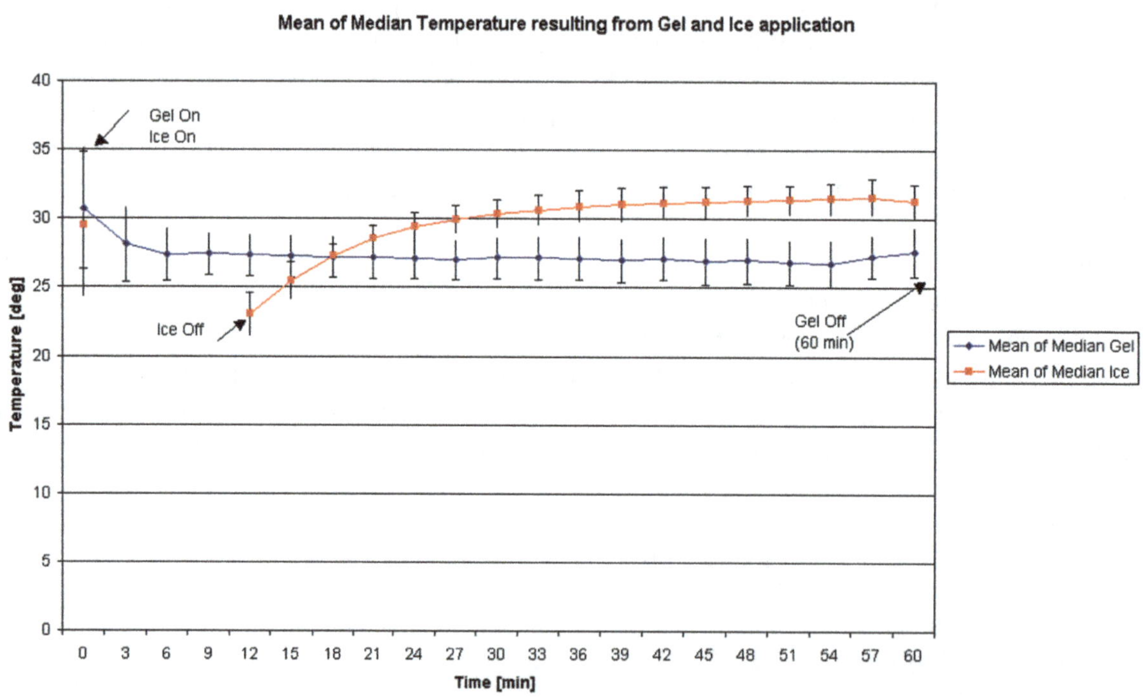

The standard deviation plots show a similar trend to those of temperature difference. The data for the mean of the median temperatures measured between 9 and 39 minutes (post ice application) were tested by student t test. The result showed a significant difference between ice and gel application (p = 0.056).

Two different assessments were recorded for each experiment and on each subject. The first was a series of boxes ranging from number: 1 - labeled warmer than normal, 2 - normal, 3 - colder than normal, 4 - cold and 5 - very cold. The data were plotted for all six subjects and presented the change in subjective assessment by the volunteer from the time of initial contact with the treatment to that of 10 minutes later.

The second assessment, a line analogue of 10 centimeters ranged from very pleasant (left part of the line) to very unpleasant (right part of the line). The intercept mark placed by the volunteer at 20 minutes and 60 minutes after treatment were measured from the left (very unpleasant) end. The measurements therefore indicate that zero is very unpleasant, 5.0 is normal and 10 is very pleasant. Therefore, the higher the score, the more pleasant the sensation recorded.

These data are shown in Figure 2 for gel and Figure 3 for ice application. The subjective score for gel in Figure 2 apparently shows only four plots, because three subjects scored at the same level.

Subject number 6, who volunteered to have a 20-minute ice treatment in addition to that for the protocol scored 3 (colder than normal) initially, 5 (very cold) after 10 minutes. After the ice removal at 10 minutes, the analogue scale (Figure 4) showed 3.0 (pleasant) at 20 minutes and 6.1(more pleasant at 60 minutes).

Figure 2. The subjective record made by the 6 subjects at 20 and 60 minutes with Deep Freeze Gel

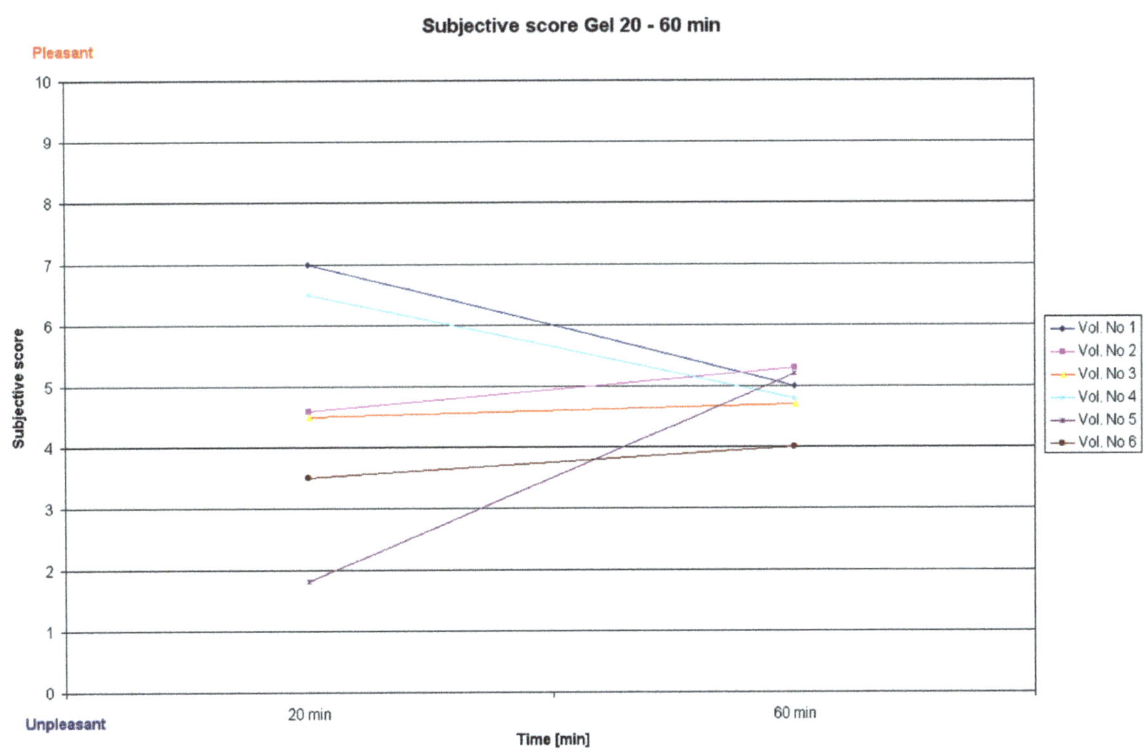

Figure 3. The subjective record made by the 6 subjects at 20 and 60 minutes with ice pack

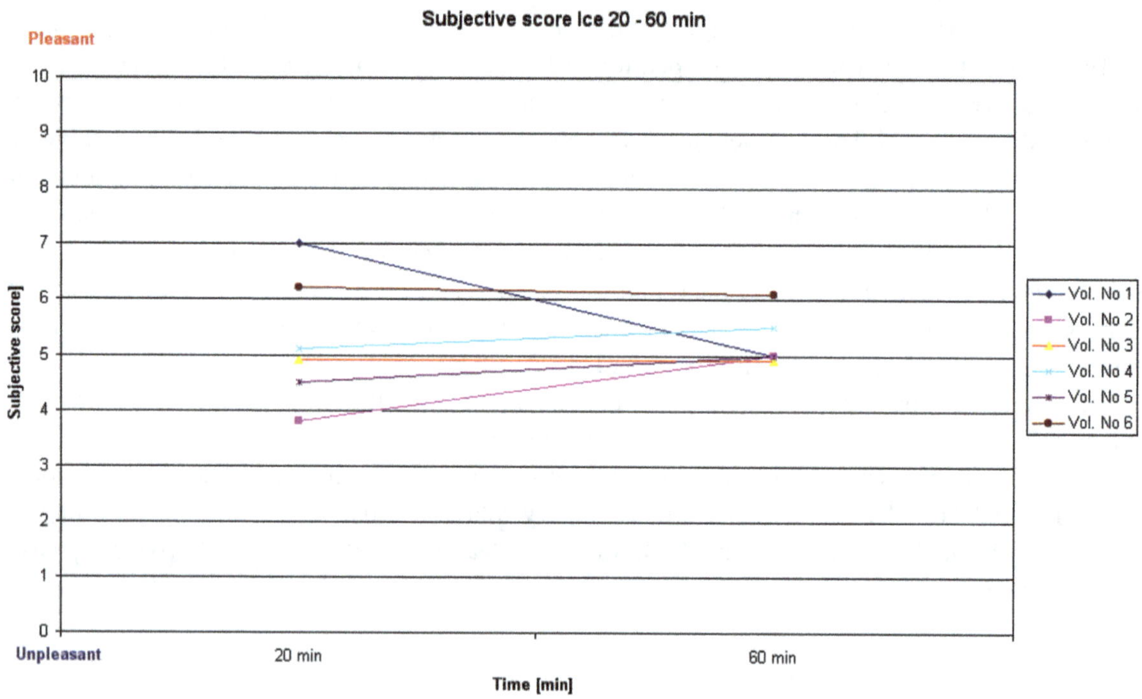

Figure 4. The subjective record made by the 6 subjects at 0 and 10 minutes with ice pack

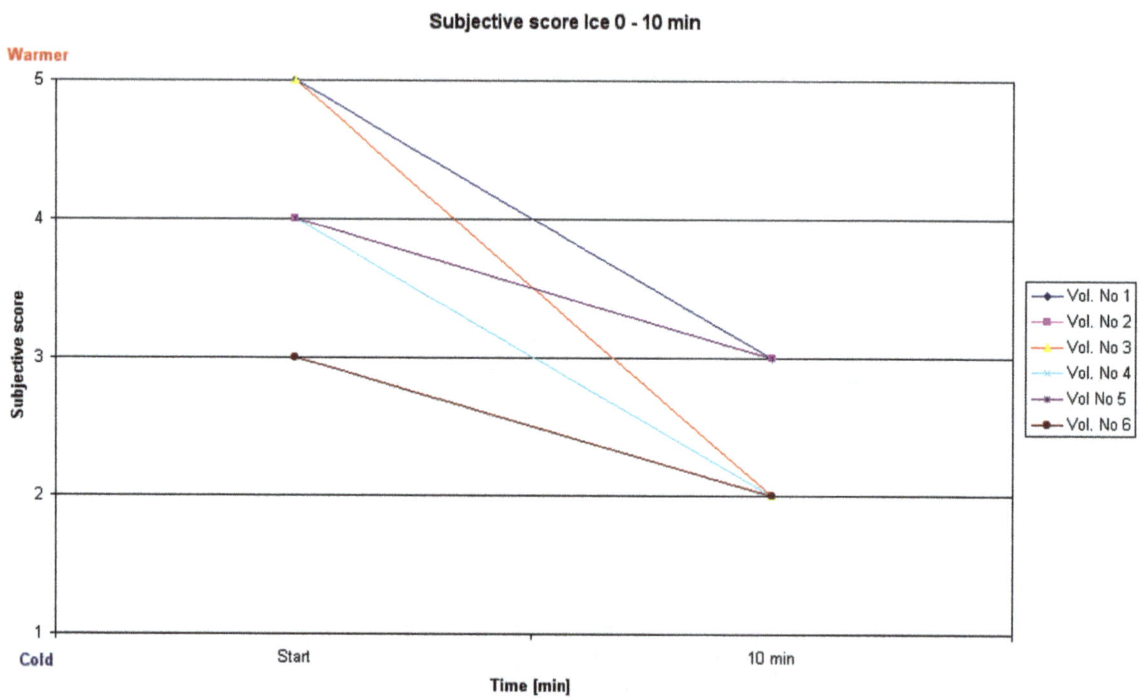

Both treatments were well tolerated, all subjects volunteered the comment that the gel method was much more pleasant than ice, and seemed to be effective. They were all conscious of the cooling effect of the gel on their skin.

Experiment 2

The temperature data extracted from the thermal images of all subject volunteers, mean of 12 subjects are summarized in Table 1 (absolute temperatures for the arm), Table 2 (temperature differences for the arm), Table 3 (absolute temperatures for the thigh) and Table 4 (temperature differences for the thigh) application sites. The data are plotted in Figures 5 and Figure 6. The thermograms from one subject are shown in Figure 7 (arm) and Figure 8 (thigh).

A single paired student t test was applied to the mean temperature differences through out the period of the study, i.e. 3 hours from application of the Deep Freeze Cold Patch. The statistical significance of temperature change between control and treated sites presented a p value of ≤ 0.05, signifying some significant difference from the control side of the body persisting at 3 hours, but rapidly reducing at that stage.

The volunteers to ascertain their subjective reactions to the application of the Deep Freeze Cold Patch (DFCP) completed a questionnaire.

The impact impression was 75% classified as cold with the other 3 subjects (25% registered as cool when DFCP was first applied to the arms). The results on the thigh were not identical with 10/12 (83%) reporting cold rather than cool.

The majority 8/9 replies felt the impact of cold between 5 and 7 minute after application. On the forearm, 11/12 considered the degree of cooling to be about right (92%), but on the thigh the subjective reply was different.

3 subjects (25%) considered the temperature to be too cold, 1 subject (8% of sample) considered the patch to not be cold enough, while 8 (67%) though the cooling effect was about right.

Overall, the comments were very favorable, all volunteers said they would use Deep freeze Cold patches for injuries, and liked the length of time it remained active in the cooling effect on the skin. All but one subject found the aroma to be pleasant.

CONCLUSION

There was generally much more reaction to the application of the ice pack than the application of the gel. The initial shock from ice contact which all found unpleasant decreased with time. However, there was a general awareness that the gel was cooling the skin in a milder, but definite way. One individual reported a sustained cooling effect on his back for one hour after the gel had been removed.

In this laboratory study, the gel was thickly applied to the skin surface and was not massaged in the way that users would probably prefer to apply it. However, the results do indicate that some gel may remain in the skin after wiping off from the surface, hence the cool sensation experienced by the subjects, the one in particular.

In contrast, the cooling of the skin made by the ice pack started to wear off immediately after the ice was removed. Almost all cooling effects were gone after 30-40 minutes.

Table 1. Mean temperatures of Deep Freeze Cold Patch applied to one arm (12 subjects). The Minimum and Mean and Standard Deviation values are obtained from the fixed region of interest (ROI) used in the image analysis, for the whole cohort of subjects

	ROI Mean Temperatures From the Arm Average (N=12)					
	Cold Patch			Control		
	Min (°C)	Mean (°C)	SD (°C)	Min (°C)	Mean (°C)	SD (°C)
Baseline	30.02	32.37	0.49	27.39	32.36	0.6
15 min	28.17	29.54	0.49	27.67	32.57	0.65
30 min	27.98	29.26	0.61	27.78	32.57	0.63
45 min	28.11	29.19	0.52	28.00	32.51	0.55
60 min	28.09	29.45	0.58	27.35	32.35	0.59
90 min	29.25	30.35	0.49	28.06	32.21	0.57
120 min	29.9	31.13	0.45	27.75	32.15	0.62
150 min	30.25	31.51	0.36	27.91	32.17	0.57
180 min	30.12	31.67	0.42	27.13	32.26	0.62

Table 2. The mean temperature differences obtained from all 12 subjects arms i.e. Treated subtracted from control untreated skin areas

	T Differences (Cold Patch-Control)	
	Min (°C)	Mean (°C)
Baseline	2.63	0.01
15 min	0.5	-3.03
30 min	0.2	-3.31
45 min	0.11	-3.32
60 min	0.74	-2.9
90 min	1.19	-1.86
120 min	2.15	-1.02
150 min	2.34	-0.66
180 min	2.99	-0.59

After both gel and ice application a feint skin reddening of the treated area was noted. However, this was a transient reaction, indicating mild superficial vasodilatation, and was usually no longer evident after 5-10 minutes.

The observations noted from the results of median temperature recordings, suggest that the gel appears to be slowly rising in temperature recovery after approximately 50 minutes. This may be an indication that the cooling action is on the decline, perhaps due to the loss of evaporative action.

A significant cooling of skin temperature compared to the contra-lateral control limb was observed over the 3-hour test period. Table 1 shows that the results were optimal on the arm for the first hour, though still significantly cooler than the control sites for the remaining two hours tested. Most of the

Table 3. The mean temperatures obtained from 12 subjects with data from the two regions of interest ROI on the treated and control thigh area

	ROI Mean Temperatures From the Thigh Average (N=12)					
	Cold Patch			Control		
	Min (°C)	Mean (°C)	SD (°C)	Min (°C)	Mean (°C)	SD (°C)
Baseline	30.39	31.25	0.34	30.26	31.31	0.35
15 min	26.66	27.66	0.39	30.15	30.98	0.29
30 min	27.06	27.86	0.37	30.56	31.51	0.31
45 min	27.08	27.86	0.38	30.47	31.44	0.31
60 min	26.77	27.62	0.44	30.19	30.98	0.31
90 min	27.66	28.56	0.48	30.22	31.16	0.31
120 min	28.38	29.31	0.45	29.92	30.84	0.32
150 min	29.36	30.19	0.37	30	30.99	0.33
180 min	30.05	30.81	0.3	30.03	31.1	0.36

Table 4. The temperature differences for minimum and mean temperatures from the 12 subjects obtained from the thermograms of the thigh

	Differences (Cold Patch-Control)	
	Min (°C)	Mean (°C)
Baseline	0.13	-0.06
5 min	-3.49	-3.32
30 min	-3.5	-3.65
45 min	-3.39	-3.58
60 min	-3.42	-3.36
90 min	-2.56	-2.6
120 min	-1.54	-1.53
150 min	-0.64	-0.8
180 min	0.02	-0.29

volunteers reported that there was a longer lasting subjective cooling of the applied site beyond 3 hours but with lessening magnitude.

The results on the thigh of the same volunteers tested on a separate occasion from the forearm tests, showed even higher significance, but again reducing at 3 hours.

In the forearm, there are blood vessels present which will have some effect on conducting local cooling away from the site. On the thigh, the dermis is thicker and the muscle mass of the quadriceps greater, which could explain the slightly more efficient cooling by the patch application. This is also shown in graphs 2 and 4 of minimum and mean temperatures, where there is homogeneity of data on the thigh, but less so on the forearm.

Figure 5. The mean and minimum temperatures obtained from the standard region of interest over the treated area of skin. The control temperatures are taken from the contra-lateral untreated limb using the same ROI

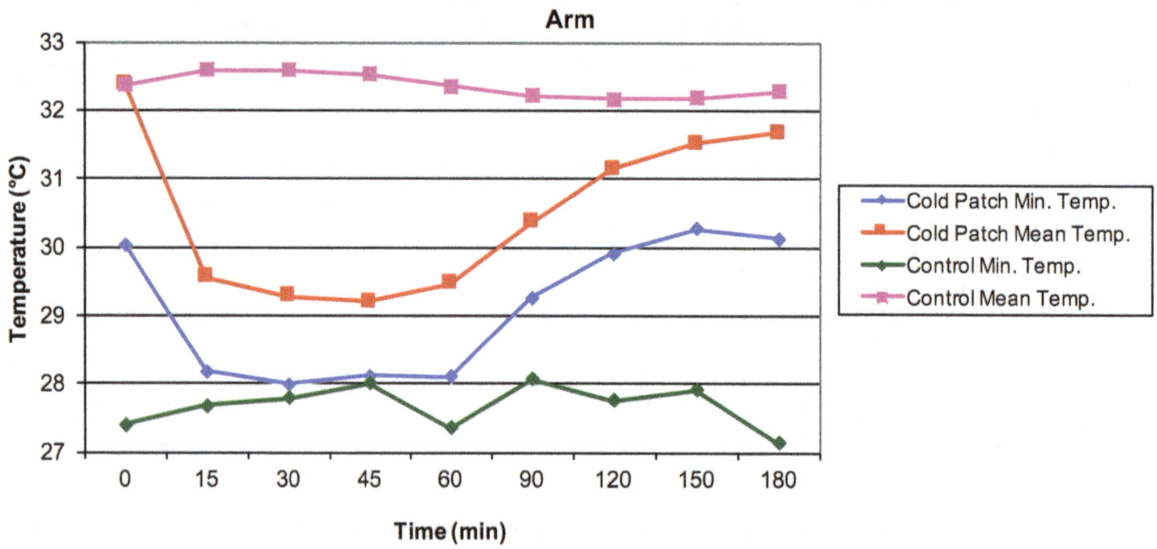

Figure 6. The mean temperatures and minimum temperatures of 12 subjects obtained from the regions of interest of the thermograms of the treated and control thigh images

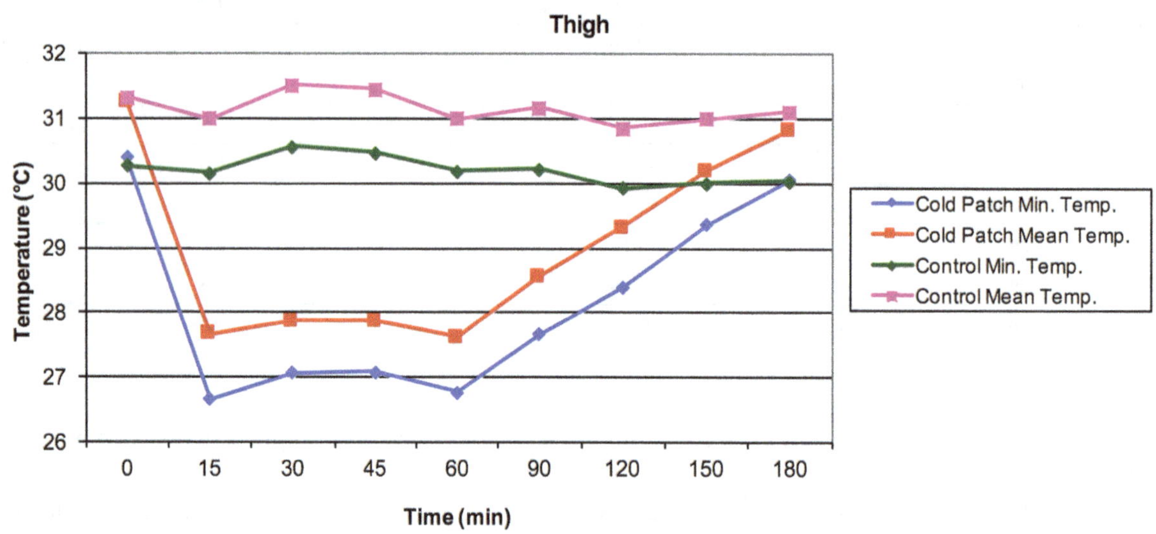

Results indicate that ice had a fall in mean temperature of the applied area of 7°C and its effect lasted for 20 minutes, the gel had a fall of 3.5°C and lasted for 50 minutes, the cold patch had a fall of 3°C in the forearm and of 3.3°C in the thigh and the effect lasted for both regions of interest for 150 minutes. The obtained results demonstrate that quantitative thermal imaging is a simple and objective tool for evaluating topical cooling treatments. The emissivity is important, so assessing the emissivity of any

Figure 7. Infrared thermograms taken throughout the study illustrating the skin cooling effect of Deep Freeze Cold Patch (DFCP) on the arm of one volunteer

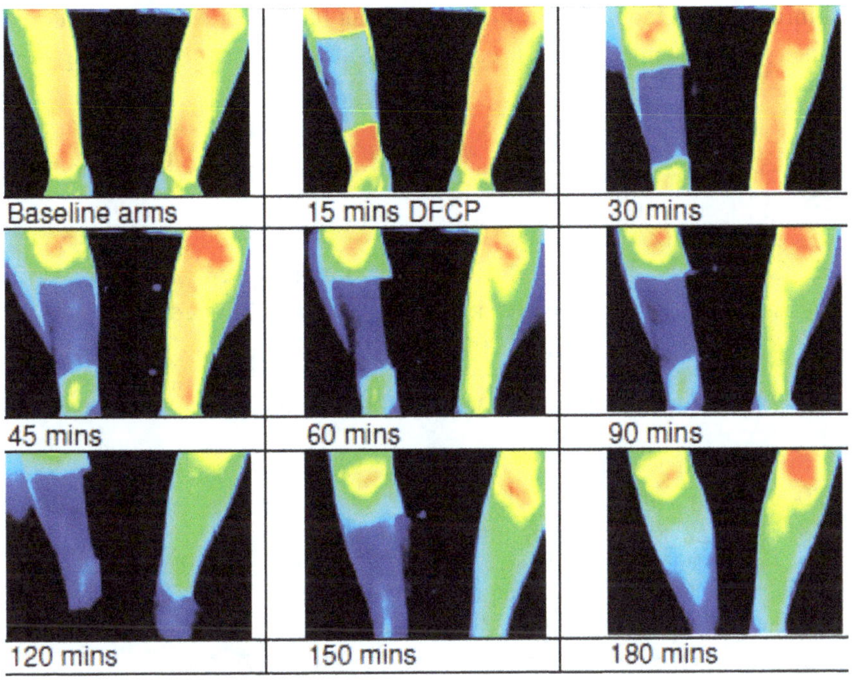

Figure 8. Infrared thermograms taken throughout the study illustrating the skin cooling effect of Deep Freeze Cold Patch (DFCP) on the thigh of one volunteer

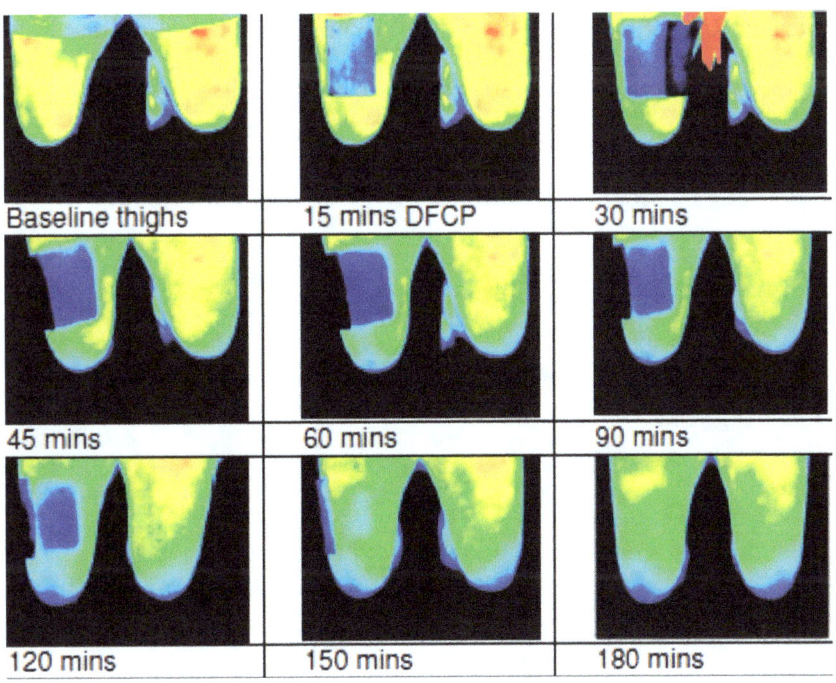

applied substance is recommended, which could have a significant effect on temperature measurement by remote sensing.

With thermal infrared imaging it is possible to assess and monitor the effect of utopic cooling solutions at skin surface through temperature, it can be a good indicator for validating new products and their performance.

REFERENCES

Airaksinen, O. V., Kyrklund, N., Latvala, K., Kouri, J. P., Grönblad, M., & Kolari, P. (2003). Efficacy of cold gel for soft tissue injuries a prospective randomized double-blinded trial. *The American Journal of Sports Medicine*, *31*(5), 680–684. PMID:12975186

Ammer, K. (2004). Temperature effects of thermotherapy determined by infrared measurements. *Physica Medica*, *20*, 64–66.

Guyton, A. C. (2006). *Body temperature, temperature regulation and fever. In Textbook of medical physiology* (11th ed.; pp. 822–833). W.B. Saunders Company.

Hug, A. M., Schmidts, T., Kuhlmann, J., Segger, D., Fotopoulos, G., & Heinzerling, J. (2012). Skin hydration and cooling effect produced by the Voltaren® vehicle gel. *Skin Research and Technology*, *18*(2), 199–206. doi:10.1111/j.1600-0846.2011.00554.x PMID:22092669

Lasanen, R., Julkunen, P., Airaksinen, O., & Töyräs, J. (2016). Menthol concentration in topical cold gel does not have significant effect on skin cooling. *Skin Research and Technology*, *22*(1), 40–45. doi:10.1111/srt.12226 PMID:25773465

Schmidt, K. L., Mäurer, R., & Rusch, D. (1979). Zur Wirkung örtlicher Wärme und Kälteanwendungen auf die Hauttemperatur am Kniegelenk. *Zeitschrift fur Rheumatologie*, *38*, 213–219. PMID:573031

Chapter 5
Whole-Body Cryotherapy as a Tool to Improving of Infrared Thermography Diagnostics

Armand Cholewka
University of Silesia, Poland

Karolina Sieroń-Stołtny
Medical University of Silesia, Poland

Agata Stanek
Medical University of Silesia, Poland

Joanna Kajewska
University of Silesia, Poland

ABSTRACT

The use of low temperature on the whole human body switched on beneficial physiological reactions. Whole-body cryotherapy is used as a part of rehabilitation. There were reported studies of thermal imaging performed due to whole body cooling in case of patients suffering from different diseases that showed a significant enhancement of the skin temperature gradient observed after cryotherapy. That explains that such therapeutic technique like whole-body cryotherapy can be used as a part of infrared thermography diagnostic procedure.

INTRODUCTION

Skin Temperature as the Physical Parameter

Body temperature is used as an indicator of diseases processes. It is usually measured by contact thermometers which must be stick to the skin or put inside the body orifices i.e. mouth, ear or rectum. It is very important factor describing our health state. But what about the skin temperature? Does it give us some important information about our health state too? Nowadays, we can say that it is very important to measure not only internal organism temperature, but also, in many cases, body surface temperature which might be sensitive indicator of metabolism changes beneath the skin what might be related to health state. This was proved by Hipocrates. However, his experiments were performed with poor precision and had only qualitative character. Can we measure it very precisely? Can we use such parameter

DOI: 10.4018/978-1-5225-2072-6.ch005

like body surface temperature to evaluate or even diagnose some diseases? Maybe it is possible to use thermal maps of the body to differentiate diseases?

However, first we should take into consideration that body surface temperature can give us very important information about tissue's health state – especially soft tissues just beneath the skin. Hippocrates was the first one who proved and showed how important skin temperature is. He did it using wet soil which was put on patient's skin in vicinity of abdomen. Wet soil while drying changing its color and Hippocrates was able to see in a sense the temperature gradient. Now it is obvious that skin temperature gradient is also a very important physical parameter that can be used in medical diagnosis. There is no doubt that the skin temperature and its variation can also be a symptom of disease in living organism. It is very important that the skin temperature change can be easily detected by infrared imaging. Temperature gradient is a very good diseases indicator because local blood flow and metabolism changes cause temperature change of the skin Therefore, infrared thermography imaging which is completely non-invasive diagnostic technique can be widely and easily used in medical diagnosis (Ring, Jung, Kalicki, Zuber, Rustecka, & Vardasca, 2013; Cholewka & Drzazga, 2006).

Maybe it will be possible to combine body cooling with thermal imaging and use it as a diagnostics method. However, before we present the achieves and possibilities of use the infrared thermography as a tool of diagnosis in whole body cryotherapy, we should first explain a little what the whole – body cryotherapy is and how it is used in medicine.

Whole Body Cooling in Sport and Medicine

In last few decades, very popular modern forms of wellness in sport has become using the whole body cooling as a part not only the rehabilitation but also as a part of normal training program as well as in recovering after injuries. Properly dosed and applied treatments renewing athletes, give a chance to reduce the negative effects of overloads and prepare the sportsman for the next train. The aim of wellness in sportsmen is to speed up the healing process and rise the efficiency level of the body (Vardasca, Ring, Plassmann, & Jones, 2012). Cryotherapy may cause circulatory and metabolic better exercise tolerance and delay the accumulation of tiredness while working muscle. In addition, the subjective feelings of the athletes after using a series of sessions in the cryochamber show a faster regeneration after training, and higher motivation to re-repetition training (Ring & Ammer, 2012). Cryotherapy has been also considered as an excellent treatment method in many fields of sports. Many clinical studies have reported that the use of cryotherapy has a beneficial effect on pain reduction and recovery of various injuries. Additionally, results of various studies are coherent on the effects on pain and neuromuscular processes (Ring, Jung, Kalicki, Zuber, Rustecka, & Vardasca, 2013). Whole-body cryotherapy, as well as the local one, are methods used for the treatment of acute soft tissue injuries. As part of the therapy can be used various methods such as ice towels, ice packs, ice massage, refrigerant gases, gel packs and inflatable splints. The chosen method of cooling the tissue directly influences the obtained therapeutic effect (Ring & Ammer, 2012).

It is known the biochemical and physiological processes in the human body are highly sensitive due to temperature change. The internal temperature of the body is constant and is kept at 37 °C with primary typical daily changes approximately 0.7 °C. But the surface temperature of the body changes in a wide range because of changes in ambient temperature.With all energy generated by the tissues mentioned, only 15-25% is converted into kinetic energy. The rest of the energy is converted into heat and distributed by the blood supply to the whole body (Ganong, 2009; Traczyk, 2007; Ronikier, 2008; Ammer, 2008). There are three main ways to heat loss: convection, conduction and infrared radiation. Instead, an important mechanism of the body's cooling process is evaporating water from the mouth and the mucous membranes of the respiratory system. The exchange of water or water vapor is an endothermic process which resulted in the body is cooled during sweating. Evaporation of one gram of water is approximately 0.6 kcal heat removal (Podbielska & Skrzek, 2014).

The average temperature of human body surface *Tsurf* is calculated based on the empirical formula (1) (Pilawski, 1983):

$$T_{surf} = 0.32 \cdot T_{tibia} + 0.18 \cdot T_{chest} + 0.14 \cdot T_{arms} + 0.07 \cdot T_{foot} + 0.07 \cdot T_{head} + 0.05 \cdot T_{hands} + 0.17 \cdot T_{back} \quad (1)$$

where: T_{tibia} is legs surface temperature; T_{chest}, chest surface temperature; T_{arms}, arms surface temperature; T_{foot}, foot surface temperature; T_{head}, head surface temperature; T_{hands}, hands surface temperature; T_{back}, back surface temperature.

Food delivered to the body is transformed by the process of digestion, which is directly related to metabolism (Ammer (2008)). The amount of heat losses ΔQ is associated with changes energy ΔE_M and the work done by the muscles ΔW, in relation to the first law of thermodynamics to biological processes, this dependence can written as (Equation 2):

$$\Delta Q = \Delta E_M + \Delta W \quad (2)$$

The moment when the body is in repose, work is not performing ($\Delta W = 0$) there is a possibility to change the Equation 2 into the Equation 3. Then the heat flux φ transferred to the environment can be calculated from Equation 3, which is called the Basal Metabolism Rate BMR0 and is presented below (Hulbert & Else, 2004; Ammer, 2008; Cholewka, Kasprzyk, Stanek, Sieroń-Stołtny, & Drzazga, 2015; Cholewka, Kasprzyk, Stanek, Sieroń-Stołtny, & Drzazga, 2015):

$$\phi = \frac{\Delta E}{\Delta t} \Leftrightarrow BMR_0 = mM^{\frac{3}{4}} \quad (3)$$

where: M – body weight; m – the factor for mammals with the value 3.4 $W*kg^{-3/4}$.

It should be also noted that many different diseases which symptoms are manifested as an increase or decrease of internal temperature as well as the skin temperature can be found (Ring, Jung, Kalicki, Zuber, Rustecka, & Vardasca, 2013; Cholewka, Drzazga, Sieroń, & Stanek, 2010). On the other hand, there are many different physical factors used in the medicine, mostly in physical medicine that can influence skin temperature of human body. This is the reason why in this chapter authors focused on some experiences of the influence of very low temperature (below -100 °C) used in the whole body cryotherapy on human organism as not only part of rehabilitation, but as a part of medical procedure used in thermovision diagnostic. It was found that the use of very low temperature before thermal imaging, can influence on thermal map by increasing the diagnostic value. When we say about cold treatment we should explain that whole body cryotherapy is a medical specialty that is widely used in medicine.

However, the main goal of whole body cryotherapy is using the lower temperature in short periods of time to stimulate different organism reactions by triggering the defense mechanisms against the cold. In this kind of treatment, whole body of patient is influenced by temperature lower than -100°C for a period of 2-3 minutes in a special room, called cryogenic chamber, in order to cause some physiological and biochemical reactions in the organism. The treatment takes usually 10-20 sessions of cryotherapy – day by day (excluded weekends). Use of extremely low temperature in such way leads to shortening the process of treatment of some diseases (Podbielska & Skrzek, 2012; Sieroń & Cieślar, 2003; Sieroń, Cieślar, & Stanek, 2010; Sieroń, Stanek, Cieślar, & Pasek, 2007). Applying of cryogenic temperature on the whole human body evokes in human body beneficial physiological reactions such as: analgesic, neuro-muscular, antiodematous and anti-inflammatory effects as well as circulatory, hormonal and immunological reactions. Moreover, whole - body cryotherapy procedures have also a beneficial influence on human psyche through relaxation action and decrease level of anxiety, as well as excretion and increase of different hormones what undoubtedly is also very important in treatment. Whole – body cryotherapy is used as a part of rehabilitation programme with kinesiotherapy (physical exercises) what leads to shortening of the recovery time and makes the rehabilitation most efficient. This therapy is applied in different motion organs diseases: degeneration and inflammatory states of joints (monoarthritis and oligoarthritis) and periarthritis, rheumatism, low back pain diseases and inflammatory, degeneration states of spinal vertebrae joints, fibromialgia and osteoporosis. It was also reported positive influence of whole – body cryotherapy on mental health what is connected with increase of concentration of some hormones and destroying the free radicals. Cold treatment may be beneficial also in tiredness and dream disturbance. Moreover, the cryotherapy has wide application in spine and nervous system diseases, like sciatica and spondyloarthrosis, as well as sclerosis multiplex. It should be underline that all of mentioned diseases are treated by used whole – body cryotherapy correlated with kinesitherapy procedures. Such procedures allow intensification of the training and extension of its duration by several times. Therefore, procedures of whole body cryotherapy and kinesiotherapy are altogether main components of so - called cryorehabilitation. Such influence is very useful in treatment of many different diseases what was reported in literature through last decades (Bauer, Hurnik, Zdziarski, Mielczarek, Skrzek, Podbielska, & Zagrobelny, 1997; Biały, Zimmer, Skrzek, & Zagrobelny, 1998).

It was also reported that whole - body cryotherapy causes only a slight change in blood morphology parameters within the range of reference values, different in patients with ankylosing spondylitis and healthy volunteers. In patients with ankylosing spondylitis after the end of a cycle of whole - body cryotherapy a significant decrease in hematocrit value and mean capacity of single blood corpuscle (MCV), as well as an increase in mean concentration of haemoglobin in blood corpuscle (MCHC) were observed. In patients with ankylosing spondylitis it seems to be a safe method leading to improvement of rheologic properties of blood. On the other hand, in healthy volunteers a significant increase in erythrocytes, hemoglobin concentration, hematocrit value and mean capacity of single blood corpuscle, decrease in mean concentration of haemoglobin in blood corpuscle as well as an increase in platelets count and proportion of monocytes in differential cell count (Stanek, Sieron, Cieslar, Matyszkiewicz, & Rozmus-Kuczia, 2005).

The whole - body cryotherapy procedures are performed in special rooms called cryochambers. There are two main types of cryochambers: closed one (two-step, so called Wroclawska cryochamber) and cryochamber with cold retention (in some papers called chamber with lingering cold). Cryochamber may be cooled by liquid nitrogen fumes and liquid synthetic air. Synthetic air is easier in exploitation and its use reduces costs of cryochamber construction up to 40%. First type of cryogenic chambers consists of two parts: a pre-chamber with temperature up to - 60ºC and a proper chamber, where main therapy takes place and temperature inside ranges from -110°C to -160°C. Pre-chamber is the place where patient adapt to extremely low temperature. Adaptation time in pre-chamber is up to 30s, then patients enter to a main chamber, where whole - body cryotherapy procedures are performed and patient is influenced at least by -100°C. Temperature and time of whole body cryotherapy procedure depends on patient's health and sometimes individual reaction to the cold. Usually the main therapy in the proper chamber lasts 3 minutes. Cryochamber operation is completely automatic and may be operated by only one person. However, there are physician as well as technician or rehabilitant always inside the chamber during the patients treatment. Moreover, cryochambers are usually covered with wood and have swing doors that a subject may easily open at any time to interrupt a procedure when a temporary indisposition occurs. In some versions of cryochambers treatment may be carried out for 4-6 subjects simultaneously. It is observed for bigger ones like two-stepped cryochambers (Stanek, Cieslar, & Sieron, 2007; Sieroń, Stanek, Cieślar, & Pasek, 2007; Stanek, Cholewka, Cieslar, Rosmus-Kuczia, Drzazga, & Sieron, 2011; Stanek, Cieslar, Strzelczyk et al., 2010). In the case of cryochamber with lingering cold, its principle of operation on the physical phenomenon of lingering cold in the basin. Therefore, the cryogenic chamber is placed underground. In this case, to get very low temperature, the liquid air with modified composition (21% to 30% oxygen) is usually used which is pumped from the tank outside the chamber by the pipes into the sprayer nozzles inside the cryogenic chamber.

There is another type of cryochamber called cryosauna which is designates for only one patient. Despite the basis of functioning being similar to the other cryochambers, there is one big difference – in this case it is possible to change the height of the platform on which patient stay, what gives possibility to take a cryotherapy by patients suffering from claustrophobia.

It was proved that that the application of 10 - days of whole – body cryotherapy sessions leads to health improvement. It was also reported that the good health state increases with the number of sessions. That is why patients sometimes take another cycle of cold treatment. Patient's health state improves relatively quickly what is manifested by the reduction of the level of pain, improvement of health condition and the feeling of well being what was reported in literature (Cholewka & Drzazga, 2005; Cholewka & Drzazga, 2006). The very important thing is that every kind of the cryochamber gives similar positive results in patients' health. The first and most important thing is that it leads to reduction of pain level what is the result of increased excretion of β-endorphins, the switching off the feeling receptors non-active due to cold and their connection with pro-prioreceptors and slower conduction in feeling fibres (Sieroń, Cieślar & Stanek, 2010; Stanek, Sieron, Cieslar, Matyszkiewicz, & Rozmus-Kuczia, 2005; Stanek, Cieslar, & Sieron, 2007). Another aspect of cold treatment, is the improvement of physical fitness what is important in sport's medicine.

It was also reported that whole – body cooling has similar positive influence on increase of the pain level for all studied patients - regardless of their age. The situation was quite different in the case of influence of whole – body cryotherapy on patients' shape. In this case, the effects are better seen for younger patients than for older ones. The cryotherapy effects for older patients were also beneficial however there were some patients that did not reported any physical shape improvement. However, body cryotherapy is beneficial and after each session patients felt better and relaxed. Thus patients took willingly the next cryotherapy sessions and there were patients that took even several times cryotherapy sessions during few years. Some studies showed that patients indicate similar reception of the whole – body cryotherapy, regardless of cryogenic chamber type what seems to be obvious when we keep strictly to the protocol and physical parameters conditions like time of treatment and magnitude of the temperature inside the chamber.

It should also be noted that there are differences in cold influence on different parts of human body. It is caused mostly by set-up and physiology of their organs as well as their geometry. That is why during whole - body cryotherapy procedures a temperature of organs in chest, abdominal cavity, skull inside and blood is steady. One only observes the changes of body surface temperature. The biggest heat losses is observed on parts of the body, which are relatively big in relation to theirs volume (mainly fingers, toes, limbs). Heat loss in fingers and toes is nearly ten times higher than in trunk what also has a meaning in diagnostic value of thermal imaging (Sieroń, Cieślar, & Stanek, 2010; Stanek, Sieron, Cieslar, Matyszkiewicz, & Rozmus-Kuczia, 2005; Stanek, Cieslar, & Sieron, 2007; Stanek, Cieślar, Mrowiec, & Sieroń, 2006; Biały, Zimmer, Skrzek, & Zagrobelny, 1998).

Every patient before whole - body cryotherapy procedures always have to be examined and qualified to procedure by a physician. For each patient qualified to whole body cryotherapy, procedure therapeutic parameters and individual program of kinesiotherapy are determined (Sieroń, Cieślar, & Stanek, 2010; Stanek, Sieron, Cieslar, Matyszkiewicz, & Rozmus-Kuczia, 2005; Stanek, Cieslar, & Sieron, 2007; Stanek, Cieślar, Mrowiec, & Sieroń, 2006; Biały, Zimmer, Skrzek, & Zagrobelny, 1998).

In a cryochamber some parts of the body that are most sensitive to extremely low temperature and mostly exposed to cryogenic temperature have to be particularly protected against injury. Hands are protected by gloves, shanks and feet - by woolen knee length socks and feet additionally by wooden clogs. Then auricles are protected by a cap or headband and mouths - by gauze - lined surgical masks. During the procedure, woman wear swimming costumes and men shorts. The main idea of whole body cooling is to expose as big as possible, body surface to cold. The above-described outfit allows for contact of bigger body area with low temperature what leads to overcooling as more as possible receptors of the body.

Before the subjects are instructed how to behave in cryochamber during whole - body cryotherapy procedure. Patient should pay special attention to the way of breathing in the chamber during the procedure. Inhaling should be two times shorter than exhaling due to decompression of cooled air in lungs. It is also forbidden to touch other subjects or rub own skin. Each time before whole - body cryotherapy procedure, patients should dry thoroughly their skin with a towel in order to remove sweat, as sweat drops turn into crystals they cause frostbite. Immediately after leaving a cryochamber, patients underwent kinesiotherapy procedures, usually lasting 30-60 minutes what is dependent on the health state of the patient and predicted by physician (Sieroń, Cieślar, & Stanek, 2010; Stanek, Sieron, Cieslar, Matyszkiewicz, & Rozmus-Kuczia, 2005; Stanek, Cieslar, & Sieron, 2007; Stanek, Cieślar, Mrowiec, & Sieroń, 2006; Biały, Zimmer, Skrzek, & Zagrobelny, 1998).

Cryotherapy treatment has rapidly developing during last 30 years. Nowadays it is being widely used in many applications, mostly in medicine i.e.: degeneration and inflammatory states of joints (monoarthritis and oligoarthritis) and periarthritis, rheumatism, low back pain diseases, inflammatory, in degeneration states of spinal vertebrae joints and fibromyalgia as well as in osteoporosis preventive treatment. It has also application in nervous system diseases like sclerosis multiplex and sciatica, discopathy and many other spine lesions that are connected with perturbations of nervous system. The very common spine diseases treated by whole- body cryotherapy are ankylosing spondylitis, sciatica and spondyloarthrosis.. Whole - body cryotherapy is also applied in sports' medicine in the treatment of both, acute and chronic injuries of soft tissue in sportsmen as well as, adjunctive method in biological regeneration (biostimulating effect, endurance and strength training, acceleration of post-endurance restitution, and prophylaxis of locomotor system overloading (Sieroń, Cieślar, & Stanek, 2010; Stanek, Sieron, Cieslar, Matyszkiewicz, & Rozmus-Kuczia, 2005; Stanek, Cieslar, & Sieron, 2007; Stanek, Cieślar, Mrowiec, & Sieroń, 2006; Gregorowiczv & Zagrobelny, 1998).

Nowadays more and more often healthy subjects start to use whole - body cryotherapy to keep good health and well-being, prevention of stresses and their consequences, revitalize and harden the body as well as a method of anti - aging (Gage & Baust, 2002).

In turn, absolute contraindications for applying whole - body cryotherapy procedures include: intolerance of cold, cold utricaria, cryoglobulinemia, cryofibrynogemia, Raynaud's symptom, hypothyroidism, severe anemia, acute diseases of respiratory tract, neoplastic disease, purulent-gangrenous skin lesions, vegetative neuropathies, local blood flow disturbances, cachexia, hypothermia, claustrophobia (Sieroń, Cieślar, & Stanek, 2010; Stanek, Sieron, Cieslar, Matyszkiewicz, & Rozmus-Kuczia, 2005; Stanek, Cieslar, & Sieron, 2007).

Assessment of Whole Body Cryotherapy by Infrared Thermography

Influence of cold on the human body leads primarily to reduce the temperature of the skin and tissues subsurface. Different parts of the body are cooling in different ways (Sieroń & Cieślar, 2003; Sieroń, Cieślar, & Stanek, 2010; Sieroń & Cieślar, 2007; Sieroń & Cieślar, 2003; Zagrobelny, 2003). Human as a warm-blooded organism - characterized by homeostasis, strives to maintain a constant temperature inside the body. Therefore, in the analysis of the thermal response to the cooling of the body must distinguish internal and surface layers' temperature. The internal temperature is necessary for the correct functioning of the body and the temperature of the surface layer depends on the ambient temperature (Cholewka, Stanek, Sieroń, & Drzazga, 2011; Sieroń & Cieślar, 2003; Sieroń, Cieślar, & Stanek, 2010; Sieroń & Cieślar, 2007; Sieroń & Cieślar, 2003; Zagrobelny, 2003; Cholewka, Drzazga, Borgieł, & Kurpas, 2005).

With some approximation, it can be assumed that the heat map observed on the surface of the body presents a thermodynamic state of the body. This state is caused by the influence of external conditions on the internal environment of the body - the metabolically active tissue producing internal heat in a living organism. This fact is illustrated on thermal images of patients treated by whole body cryotherapy (Figures 1-3). One can see that thermal images performed immediately after body cooling are different and show some detailes not seen before one what was discussed in literature (Cholewka, Stanek, Sieroń, & Drzazga, 2011; Cholewka & Drzazga, 2005; Cholewka, Drzazga, & Sieroń, 2006; Cholewka, Drzazga, Kajewski, Bogucki, & Wiśniowska, 2004; Cholewka, Drzazga, Kajewski, Bogucki, & Wiśniowska, 2004; Cholewka, Drzazga, Sieroń, Stanek, Knefel, Kawecki, & Nowak, 2010; Cholewka, Drzazga, Borgieł, & Kurpas, 2005; Cholewka, Drzazga, Kajewski, Sieroń, & Wiśniowska, 2004).

Analysis of thermal images and temperature parameters collected in the tables draws (Figure 1) attention to decrease in the surface temperature of the body as a result of cryotherapy and changing the temperature gradient by cooling the body. On thermograms can be seen a slight thermal asymmetry of the body related to the anatomical asymmetry. Also, by comparing the average temperature obtained for the extremities from thermal parameters of thorax it is easy to see greater decreases of the temperature of these parts of the body where the surface to volume ratio is relatively large. It is easy to notice that the higher temperature with skin areas directly with blood vessels and blood flow, which will have a temperature close to 37°C (e.g. subclavian veins, around the mediastinum). The average temperature is lower in areas where blood flow and metabolic processes are less intensive e.g. knees. Analysis of the thermal images of the chest taken before, and immediately after cooling of the body showed that the greatest cooling was observed on large batches of muscles: musculus pectoralis major and minor and the musculus rectus abdominis as opposed to the area of the breastbone where the pulmonary trunk and large blood vessels (Cholewka, Stanek, Sieroń, & Drzazga, 2011; Cholewka, Drzazga, Sieroń, & Stanek,

Figure 1. Representative thermal images of the chest and tables of temperatures from areas of interest received for a healthy man made before and after cryotherapy

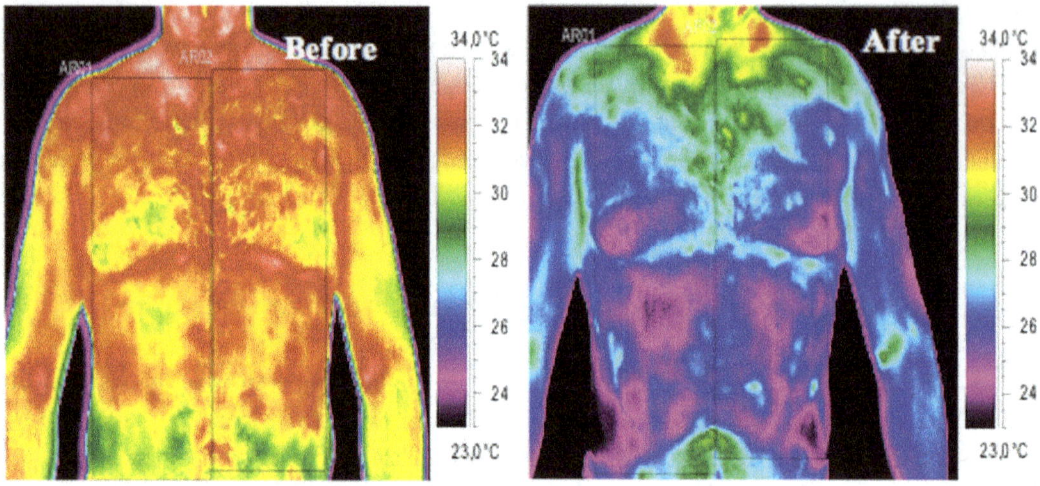

Area	Temperature °C Before cryotherapy	Temperature °C After cryotherapy
AR01 : T_{mean}	31,2	26,4
AR02 : T_{mean}	31,4	26,6
AR01: T_{max}	33,9	31,9
AR01: T_{min}	28,9	22,7
AR02: T_{max}	33,5	22,8
AR02: T_{min}	29,0	32,0

2010; Cholewka, Drzazga, & Sieroń, 2006; Cholewka, Drzazga, Sieroń, Stanek, Knefel, Kawecki, & Nowak, 2010; Cholewka, Drzazga, Sieroń, & Wiśniowska, 2004; Cholewka, Drzazga, Kajewski, Sieroń, & Wiśniowska, 2004). The study showed that the internal temperature of the body due to cryotherapy decreases slightly (ΔT_{org} = 0.8 °C) which proves that a short stay in a cryochamber may not cause any negative effects (Cholewka, Drzazga, Michalik, & Sieroń, 2006; Cholewka & Drzazga, 2006; Ring, 1999). The use of thermal imaging allowed the calculation of the average temperature from the selected areas of the body surface to estimate the average temperature of the total body surface area (T_{body}) before and after cryotherapy based on empirical Equation 1. It was the subject of the researches presented in literature (Cholewka, Stanek, Sieroń, & Drzazga, 2011; Cholewka, Drzazga, Kajewski, Bogucki & Wiśniowska, 2004). According to the empirical formula (1) the main role in the mean temperature of the total body have the back, legs, chest and arms.

The calculations of average temperatures of regions of interest are summarized in Table 1.

The temperature parameters summarized in Table 1 show that, as a result of cryotherapy, surface of the body is cooling what is obvious but the average temperature of the whole body surface calculated from the equation (1) decreased almost 6°C. Different body parts got cooled at different rates. The oc-

Table 1. The average skin surface temperature before (Ta ± SD) and after (Tb ± SD) cryotherapy for research group

Temperature (°C)	**Temperature ± SD (°C)** *Before Cryotherapy*	**Temperature ± SD (°C)** *After Cryotherapy*	$\Delta T = T^{before} - T^{after}$ (°C)
T_{head}	30.0 ± 0.9	27.7 ± 0.9	2.3
T_{chest}	31.9 ± 1.0	27.0 ± 1.8	4.9
T_{back}	31.6 ± 1.1	27.5 ± 1.8	4.1
T_{arms}	30.1 ± 1.3	24.5 ± 2.6	5.6
T_{shin}	28.0 ± 1.8	19.3 ± 3.9	8.7
T_{hands}	24.2 ± 2.7	20.7 ± 2.8	3.5
T_{feet}	23.4 ± 2.8	18.2 ± 2.2	5.2
T_{body}	29.2 ± 0.9	23.4 ± 2.0	5.8
$T_{internal\ body}$ ($T_{int.}$)	35.6 ± 0.6	34.8 ± 0.6	0.8

Source: Cholewka, Drzazga, Kajewski, Bogucki, & Wiśniowska, 2004; Cholewka, Stanek, Sieroń, & Drzazga, 2011

currence of high standard deviation (SD) providing for differences between individuals in terms of the body's response to cryotherapy.

Analyzing the changes of the average of whole body surface temperature due to cryotherapy, an interesting effect associated with varying degrees of cooling the body depending on obesity factor (Body mass index) was observed and discussed in literature (Cholewka, Stanek, Sieroń & Drzazga, 2011; Cholewka, 2005). It was obtained that the average temperature decrease (ΔT) of whole surface of the body is correlated with the BMI (Cholewka, Stanek, Sieroń, & Drzazga, 2011; Cholewka, 2005).

The obtained positive correlation indicates that the body's response to low temperature depends on the physical characteristics (weight and height) of the patient. Obtained result may suggest that parameters such as exposure time and the absolute value of the temperature in the cryogenic chamber should be selected according with the BMI. It can have a potential impact on the therapeutic effect carried out cryotherapy.

Thermal imaging performed immediately after cooling the body in a cryogenic chamber have reflected some anatomical details that were not visible on the thermograms taken before cryotherapy at standard conditions. It is easier to observe some of the muscles on the thermograms of the chest and back. For example, on the back thermograms (Figure 2 and Table 2) it can be seen the entire range of dorsal region of upper back with the lumbar area allows to see trapezius muscle and monotonic changes in temperature along the spine. In this case, it can be seen areas with significantly lower (cold spot) or higher temperature (hot spot) on the line of the spine, which can be linked to the vertebrae, or whole sections of the spine and surrounding area. The effect of increasing the accuracy of the thermal images is associated with a nearly double increase in the temperature gradient (ΔT = Tmax - Tmin) between the maximum and minimum temperatures obtained from selected areas (Cholewka, Stanek, Sieroń, & Drzazga, 2011; Cholewka, Drzazga, Sieroń, & Stanek, 2010; Cholewka, Drzazga, & Sieroń, 2006; Cholewka, Drzazga, Sieroń, Stanek, Knefel, Kawecki, & Nowak, 2010; Cholewka, 2005; Cholewka, Drzazga, Sieroń, & Wiśniowska, 2004). This is caused by the intensification of metabolic processes of various tissues or whole muscle groups. Therefore, the low temperature impact differentiates a thermal map of the body showing details not visible or less visible in the classical thermography (Cholewka,

Figure 2. Representative thermograms of the back

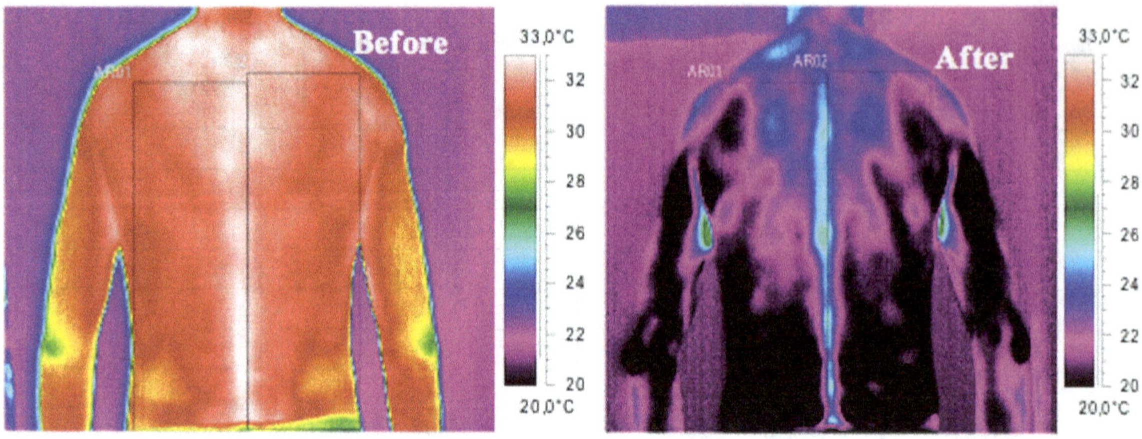

Table 2. Temperatures of regions of interest received for healthy patients taken before and after cryotherapy

Area	Temperature °C Before Cryotherapy	Temperature °C After Cryotherapy
AR01: T_{mean}	31.5	21.0
AR02: T_{mean}	31.1	20.9
AR01: T_{max}	33.7	25.9
AR01: T_{min}	27.7	14.3
AR02: T_{max}	33.1	25.6
AR02: T_{min}	28.1	15.1

Stanek, Sieroń, & Drzazga, 2011; Cholewka, Drzazga, Sieroń, & Stanek, 2010; Cholewka, Drzazga, & Sieroń, 2006; Cholewka, Drzazga, Sieroń, Stanek, Knefel, Kawecki, & Nowak, 2010; Cholewka, 2005; Cholewka, Drzazga, Sieroń, & Wiśniowska, 2004).

Thermography as a technique for imaging the surface of the body presents a temperature gradient on the patients skin. Heat map of the skin is connected with changes in blood supply and metabolism changes in soft tissues. Imaging is more accurate if these changes are related to the tissues located closer to the surface of the skin (Cholewka, Stanek, Sieroń, & Drzazga, 2011; Cholewka, Drzazga, Sieroń, & Stanek, 2010; Cholewka, 2005; Nowakowski et al., 2001; Żuber & Jung, 1997). This allows to use in the evaluation of various diseases. Thermal imaging performed before and after cryotherapy is a one of application in various disease entities. An example might be palm thermograms of a patient with a chronic bacterial infection left hand performed before and after cryotherapy (Figure 5) (Cholewka, Stanek, Sieroń, & Drzazga, 2011; Cholewka, Drzazga, Sieroń, & Stanek, 2010; Cholewka, 2005; Nowakowski et al., 2001; Żuber & Jung, 1997; Ring, 2001; Ammer, 2004).

The evaluation of thermal images after performing cryotherapy allows to see a strong asymmetry in the temperature of both hands. Analysis of the temperature data presented in the tables shows that, prior to cryotherapy, the difference in average temperatures between selected areas was only 0.2°C.

Figure 3. The thermograms lower extremity with marked areas the lower leg and tables temperatures of the areas of interest for the health of the patient taken before and after cryotherapy
Source: Cholewka & Drzazga, 2005; Cholewka, Drzazga, Sieroń, Stanek, Knefel, Kawecki, & Nowak, 2010

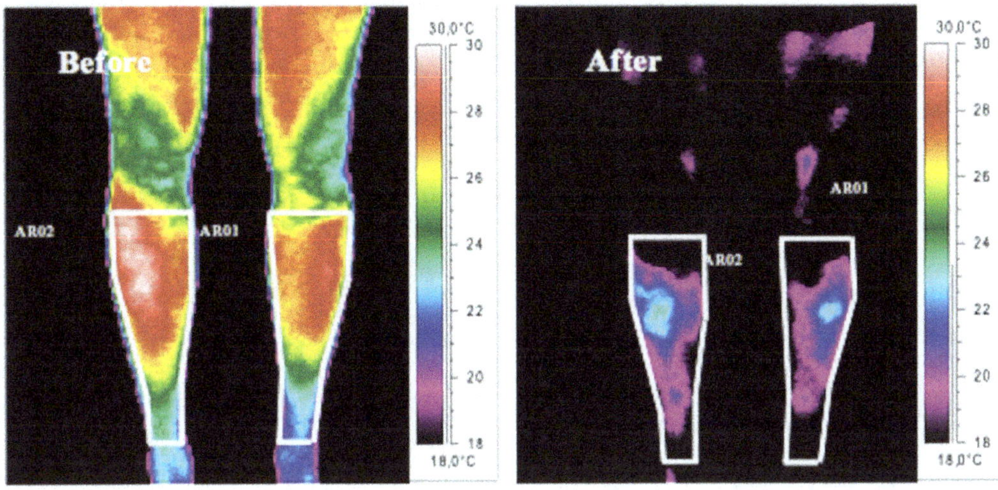

Area	Temperature (°C) Before cryotherapy	Temperature (°C) After cryotherapy
AR01 : T_{mean}	26.2	19.1
AR02 : T_{mean}	27.0	18.5
AR01: T_{max}	28.9	23.6
AR01: T_{min}	19.8	12.6
AR02: T_{max}	30.1	23.1
AR02: T_{min}	21.3	12.6

While the difference after cryotherapy increases more than 10 times to the value 2.7°C. Healthy hand has cooled as a result of staying in a cryogenic chamber while the hand with a bacterial infection did not show significant cooled. This confirms inflammation of patient hand (Cholewka, 2005; Cholewka, Drzazga, Kajewski, Sieroń, & Wiśniowska, 2004; Cholewka, Drzazga, Sieroń, Stanek, Knefel, Kawecki, & Nowak, 2010; Cholewka & Drzazga, 2005).

Another very interesting example of application of thermography and cryotherapy is related to venous insufficiency and has been discussed in literature (Cholewka, 2005; Cholewka, Drzazga, Kajewski, Sieroń, & Wiśniowska, 2004; Cholewka, Drzazga, Sieroń, Stanek, Knefel, Kawecki, & Nowak, 2010; Cholewka & Drzazga, 2005). The case refers to a patient complaining about the pain in the left thigh. The patient was diagnosed as saphenous vein insufficiency of the left thigh. In this case, classic thermography performed before cooling the body revealed an elongated area characterized by higher temperature near the medial left thigh. Such a thermal asymmetry in relation to the other limb may indicate the existing inflammatory state of soft tissue or other lesion associated with venous stasis of blood in the area of the limb. Owever the thermogram taken after the cooling of the body is much more detailed and shows

Figure 4. A scatterplot parameters presented dependence of temperature decrease as a function of body mass index

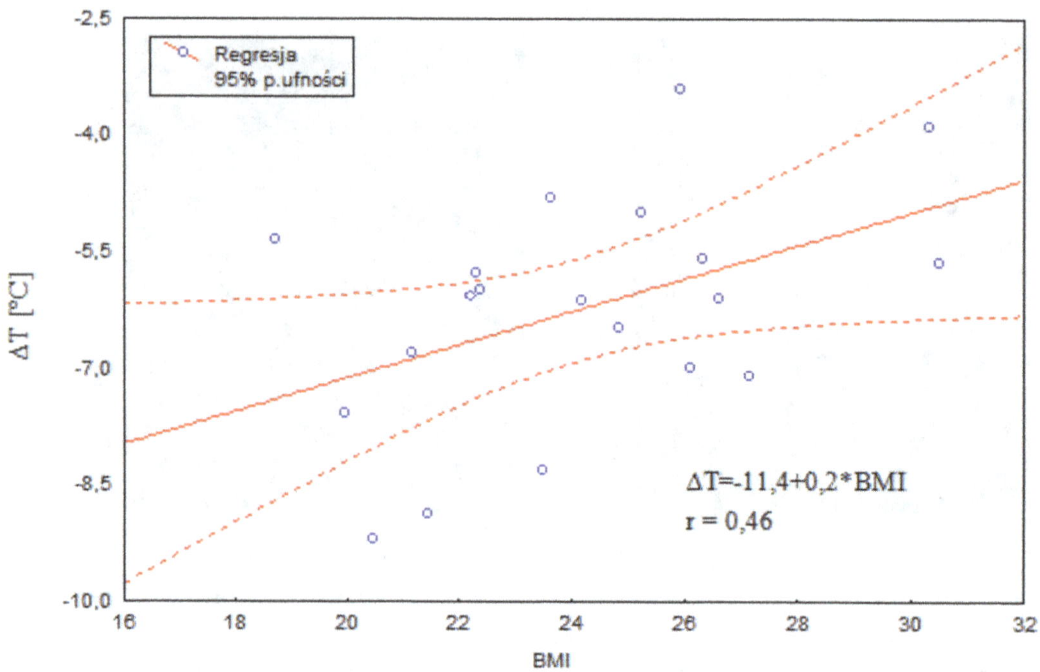

Figure 5. The thermograms of hands (left with chronic bacterial infection) performed before and after cryotherapy

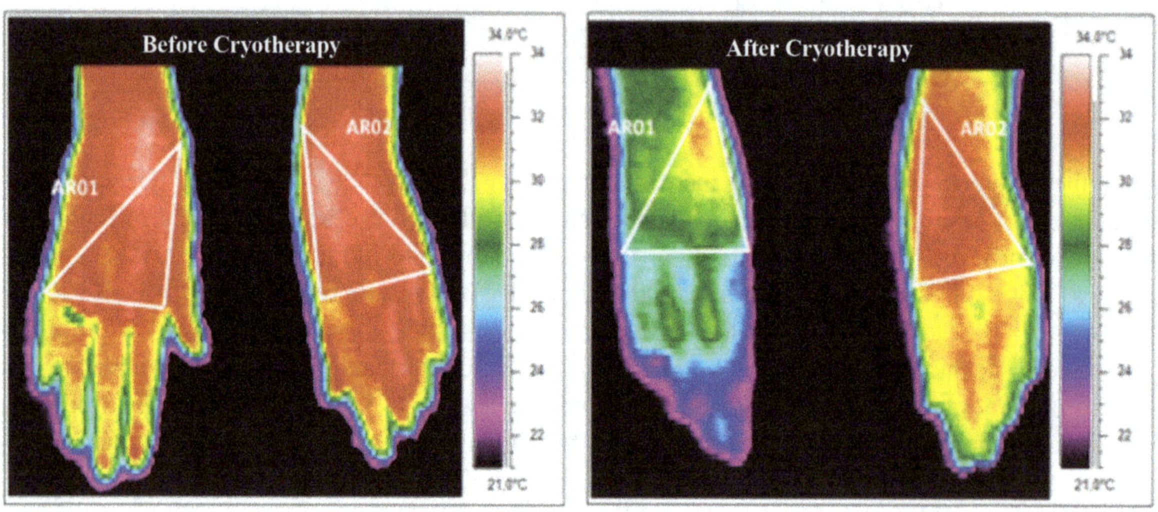

Parameter	$\Delta T = T_{mean}^{AR01} - T_{mean}^{AR02}$
ΔT_{befor}	0.2
ΔT_{after}	2.7

three additional areas of high temperature - indicated in Figure 6 by arrows. They are probably the areas of location of bad working venous valves in the saphenous vein of the left thigh (bad blood flow) which results in a local increase in the surface temperature of the body. In the examined patients it was diagnosed inflammation of the saphenous vein in the course of its valves insufficiency. Saphenous vein in the thigh has 2 to 5 valves, which may lead to malfunction of the deformation and extension of the vessel as a result of stagnation in the blood.

This example shows that thermal imaging diagnostics in combination with cooling the body can bring helpful information, for example, to a vascular surgeon. This is a quick and completely safe method that can be used in the screening of venous diseases.

This research used thermal imaging for the diagnosis of various diseases in combination with cooling body and the assessment of the effects of cryotherapy. Performed studies showed that the application of a short-term (up to 3 minutes) pulse cold affecting the entire human body significantly increases the temperature range of the analyzed areas. This leads to a better differentiation of the surface temperature of the skin and thus increase the contrast of temperature demonstrating the details of which the classic thermography is not able to see accurately.

Figure 6. The thermograms of the lower limbs of the patient diagnosed with insufficiency saphenous vein left thigh performed after whole – body cryotherapy
Source: Cholewka & Drzazga, 2005; Cholewka, Drzazga, Sieroń, Stanek, Knefel, Kawecki, & Nowak, 2010

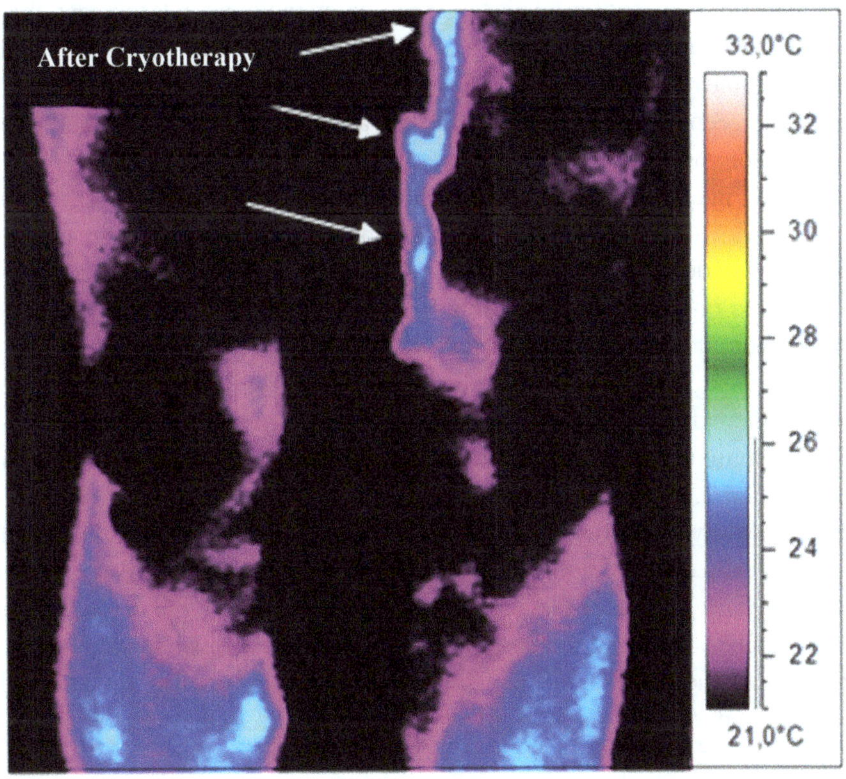

WHOLE BODY COOLING AS A TOOL TO IMPROVING OF THERMOVISION DIAGNOSTICS

Most of the diseases that are treated by whole – body cryotherapy – especially locomotory diseases are connected with metabolism changes so they can be seen in thermal imaging. Moreover, it was proved that decrease of body surface temperature differentiates thermal map of the body what reveals the details. When we consider metabolism increase or decrease of some tissues especially in the very superficial layers of the body it is possible to see then very clearly on thermograms performed just after body cooling. One can find that there have been many papers about cold treatment and application of whole body cryotherapy (Podbielska & Skrzek, 2012; Jiménez-Balderas & Mintz, 1993). However, there are not so many papers concerning data of using the thermal imaging due to cold impact on human body to determine diagnostics value of thermovision (Cholewka, 2005; Cholewka, Ciszek, & Drzazga, 2012). That is why this chapter concerns the use of body cooling as a tool to improving of thermovision diagnostics.

It was found that the use of thermal imaging after whole-body cryotherapy for patients with different diseases indicate the marked changes of thermal map of the body surface. The increase of difference between maximum and minimum (ΔT), called temperature contrast, derived from chosen Region of Interest obtained after cold impact point out significant increase of thermal imaging diagnostics value what was reported in literature mostly for patients with spine diseases (Cholewka, Stanek, Sieroń, & Drzazga, 2011; Cholewka, Drzazga, Sieroń, & Stanek, 2010).

The effect of increase the diagnostic value of thermal imaging can be easily shows on thermograms performed before and after body cooling. This fact is presented in Figure 7. Representative thermograms of patients suffering from spine diseases (low back pain) performed before and after whole - body cryotherapy session in the same temperature scale are presented in Figures 7 and 8. The bigger differentiation of thermal maps is easy seen on thermograms performed after whole – body cryotherapy (images on the right side) in comparison to thermograms performed before one.

It is clearly seen in Figure 7 that the body surface thermal maps obtained after extremely low temperature impact on whole human body reveal significant temperature differentiation on it. It was reported in literature that there are details not seen in classic thermography which become more visible on the thermograms performed only after body cooling. It led to increase the diagnostics value of thermal imaging what was reported in some papers (Cholewka, Stanek, Sieroń, & Drzazga, 2011; Cholewka, Drzazga, Sieroń, & Stanek, 2010). On the other hand, it follows from comparison of temperature variation along spine that there are no temperature anomalies along spinal column for healthy (both before and after cold impact) unlike patient with spine diseases (Cholewka, Stanek, Sieroń, & Drzazga, 2011; Cholewka, Drzazga, Sieroń, & Stanek, 2010). This is other interesting fact that gives opportunity to differentiation between healthy and patients – in this case patients with spine diseases. It is also important that thermograms performed after whole body cryotherapy, while taking into consideration all tissues observed on the whole back, reveal the decrease of whole body surface temperature. There are hot spots observed in thermograms suggest inflammatory states connected with strict vertebrates. It seems that important advantages of thermal diagnostics connected with body cooling gives possibilities to see some temperature gradient changes in different part of the body i.e. occurred on the both side of spinal cord what may suggest the inflammatory states of soft tissues characterized sciatica. That fact was also reported in literature (Cholewka, Stanek, Sieroń, & Drzazga, 2011; Cholewka, Drzazga, Sieroń, & Stanek, 2010). It was also reported that of temperature variations depends on severity as well as the kind of illness. Moreover, the temperature plots performed on thermograms obtained after cold impact

Figure 7. Representative thermograms of patient's backs suffering from back pain performed before (left column) and after (right column) 3 minutes of body cooling with temperature inside the cryochamber set as -120°C. There are no lines marked along spinal for Patient No. 1 opposite for Patients No. 2 for whom in the range of Th1/Th2 – L5/S1 was marked line. Moreover thermograms are performed in two common scales of pseudocolors – rain and medical, for Patient No. 1 and 2, respectively

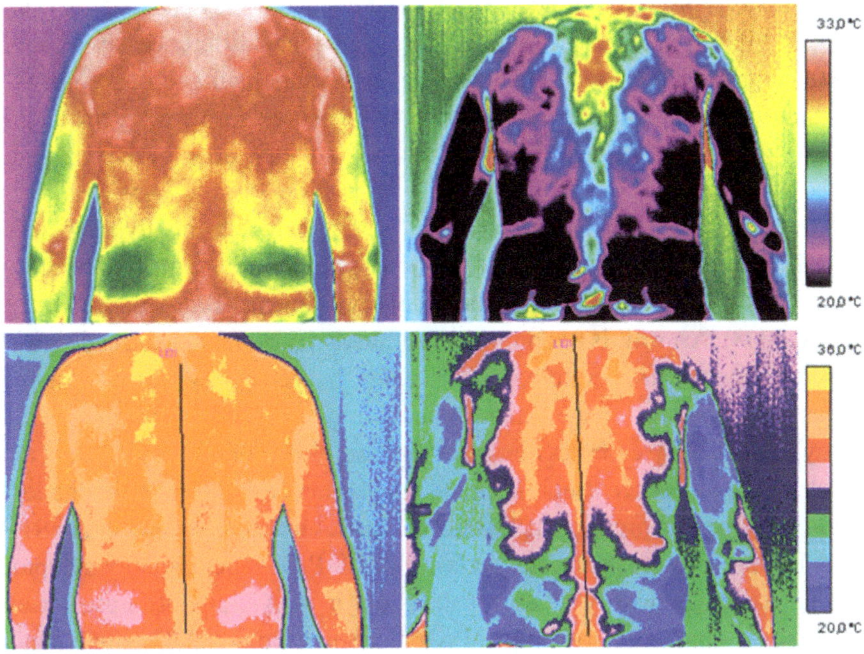

give additional and important information. The temperature plots obtained i.e. along spinal cord indicate very clearly the inflammatory states connected with concrete vertebrates (Cholewka, Stanek, Sieroń, & Drzazga, 2011; Cholewka, Drzazga, Sieroń, & Stanek, 2010). What seems to be interesting diagnostic fact for physician or rehabilitation.

We can influence on skin thermal map by using cold impact on human body but the question was - can we see significant differences in thermal images performed after body cooling for different spine diseases and differentiate them just using thermograms? That was the aim of the different work where authors focused on possibilities of differentiation between thermal maps of patients suffering from ankylosing spodylitis, sciatica and spondyloarthrosis (Cholewka, Drzazga, Sieroń, & Stanek, 2010).

In those studies chosen spine region (Th1/Th2 – L5/S1) was taken into consideration for all groups of patients and healthy. Representative thermograms of the back for healthy man (H), patient suffering from ankylosing spodylitis (AS), suffering from sciatica (Sc) and spondyloarthrosis (Sp) performed after whole body cryotherapy in the same time of rehabilitation cycle (in presented results it was after 5th day of treatment) are presented in Figure 8. We should focus on thermograms performed after body cooling. These thermograms are more clear and reveal some hot spots not seen in thermograms performed in classic thermography what undoubtedly increase a diagnostic value of thermal imaging. Such effect was presented and commented widely in literature. But the more important thing which seemed to conclude from thermograms analysis that obtained thermal maps seem to be specific for studied back diseases. It could be seen that obtained thermograms suggest standard maps for chosen spine diseases

(Cholewka, Stanek, Sieroń, & Drzazga, 2011; Cholewka, Drzazga, Sieroń & Stanek, 2010). That is why it was interesting to compare the thermograms of the back of patient suffering from ankylosing spodylitis (Figure 8 AS) with representative thermograms of patients suffering from sciatica (Figure 8 Sc) and spondyloarthrosis (Figure 8 Sp) all performed after cold impact.

Thermal studies are a useful diagnostic tool in many fields of medicine, including arthritis, venous insufficiency spine diseases or even in cancer diagnosis. The idea of thermal diagnosis in different diseases relies on bigger differentiation of the thermal body map due to differences in metabolism intensity in soft tissues in the region of interest. Usually the biggest metabolism is observed in the areas where the inflammatory state or intensity blood supply occurred. When these processes are amplified by some physical factor, like cold influenced on the body, it leads to a wider range of thermal maps and allows to see more details.

For example, the thermograms obtained for patients with ankylosing spondylitis points out the areas of higher temperature are observed almost along the whole spinal column. This is a chronic inflammatory arthritis connected with almost all vertebrates in spinal column (Jiménez-Balderas & Mintz, 1993; Brooks, Bogduk, & Bellamy, 2003). Arthritis is a common condition that apart from pain, causes inflammation of the joints and tissue around them. Therefore, the area characterized by higher temperature is connected with whole spine and has elongated shape. On the other hand, sciatica is the disease where all symptoms including pain may be caused by compression and irritation of one of five nerve roots that give rise to the sciatic nerve, or the sciatic nerve itself. The pain is felt usually in lower back, one leg or even foot. It is generally caused by the compression of lumbar nerves L4 or L5 or sacral nerves S1, S2 or S3 and far less commonly by compression of the sciatic nerve itself. Pain is not the only symptom of sciatica. There could be seen also inflammatory states of soft tissues in the vicinity of loins. It usually occurs on the both sides of the spine what seems to be typical symptom of this disease. Thermal imaging of patients back with sciatica showed temperature anomalies mainly in the lower lumbar region. The increase of skin temperature occurred not only along the spine in lumbar region but also in the areas over the tissues adjacent to the spine on both sides in the lower lumbar region (Cholewka, Drzazga, Wiśniowska, & Sieroń, 2002; Cholewka, Drzazga, Kajewski, Sieroń, & Wiśniowska, 2004; Cholewka, Drzazga, & Sieroń, 2006; Cholewka, Drzazga, Sieroń, & Stanek, 2010). This fact is presented in Figure 8*Sc* where the hot spots are clearly seen in the lower lumbar region on the both sides of the spine. Such thermal maps seem to correspond with medical report. However, in the case of spondyloarthrosis, the inflammatory state also occurs mainly in the lumbar region of spine and in the cervical. From medical point of view, this is a progressive destruction of the facet joint sand and is characterized by loss of articular cartilage and production of osteophytes. This disease can lead to narrowing of the neural foramina in the lumbar regions and a stenosing of spinal canal causing inflammatory state and back pain (Jiménez-Balderas & Mintz, 1993; Brooks, Bogduk & Bellamy, 2003). Probably that is why the situation is similar to that observed in the thermograms of patients suffering from sciatica but in the case of spondyloarthrosis the inflammatory state as well as the area characterized by higher temperature of the spine (Figure 8, *Sp*) is usually observed in wider/longer area than in sciatica but is also connected with lower lumbar region. However, the tissues adjacent to the spine are less affected than in sciatica what can be also clearly seen in Figure 8*Sp* in comparison to the Figure 8*Sc*.

Thermal images of other diseases i.e. crura ulceration can also give bigger differentiation due to processes that are localized in very superficial tissue or even on the skin surface. However, thermal map evaluation may be difficult to describe when we consider oncology changes like breast cancer due to different depth of localized the cancerous tissue what influences on heat transfer to the body surface, so

Figure 8. Thermograms of patients' backs of healthy man (H) and patient suffering from ankylosing spodylitis (AS), sciatica (Sc) and spondyloarthrosis (Sp) performed after whole body cryotherapy at the same period of rehabilitation cycle

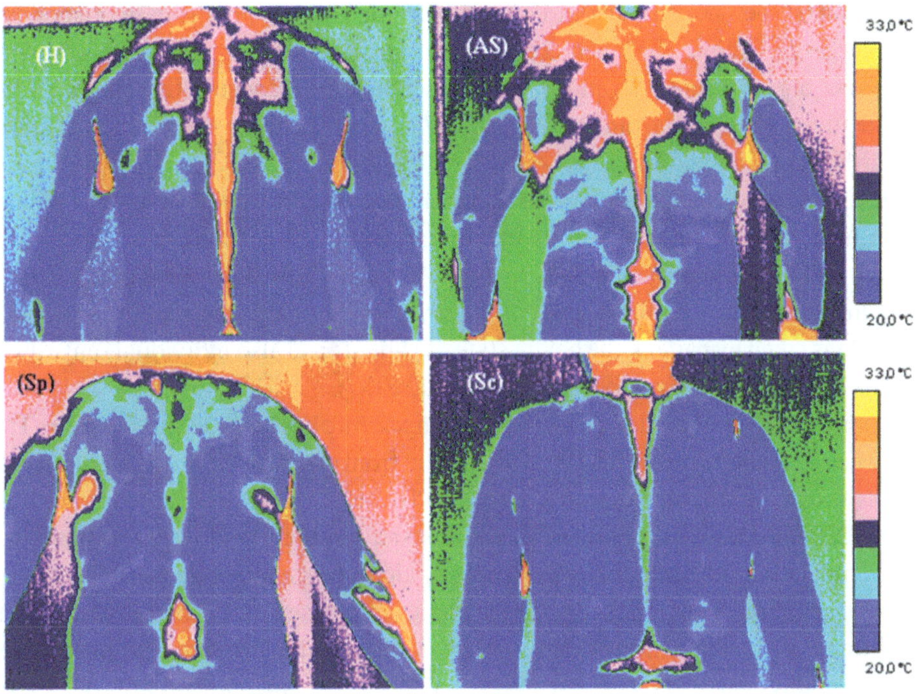

the temperature map observed in thermovision. The similar situation may be seen in the case of blood supply system evaluation. That is why the easiest to see in thermal imaging are superficial veins.

It was reported in literature that temperature plots derived from the thermograms show changes of skin temperature more clearly than plots derived from thermograms performed before body cooling in normal conditions – from classic thermograms. It was wide discussed in previous papers (Cholewka, 2012; Cholewka, Drzazga, Kajewski, Sieroń, & Wiśniowska, 2004; Cholewka, Drzazga, Sieroń, & Stanek, 2010). Such phenomenon confirms the increase of thermal imaging diagnostic value. The anomalies of temperature (increase and decrease) in different ranges of vertebrates seen, in the cases of patients with spondyloarthrosis and ankylosing spondylitis, or seen in the soft tissues on both sides of spine in vicinity of loins, in the case of patient with sciatica, can be treated as connected with different pathology states. Thermogram of patient with sciatica (Sc) reveals increase of temperature only in the lower lumbar region. So the temperature plots performed for patient with spondyloarthrosis also point out the marked inflammatory states in the corresponding range. For example, in patient thermogram presented in Figure 8 Sc, the inflammatory state will be seen from L2/L3 to L5/S1, the degeneration state in the vicinity of Th11/Th12 and the weak inflammatory state from Th6/Th7 to Th9/Th10. Moreover, the temperature plots along the lines performed perpendicular to spinal column will be corresponding with specific of the disease as well as health state of patient showing increase of temperature on both sides of spine. It was also presented on thermogram of patient with sciatica. Increased temperature on both sides of spine confirms the inflammatory state of tissues adjacent to the spine, what is a characteristic symptom for this kind of disease. Thermogram after body cooling in the case of patient with ankylosing spondylitis revealed increased temperature on almost all spinal column, however the levels Th5/Th6 – Th8/Th9 and Th11/Th12 – L2/L3 seem to indicate bigger inflammatory states thanother spine regions. It was also showed and discussed in previous papers that such increased temperature in adjacent tissues in the vicinity of loins can be seen not only for patients with sciatica but also in the case of spondyloarthrosis (Cholewka, Drzazga, Sieroń, & Stanek, 2010). However, the inflammatory state in spondyloarthrosis seems to have a bigger range than in the case of sciatica. In presented thermograms the range of increased temperature is observed from Th12/L1 to L5/S1 what is clearly seen in thermogram of patient with spondyloarthrosis (Figure 8 Sp).

Moreover it follows from the results of the thermal imaging in spine diseases that using only such parameters like mean temperature as well as maximum or minimum temperature seem to be not adequate to analyze and differentiation the diseases. This is because diseases are dependent on magnitude of temperature inside the cryochamber, level of decrease of the body surface temperature, number of cryotherapy sessions taken by patient, the health state of patients and also individual sensitivity of patient to body cooling (Cholewka, Drzazga, Sieroń, & Stanek, 2010).

For the better inside into the problem, the contrast temperature has been defined as $\Delta T = Tmax - Tmin$ (difference between maximum and minimum temperature from chosen Region of Interest). Moreover the relative contrast ratio defined as temperature contrast and mean temperature derived from chosen Region of Interest ratio $(\Delta T)/(Tmean)$ was introduced. Results showed that the difference between maximum and minimum temperature obtained from chosen lines along the spine is about 3°C for healthy while for patients with back diseases is markedly larger and even crossed 4.5°C and it was statistically significant. The differences become more visible when we consider the relative contrast ratio $\Delta T/Tmean$. For the group of healthy people its value was 0.12 ± 0.03 while it increases up till 0.19 ± 0.06 for the patients with back pain. Such increase of this parameter was also statistically significant for all groups of patients. It seems that the temperature contrast and relative contrast ratio should be more proper in thermal characteristics of back pain diseases due to theirs independency of conditions of body cooling (Cholewka, Drzazga, Sieroń, & Stanek, 2010).

Thermal imaging as a completely noninvasive and safe for patients diagnostic technique can be used not only to diagnosis, but also to evaluate the effects of therapy. In this case thermal imaging was the tool to lead the study on back's temperature changes along the spinal column in the case of patients with spine diseases treated by whole body cryotherapy and kinesiotherapy.

The region of increased temperature in the lower lumbar region connected with inflammatory state is observed during the whole therapy cycle when it is considered patients suffering from Spondyloarthrosis. The other important thing is that when we take into consideration the temperature plots as a function of number of rehabilitation cycles (2, 5 and 10) obtained results suggest that a wide peak connected with the inflammatory state observed after 2nd day of whole body cryotherapy becomes more clear and better visible and reveals not one big area but two smaller peaks what may be connected with the shrink inflammatory states or points out that bigger decrease of body surface temperature lead to better differentiation of thermal maps. However, it is noteworthy that temperature plots did not show the significant differences in size of area characterized with higher temperature with number of cryotherapy sessions although people reported decrease of pain and increase of fitness (Cholewka, Drzazga, Sieroń, & Stanek, 2010; Cholewka & Drzazga, 2005; Cholewka & Drzazga, 2006).

Avail oneself of possibility of thermal imaging it was checked the correlation between the whole body skin temperature decrease caused by whole body cryotherapy and body mass index (BMI), what was presented and discussed in literature (Cholewka, Drzazga, Sieroń, & Stanek, 2010; Cholewka & Drzazga,

2005; Cholewka & Drzazga, 2006). Obtained results showed medium positive correlation between BMI and the decrease of mean body temperature due to cold impact in cryogenic chamber. The results gave clear information that the response of organisms on whole body cryotherapy depends on the physical conditions of the organism (i.e. mass and height). Moreover, the magnitude of body temperature response on cooling is also dependent on the state of health as well as the individual features of the patient. By analyzing such results, it comes one important question - do such parameters like the magnitude of the low temperature used in the cryogenic chamber or time of stay in cryogenic chamber should be selected with regards to body mass index. It may have a potential meaning on the range of body cooling as well as the therapy effects. It seems that due to wider application of thermovision in medicine it could be possible to match the time of lasting and the magnitude of temperature inside the cryochamber according to body mass index of patient as well as health state (Cholewka, Drzazga, Sieroń, & Stanek, 2010; Cholewka & Drzazga, 2005; Cholewka & Drzazga, 2006).

CONCLUSION

The results of discussed works and presented representative analysis showed clearly that the thermal imaging performed after whole-body cryotherapy has a potential diagnostics value in case of back diseases i.e. spondyloarthrosis, ankylosing spondylitis and sciatica. Moreover, it seems that thermovision is not only the qualitative technique but also can give some quantitative data. Temperature plots performed along, as well as, perpendicular to spine and temperature parameters such as temperature contrast and relative contrast ratio are objective and useful in differentiating between some spine diseases. Additionally, thermal imaging studies in combination with cryotherapy show improved diagnostic possibilities of many diseases. The combination of these two methods is perfect for sportsmen - improves the athlete performance and allows him to faster recovery.

REFERENCES

Ammer. (2004). Temperature effects of thermotherapy determined by infrared measurements. *Physica Medica, 20*(S1), 64-66.

Ammer. (2008). The Glamorgan Protocol for recording and evaluation of thermal images of the human body. *Thermology International.*

Banfi, L., Lombardi, G., Colombini, A., & Melegati, G. (2010). Whole-body cryotherapy in athletes. *Sports Medicine (Auckland, N.Z.), 40*(6), 509–517. doi:10.2165/11531940-000000000-00000 PMID:20524715

Bauer, Hurnik, & Zdziarski, Mielczarek, & Podbielska. (1997). Thermovision and its applications in medicine. *Acta Bio-Optica et Informatica Medica, 3*(2-4), 121–131.

Bauer, Hurnik, Zdziarski, Mielczarek, & Skrzek, Podbielska, & Zagrobelny. (1997). Thermovison evaluation of cryotherapy effects. *Acta Bio-Optica et Informatica Medica, 3*(2-4), 133–140.

Bauer & Skrzek. (1997). Physiological basis of cryotherapy. *Acta Bio-Optica et Informatica Medica, 3*(2-4), 115–120.

Bauer & Skrzek. (1999). Fizjologiczne podstawy krioterapii. *Medycyna sportowa, 94*, 3-7. (in Polish)

Biały, Zimmer, Skrzek, & Zagrobelny. (1998). Cryogenic Chamber – Possibilities Of Use In Rehabilitation. *Baln. Pol*, *40*(3-4), 44–47.

Biały, Zimer, & Zagrobelny. (1999) Acta Bio-Optica et Informatica Medica. *Inżynieria Biomedyczna Wpływ ogólnoustrojowej krioterapii na parametry krwi obwodowej zawodników kadry narodowej lekkoatletów, 5*(1-2), 7-10. (in Polish)

Birkner, Sieroń, Beck, Jagodziński, & Romuk, Skrzep-Poloczek, & Stanek. (2003). Application of cryogenic temperatures in medicine. *Wiadomosci Lekarskie (Warsaw, Poland)*, *56*(1-2), 53–56. PMID:12901269

Brengelmann. (1989). Body temperature regulation In H. D. Patron, A. F. Fuchs, B. Hill, A. M. Scher, & R. Steiner (Eds.), *Textbook of Physiology*. Academic Press.

Brooks, Bogduk, & Bellamy. (2003). *Evidence based – Management of acute muscosceletal pain.* Australian Academic Press.

Cholewka, Ciszek, & Drzazga. (2012). Cryogenic chamber used in physical medicine and their comparison. *W: Zastosowanie niskich temperatur w medycynie, redakcja: Anna Skrzek i Halina Podbielska 2012*. Oficyna Wydawnicza Politechniki Wrocławskiej, Wrocław.

Cholewka, Drzazga, Wiśniowska, & Sieroń. (2002). The temperature changes of the skin surface during whole body cryotherapy. *IFMBE Proceedings of 2nd EMBEC, 2*, 1330-31.

Cholewka, Drzazga, Sieroń, & Wiśniowska. (2004). Temperature effect of whole body cryotherapy determined by thermography. *Thermology International*, 57-63.

Cholewka, Drzazga, Borgieł, & Kurpas. (2005). Cold penetration of the fourth layer tissue model in the whole body cryotherapy conditions. *IFMBE Proceedings of 3rd EMBEC.*

Cholewka, Drzazga, Michalik, & Sieroń. (2006). Whole Body Cryotherapy and Magnetotherapy Influence on Some Cardiac Parameters. *Pol J of Environ Stud, 15*(4A), 19-21.

Cholewka, Drzazga, Sieroń, & Stanek. (2010). Thermovision diagnostics in chosen spine diseases treated by whole body cryotherapy. *Journal of Thermal Analysis and Calorymetry.*

Cholewka, D., Drzazga, Z., & Sieroń, A. (2006). Monitoring of whole body cryotherapy effects by thermal imaging – preliminary report. *Physica Medica*, *22*(2), 57–62. doi:10.1016/S1120-1797(06)80054-2 PMID:17643893

Cholewka, D., Drzazga, Z., Sieroń, A., & Stanek, A. (2010). Thermovision diagnostics in chosen spine diseases treated by whole body cryotherapy. *Journal of Thermal Analysis and Calorimetry*, *102*(1), 113–119. doi:10.1007/s10973-010-0873-y

Cholewka, Drzazga, & Kajewski, Bogucki, & Wiśniowska. (2004). The thermal imaging of skin body surface due to whole body cryotherapy – preliminary report. *Physica Medica*, *20*(Suppl. I), 70–72.

Cholewka, Drzazga, Kajewski, Sieroń, & Wiśniowska. (2004). Thermographic assessment of cryotherapy effects. *VI Konferencja Krajowa TTP2004 Ustroń-Jaszowiec, Proceedings*, (pp. 143 – 148).

Cholewka, Drzazga, Knefel, Kawecki, & Nowak. (2010). Thermal Imaging In Hyperbaric Oxygen Therapy (HBO). *Inżynieria Biomedyczna.*

Cholewka, Drzazga, Sieroń, Stanek, Knefel, Kawecki, & Nowak. (2010). Some Applications Of Thermal Imaging In Medicine. *Monographs of Polish Journal of Environmental Studies.*

Cholewka, Knefel, Stanek, Kawecki, & Nowak, Sieroń, & Drzazga. (2011). Thermal imaging and TC oximetry measurements of hyperbaric oxygen therapy (HBO) effects on trophic ulceration of the crura. *Journal of Thermal Analysis and Calorimetry*. doi:10.1007/s10973-011-1934-6

Cholewka, Kasprzyk, & Stanek, Sieroń-Stołtny, & Drzazga. (2015). May thermal imaging be useful in cyclist endurance tests? *Journal of Thermal Analysis and Calorimetry*. doi:10.1007/s10973-015-4662-5

Cholewka, Stanek, Sieroń, & Drzazga. (2011). Thermography study of skin response due to whole-body cryotherapy. *Skin Research and Technology*. PMID:21507075

Cholewka, Sieroń, & Drzazga. (2014). Application thermal imaging in diseases of the blood vessels. W: Biomedyczne zastosowania termowizji, pod redakcją H. Podbielska i A. Skrzek, Biomedyczne zastosowania termowizji. Oficyna Wydawnicza Politechniki Wrocławskiej.

Cholewka, Stanek, Kasprzyk, Urbańczyk, Jagodziński, Sieroń, & Drzazga. (2013). The application of thermography in research efficiency athletes, pilot studies. *PAK, 9*, 871-874.

Cholewka, S., & Klimas, S. (2014). Thermal imaging application in chronic venous disease: Pilot study. *Journal of Thermal Analysis and Calorimetry, 115*(2), 1609–1618. doi:10.1007/s10973-013-3356-0

Cholewka, Stanek, Kwiatek, Sieroń, & Drzazga. (2011). The use of thermography in the diagnosis of selected changes to skin cancer - preliminary study. *Application of thermovision to diagnosis of chosen skin cancer changes – preliminary studies*. PAK.

Cholewka, S., & Kwiatek, S. (2013). Does the temperature gradient correlate with the photodynamic diagnosis parameter numerical colour value (NCV)? *Photodiagnosis and Photodynamic Therapy, 10*(1), 33–38. doi:10.1016/j.pdpdt.2012.07.001 PMID:23465370

Cholewka & Drzazga. (2005a). Diagnostic value of thermal imaging due to whole body cryotherapy. *IFMBE Proceedings of 3rd EMBEC.*

Cholewka & Drzazga. (2005b). Krioterapia ogólnoustrojowa w kriokomorze dwu-stopniowej oraz kriokomorze z zaleganiem zimna. *Acta Bio-Optica et Informatica Medica*, 57-63. (in Polish)

Cholewka & Drzazga. (2006). Comparison Of Some Parameters Of Two-Stepped Cryogenic Chamber And Chamber With Lingering Cold. *Biomedical Engineering Acta Indygo, 11*, 103–110.

Cholewka. (2005). *The impact of low temperatures on the body - in vivo and in vitro studies*. Rozprawa doktorska Uniwersyetet Śląski w Katowicach, Katowice.

Cholewka. (2012). Meaning of thermal diagnostic analysis of the whole body cryotherapy. *W: Zastosowanie niskich temperatur w medycynie*. Redakcja: Anna Skrzek i Halina Podbielska.

Chwalbińska-Moneta. (2003). Wpływ kriostymulacji ogólnoustrojowej na niektóre reakcje wysiłkowe u sportowców. *Sport Wyczynowy, 5/6*, 50-54. (in Polish)

Ganong. (2009). FizjologiaPZWL.

Gage & Baust. (2002). Cryosurgery – a review of recent advances and current issues. *Cryo Letters, 23*(2), 30–32. PMID:12050774

Goodman, Murphy, Siltanen, Kelley, & Rucker. (1986). Normal temperature asymmetry of the back and extremities by computer-assisted infrared imaging. *Thermology, 1*, 195-202.

Góralczyk, Mikuła, & Jagodzińska. (2002). Osteoarthritis. Choroba zwyrodnieniowa stawów. *Medycyna Rodzinna, 10*, 2.

Gregorowicz & Dalidowski. (1998). Cryotherapy In Sclerosis Multiplex (Sm) Treatment Acta Bio-Opt. *Inform. Med., 4*(4), 173 – 174.

Gregorowicz. (1992). *The influence of whole body cryotherapy on chosen haemodynamic and lungs ventilation markers in rheumatoid diseases*. Praca Doktorska AM.

Gregorowiczv & Zagrobelny. (1998). Whole body cryotherapy, indications and contraindications, treatment and its physiological and clinical effects. Acta Bio-Optica et Informatica Media, 4, 120-131.

Hoffman & Bischo. (2002). The cryobiology of cryosurgical injury. *Urology, 60*(2), 40-49.

Hrycaj & Łącki. (2002). Od zwyrodnienia do zapalenia – współczesne poglądy na patogenezę choroby zwyrodnieniowej stawów. *Nowa Medycyna*, (2), 115.

Hulbert & Else. (2004). Basal Metabolic Rate: History, Composition, Regulation and Usefulness. *Physiol Biochem Zool., 77*(6), 869-76.

Jagodziński, Kubacka, & Wiśniowska, Puszer, & Stanek. (2001). Whole Body Cryotherapy Part 1 Priv. [In Polish]. *Cab, 4*(92), 10–11.

Jagodziński, S., & Gmyrek, C. (2007). Evaluation of whole - body cryotherapy on the circulatory system in patients with ankylosing spondylitis by analysis of duration and QT interval dispertion. *Fizjoterapia Polska, 7*(3), 362–369.

Jazienicka, Pietrzak, & Toruniowi. (1991). New indications for cryotherapy. *Przeglad Dermatologiczny, 78*(3), 190–194.

Jiménez-Balderas & Mintz. (1993). Ankylosing Spondylitis: Clinical Course In Women And Men. *J Rheumatol, 20*(12), 2069–72.

Johnston, S., Schoenfeld, P., Mysore, J. V., & Dubois, A. (1999, July). Endoscopic spray cryotherapy: a new technique for mucosal ablation in the esophagus. *Gastrointestinal Endoscopy, 50*(1), 86–92. doi:10.1016/S0016-5107(99)70352-4 PMID:10385730

Jonderko. (1990). Current state of knowledge about the application of cryotherapy for treatment of musculoskeletal diseases. *Chir Narzadow Ruchu Ortop Pol, 55*, 31-5.

Kasprzyk, Wójcik, Cholewka, Sieroń-Stołtny, Piętka, Drzazga, & Stanek. (2015). *The applications of thermal imaging in energy cost rating during Aerobic Circuit Training*. QIRT.

Kerschan-Schindl, Uher, Zauner-Dungl, & Fialka-Moser. (1998). V Cold And Cryotherapy. A Review Of The Literature On General Principles And Practical Applications Acta Med. *Austriaca, 25*(3), 73 – 8.

Knight. (1995). *Cryotherapy in sport injury management*. Human Kinetics.

Korzonek-Szlacheta, Wielkoszynski, & Stanek. (2007). Influence of whole - body cryotherapy on the levels of some hormones in professional footballers. *Endokrynologia Polska, 58*(1), 27–32. PMID:17354202

Kozielski & Ziora. (1997). Bronchoscopic cryotherapy. *Pneumonologia i Alergologia Polska, 65*(5-6), 411–416. PMID:9340073

Księżpolska-Pietrzak. (1998). Krioterapia W Osteoporozie: Polski Merkuriusz Lekarski, D.[In Polish]. *Polski Tygodnik Lekarski, 28*, 222–224.

Księżpolska-Pietrzak, Cygler, Lesiak, & Noniewicz. (1993). The Influence Of Low Temperature Treatment On Reumatoid Arm. *Reumatologia, 31*(2), 179–183.

Leppaluto, W. (2008). Effect of long-term whole-body cold exposures on plasma concentrations of ACTH, beta-endorphin, cortisol, catecholamines and cytokines in healthy females. *Scandinavian Journal of Clinical and Labolatory Investstigation, 68*(2), 145–153. doi:10.1080/00365510701516350

Maraso, B., Gai, G., & Massaglia, O. (1998). Radiofrequency resection of bronchial tumours in combination with cryotherapy: Evaluation of a new technique. *Thorax, 53*(2), 106–109. doi:10.1136/thx.53.2.106 PMID:9624294

Meeusen & Lievens. (1986). The use of cryotherapy in sports injuries. *Sports Med., 3*(6), 398-414.

Metzger, Zwingmann, Protz, & Jackel. (2000). Die Bedeutung Der Ganzkorperkaltetherapie Im Rahmen Der Rehabilitation Bei Patienten Mit Rheumatishen. *Erkrank. Rehabil., 39*, 93–100. doi:10.1055/s-2000-14442

Misztela, Kuliński, & Rybak. (1995). Ocena Krioterapii Miejscowej W Reumatoidalnym Zapaleniu Stawów Baln.[In Polish]. *Pol, 37*(3-4), 38–41.

Mraz, Skrzek, & Gruszka, Chamela-Bilińska, Drak-Wojakiewicz, & Dutkiewicz. (2001). The influence of physiotherapy and whole body cryotherapy on standing position balance of patients with sclerosis multiplex. *Physiotherapy, 9*(1), 26–29.

Nowakowski. (2001). *Postępy termografii – aplikacje medyczne*. Gdańsk: Academic Press.

O'Keefe, M., OReilly, J., & Lanigan, B. (1998). Longer term visual outcome of eyes with retinopathy of prematurity treated with cryotherapy or diode laser. *The British Journal of Ophthalmology, 82*(11), 1246–1248. doi:10.1136/bjo.82.11.1246 PMID:9924326

Pasricha, Hill, Wadwa, Gislason, & Okolo. (1999). Endoscopic cryotherapy: experimental results and first clinical use. *Gastrointest. Endosc., 49*(5), 627-631.

Pilawski. (1983). *Podstawy biofizyki*. PZWL. (in Polish)

Podbielska & Skrzek. (Eds.). (2012). The application of low temperatures in biomedicine. Oficyna Wydawnicza Politechniki Wrocławskiej, Wrocław.

Podbielska & Skrzek. (2014). *Biomedical application of thermography, Biomedyczne zastosowania termowizji, praca zbiorowa*. Wrocław: Oficyna Wydawnicza Politechniki Wrocławskiej.

Raczkowski & Zagrobelny. (1990). *Technical and physiological aspects of whole body cooling*. Materials of IV Science and Training Conference of Polish Cryomedical Society.

Ring, Jung, Kalicki, Zuber, Rustecka, & Vardasca. (2013). New Standards For Fever Screening With Thermal Imaging Systems. *Journal of Mechanics in Medicine and Biology, 13*(2).

Ring & Ammer. (2000). The technique of infrared imaging in medicine. *Thermol. Intern., 10*(1), 7-14.

Ring & Ammer. (2012a). Infrared thermal imaging in medicine. *Physiological Measurement, 33*(3), R33-46.

Ring & Ammer. (2012b). Thermal imaging in rheumatology - An overview. *Thermology International, 22*(2), 68-69.

Ring. (1999). Thermal Symmetry of Human Skin Temperature. *Thermology International, 9*(2), 53-55.

Ring. (2001). Provocation tests in thermal imaging. *Abs. Thermology Int., 11*, 2.

Ronikier. (2008). *Physiology of exercise in sports, physiotherapy and recreation*. Centralny Ośrodek Sportu, Warszawa.

Rybak, Kuliński, Misztela, & Podgórski. (1995). Zastosowanie Krioterapii W Leczeniu Następstw Blizn Kanału Kręgowego Baln.[In Polish]. *Pol, 37*(3-4), 29–30.

Rymaszewska, Biały, Zagrobelny, & Kiejna. (2000). The Influence Of Whole Body Cryotherapy On Mental Health. *Psychiatria Polska, 34*(4), 649 – 653.

Rymaszewska, R., Ramsey, D., & Chładzińska-Kiejna, S. (2008). Whole - body cryotherapy as adjunct treatment of depressive syndrome and anxiety disorders. *Archivum Immunologiae et Therapiae Experimentalis, 56*(1), 63–68. doi:10.1007/s00005-008-0006-5 PMID:18250970

Schroder & Anderson. (1995). *Kryo- und Thermotherapie. Grundlangen und praktische Anwendung*. New York: Gustaw Hischer Verlag.

Sieroń, Cieślar, & Stanek. (2010). *Cryotherapy. Theoretical bases, biological effects, clinical applications*. α-Medica Press Bielsko Biała.

Sieroń, Pastuszka, Marniok, Wiśniowska, & Jagodziński, Ślusarczyk, … Stanek. (2004). Influence of low temperature on lymph formation and lymph flow velocity in mice. *Thermol. Int., 14*, 127–130.

Sieroń, Stanek, Cieślar, & Pasek. (2007). Cryorehabilitation - the role cryotherapy in modern rehabilitation. *Fizjoterapia, 15*(2), 3–8.

Sieroń, Stanek, & Cieślar. (Eds.). (2014). *Wellness, Spa, Anti-aging*. PZWL.

Sieroń & Cieślar. (2003a). *The Application Of Cold In Medicine - Cryosurgery And Cryotherapy*. A-Medica Press Bielsko-Biala Poland. (in Polish)

Sieroń & Cieślar. (2003b). The theoretical basis for cooling treatment. The application of cold medicine - cryosurgery and cryotherapy. α-Medica Press.

Sieroń & Cieślar. (2007). Cryotherapy – cold treatment. α-Medica Press.

Silverman, Tuncali, Adams, von Sonnenberg, Zou, Kacher, ... Jolesz. (2000). MR imaging-guided percutaneous cryotherapy of liver tumors: Initial experience. *Radiology, 217*, 657-664.

Stanek, Cieslar, & Matyszkiewicz. (2005). Subjective estimation of therapeutic efficacy of whole - body cryotherapy in patients with ankylosing spondylitis. *Balneolologia Polska*, *47*(1-2), 24–32.

Stanek, Cieślar, & Matyszkiewicz. (2006). Changes in antioxidant status in patients with ankylosing spondylitis during cryotherapy. *European Journal of Clinical Investigation*, *36*(Suppl.1), 20.

Stanek, Cieslar, & Rosmus-Kucza. (2006). Influence of whole - body cryotherapy on blood morphology parameters in patients with ankylosing spondylitis and in healthy volunteers. *Acta Bio-Optica et Informatica Medica*, *12*(3), 207-210.

Stanek, Cieślar, Mrowiec, & Sieroń. (2006). Cryotherapy in clinical practice. *Rehabilitacja w Praktyce*, *1*, 27–31.

Stanek, Cieslar, & Sieron. (2007). Therapeutic application of cryotherapy in clinical practice. *Balneologia Polska*, *49*(1), 37–45.

Stanek, Cieślar, & Sieroń. (2008). Application of cryotherapy in sport medcine. *Rehabilitacja w Praktyce*, *2*, 34–35.

Stanek, Cieslar, & Strzelczyk. (2010). Influence of cryogenic temperatures on inflammatory markers in patients with ankylosing spondylitis and healthy volunteers. *Polish Journal of Environmental Studies*, *19*(1), 167–175.

Stanek, Cholewka, & Cieslar, Rosmus-Kuczia, Drzazga, & Sieron. (2011). The assessment of the analgesic action of whole - body cryotherapy in patients with ankylosing spondylitis. *Fizjoterapia Polska*, *11*(1), 49–55.

Stanek, Sieron, & Cieslar, Matyszkiewicz, & Rozmus-Kuczia. (2005). Influence of whole-body cryotherapy on parameters of spine mobility in patients with ankylosing spondylitis. *Ortopedia, Traumatologia, Rehabilitacja*, *5*(7), 549–554. PMID:17611448

Stanek, Wielkoszynski, & Cholewka. (2011). Influence of whole - body cryotherapy on some chosen non - enzymatic parameters of antioxidant status in patients with ankylosing spondylitis. *Acta Balneolgica*, *53*(4), 264–269.

Styczyński, Gasik, Krzemińska-Dąbrowska, & Pyskło. (2001). Ocena Przydatności Krioterapii U Chorych Na Bóle Krzyża Związane Z Dyskopatią I Zmianami Zwyrodnieniowymi Kręgosłupa Baln. *Pol.*, *43*(1-2), 50 – 55. (in Polish)

Swenson, S., Swärd, L., & Karlsson, J. (1996). Cryotherapy in sports medicine. *Scandinavian Journal of Medicine & Science in Sports*, *6*(4), 193–200. doi:10.1111/j.1600-0838.1996.tb00090.x PMID:8896090

Traczyk. (2007). *Fizjologia człowieka w zarysie*. PZWL.

Vardasca, Ring, Plassmann, & Jones. (2012). Thermal symmetry of the upper and lower extermities in healthy subjects. *Thermology International, 22*(2), 53-60.

Wiącek, Rzymska-Klicha, Kaszuba, & Drobnik. (1999). The use of cryosurgical techniques in dermatology – own experiences. *Nowa. Klin.*, *6*(12), 1178–1184.

Wozniak, M.-K., Drewa, D., & Wozniak, O. (2001). Activity of chosen lisosome′s enzymes in plasma of canoeists after whole - body cryotherapy. *Med Sport*, *17*, 322–327.

Yamauchi, Nogami, & Miura. (1981). Various applications of extreme cryotherapy and strenuous exercise program - focusing on chronic rheumatoid arthritis. *Physiother Rehab*, *5*, 35–39.

Zagrobelny, Halawa, Jegierski, & Wawrowska. (1993). The influence of whole body cooling in cryogenic chamber on chosen haemodynamic markers and hormone concentration in serum of healthy people. *Physician Polish Weekly, 48*(14-15), 303-305.

Zagrobelny & Zimmer. (1999). The application of of cryogenic temperatures in medicine and physical sports therapy. *Med. Sport.*, *15*(94), 8–13.

Zagrobelny. (Ed.). (2003a). *Whole-body and local cryotherapy*. Urban & Partner.

Zagrobelny. (Ed.). (2003b). *Local and wholebody cryotherapy*. Urban & Partner.

Żuber & Jung. (1997). *Thermographic methods in medical diagnostics*. Warszawa: Academic Press.

Chapter 6
Thermal Evaluation of Myogenous Temporomandibular Disorders and Myofascial Trigger Points in the Masticatory Muscles

Denise Sabbagh Haddad
University of São Paulo, Brazil

Marcos Leal Brioschi
University of São Paulo, Brazil

Emiko Saito Arita
University of São Paulo, Brazil

ABSTRACT

It is known that the myofascial trigger points (MTP) and myogenous temporomandibular disorders (TMDs) cause regional sympathetic hyperactivity in local temperature due to the cutaneous vasomotor activity and, for detection of functional changes, thermography is used as an complementary diagnostic imaging method. This chapter intends to study two masticatory muscles, masseter and anterior temporalis, in measurement of the cutaneous temperature of volunteers with and without myogenous TMD and MTP. Results: The temperature levels measured at both muscles regions in myogenous TMD volunteers were significantly lower than those measured in controls. Infrared imaging indicated differences between referred and local pain in MTPs of 0.5°C. Conclusions: Infrared imaging measurements seem to indicate that it can be used as an aid in complimentary diagnosing of TMDs and MTPs in masticatory muscles.

DOI: 10.4018/978-1-5225-2072-6.ch006

INTRODUCTION

Temperature is a long established as a diagnostic sign and thus an indicator of health. In 400 B.C., Hippocrates wrote "In whatever part of the body excess of heat or cold is felt, the disease is there to be discovered" (Brioschi et al., 2010). The beginning of the infrared temperature measurement started, in 1800, with the discovery of the infrared radiation by Sir William Herschel (Brioschi et al., 2010; Haddad, 2001).

During the World War II, military research in monitoring infrared systems allowed the beginning of a new era in thermal diagnosis. In the 50s was developed the first generation of infrared tracking for military applications, named FLIR (Forward Looking InfraRed) (Sanches, 2009). However, the first medical publication using infrared thermography was in 1956, by Dr. Ray N. Lawson of McGill University (Montreal, Canada) (Lawson, 1956). The first dental research using infrared thermography was done by Crandell and Hill in 1966 (Crandell & Hill, 1966). Since that time, many researches were done in Dentistry (Haddad, Brioschi & Arita, 2012; Haddad et al., 2014; Canavan & Gratt, 1995; Johansson, Kopp & Haraldson, 1985; Gratt et al., 1989; Gratt & Sickles, 1993; Gratt & Sickles, 1995; Gratt & Anbar, 1998; Dworkin et al., 1990; Fillingim et al., 1996; Pogrel et al., 1989; Christensen, Vaeth & Wenzel, 2012; Kawano et al., 1993; Gratt et al., 1994; Leonardi et al., 1991; Anbar, Gratt & Hong, 1998; Weinstein et al., 1991; Biagioni et al., 1996; Berry & Yemm, 1971; Berry & Yemm, 1974; Mongini et al., 1990; Gratt et al., 1996; Dibai-Filho et al., 2014; Dibai-Filho et al., 2015].

Medical infrared thermography is a nonionizing and noninvasive imaging technique that allows the real-time representation of the skin surface thermal distribution into images (Brioschi et al., 2010; Haddad, Brioschi & Arita, 2012; Haddad et al., 2014). The skin temperature distribution depends on the heat exchange processes between skin tissue, local vasculature and metabolic activity (Brioschi et al., 2010; Haddad, Brioschi & Arita, 2012; Haddad et al., 2014; Merla & Romani, 2008). Natural vascular heat emissions that present on the human face can provide physiologic indicators of underlying health or disease. All of these processes are mediated and regulated by the autonomous nervous system to maintain the thermal homeostasis (Brioschi et al., 2010; Haddad, Brioschi & Arita, 2012; Haddad et al., 2014; Merla & Romani, 2008). The resultant thermal image indicates the amount of heat given off by blood flowing within and beneath the skin and muscles. As the amount of blood circulating within and beneath the skin layers varies, so does the skin temperature. Only the body surface and a superficial layer 6 to 10 mm in depth is surveyed and recorded using thermography

The literature clearly documents that, in a normal situation, blood flow through the skin of most body parts produces a nearly symmetrical thermal pattern (Haddad, Brioschi & Arita, 2012; Canavan & Gratt, 1995; Gratt & Sickles, 1993; Gratt & Sickles, 1995; Gratt & Anbar, 1998; Vardasca et al., 2012). The presence of biological dysfunctions can affect the heat balance or exchange processes, resulting in an increase or a decrease of the local skin temperature. Quantitative and qualitative changes in infrared heat emission by the skin have been reported to occur in a variety of diseases. These changes include conditions involving facial structures, such as temporomandibular joint (TMJ) disorders, atypical facial pain (atypical odontalgia), nerve damage and repair following oral surgery, headache, inflammation of the lacrimal drainage system, and psychogenic facial pain (Merla & Romani, 2008).

Anatomical and functional information of the structures of interest are the basis of radiology interpretation. For recognizing diseases it is necessary to understand and identify the anatomical structures and its variations. Many diagnosis of some facial diseases (e.g.: bone alterations, caries, temporomandibular joint disorders, etc) may be done through medical imaging techniques, however the most conventional present lack of information in analyzing physiological functional aspects such as microcirculation and autonomous nervous system. The measurements of facial skin temperature may be used to investigate and assess lesions of peripheral branches of cranial nerves supplying the face.

The literature reports different methods of evaluating skin facial surface but all authors affirm that infrared thermography is a promising imaging method in Dentistry (Haddad, Brioschi & Arita, 2012; Haddad et al., 2014; Gratt & Sickles, 1995; Merla & Romani, 2008). This method can provide new complementary information on the anatomy of the vasculature, neuronal systemic and local control of vascular blood flow and perfusion of the capillary bed (Anbar, 2008) and therefore it can be correlated with the patient complains (e.g.: pain in the area of masticatory muscles, headaches, athypical odontalgias, etc).

Temporomandibular disorders are characterized by pain and mobility dysfunction in the temporomandibular joint area, masticatory muscles and associated musculoskeletal structures in the head and neck (Dworkin et al., 1990). The aetiology and pathogenesis of TMD have been suggested as indicative of a psychophysiological disorder involving changes in regulatory pain pathways, resulting in maladaptive emotional, physiological and neuroendocrine responses to physical and psychological stressors (Fillingim et al., 1996).

Numerous complementary diagnostic methods have been proposed for TMDs. The current diagnostic imaging methods for the assessment of the TMDs include plain film radiography, panoramic radiography, tomography, arthrotomography, arthroscopy, computerized tomography and magnetic resonance imaging. Most of these techniques require ionizing radiation, are invasive, or are costly.

The research diagnostic criteria for TMDs (RDC/TMD) (Dworkin & LeResche, 1992) are the gold standard available for TMD diagnostic system and are empirically based. It uses operationally defined measurement criteria to generate computer-derived diagnostic algorithms for the most common TMD forms (Dworkin & LeResche, 1992) and provides specifications for conducting a standardized clinical physical examination (John, Dworkin & Mancl, 2005).

Physical disorders that are related to the TMDs and have been reported to produce abnormal facial thermograms include (but are not limited to) myofascial pain syndromes, myositis, musculoligamentous injury, temporomandibular joint disorders, motor and sensory radiculopathy, and the inflammation of arthritis and bursitis. Hence, the TMD can be evaluated morphologically and dynamically through medical imaging techniques; however, the most conventional present lack of information in analyzing physiological functional aspects such as microcirculation and autonomous nervous system. This information would be of major importance for clinical conditions such as trigeminal neuralgia and facial musculoskeletal pain.

Myofascial pain syndrome (MPS) is characterized by diffuse muscle pain and the presence of myofascial trigger points (MTPs) (de Leeuw, 2008). MPS is much more common than is generally recognized (Simons, Travell & Simons, 1999), affecting the quality of life of patients with this condition. Simons (Simons, 1988) found that 85% of patients admitted to a chronic pain center were suffering primarily from MPS. Early identification of the disease, using precise diagnostic methods, improves the effectiveness of treatment and, consequently, leads to a reduction in the cost of public health.

MPS is not limited to the masticatory muscles. It can occur anywhere in the body, most commonly involving muscles in the neck and back.

Clinically, an MTP can be defined as a hyperirritable nodule of spot tenderness in a palpable taut band of skeletal muscle. The spot is a site of exquisite tenderness to palpation, from which a local twitch response can be elicited when appropriately stimulated, which refers pain to a distance. That response can cause distant motor and autonomic effects (Simons, Travell & Simons, 1999; Simons, 2004). Algometry, or the measurement of the pressure threshold meter (PTM), is a diagnostic method used to document the sensitivity of MTPs quantitatively. The pressure pain threshold (PPT) for the examination of MTPs is the minimal force that induces pain (Fischer, 1983; Fischer & Chang, 1986; Jaeger & Reeves, 1986; Fischer, 1987).

This chapter intends to summarize significant studies in measurement of the cutaneous temperature not just in asymptomatic masticatory muscles, but also in myogenous temporomandibular disorder (TMD) and myofascial trigger points (MTP). In addition, the authors proposed a new facial protocol evaluation of the superficial facial anatomy (facial thermoanatomy) and how the medical infrared imaging can be used.

FACIAL THERMOANATOMY

It is essential to know the pattern of facial skin temperatures in normal subjects to be able to objectively assess differences in cases of illness. It is widely accepted that injuries of the peripheral nervous system result in disturbance of sympathetic innervation, causing changes in cutaneous blood flow, surface temperature, sweat secretion and piloerection.

Two types of thermographic projections can be done for analyzing the face: frontal and lateral views. In the assessment of asymptomatic volunteers for orofacial pain, some regions are considered colder than others, for example, nose, chin and cheek (Figure 1). It depends on the regional vasculature anatomy. On the other hand, hottest areas can be detected over superficial arteries regions as temporal, frontal, lips, temporomandibular joint and eyelid medial and lateral commissure (Figure 1).

Due to the lack of facial protocol in the dental literature, the authors proposed three different methods to explore the facial skin temperature surface based on the vascular and nervous systems.

Vascular Division

The vascular division was based on the facial vascular regions. The Figure 2 shows all the regions of interest (ROIs):

Figure 1. Facial thermograms (frontal and lateral views) showing the superficial vasculature regions, which hottest areas can be detected over temporal, frontal, lips, temporomandibular joint, eyelid medial and lateral commissure regions. Cold regions can be seeing over the nose, chin and cheek regions.

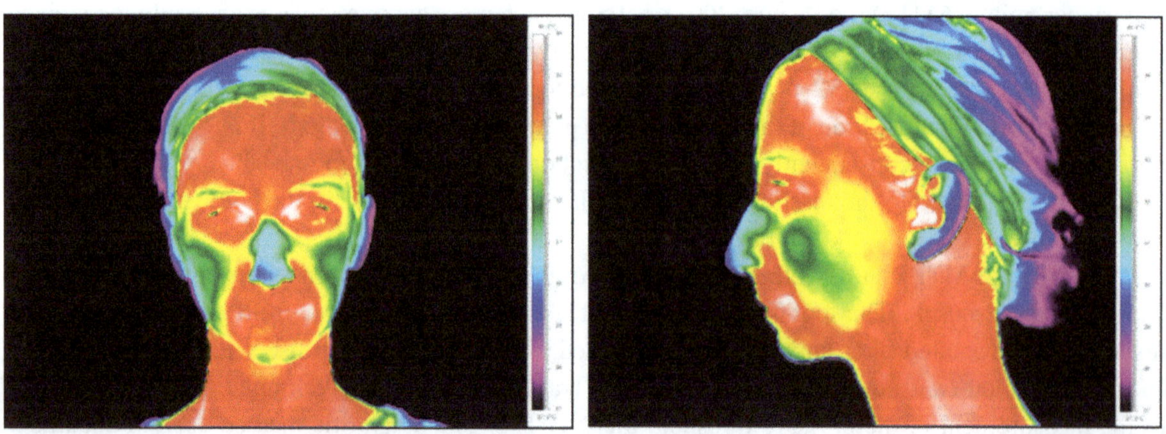

Figure 2. Facial thermograms (frontal and lateral views) with the vascular ROIs proposed by the authors: 1- Supratrochlear; 2- Supraorbital; 3- Frontal; 4- Temporal; 5- Superior eyelid; 6- Eyelid medial commissure ; 7- Dorsal nose; 8- Infraorbital; 9- Lateral palpebral commissure; 10- Superior-anterior buccal; 11- Superior-posterior buccal; 12- Parotid-masseteric; 13- Upper lip; 14- Oral rhyme; 15- Lower lip; 16- Mental; 17- Inferior buccal; 18- Temporomandibular Joint.

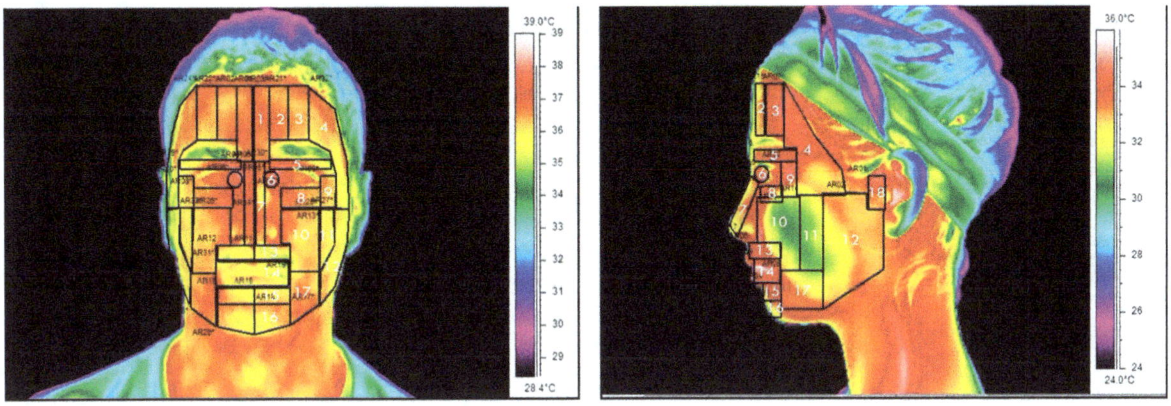

1. Supratrochlear;
2. Supraorbital;
3. Frontal;
4. Temporal;
5. Superior eyelid;
6. Eyelid medial commissure;
7. Dorsal nose;
8. Infraorbital;
9. Lateral palpebral commissure;
10. Superior-anterior buccal;
11. Superior-posterior buccal;
12. Parotid-masseteric;
13. Upper lip;
14. Oral rhyme;
15. Lower lip;
16. Mental;
17. Inferior buccal;
18. Temporomandibular Joint.

Trigeminal Nerve Division

The proposed of the trigeminal nerve division was based on the trigeminal nerve branches and the Figure 3 shows all ROIs:

1. Ophthalmic;

2. Maxillary;
3. Mandibular.

Facial Nerve Division

The proposed of the facial nerve division was based on the facial nerve branches and the Figure 4 shows all ROIs:

1. Temporal;
2. Zygomatic;
3. Buccal;
4. Marginal mandibular.

Figure 3. Facial thermograms (frontal and lateral views) with the trigeminal ROIs proposed by the authors: 1- Ophthalmic; 2- Maxillary; 3- Mandibular (trigeminal nerve assessment).

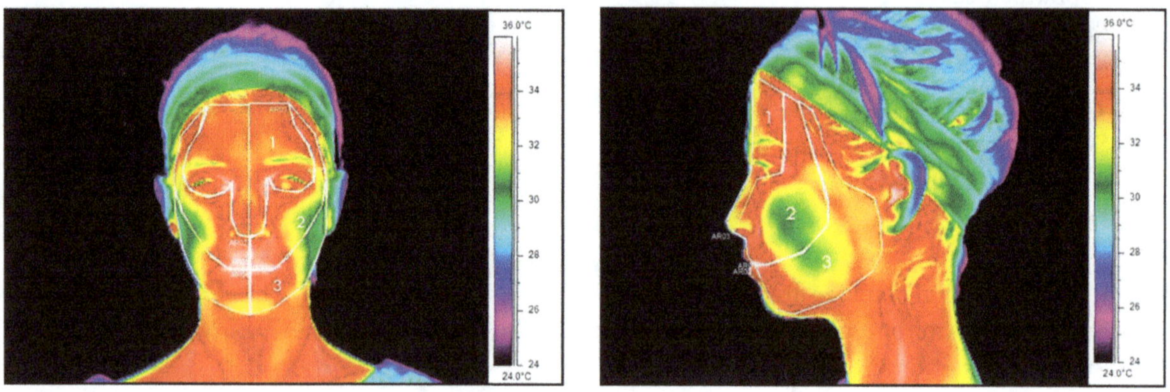

Figure 4. Facial thermograms (frontal and lateral views) with the facial ROIs proposed by the authors: 1- Temporal; 2- Zygomatic; 3- Buccal; 4- Marginal mandibular (facial nerve assessment).

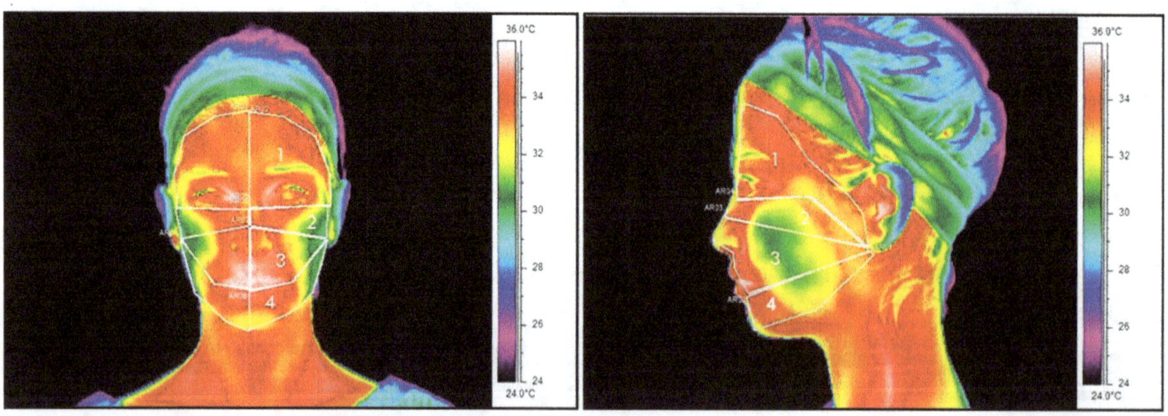

METHODS AND MATERIALS

This diagnostic study was lead in 2013 after approved by the Research Ethics Committee, School of Dentistry, University of São Paulo, São Paulo, Brazil. The Standards for Reporting of Diagnostic Accuracy (STARD) guidelines were followed in this investigation. All volunteers gave their signed informed consent (Haddad, 2001; Haddad, Brioschi & Arita, 2012; Haddad et al., 2014).

Volunteers

The volunteers were recruited at the clinic of Dentistry Faculty, University of São Paulo, São Paulo, Brazil. Patients with and without TMD and MPS were recruited during a period of 2 months.

Only adult females were investigated in this study because masticatory pain disorders are more prevalent in females than in males (de Leeuw, 2008). Twenty-six volunteers, with a mean age of 41 years, were included in the MTP study and 23 volunteers were included in the TMD study. All subjects underwent clinical and dental examinations. The selection criteria for this research included a negative history for systemic problems (e.g. hypothyroidism, diabetes, hypertension, fibromyalgia), headaches, toothache pain, history of eye surgery, impaired vision, contact lenses, hearing aids, facial blemishes, arthritis, sinusitis, rhinitis, dry mouth, sensitivity to cosmetics, wisdom tooth extraction, or previous use of orthodontic appliances (braces), scars or wheals on the face, articular temporomandibular disorders (TMDs), premenopausal females should be in the second phase of the menstrual cycle and the menopause females were absent of hot flushes (Keith, Thomas & Ferganson, 1973).

In order to detect the presence of TMDs, Research Diagnostic Criteria for Temporomandibular Disorders (RDC/TMD) were applied (Dworkin & LeResche, 1992). The subjects were instructed in the use of a visual analogue scale (VAS).

Facial Thermography: Measurement Procedure

Thermographic images were recorded following a standard protocol, recommended by the Brazilian Association of Medical Thermology and Academy of Neuro-Muscular Thermography (Schwartz, 2006). The subjects were instructed not to apply any lotion, makeup or powder to the skin; not to use a dryer or flat iron on the hair; and not to smoke for 2 h before the recording. Also, they were instructed to avoid skeletal manipulation, acupuncture, physical therapy, the use of transcutaneous neural stimulation units or electrodiagnostic testing for 12 h prior to the test and for at least 24 h after the test; not to drink coffee or alcoholic drinks; and not to use nasal decongestants, analgesics, anti-inflammatory drugs or any substance that alters sympathetic function.

Patients were acclimatized in a room with a mean temperature of 23 °C and a relative humidity of 80% for 15 min. They were instructed not to palpate, press, rub or scratch the facial skin at any time up to the completion of the entire thermographic examination. Ambient temperature and humidity were controlled in a draught-free environment. Air flow was maintained at less than $0.2ms^{-1}$, to avoid loss of heat through forced convection. Ambient temperature was measured using a reliable digital thermohygrometer that was visible and easy to read. Thermographic images were taken by an experienced physician who also evaluated them.

To facilitate image acquisition, the hair was held in place with a head band and a disposable head covering.

The examiner had the patient sit on the examination chair. A cephalostat (Figure 5) (Haddad, 2001; Haddad, Brioschi & Arita, 2012; Haddad et al., 2014), constructed specifically for these studies, was used in order to standardize the positioning of the patients during the thermal and photographic acquisitions. The Frankfurt plane parallel to the horizontal plane was used to assist in proper placement. The subject was asked to relax the muscles with the teeth apart. In a randomized order, two series of colour thermograms were taken, from the right and left perpendicular projections.

Skin temperature of all muscles (masseter and anterior temporalis muscles) was registered using a computer assisted infrared thermograph (ThermaCAM® T400, FLIR Systems, Inc., Wilsonville, OR). The infrared detector has a thermal sensitivity of 0.05 °C at 30 °C; spectral range between 7.5 μm – 13 μm; and the built-in digital video with 320x240 pixels resolution. Data were obtained using high-speed (30 Hz) analysis and recording systems coupled to a desktop computer. This equipment allows images with spatial resolution (IFOV) of 1.4 mrad to be obtained for the visualization of hot spots of 1.4 mm at 1 m distance, using a standard lens of 25° with no additional lenses.

The infrared camera produces a high definition matrix of temperature values. Each pixel represents a correct calibrated temperature in the picture measured.

The thermograph allows quantitative and qualitative mapping of superficial temperature, which can be related to different pathological conditions and blood flow. It was possible to show the images in greyscale or in colour scales available within the software. All images were analysed and showed at least one palette of 256 colours, with a 0.15 °C thermal window for each colour. Thermal sensitivity of 0.51°C per colour tone was used, based on a rainbow-type colorimetric scale (colour palette), in which the colours were, from hottest to coldest: white, pink, red, orange, yellow, light green, dark green, light

Figure 5. The cephalostat constructed specifically for these studies A- Frontal view, B- Lateral view
Source: Haddad, 2001; Haddad, Brioschi, & Arita, 2012; Haddad et al., 2014

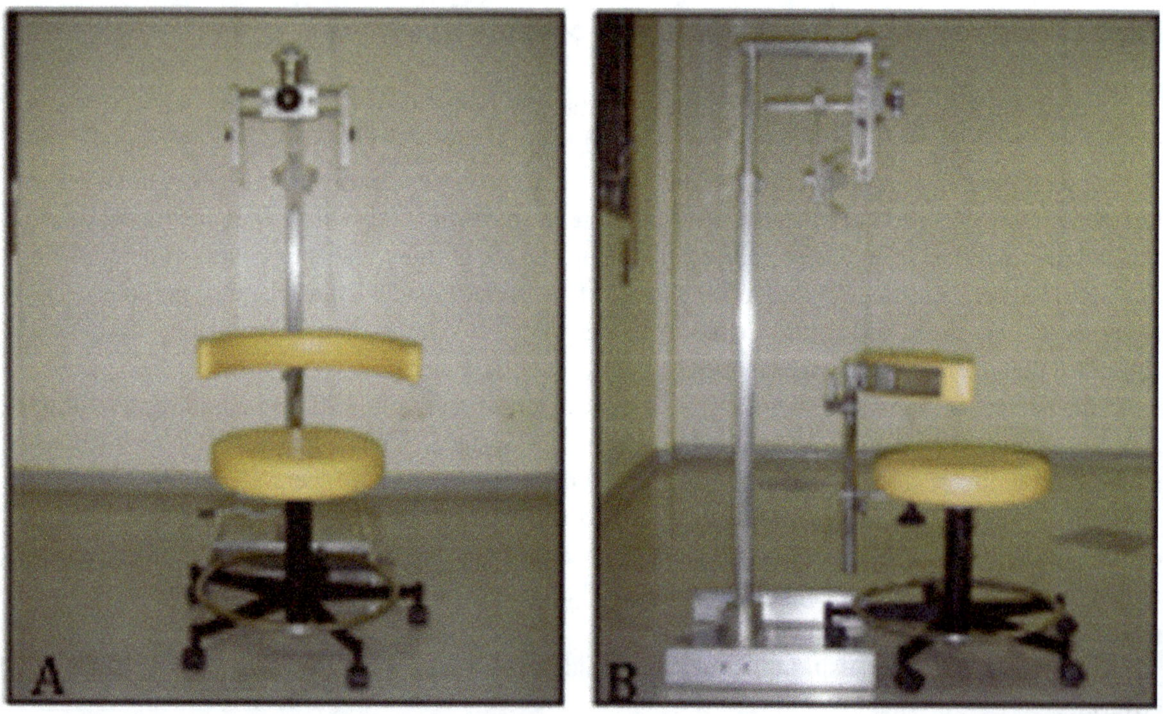

blue, dark blue, purple and black (FLIR QuickReport® v. 1.2 and FLIR Reporter® v. 8.5, FLIR Systems, Inc.). The colours indirectly indicated the degree of distribution of local cutaneous blood perfusion. All images were displayed with the palette beside the image, for reference.

The distance between the camera and the lateral face measured was adjusted to 0.75 m, at an angle of 90°, with the lens of the camera parallel to the assessed region. The emissivity value of the skin considered for this study was 0.987.

The core body temperatures of volunteers were measured using an infrared, digital thermometer ThermoScan® Instant Ear Thermometer IRT 1020 (Braun®; BraunAG, Frankfurt am Main, Germany). This thermometer measures temperature values of the eardrum and the surrounding tissues, the location most frequently indicated for measuring body temperature owing to its proximity to the hypothalamus and the perfusion of the arterial labyrinth (Vargas et al., 2009).

Clinical Examination and Algometry (MTP Study)

A trained specialist in TMD management area divided the surface facial area over the masseter and anterior temporalis muscles into 15 ROIs (Figure 6) on each side (n=780), with an area of approximately 1 cm^2 (Haddad, 2001; Haddad, Brioschi & Arita, 2012). This marking was based on Pogrel et al. study (Pogrel et al., 1989). The reference for defining regions of the masseter muscle was the zygomatic arch (proximal insertion) and the lateral surface of the mandibular angle (distal insertion). The temporalis muscle was evaluated only in its exposed anterior part not hidden by hair. Examination of MTPs was performed according to the Fischer protocol (Fischer, 1983; Fischer & Chang, 1986; Jaeger & Reeves, 1986), which uses the PPT to evaluate the minimal force that induces pain, expressed in kilograms of pressure. PTM is a hand force gauge calibrated to 10x0.01kgf and the area of the algometer tip was 1 cm^2. Before the test, the subject was instructed to relax the masticatory muscles with the teeth apart. First, the presence and location of the MTP was confirmed via palpation and was marked using a coloured pencil. Next, the pressure threshold was measured. The PTM was applied directly onto the location of tenderness, with the axis of the shaft maintained at 90° to the examining surface. The subject was instructed to inform verbally when pain or discomfort was initially felt. At this moment, the compression lasted for 5 seconds in the same location, with the same pressure maintained. The patient was asked if the pain was felt only in this location, or if it extended to another region. Finally, digital photographs (Nikon Coolpix S51® 8.1 megapixels; Nikon, Sendai, Japan) of the lateral face with the head in the same position as the infrared thermography examination were taken (Haddad, 2001; Haddad, Brioschi & Arita, 2012).

In order to correlate the PPT values with the values obtained from the thermographs of the ROI, the thermographs were superimposed on the digital photographs using dedicated infrared imaging software (Reporter 8.5—SP3 Professional Edition and QuickReport 1.2). The standardized reference points of the superimposition were:

1. Midpoint of the median sagittal plane between the chin and the hyoid bone;
2. Lowest portion of the earlobe; and
3. The apex of the nasal pyramid (Haddad, 2001; Haddad, Brioschi & Arita, 2012).

The averages of the temperature of the ROI of the muscles were calculated individually (T), and thermal asymmetry between the corresponding opposite sides, also called the conjugated gradient of the absolute temperature (xT).

Figure 6. Schematic design of the ROI (MTP study), restricted to the masseter and anterior part of the temporalis muscles, on both sides
Source: Haddad, Brioschi, & Arita, 2012

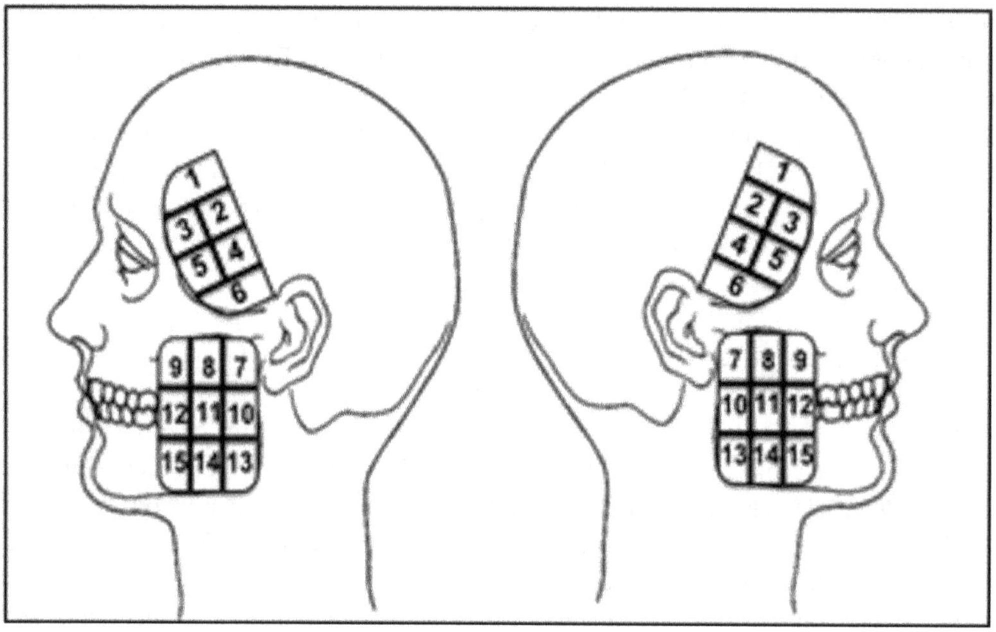

In order to normalize the temperature results, it was used an adimensional variable (θ) proposed by Vargas and Brioschi for quantitative thermography analysis (Vargas et al., 2009).

Thus, the interpretation of the infrared camera readings was done using an adimensional temperature (θ) which combines the measured local skin temperature with the core body (T_b) and ambient temperatures (T_∞) during the infrared imaging caption, according to the following equation 1 (Vargas et al., 2009):

$$\theta = \frac{T - T_\infty}{T_b - T_\infty} \tag{1}$$

The gradient of the normalized temperature was also used to calculate the thermal asymmetry with the corresponding opposite ROIs:

$$x\theta = |\theta_{right} - \theta_{left}| \tag{2}$$

After obtaining all the data (PPT, T, θ) and calculating the gradients of temperature and normalized temperature (xT and xθ), the assessed points were divided into three groups: no MTP, MTP with local pain and MTP with referred pain (Haddad, 2001; Haddad, Brioschi & Arita, 2012).

Clinical Examination (TMD Study)

The RDC/TMD is an instrument widely used in research and clinical practice for identifying TMDs and was applied to detect the presence of TMD in this study (Dworkin & LeResche, 1992). After that, a trained specialist in TMD management divided the facial surface area over the anterior temporalis and masseter muscles into four regions to facilitate the palpation (Figure 7) (Haddad et al., 2014). The temporalis muscle region was defined as the anterior portion, not covered by hair, whereas the reference points used to define the masseter muscle region were the zygomatic arch (proximal insertion) and the lateral surface of the mandibular angle (distal insertion).

The ROIs were marked with a dermatographic pencil on the patient's skin after the thermal images and before the palpation examination. Digital photographs of the lateral face were taken after the thermal images in the same position as that used for the infrared thermographic examination. The positioning of the volunteer during the thermal and photographic images was standardized by the same cephalostat (Haddad, Brioschi & Arita, 2012) as used in the MTP study.

For precise evaluation of the ROIs, the same technique of thermograms and digital photographs superimposition was done (Haddad, 2001; Haddad, Brioschi & Arita, 2012; Haddad et al., 2014).

The mean absolute temperatures (T) were averaged according to the landmarks (ROIs) recorded on photographic images, and the normalized temperature (θ) (Vargas et al., 2009) of each ROI was calculated individually. During the data analysis, all volunteers were separated into two groups: symptomatic and asymptomatic for myogenous TMD.

Figure 7. Regions of interest (ROI) of the TMD study, restricted to the masseter and anterior part of the temporalis muscles, on left (L) and right (R) sides (ROI 1- anterior temporalis, ROI 2- superior masseter, ROI 3- middle masseter, ROI 4- inferior masseter, ROI 5- masseter)
Source: Haddad et al., 2014

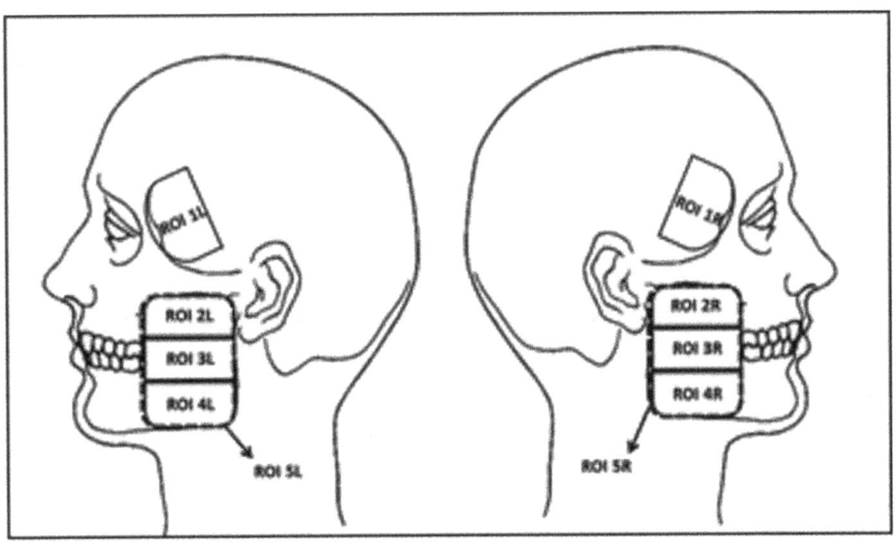

Statistical Analyses

The data were tabulated using Microsoft Excel (Microsoft Corporation, Redmond, WA). The analyses were performed using SPSS® 19 (IBM Corporation, Armonk, NY). Pearson's x^2 test and the non-parametric Kruskal–Wallis test with Bonferroni correction were used when necessary.

The sensitivity and specificity of the ratings were calculated using receiver operating characteristic (ROC) curve analysis. The receiver operating characteristic curve is a plot of the true-positive rate (sensitivity) against the false-positive rate (specificity) for the different possible cut-off points of a diagnostic test. It shows the trade-off between sensitivity and specificity. A level of $p<0.05$ was considered to be statistically significant. The correlation coefficient for the entire sample was calculated using Spearman's non-parametric method.

RESULTS

MTP Study

The sample consisted of 26 female volunteers (mean age 41±15 years, range 22–82 years). Of the 780 ROIs assessed over the masseter and anterior temporalis muscles (15 ROI on each side), MTPs were found in 395 ROIs (50.6%). All volunteers were asymptomatic on the day of the examination (VAS=0) (Haddad, 2001; Haddad, Brioschi & Arita, 2012).

Of the entire sample of 395 MTPs, physical examination findings characterized 264 as points of local pain, consisting of 74 (18.7%) anterior temporalis and 190 (48.1%) masseter muscles, and 131 were points of referred pain, consisting of 35 (8.9%) anterior temporalis and 96 (24.3%) masseter muscles (Haddad, 2001; Haddad, Brioschi & Arita, 2012).

When the right ($T = 33.71 \pm 1.21$ °C; $\theta = 0.805 \pm 0.087$) and left ($T = 33.76 \pm 1.13$ °C; $\theta = 0.803 \pm 0.082$) hemifacials were compared, no thermal predominance was found for either side, either for T or for θ ($p>0.05$) (Haddad, 2001; Haddad, Brioschi & Arita, 2012).

The temporalis muscle showed higher temperature ($T = 34.63 \pm 0.73$ °C; $\theta = 0.861 \pm 0.768$) than the masseter muscle ($T = 33.18 \pm 1.05$ °C; $\theta = 0.768 \pm 0.078$), for all subjects ($p<0.05$). The masseter muscle (1.54±0.58 kgf) showed greater sensitivity to pain sensations of the PPT than the temporalis muscle (1.67±0.62 kgf) ($p<0.05$) (Haddad, 2001; Haddad, Brioschi & Arita, 2012).

The correlations between the PPT (kgf) and temperature (T) were positive and moderate ($0.4 \leq r < 0.7$), with the higher the PPT value (kgf) applied to the ROI, the higher the local temperature.

The values for temperature (T), normalized temperature (θ) and the PPT were greater for the points of local pain than for the points of referred pain ($p<0.05$), i.e. the greater the pain sensitivity of the point, the lower the value of temperature and normalized temperature. The cut-off points found for T, θ, xT and xT are shown in Table 1; the gradient temperature in all muscles, with and without MTP, was greater than 0.3 °C (Haddad, 2001; Haddad, Brioschi & Arita, 2012).

The area under the ROC curve is interpreted as the probability that the individual with MTPs has a diagnostic test result of greater magnitude than the individual without MTPs. A test that can distinguish them has an area under the ROC curve above 0.5 and is described in Table 2. For both T and θ, the sensitivity of the method to identify MTPs with referred pain was average (50%), although the specificity

Table 1. Cutoff points found for temperature (T), normalized temperature (θ), gradient temperature (xT) and gradient of the normalized temperature (xθ)

	T (°C)	*θ*	*xT (°C)**	*xθ*
Without MTP	*>34*	*>0.810*	*<0.3*	*<0.036*
Local Pain	*34-33.3*	*0.810-0.756*	*0.4*	*0.037*
Referred Pain	*<33.3*	*<0.756*	*0.5*	*0.048*

MTP: Myofascial Trigger Points
* values considered only when the contralateral side showed no MTP
** in the situation in which local pain exists on one side, and referred pain on the other side, the observed values were xT=0.5 °C and xθ=0.045

Table 2. Areas under the ROC curve (AUC) and the confidence interval (CI) of the myofascial trigger points (MTP)

MTP - Local Pain x Referred Pain	**AUC**	**CI95%**	
T	**0.564**	**0.504**	**0.623**
xθ	**0.578**	**0.041**	**0.743**
xT	**0.609**	**0.451**	**0.766**
θ	**0.617**	**0.559**	**0.674**
PPT	**0.737**	**0.685**	**0.789**

T: temperature; xθ: gradient of the normalized temperature; xT: gradient temperature; θ: normalized temperature; PPT: Pressure Pain Threshold; CI: confidence interval.

was low (17%). By evaluation of the cut-off points, the value of the conjugated gradient (xT) was higher than 0.3 °C and the normalized temperature value (xθ) was greater than 0.036. Regarding the presence of MTPs, sensitivity and specificity for both xT and xθ were 62.5% and 71.31%, respectively (Haddad, 2001; Haddad, Brioschi & Arita, 2012).

TMD Study

The sample consisted of 23 female volunteers (mean age, 41 years; range, 33–49 years). They were divided into two groups according to the RDC/TMD: asymptomatic and symptomatic (Haddad, 2001; Haddad et al., 2014).

On the day of the examination, all volunteers had no pain (visual analogue scale = 0). For all ROIs used, it can be seen that there was no statistical evidence ($p>0.05$) of dependence between the asymptomatic and symptomatic groups of participants considering the bilateral mean temperature differences.

Absolute mean temperatures (Table 3) and normalized mean temperatures (Table 4) for asymptomatic and symptomatic participants were calculated for all muscle ROIs ($p<0.05$). The absolute mean temperature (Table 3) and the normalized mean temperature over the temporalis muscle (Table 4) was higher than that over the masseter muscle for all participants ($p<0.05$). The absolute (Table 3) and normalized (Table 4) mean temperatures of the muscle ROIs of asymptomatic and symptomatic subjects were compared (Haddad, 2001; Haddad et al., 2014).

Table 3. Analysis of absolute mean temperature (°C) for asymptomatic and symptomatic participants

Muscle ROIs	Asymptomatic (n = 26)		Symptomatic (n = 20)		*p*-value
	xT (°C)	s.d.	xT (°C)	s.d.	
Anterior Temporalis (ROI 1)	34.78	0.44	34.37	0.64	0.0016
Superior Masseter (ROI 2)	33.49	1.00	32.81	0.83	0.0116
Middle Masseter (ROI 3)	33.54	0.92	32.91	0.85	0.0093
Inferior Masseter (ROI 4)	33.45	0.89	32.82	0.94	0.0050
Masseter (ROI 5)	33.49	0.92	32.85	0.86	0.0067

xT: absolute mean temperature; s.d.: standard deviation

Table 4. Analysis of normalized mean temperature (θ) for asymptomatic and symptomatic participants

Muscle ROIs	Asymptomatic (n = 26)		Symptomatic (n = 20)		*p*-value
	xθ	s.d.	xθ	s.d.	
Anterior Temporalis (ROI 1)	0.877	0.04	0.831	0.04	0.0001
Superior Masseter (ROI 2)	0.795	0.08	0.732	0.05	0.0014
Middle Masseter (ROI 3)	0.798	0.07	0.738	0.05	0.0008
Inferior Masseter (ROI 4)	0.791	0.06	0.733	0.06	0.0004
Masseter (ROI 5)	0.795	0.07	0.734	0.05	0.0006

xθ: normalized mean temperature; s.d.: standard deviation

The absolute mean temperature in symptomatic participants was lower than that in the control group ($p<0.05$). In the assessment of the absolute mean temperature of the anterior temporalis ROI, it showed higher sensitivity and lower specificity (respectively, 80% and 62%), when compared with the sensitivity and specificity observed for the masseter ROI (70% and 73%, respectively). Assessing the normalized muscle mean temperature for the anterior temporalis and the masseter ROI showed almost the same sensitivity and specificity when compared with the absolute mean temperature (Haddad, 2001; Haddad et al., 2014).

DISCUSSION

Solutions and Recommendations

Only adult females were investigated in these studies because masticatory pain disorders are more prevalent in females than in males (de Leeuw, 2008).

Medical infrared thermography is a non-invasive and non-ionizing bidimensional imaging technique that maps the distribution of body surface thermal radiation into images. It is based on the capture and transformation of infrared radiation emitted by the human skin to form images that reflect the local vasomotor response. Although it is not standardized at all, qualitative and quantitative changes in symmetrical thermal patterns have been reported as indicators of changes in metabolism, hemodynamics or neuronal thermoregulatory processes in the ROI [Haddad, Brioschi & Arita, 2012; Gratt et al., 1989; Gratt & Sickles, 1993; Gratt & Sickles, 1995; Christensen, Vaeth & Wenzel, 2012; Kawano et al., 1993; Vardasca et al., 2012; Vargas et al., 2009).

Different results about temperature values in skin facial surface were present in the literature. This can be owing to the usage of distinct capture methodologies (Gratt & Anbar, 1998; Gratt et al., 1994; Leonardi et al., 1991). Despite numerous articles addressing infrared thermography as a promising method in the diagnosis of TMD (Haddad, Brioschi & Arita, 2012; Canavan & Gratt, 1995; Gratt et al., 1989; Gratt & Sickles, 1993; Gratt & Sickles, 1995; Gratt & Anbar, 1998; Pogrel et al., 1989; Anbar, Gratt & Hong, 1998; Weinstein et al., 1991; Biagioni et al., 1996), so far, no study has specifically used superimposition of ROI images, as performed in these studies.

MTPs are one of the diagnostic criteria of MPS. However, they are commonly overlooked as sources of pain because the sensory experience may be local or widespread, owing to pain referral mechanisms being not yet fully understood. MTPs are thought to be initiated by a muscle or connective tissue change that sets up positive feedback with the central nervous system, resulting in sensory, motor and autonomic changes (Kruse & Christiansen, 1992).

Algometry provides us with a means to gauge the pain sensitivity of trigger points quantitatively. The results of many studies confirm that MTPs are more sensitive than contralateral, MTP-free muscle areas (Simons, 1988; Fischer & Chang, 1986; Kruse & Christiansen, 1992). The MTP study confirms those findings, and the pressure threshold for MTPs was lower in points of referred pain (1.28 kg cm^{-2}) than in points of local pain (1.73 kg cm^{-2}), i.e. the greater the pain sensitivity of the point, the lower the value of PPT (Haddad, 2001; Haddad, Brioschi & Arita, 2012).

When right–left sensitivity to pain was compared with the PPT no statistically significant difference was found between the temporalis muscles, only between the masseter muscles ($p<0.05$). Visscher et al (Visscher, Lobbezoo & Naeije, 2004) demonstrated that the PPT test result was greater on the right side of the face than on the left. According to them, a possible explanation for this fact is that the side with the greater value is related to the dominant side of the body. However, in this study, a statistical difference ($p<0.05$) was found when the sensitivity to pain between the temporalis and masseter muscles on the same side was compared. The masseter muscle was more sensitive than the temporalis muscle. These results are also in agreement with those found by Visscher et al (Visscher, Lobbezoo & Naeije, 2004).

The sensitivity and specificity to the PPT in the assessment of referred muscle pain were 0.66 and 0.73, respectively (Haddad, 2001; Haddad, Brioschi & Arita, 2012). Farella et al (Farella et al., 2000) found the sensitivity of the temporalis and masseter muscles to be 0.85 and 0.67, respectively, and the specificity to be 0.87 and 0.77, respectively. Similar results for sensitivity and specificity were observed by Visscher et al (Visscher, Lobbezoo & Naeije, 2004), respectively, for groups both without temporomandibular disorders (0.64 and 0.68), and with temporomandibular disorders (0.7 and 0.72).

Thermal symmetry is present in many parts of the body in a normal population. Skin temperature is a function of blood flow, controlled by the autonomic nervous system. This affects both sides of the body uniformly and simultaneously, resulting in near symmetry of thermal patterns (Gratt et al., 1989; Gratt et al., 1994; Weinstein et al., 1991; Berry & Yemm, 1971; Berry & Yemm, 1974; Mongini et al., 1990).

The literature describes the infrared hyper-radiation presence in the regions of muscle tension when compared with the unaffected opposing muscle (Kawano et al., 1993; Berry & Yemm, 1971; Berry & Yemm, 1974; Fischer & Chang, 1986; Fischer, 1988; Fischer, 1991). However, all authors evaluated large ROIs. Owing to its size and functionality, a single masticatory muscle can have more than one MTP. When calculating the average temperature of the entire muscle, without individualizing the MTP, a false thermal symmetry of the face might be observed because the values obtained may be dissipated by calculating the average temperature. However, when evaluating smaller areas corresponding to the size of an MTP this tends not to occur. This makes the results of thermal studies of smaller ROIs much more reliable, in relation to the study of a single ROI corresponding to an entire muscle. In addition, the higher the image resolution of the infrared sensor (in this case, 76 000 pixels), the more precise will be the thermal assessment of smaller ROIs. It is important to take into consideration that the thermal assessment protocol is very important to assist in the conclusion of the exam. So, using this methodology based on Pogrel et al's study (Pogrel et al., 1989), it was possible to observe the thermal behavior of the cutaneous region exactly at the location of the area of muscular tension.

In these studies, infrared imaging revealed a difference of 1.4 °C between mean anterior temporalis and masseter muscle temperatures and a difference of 0.09 between the corresponding normalized temperatures in asymptomatic subjects for TMD, indicating that the temporalis muscle was significantly more hyper-radiant than the masseter ($p<0.05$) (Haddad et al., 2014). Similar results were found in the literature [Pogrel et al., 1989; Kawano et al., 1993; Weinstein et al., 1991; Berry & Yemm, 1971). This difference in temperature between these muscles is explained on the basis of anatomy: the temporalis muscle, in addition to being thinner than the masseter, is influenced by the superficial path of the temporal artery, which makes the region more hyper-radiant. In the thermal comparison (xT; xθ) between the opposing sides, the temporalis and masseter muscles showed no significant difference.

Although the PPT and thermographic examinations serve totally different purposes, in which the first assesses tenderness to compression and the second evaluates the local vasomotor response, moderately significant correlations were observed between the PPT values (kgf) and the temperature (T and θ), suggesting that the greater the force applied, the greater the local temperature recorded. Also, the temperatures (T, θ) at the points of local pain were higher than those at areas of referred pain ($p<0.05$). Therefore, the temperature decreases according to the severity of myofascial dysfunction. Similar results of the chronicity of myogenous TMD changes the skin temperature over the anterior temporalis muscle was found in the literature (Dibai-Filho et al., 2014; Dibai-Filho et al., 2015).

The most heated areas of the face were correlated with regions without MTP, seen in the ROC curve as cut-off points with T above 34 °C and θ above 0.810, between the corresponding ROIs. At the same time, PPT values below 1.35 kgf, T below 33 °C, and θ under 0.756 were related to MTPs with referred pain. In a middle range, values of T between 34 °C and 33.3 °C and θ between 0.810 and 0.756 were present in cases of MTPs with local pain (Haddad, 2001; Haddad, Brioschi & Arita, 2012). These results are apparently different from those found in the literature, which state that an MTP is always hotter than the unaffected side (Simons, Travell & Simons, 1999; Simons, 1988; Fischer & Chang, 1986; Kruse & Christiansen, 1992; Fischer, 1988; Diakow, 1992; Fischer, 1991a). A single study also found no relationship between hyper-radiant points and active MTPs when studying the upper trapezius muscle (Swerdlow & Dieter, 1992). In the present studies, an inverse behavior of the vasomotor response was observed in the ROIs, corresponding to the MTP and myogenous temporomandibular disorder of the masseter and temporalis muscles. That is, they were cooler than the corresponding contralateral asymptomatic region.

The explanation formulated for this result is given on the basis of studies conducted by Simons (Simons, 1988) elucidating on autonomic disorders in myofascial dysfunction. Cutaneous temperature is a function of blood flow, controlled by the autonomic sympathetic small nervous fibers. In the presence of a sarcomeric contraction of the muscle fiber, there can be a response of reduced blood flow, thus reducing local muscle oxygenation (hypoxia) (Berry & Yemm, 1974; Simons, Travell & Simons, 1999; Simons, 2004; Gerwin, Dommerholt & Shah, 2004; Shah et al., 2008). This hypoxia can trigger a regional sympathetic hyperactivity in the cutaneous projection area of the muscle, also decreasing the local temperature through skin vasoconstrictive activity sometimes as a referred pain (Haddad, 2001; Haddad, Brioschi & Arita, 2012). Pogrel et al (Pogrel et al., 1989) also described that ischemic areas and areas of increased sympathetic tone would show as cold areas on a thermogram, thus myogenic facial pain may in part be attributed to muscle ischemia.

The parameter most used in the evaluation of infrared thermography is thermal asymmetry, also known as the conjugated gradient (xT) between the corresponding opposite sides. According to the literature, right–left thermal differences greater than 0.3 °C can define a myofascial dysfunction (Canavan & Gratt, 1995; Gratt & Sickles, 1993; Kawano et al., 1993; Gratt et al., 1994; Weinstein et al., 1991; Gratt et al., 1996; Vargas et al., 2009; Gerwin, Dommerholt & Shah, 2004). By the evaluation of the cut-off points, the value of the conjugated gradient (xT) was higher than 0.3 °C and the normalized temperature value (xθ) was greater than 0.036. When the MTPs were separated into local and referred pain, the values of xT = 0.4 °C and xθ = 0.037 were found to detect the point of local pain, and xT = 0.5 °C and xθ = 0.048 to detect ROIs with referred pain. In cases in which there was local pain on one side and referred pain on the other, the values recorded were xT = 0.5 °C and xθ = 0.045. Except for Fischer and Chang (Fischer & Chang, 1986), who described MTPs with xT much higher, ranging from 0.5 °C to 1 °C, all other authors agree with the variations between 0.3 °C and 0.5 °C. However, they all agree in saying that the thermal image formed in the projection region of the MTP is a local vasomotor response (Haddad, 2001; Haddad, Brioschi & Arita, 2012).

In this study, the presence of an MTP in the ROI showed progressive positive predictive values of T, θ and the PPT as 36.8%, 39.3% and 53.4%, respectively. For both T and θ, the sensitivity of the method to identify an MTP with referred pain was average (50%), although the specificity was low (17%). Regarding the presence of an MTP, sensitivity and specificity for both xT and xθ were 62.5% and 71.31%, respectively. These results suggest greater diagnostic accuracy when different temperatures (xT; xθ), rather than absolute temperature (T), are used, even when corrected for each individual core temperature (θ) for the identification of MTPs. The results of sensitivity and specificity of the thermographic assessment for masticatory muscle regions suggest greater diagnostic accuracy when absolute mean temperature (T) is used, even when converted to dimensionless temperature (θ) (Haddad, 2001; Haddad, Brioschi & Arita, 2012).

These results suggest that thermal values, if used in conjunction with physical assessment, can serve as a means of screening and improved diagnostic accuracy in myogenous TMDs and MTP.

FUTURE RESEARCH DIRECTIONS

The literature reports different methods of evaluating facial skin surface but there is not a consensus. Due to this fact, the authors proposed a new facial protocol to facilitate the thermal evaluation of the vascular and nervous systems. Further investigations is needed for testing this proposed, which this protocol may prove helpful in the objective evaluation of diseases that could occur or refer to the facial region.

Further investigation is needed of MTPs and myogenous TMD in masticatory muscles, but these findings suggest that thermography may prove helpful in the objective evaluation of MTPs and temporomandibular disorders, especially if it is used in conjunction with physical assessment, as a means of screening and of improved diagnostic accuracy in clinical practice. In order to highlight the findings of this research, the use of a stimulus (thermal, mechanical and chemical) with dynamic thermal imaging is advised. It will provide important and new pathophysiological information characterization for TMD patients, myofascial pain syndrome and healthy individuals.

CONCLUSION

In conclusion, there is a statistically significant and directly proportional correlation between algometry and thermography in the assessment of MTPs, in which the greater the force applied, the greater the local temperature recorded. Thus, the temperature of facial cutaneous areas over the masseter and anterior temporalis muscles decreases in the presence of myogenous TMD and MTP.

The facial protocol proposed also can provide new information on the anatomy of the vasculature, on systemic changes in blood flow, or neuronal systemic changes.

These findings suggest that infrared thermography is helpful in evaluating myogenous TMD and MTP. It could be used as a complementary diagnostic imaging method and improved diagnostic accuracy in clinical practice.

REFERENCES

Anbar, M. (2008). Dynamic Thermal Assessment. In N. A. Diakides & J. D. Bronzino (Eds.), *Medical infrared imaging* (pp. 8.1–8.17). Boca Raton, FL: CRC Press.

Anbar, M., Gratt, B. M., & Hong, D. (1998). Thermology and facial telethermography. Part I: History and technical review. *Dento Maxillo Facial Radiology*, *27*(2), 61–67. doi:10.1038/sj.dmfr.4600314 PMID:9656868

Berry, D. C., & Yemm, R. (1971). Variations in skin temperature of the face in normal subjects and in patients with temporomandibular dysfunction. *The British Journal of Oral Surgery*, *8*(3), 242–247. doi:10.1016/S0007-117X(70)80086-5 PMID:5282910

Berry, D. C., & Yemm, R. (1974). A further study of facial skin temperature in patients withmandibular dysfunction. *Journal of Oral Rehabilitation*, *1*(3), 255–264. doi:10.1111/j.1365-2842.1974.tb01437.x PMID:4530064

Biagioni, P. A., Longmore, R. B., McGimpsey, J. G., & Lamey, P. J. (1996). Its role in dental research with particular reference to craniomandibular disorders. *Dento Maxillo Facial Radiology*, *25*(3), 119–124. doi:10.1259/dmfr.25.3.9084259 PMID:9084259

Brioschi, M. L., Teixeira, M. J., Silva, F. M., & Colman, D. (2010). *Princípios e Indicações da Termografia Médica*. São Paulo: Andreoli.

Canavan, D., & Gratt, B. M. (1995). Electronic thermography for the assessment of mild and moderate temporomandibular joint dysfunction. *Oral Surgery, Oral Medicine, Oral Pathology, Oral Radiology, and Endodontics*, *79*(6), 778–786. doi:10.1016/S1079-2104(05)80316-6 PMID:7621039

Christensen, J., Vaeth, M., & Wenzel, A. (2012). Thermographic imaging of facial skin-gender differences and temperature changes over time in healthy subjects. *Dento Maxillo Facial Radiology*, *41*(8), 662–667. doi:10.1259/dmfr/55922484 PMID:22554986

Crandell, C. E., & Hill, R. P. (1966). Thermography in dentistry: A pilot study. *Oral Surgery, Oral Medicine, and Oral Pathology*, *21*(3), 316–320. doi:10.1016/0030-4220(66)90064-8 PMID:5216735

de Leeuw, R. (2008). *Orofacial pain: guidelines for assessment, diagnosis and management. The American Academy of Orofacial Pain* (4th ed.). Chicago, IL: Quintessence.

Diakow, P. R. (1992). Differentiation of active and latent trigger points by thermography. *Journal of Manipulative and Physiological Therapeutics*, *15*(7), 439–441. PMID:1431631

Dibai-Filho, A. V., Packer, A. C., Costa, A. C., & Rodrigues-Bigaton, D. (2014). The chronicity of myogenous temporomandibular disorder changes the skin temperature over the anterior temporalis muscle. *Journal of Bodywork and Movement Therapies*, *18*(3), 430–434. doi:10.1016/j.jbmt.2013.11.001 PMID:25042314

Dibai-Filho, A. V., Packer, A. C., Costa, A. C., & Rodrigues-Bigaton, D. (2015). Women with more severe degrees of temporomandibular disorder exhibit an increase in temperature over the temporomandibular joint. *The Saudi Dental Journal*, *27*(1), 44–49. doi:10.1016/j.sdentj.2014.10.002 PMID:25544814

Dworkin, S. F., Huggins, K. H., LeResche, L., Von Korff, M., Howard, J., Truelove, E., & Sommers, E. (1990). Epidemiology of signs and symptoms in temporomandibular disorders: Clinical signs in cases and controls. *The Journal of the American Dental Association*, *120*(3), 273–281. doi:10.14219/jada.archive.1990.0043 PMID:2312947

Dworkin, S. F., & LeResche, L. (1992). Research diagnostic criteria for temporomandibular disorders: Review, criteria, examinations and specifications, critique. *Journal of Craniomandibular Disorders*, *6*(4), 301–355. PMID:1298767

Farella, M., Michelotti, A., Steenks, M. H., Romeo, R., Cimino, R., & Bosman, F. (2000). The diagnostic value of pressure algometry in myofascial pain of the jaw muscles. *Journal of Oral Rehabilitation*, *27*(1), 9–14. doi:10.1046/j.1365-2842.2000.00526.x PMID:10632838

Fillingim, R. B., Maixner, W., Kincaid, S., Sigurdsson, A., & Harris, M. B. (1996). Pain sensitivity in patients with temporomandibular disorders: Relationship to clinical and psychosocial factors. *The Clinical Journal of Pain*, *12*(4), 260–269. doi:10.1097/00002508-199612000-00005 PMID:8969871

Fischer, A.A. (1983). Advances in documentation of pain and soft tissue pathology. *J Fam Med*, 24–31.

Fischer, A. A. (1987). Pressure algometry over normal muscles. Standard values, validity and reproducibility of pressure threshold. *Pain*, *30*(1), 115–126. doi:10.1016/0304-3959(87)90089-3 PMID:3614975

Fischer, A. A. (1988). Documentation of myofascial trigger points. *Archives of Physical Medicine and Rehabilitation*, *69*(4), 286–291. PMID:3281631

Fischer, A. A. (1991). Muscle spasm: Documentation by thermography and by clinical methods. *Thermology*, *3*, 276.

Fischer, A. A. (1991a). Trigger points: Visualization by thermography. *Thermology, 3*, 276.

Fischer, A. A., & Chang, C. H. (1986). Temperature and pressure threshold measurements in trigger points. *Thermology, 1*, 212–215.

Gerwin, R. D., Dommerholt, J., & Shah, J. P. (2004). An expansion of Simons integrated hypothesis of trigger point formation. *Current Pain and Headache Reports, 8*(6), 468–475. doi:10.1007/s11916-004-0069-x PMID:15509461

Gratt, B. M., & Anbar, M. (1998). Thermology and facial telethermography: Part II. Current and future clinical applications in dentistry. *Dento Maxillo Facial Radiology, 27*(2), 68–74. doi:10.1038/sj.dmfr.4600324 PMID:9656869

Gratt, B. M., Graff-Radford, S. B., Shetty, V., Solberg, W. K., & Sickles, E. A. (1996). A 6-year clinical assessment of electronic facial thermography. *Dento Maxillo Facial Radiology, 25*(5), 247–255. doi:10.1259/dmfr.25.5.9161178 PMID:9161178

Gratt, B. M., Pullinger, A., Sickles, E. A., & Lee, J. J. (1989). Electronic thermography of normal facial structures: A pilot study. *Oral Surgery, Oral Medicine, and Oral Pathology, 68*(3), 346–351. doi:10.1016/0030-4220(89)90222-3 PMID:2771378

Gratt, B. M., & Sickles, E. A. (1993). Thermographic characterization of the asymptomatic temporomandibular joint. *Journal of Orofacial Pain, 7*(1), 7–14. PMID:8467300

Gratt, B. M., & Sickles, E. A. (1995). Electronic facial thermography: An analysis of asymptomatic adult subjects. *Journal of Orofacial Pain, 9*(3), 255–265. PMID:8995925

Gratt, B. M., Sickles, E. A., Ross, J. B., Wexler, C. E., & Gornbein, J. A. (1994). Thermographic assessment of craniomandibular disorders: Diagnostic interpretation versus temperature measurement analysis. *Journal of Orofacial Pain, 8*(3), 278–288. PMID:7812225

Haddad, D. S. (2001). *Correlação clínica e termográfica do ponto-gatilho miofascial nos músculos da mastigação* (dissertação). São Paulo: Universidade de São Paulo, Faculdade de Odontologia.

Haddad, D. S., Brioschi, M. L., & Arita, E. S. (2012). Thermographic and clinical correlation of myofascial trigger points in the masticatory muscles. *Dento Maxillo Facial Radiology, 41*(8), 621–629. doi:10.1259/dmfr/98504520 PMID:23166359

Haddad, D. S., Brioschi, M. L., Vardasca, R., Weber, M., Crosato, E. M., & Arita, E. S. (2014). Thermographic characterization of masticatory muscle regions in volunteers with and without myogenous temporomandibular disorder: Preliminary results. *Dento Maxillo Facial Radiology, 43*(8), 20130440. doi:10.1259/dmfr.20130440 PMID:25144605

Jaeger, B., & Reeves, J. L. (1986). Quantification of changes in myofascial trigger point sensitivity with the pressure algometer following passive stretch. *Pain, 27*(2), 203–210. doi:10.1016/0304-3959(86)90211-3 PMID:3797015

Johansson, A., Kopp, S., & Haraldson, T. (1985). Reproducibility and variation of skin surface temperature over the temporomandibular joint and masseter muscle in normal individuals. *Acta Odontologica Scandinavica, 43*(5), 309–313. doi:10.3109/00016358509046513 PMID:3866482

John, M. T., Dworkin, S. F., & Mancl, L. A. (2005). Reliability of clinical temporomandibular disorder diagnoses. *Pain*, *118*(1-2), 61–69. doi:10.1016/j.pain.2005.07.018 PMID:16154702

Kawano, W., Kawazoe, T., Tanaka, M., & Hikida, Y. (1993). Deep thermometry of temporomandibular joint and masticatory muscle regions. *The Journal of Prosthetic Dentistry*, *69*(2), 216–221. doi:10.1016/0022-3913(93)90143-C PMID:8429516

Keith, L. E., Thomas, W. D., & Ferganson, J. L. (1973). Effects of activity, alcohol, smoking, and the menstrual cycle on liquid crystal breast thermography. *The Ohio Journal of Science*, *73*, 55–58.

Kruse, R. A., & Christiansen, J. A. (1992). Thermographic imaging of myofascial trigger points: A follow-up study. *Archives of Physical Medicine and Rehabilitation*, *73*(9), 819–823. PMID:1514891

Lawson, R. N. (1956). Implications of surface temperatures in the diagnosis of breast cancer. *Canadian Medical Association Journal*, *75*(4), 309–311. PMID:13343098

Leonardi, R., Zaborra, G., Li Pera, A. M., & Tripi, T. R. (1991). Comparison of telethermography and electromyography in instrumental symptomologic evaluation of the anterior temporalis and the masseter. [In Italian.]. *Stomatologia Mediterranea*, *11*(1), 5–10. PMID:1871658

Merla, A., & Romani, G. L. (2008). Biomedical appplications of functional infrared imaging. In N. A. Diakides & J. D. Bronzino (Eds.), *Medical infrared imaging* (pp. 15.1–15.20). Boca Raton, FL: CRC Press.

Mongini, F., Caselli, C., Macri, V., & Tetti, C. (1990). Thermographic findings in cranio-facial pain. *Headache*, *30*(8), 497–504. doi:10.1111/j.1526-4610.1990.hed3008497.x PMID:2228600

Pogrel, M. A., Erbez, G., Taylor, R. C., & Dodson, T. B. (1989). Liquid crystal thermography as a diagnostic aid and objective monitor for TMJ dysfunction and myogenic facial pain. *Journal of Craniomandibular Disorders*, *3*(2), 65–70. PMID:2606998

Sanches, I. J. (2009). *Sobreposição de Imagens de Termografia e Ressonância Magnética: uma nova modalidade de imagem médica tridimensional*. Curitiba: Universidade Tecnológica Federal do Paraná, Engenharia Elétrica e Informática Industrial.

Schwartz, R. G. (2006). Guidelines for Neuromusculoskeletal Thermography. Wheeling. *Thermol Int*, *16*(1), 5–9.

Shah, J. P., Danoff, J. V., Desai, M. J., Parikh, S., Nakamura, L. Y., Phillips, T. M., & Gerber, L. H. (2008). Biochemicals associated with pain and Inflammation are elevated in sites near to and remote from active myofascial trigger points. *Archives of Physical Medicine and Rehabilitation*, *89*(1), 16–23. doi:10.1016/j.apmr.2007.10.018 PMID:18164325

Simons, D. G. (1988). Myofascial pain syndromes: Where are we? Where are we going? *Archives of Physical Medicine and Rehabilitation*, *69*(3 Pt 1), 207–212. PMID:3279935

Simons, D. G. (2004). Review of enigmatic MTP as a common cause of enigmatic musculoskeletal pain and dysfunction. *Journal of Electromyography and Kinesiology*, *14*(1), 95–107. doi:10.1016/j.jelekin.2003.09.018 PMID:14759755

Simons, D. G., Travell, J. G., & Simons, L. S. (1999). *Travell & Simons' myofascial pain and dysfunction: the trigger point manual* (2nd ed.; Vol. 1). Baltimore, MD: Williams & Wilkins.

Swerdlow, B., & Dieter, J. N. I. (1992). An evaluation of the sensitivity and specificity of medical thermography for the documentation of myofascial trigger points. *Pain*, *48*(2), 205–213. doi:10.1016/0304-3959(92)90060-O PMID:1589239

Vardasca, R., Ring, E. F. J., Plassmann, P., & Jones, C. D. (2012). Thermal symmetry of the upper and lower extremities in healthy subjects. *Thermol Int*, *22*(3), 53–60.

Vargas, J. V. C., Brioschi, M. L., Dias, F. G., Parolin, M. B., Mulinari-Brenner, F. A., Ordonez, J. C., & Colman, D. (2009). Normalized methodology for medical infrared imaging. *Infrared Physics & Technology*, *52*(1), 42–47. doi:10.1016/j.infrared.2008.11.003

Visscher, C. M., Lobbezoo, F., & Naeije, M. (2004). Comparison of algometry an palpation in the recognition of temporomandibular disorder pain complaints. *Journal of Orofacial Pain*, *18*(3), 214–219. PMID:15509000

Weinstein, S. A., Weinstein, G., Weinstein, E. L., & Gelb, M. (1991). Facial thermography, basis, protocol, and clinical value. *Cranio*, *9*(3), 201–211. doi:10.1080/08869634.1991.11678368 PMID:1810666

KEY TERMS AND DEFINITIONS

Algometer: It is an instrument for measuring the degree of pain caused by pressure.

Masticatory Muscles: They are responsible for the mastication. They are characterized by four muscles: temporalis, masseter, lateral pterygoid and medial pterygoid.

Medical Infrared Thermography: It is a noninvasive and nonionizing imaging technique that allows the real-time representation of the thermal skin surface distribution into thermograms.

Myofascial Pain Syndrome (MPS): It is characterized by diffuse muscle pain and the presence of myofascial trigger points (MTPs).

Myofascial Trigger Point (MTP): It is a hyperirritable nodule of spot tenderness in a palpable taut band of skeletal muscle. The spot is a site of exquisite tenderness to palpation, from which a local twitch response can be elicited when appropriately stimulated, which refers pain to a distance.

Temporomandibular Disorder (TMD): They are characterized by orofacial pain and mobility dysfunction of the masticatory structures.

Thermology: It is the medical science that derives diagnostic indications from highly detailed and sensitive infrared images of the human body.

Chapter 7
Thermal Imaging in Evaluation of the Physical Fitness Level

Teresa Kasprzyk
University of Silesia, Poland

Karolina Sieroń-Stołtny
Medical University of Silesia, Poland

Agata Stanek
Silesian Medical University, Poland

Armand Cholewka
University of Silesia, Poland

ABSTRACT

The thermoregulation mechanisms during the physical effort can be easily study by using the thermovision. The thermoregulation mechanisms in human body keep the body core temperature on basic level 37 ± 2 ° C. However, the question is if there are any differences in skin surface temperature distribution between trainee sportsmen and amateur. Is there any possibility to show the sportsman level of practise using the thermal imaging? Would it be possible to evaluate the efficiency of athlete or evaluate the level of sports possibilities in average amateur who just wants to start cycle training. To find how the thermoregulation mechanisms work the different measurements were done i.e. during the cyclist endurance test for group of male cyclist (intermediate level of cycling skill) and during the Aerobic Circuit Training (ACT) for trainee and amateur group of women.

INTRODUCTION

The Mechanisms of Organism Thermoregulation

It is known that body core temperature is kept on basic level 37,0 ± 2,0 °C due to the thermoregulation mechanisms in human body. All living processes are dependent upon the temperature. The optimal core temperature is maintaining the normal heart beating, muscles working and nervous system functioning. The correct living organism functioning due to normal metabolism and organs functioning is possible thanks to optimal temperature conditions called thermal homeostasis (Górski, 2010). However, the temperature of human body (core as well as the surface) can change due to diseases, fever, stress and physical effort (Wendt, 2007; Pilawski, 1983).

DOI: 10.4018/978-1-5225-2072-6.ch007

The human body raises the energy needed for living from nutrition (oxygen and food metabolism). Part of this energy is used for work and the rest is radiated as a thermal energy (heat) (Herman, 2007). To keep the thermal homeostasis the overcapacity of energy has to be removed from the organism. Heat transfer between human body and environment can be done by mechanisms like: conducting, convection, radiation and evaporation. It can be noticed that the fragmented streams from convection Φ_K, radiation Φ_R and evaporation Φ_E have contribution to the total heat flow Φ (Equation 1):

$$\Phi = \Phi_k + \Phi_r + \Phi_p \tag{1}$$

However the heat transfer due to the conducting is observed only in the thermal energy transport between the tissues and skin (Pilawski, 1983; Herman, 2007).

Human body as a subject with temperature higher than absolute zero (0°K) transfers heat also by radiation (Usamentiaga, 2014). The power of radiation loss can be estimated from the surface of the body using the Stefan-Boltzmann law for biological object (Pilawski, 1983; Cholewka, 2004; Cholewka, 2005; Tuszynski, 2002; Wiśniewski, 2009):

$$\Phi_R = \sigma \cdot a \cdot A \cdot (T_S^4 - T_0^4) \tag{2}$$

where:

σ – black body radiation constant,

$$\sigma = 5,67 \cdot 10^{-8} \frac{W}{m^2 K^4},$$

a – radiation surface emissivity,
A – body surface.

Another way of heat transfer occurring in the human organism is sweating and evaporation, which should be taken into consideration from the thermal imaging point of view. It is known that the human body excretes the water due to sweating. In normal conditions the 50 ml of water is lost per hour in evaporation way. Obviously the evaporation speed depends on the level of environment humidity and the heat exerted by the body i.e. during training (Pilawski, 1983; Cholewka, 2013; Cholewka, 2015).

The first thermodynamics rule is interrelated with the biological processes. For the human body it can be written as:

$$\Delta U = \Delta Q - \Delta W \tag{3}$$

where:

ΔU – exchanged energy,
ΔQ – change of thermal energy,

ΔW – performed work (by the muscles).

When the work is done ($\Delta W > 0$) the heat is transferred out of the body ($\Delta Q < 0$) and the stored energy is rising down ($\Delta U < 0$). The heat from metabolic processes Q_{met} (called also the metabolic rate, *MR*) and the heat loss due to the heat transfer Q_{loss} contributes to the total heat Q inside the body. The body temperature is regulated by increase of heat production (thermogenesis) when the heat is losing passive and active heat loss (thermolysis) when the organism is overheated (Pilawski, 1983; Herman, 2007; Kasprzyk, 2014).

However the thermoregulation system in human body is working to keep the constant temperature of body core and not to keep the constant level of heat in organism (Górski, 2010).

Thermoregulation Processes During the Physical Activity

During the physical effort thermoregulation mechanisms are activated due to energy loss what simultaneously leads to temperature increase. However, to remove the surplus of heat energy it is transported from body core to body surface. The heat transfer is done compatible with the temperature gradient. As long as the organism is in rest the heat energy is transported from the body core to the skeletal muscles. On the other hand when physical activities were done the temperature of skeletal muscles increases and the temperature gradient between muscles and artery blood becomes diverted. The heat is produced and the body core as well as the body surface temperature rises up. During the physical activities the body energy increases and the metabolism speeds up. In consequence the temperature gradient between the body and environment is changing and the proper thermoregulation mechanisms are switched on what leads to take back the body thermodynamic equilibrium (Górski, 2010; Wendt, 2007).

For effective thermoregulation the blood circulation is important phenomenon. The heart rate rises up during the physical effort, and so the blood circulation is faster and heat is transferred to the body surface more effectively (Cholewka, 2013; Cholewka, 2015; Kasprzyk, 2014). It leads to heat transport to the environment and the body is cooled down. However during the physical effort the temperature of environment may be close to the body surface temperature and the convection and radiation heat transfer has become inefficient. The only way to protect body from overheating is water evaporation during sweating. In case of dynamic and intense training, excretion of water through sweat increases from 50 ml per hour to 2 liters per hour and in extreme situation even to 4 liters per hour (Pilawski, 1983). In the case of too intensive and prolonged exercise, sweating body intensifies and evaporation process also can become not effective what can lead to human body hyperthermia or even significant health problems (Górski, 2010).

Body Surface Temperature

The body surface temperature follows the environment conditions much faster than the core temperature. The heat produced in body core is transported to the skin mostly by blood circulation so the convection however it should be also consider the radiation and the conduction occurred between tissues in the contact. The verification of heat stream flowing to the surface is caused by the skin perfusion change by adjusting the mobility of skin's blood vessels (Górski, 2010; Pilawski, 1983). In normal conditions the average temperature of skin in different regions of body is located between 29 °C and 35 °C (Cholewka, 2013; Kasprzyk, 2014).

It is possible to calculate the average body surface temperature from the empirical equation (Górski, 2010; Pilawski, 1983):

$$T_{surf} = 0,07 \cdot T_{feet} + 0,32 \cdot T_{legs} + 0,17 \cdot T_{back} + 0,18 \cdot T_{chest} + 0,14 \cdot T_{shoulders} + 0,05 \cdot T_{arms} + 0,07 \cdot T_{head} \quad (4)$$

where: T_{tibia}, legs surface temperature; T_{chest}, chest surface temperature; T_{arms}, arms surface temperature; T_{foot}, foot surface temperature; T_{head}, head surface temperature; T_{hands}, hands surface temperature; T_{back}, back surface temperature.

Such analysis and calculation can be useful in evaluation of energy cost during different sport activities what are the goals of this chapter.

The thermoregulation mechanisms during the physical effort can be easily studied by using the thermovision. The question is, if there are any differences in skin surface temperature distribution between trainee sportsmen and amateurs that are studied during the training. Is there any possibility to show the sportsman level of practice using the thermal imaging? Would it be possible to evaluate the efficiency of athlete or evaluate the level of sports possibilities in average amateur who just wants to start a cycle training.

To find how the thermoregulation mechanisms work the different measurements were done i.e. during the cyclist endurance test for group of male cyclist (intermediate level of cycling skill) and during the Aerobic Circuit Training (ACT) for trainee and amateur group of women what is presented in details in further parts of this chapter.

THE THERMAL IMAGING OF CYCLISTS BODY SURFACE

Physiology and Bases of Training in Cycling

Cycling as a very complex sport discipline is played in difference conditions. Cycling can be divided as a multiple forms, from mountain biking (MTB) with short and dynamic Cross-Country races (XC) and long marathons to the road cycling with endurance mountain stages or dynamic time-trials.

In fact during the XC race the average heart beat is about 171 bpm and this constitutes 86-90% of the maximum heart rate (Zatoń, 2011).

Professional road cyclist have to do about 35 000 km during the trainings and races. This amount seems to be unreal however for example during the 21 day stage race Giro d'Italia in 2014 the total distance was 3457 km with more than 35 km height difference. That's why training in cycling should be well-fitting to the specific forms of this discipline. However cycling is an endurance sport, which means that training cycle is divided into periods (Friel, 2000; Van Den Bosh, 2006). The classic division of year training plan contains three main periods: the preparatory, initiation and temporary phase (Table 1). Each of them differ toward others with ratio between training volume and endurance (Zatoń, 2011).

In overall the preparatory period volume training is the most important, however the intensity of exercising increases slowly. Although in a specific preparatory phase the intensity dominates. The preparatory phase goal is to economization the effort in initiation phase, when the races season is beginning. In initiation stage the cyclist has to keep the training intensity on constant level, which is needed to reach the best results. The last one, temporary phase is the regeneration period. Low intensity exercises are

Table 1. Example periodization of the year cycling plan

<table>
<tr><th>MACRO PERIOD</th><th colspan="19">TRAINING YEAR</th></tr>
<tr><td rowspan="3">MEZO PERIOD</td><td colspan="8">PREPARATION</td><td colspan="6">COMPETITION</td><td colspan="5" rowspan="3">TEMPORARY PHASE</td></tr>
<tr><td colspan="7">OVERALL PREPARATION</td><td>SPECIFIC PREPARATION</td><td>BEFORE</td><td colspan="5">COMPETITION</td></tr>
<tr><td>PREPARATION</td><td colspan="6">BASE</td><td>EXTENSION</td><td>PEAK</td><td colspan="5">RACES</td></tr>
<tr><td>MICRO PERIOD (Week No)</td><td>1 2</td><td>3</td><td>4</td><td>5</td><td>6</td><td>7</td><td>8</td><td colspan="2">9 - 42</td><td>43</td><td>44</td><td>45</td><td>46</td><td>47</td><td>48</td><td>49</td><td>50</td><td>51</td><td>52</td></tr>
</table>

Source: Friel, 2000

preferred in this stage. This is the time when sportsmen should take a break and have an active recovery (Friel, 2000).

There are two selected times for efficiency test in cycling: at the beginning of temporary phase to check the level of exhaustion after the start season and in the middle of specific preparatory phase to monitoring the progress of sportsmen.

Efficiency Test in Cycling

The organism physical parameters, i.e. pulse, power or oxygen capacity, are the base of correct training plan. The threshold from these parameters is obtained from the efficiency tests. Heart rate zones are calculated from the heat rate changes during the progressive effort. The main heart rate zones are showed in Table 2 (Baker, 1998).

During the efficiency test the lactic acid level in muscles is measured. Lactate level is a basic parameter to determine the organism oxygen capacity (Zatoń, 2011; Van Den Bosh, 2006). It is known that the overfill of lactate is toxic for the body cells. Lactate gain above some base concentration could result as discomfort in athlete's muscles. That's why sportsmen cannot continue effort when lactate level increases rapidly. However the lactic acid is the substance, which protect athlete's body from the overtraining (Friel, 2000; Van Den Bosh, 2006). The metabolic conversion thresholds are determined to estimate the base of the changes of lactic acid during the effort (Table 3) (Zatoń, 2011; Friel, 2000; Van Den Bosh, 2006; Baker, 1998).

Table 2. Heart rate zones in cycling

ZONE	1	2	3	4	5	6
NAME	RECOVERY	BASE ENDURANCE	STRENGTH	INTERVAL	INTENSITY	HIGH INTENSITY
$\%HR_{max}$	60 – 65%	65 – 75%	75 – 82%	82 – 89%	89 – 94%	>94%
DESCRIPTION	Equable training, active recovery.	Longer but not dynamic training.	The increasing of respiratory and blood circulation system capacity	Training over lactate threshold. So called extensive intervals method.	Anaerobic training, intensive intervals.	High intensive intervals, usually during the races.

Table 3. Metabolic conversion threshold in organism

Threshold	Description
AT *(anaerobic treshold)*	Start of lactic acid accumulation in muscles. The anaerobic processer are outweighted the aerobic processes. Training over the AT allowed increasing the oxygen capacity, buildup the endurance of cardiovascular and respiratory systems. Exercising under AT run the recovery and adaptive processes.
RPC *(respiratory compensation point)*	The point when hiperventilation is started. Over the RCP CO_2 cannot be remove from body. The energy produce from muscles is came from anaerobic transformation. Lactate level is increasing and the blood pH level is decreasing.
LT *(lactate treshold)*	The dynamic lactate accumulation in blood is proceeded over LT. Symptoms of strong exhausted are observed. The pace of removing lactic acid from blood is an indicator of this threshold.

All mentioned above parameters checked during effort are used in sport medicine for a very long time and all of them are charging or uncomfortable in some way for the studied sportsmen i.e. mask on the face or taking a blood sample during training may be distracting. That is why it is interesting to find out if there are any other methods that can give similar information that standard used methods which can be not so distractible or even unnoticeable for the sportsman during tests.

Maybe the thermovision may be the solution and next subchapters will try to point the attention on this totally non-invasive technique.

The Analyze of Temperature Distribution During the Cycling Efficiency Test

In the paper (Cholewka, 2015) the group of male cyclists participated in progressive efficiency test. Studied subjects were healthy and without any coexisting illnesses or injuries. Studies were performed in the Sport Diagnostic Centers Diagnostic in Katowice and Wisła, Poland, which provided services regarding effort tests for sportsmen. Imaging was done during typical protocol of cyclist efficiency test. Each cyclist was wearing the Cortex Metamax 3b ergospirometry mask with telemetry system CPET „BREATH-BY-BREATH“. Mask was needed to measures parameters like VO_2 (the amount of intake oxygen) and VE (ventilation per minute, which is the volume of air flowing through the lungs per 1 minute). The correlations between spirometric parameters and the body surface or body core temperature were done to check if the metabolism changes can be counted through the thermal parameters.

A thermal imaging was performed by camera Flir Systems E60 (with sensivity 0,05 K). Each of subjects had to pass a temperature adaptation process, which takes about 30 minutes. The temperature of the environment in test room was monitored and kept at a basis level 21 ± 1°C.

The measured areas of the body remained unclothes. Measurements were done for face, arms, chest, back and legs. Thermal imaging was done every 3 minutes started with a measure before the efficiency test. The protocol of endurance test is showed in Figure 1.

Figure 1. The protocol of endurance test. Dependence between power and time of the test
Source: Cholewka, 2015

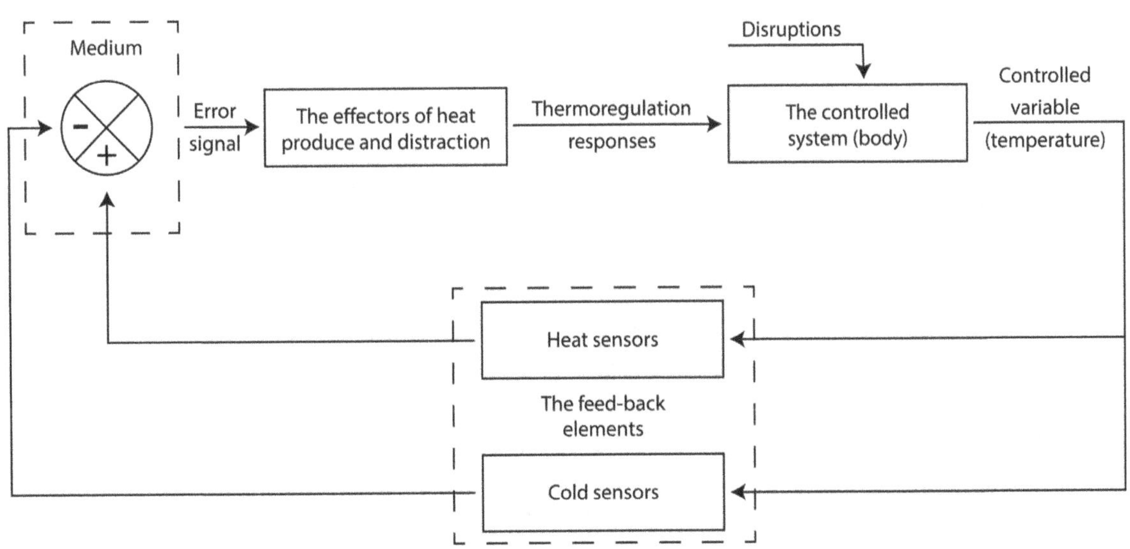

Based on the Equation 4 the average body surface temperature can be calculated according to the surface temperatures of individual body parts. The body temperature changes can be estimated during the effort test. However in the formula 4 some body parts (tibia, chest, arms and back) have a bigger influence on the average body surface temperature. The surface temperature of the face (instead of the heat temperature) and calf temperature (instead of tibia area) was measured.

Moreover, lactate sample, thermal imaging and load increases were timing as well – every measure was done with 3 minutes step. The measurements were such precise because of this parameters fitting. The load was increase in every 3 minutes and the thermal images were done exactly at the end of each power level. It is evident that the temperature distribution for every power level can be measured and based on this it was possible to evaluate the thermoregulation mechanisms for each power threshold.

However, measurements of some body parts were difficult to perform, i.e. leaning position of the body and movement of the limbs made some problems. Thermal camera was placed as much perpendicular to body as it was possible. All the measurements were performed in a similar way to *Glamorgan Protocol*, which included thermal imaging in its medical standards and rules (Ammer, 2008; Ring, 2000). Consequently, the researchers had to adapt to the conditions with which the athletes found themselves during the efficiency test. Very important thing was not to bother the sportsman during the efficiency test and try to provide as much comfort as possible.

Effort tests target is to check the limit of physical efficiency, which can be done when cyclists put themselves in similar conditions as in training or race.

Moreover, bikes were connected to device, which provides power measurement. Efficiency test started from 50 W threshold, which increased by 40 W after 3 minutes and next rose up every 3 minutes by 30 W (Figure 1). The test ended when the cyclist could not continue his effort due to reaching maximum exertion. Every test took about 30 minutes.

In chapter's Autors paper high correlations were obtained between ventilation parameters and temperature parameters, which may suggest possibilities for using the thermovision as a helpful method in planning of training cycles.

Moreover the goal of the work (Kasprzyk, 2014) by Teresa Kasprzyk was to compare amateur and professional group of cyclists. Obtained results showed visible changes in temperature distribution between mentioned groups. Thermal images for professional and amateur cyclists obtained in the work are shown in Figure 2 and Figure 3.

Changes in the body surface temperature during effort test are clearly visible (Figure 2, Figure 3). In fact, there was no possibility to measure feet and hands during the test. The region of interest was reduced to face, chest, arms, back and legs (tibias). The measures from face thermal images were done excluding areas covered by the spirometry mask. However, regions, which were excluded from calculations of the average body surface temperature, had the small contribution to the result according to formula 4.

The average body surface temperature for the amateur group (AM) and professional group (PRO) was calculated based on formula 4. Results are shown in Figure 4. The sportsmen division for the two group were done based on the level of training define by the sportsmen.

At the beginning of training the decreasing of surface temperature can be visible, for both of groups. However, for PRO group the decreasing is observed till the end of the test and for AM group the temperature is rising up after the 12th minute of training. Based on the analyze of Figure 3 it can be observed that increase of body surface temperature for AM group is bigger than for PRO. However the minimum value of surface temperature has been achieved in 27th minute of training. For the PRO group the minimum value of surface temperature was 26,5 ^{o}C and for AM group it was 27,2 ^{o}C. The greater

Figure 2. Thermal images of standard cyclists' body parts performed at the test beginning (a), after 6 min (b), 12 min (c), 18 min (d), 24 min (e) and 30 min (f). Images of cyclist from professional group
Source: Kasprzyk, 2014

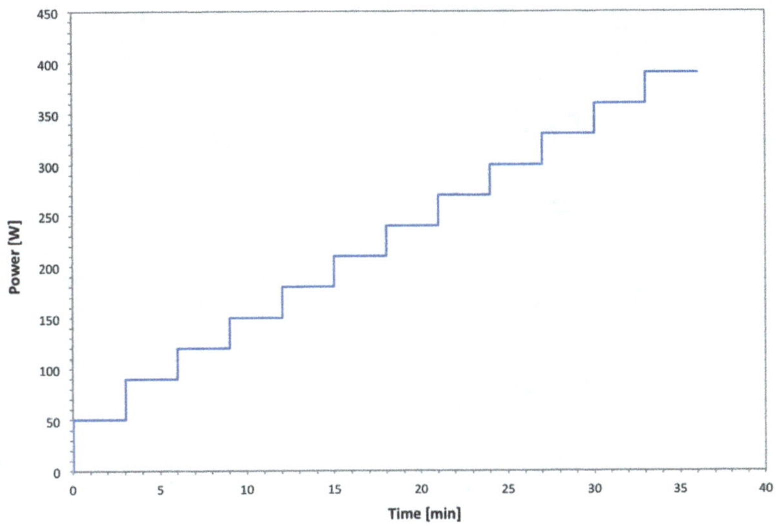

Figure 3. Thermal images of standard cyclists' body parts performed at the test beginning (a), after 6 min (b), 12 min (c), 18 min (d), 24 min (e) and 30 min (f). Images of cyclist from amateur group
Source: Kasprzyk, 2014

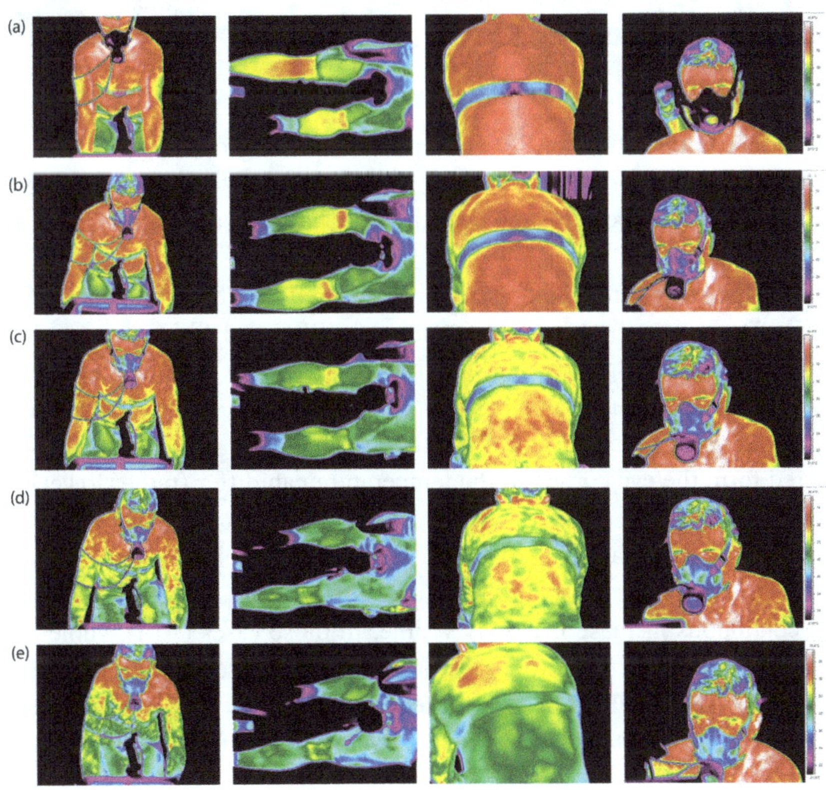

Figure 4. Average body surface temperature changes during training for AM group and PRO group

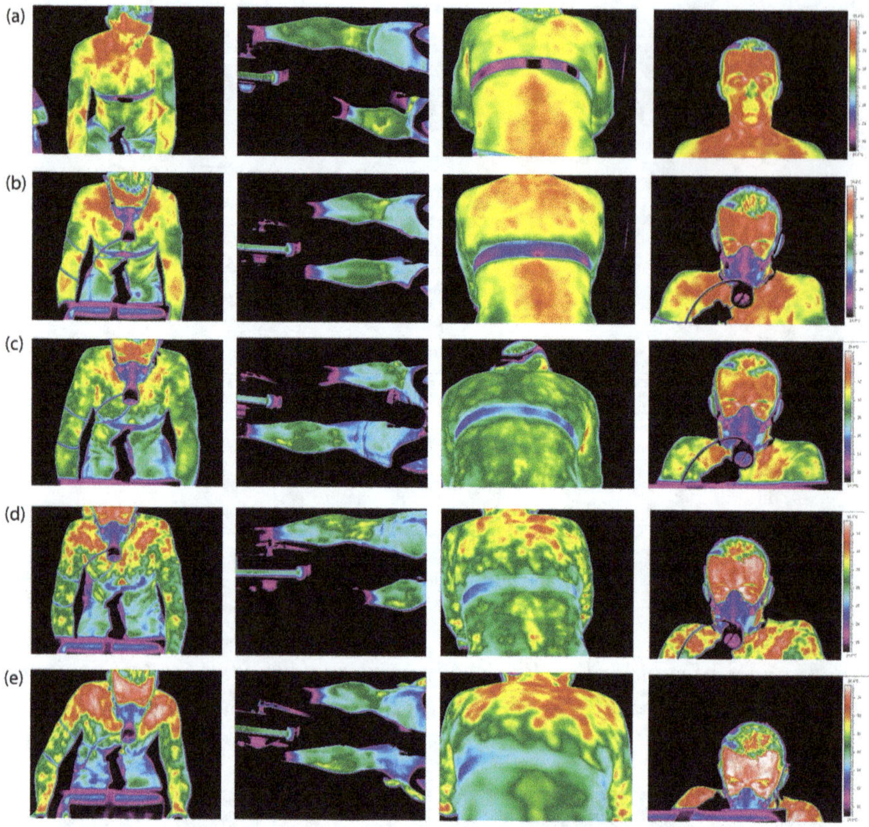

decrease of body surface temperature for PRO group than for AM group suggest that thermoregulation mechanisms are more effective for sportsmen with higher physical activity level. The body is cooling down during progressive effort because the sweating mechanisms are adjust and water evaporation removing heat from organism.

For better analysis the body core temperature was measured and the values were taken from the eye corner (Ring, 2007). The average body core temperature for PRO and AM group are shown in Figure 5.

It can be easily to see from Figure 5 that the difference in body core temperature varies between PRO and AM group. The maximum value of body core temperature is 36,8 °C for AM group but for PRO group the body core temperature values oscillate around 34,9 ± 0,3 °C. It should be underlined that it was measured form the eye corner so the temperature can differ (rather lower) from the proper core temperature.

The obtained results confirm that the thermoregulation mechanisms are more effective for PRO group. We can see that for professional cyclists the body core temperature is only oscillated unlike amateur group, where the continuous increase is clearly visible. In those cases (AM) whole thermoregulation processes (including evaporation) seem to be the not effective – it seems that the heat isn't removing from body effectively unlike the PRO ones. In consequence the body core temperature is rising up.

Figure 5. Average body core temperature for AM group and PRO group

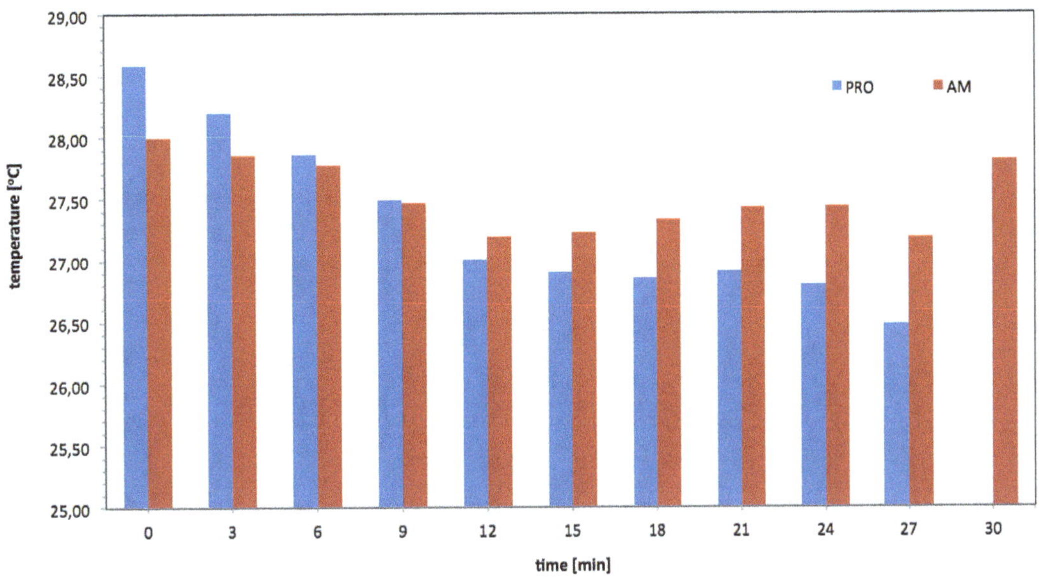

The obtained results confirmed expected thesis. Firstly, the thermal imaging during the training shows the thermoregulation mechanisms efficiency level. Secondly, the body core as well as body surface temperature changes are changing during the physical effort.

During the efficiency test, as has already been mentioned, the measurement of standard athlete's parameters were done. In result researchers get information about: heart rate (HR), intake oxygen volume (VO2), ventilation (VE) and lactic acid level (LA).

The standard efficiency parameters show minimal differences between amateur and professional groups. For VO_2 parameter the biggest difference is visible at the beginning (till 9th minute of training) and at the end (from 24th test minute) of the effort test. In the middle of the training the oxygen capacity level is similar for both group. Although, for HR parameter the difference at the end of the test is about 10 bpm. For professional group the HR_{max} is lower than amateur HR_{max}. For amateur group the average HR is 143,8 bmp and for professional group HR_{av} = 139,7 bpm. It is expected situation – the professional cyclist has lower HR_{max} and average HR than amateur. Lactic acid maximum level is lower for professional group too. However, the shape of lactate changes are similar for both groups. In fact, the professional cyclist has got better acid-alkaline organism management. The pH level is kept on basic threshold because the body get used to the physical effort. Also the hydro balance is more efficiency for professional cyclist and as it is known the hydro-management is helpful in pH increase protection. The changes of ventilation parameter also have got similar shapes for both group. However the highest values of VE are noticed for amateur group. It is very probably that biggest oxygen capacity is needed for amateur cyclist.

So, the question was - is it possible to use thermal imaging to evaluate the energy of power of athletes?

The power from a bicycle ergometer is calculated from load applied on bike. The load rising up until cyclist stopped the training. That's why the correlations between power from bicycle ergometer, HR and VO_2 and temperature changes during test were calculated (Figure 6 and Figure 7). The statistical significance factor $p < 0,05$ was obtained.

Figure 6. Correlation between VO_2 and body surface temperature for AM group. The Pearson coefficient r = -0,57
Source: Kasprzyk, 2014

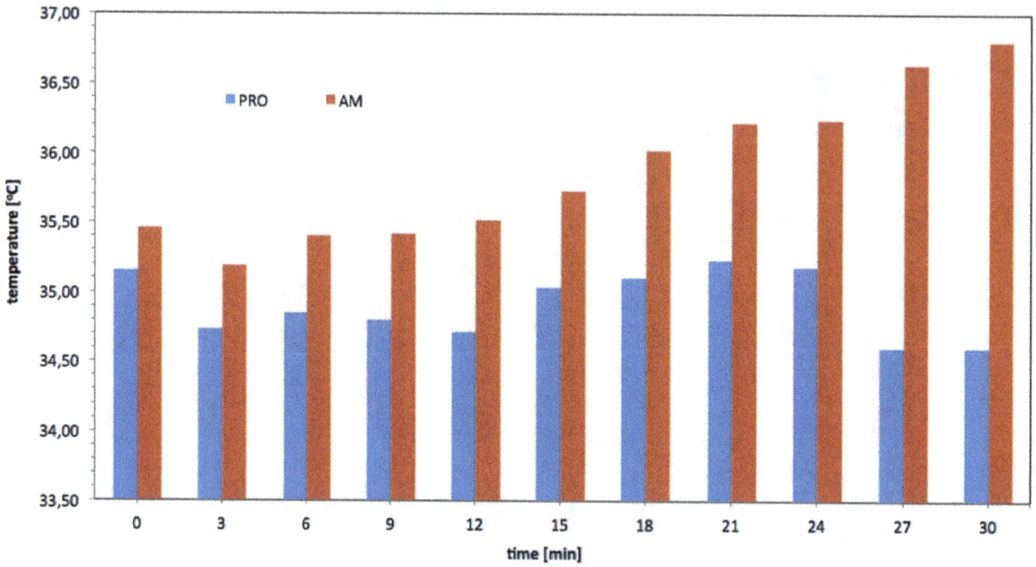

Figure 7. Correlation between ergometer power and body surface temperature for PRO group. The Pearson coefficient r = -0,95
Source: Kasprzyk, 2014

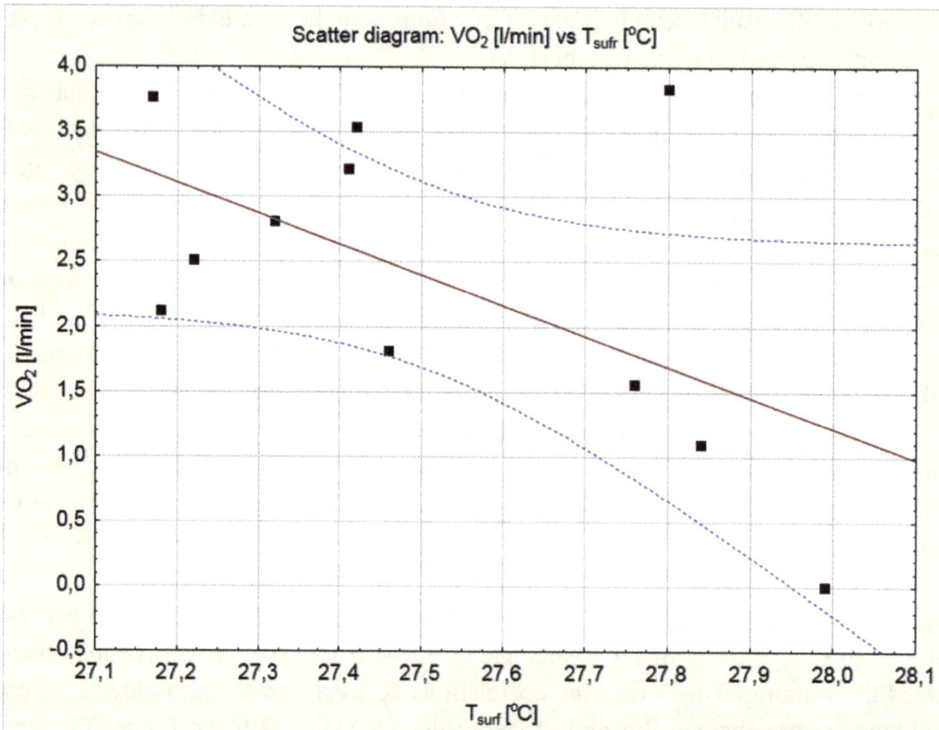

Obtained graphs show that ergometer power and the body surface temperature correlation for PRO group is negative and very strong (Pearson coefficient r = - 0,95, statistic significant). On the other hand good correlation between VO_2 and body surface temperature for amateur (r = -0,57) was obtained. In this case the correlation was also negative. These analysis show that the relation between standard athlete's organism parameter and body surface temperature changes and distribution are existing and they are strong.

Obtained high values of correlation coefficients may point a possibility to estimation the sportsmen performance based on thermal imaging, which might prove not so expensive like traditional methods and also fast and may be performed during normal program of exercising. Moreover it seems that thermal imaging can give similar information that standard used methods and can be not so distractible or even unnoticeable for the sportsman during tests.

Thermovision is a completely non-invasive and non-contact method, so sportsmen might focus only on training. Nowadays to calculate the lactate level the blood sample it is necessary to be taken blood sample from finger in every 3 minutes, which can diffuse athlete. In the case of thermal imaging, sportsmen may not even be aware that the study is in progress what is undoubtedly the main advantage.

Thermal imaging may be use not only as a diagnostic method in medicine but also in sport to check the metabolic changes during sport training. It may be possible in future to use information from thermal imaging for planning the training schedules for players.

THE THERMAL IMAGING DURING AEROBIC CIRCUIT TRAINING

A Few Fact About Fitness

Fitness is understood as a kind of Physical Function. A „fit" term meaning is healthy and physical efficient. Due to the physical activities human is going to be more resistance for the stressful situations, diseases or injuries and also can adapted to the every-day life. Fitness is a kind of activity between the high-performance sport and a stillness. It is based on three main factors: physical activity, health diet and recovery. Endurance activities, which have to reduce the fat tissue, strength training to build muscle mass and the suppleness exercising are collapsed to the fitness. Increasing of the oxygen capacity, decreasing the rest Heart Rate (HR_{rest}) and blood pressure, improvement of blood circulation system or decreasing of fat tissue and cholesterol level are a physiology profits from regular activities. Also there are a lot physiological profits, i.e. exhausting decline, better mood or increasing of pain threshold (Clover, 2008; Olex-Zarychta, 2009).

The Aerobic Circuit Training (ACT) is a form of training using in a Physical Function building-up. On ACT the strength, rapid-fire and endurance exercising are using (Mulak, 1982). ACT can be employed i.e. as a endurance-strength training or endurance-rapid fire training. The character of ACT is determined based on the main part of training (strength, rapid-fire or endurance). From 10 to 20 repetition in time should be done by athlete. Every exercise (so called station) should take from 15 to 60 seconds, due to physical activity level (Ważny 1994).

The main goal of presented results in this chapter was to find out if it is possible to use thermal imaging to evaluate the physical fitness level of the trained sportsmen or amateur and if there are any differences in body thermal map between studied groups of amateurs and trainee sportsmen.

Temperature Distribution Analysis During Aerobic Circuit Training

In the other studies of the chapter's Authors only women participated in thermal imaging. The age of subjects was between 21 and 47 years old. Studies were done in The Energy Studio in Ruda Śląska, Poland. Thermal imaging were performed by using the thermal camera FLIR Systems E60, with the 0,05 K sensitivity.

Measured Women had to exercise in short ACT (Aerobic Circuit Training) which took about 5 min ± 1 min. The aim of proposed ACT was to engaged different muscles parts. In our research ACT was composed with:

- **Jumping Jack (30 sec)**
    - **Start Position:** Straight figure, taut belly, arms loosely at your sides. Jump up with straddle position landing (flexed knee, arms over head), next jump up with landing in start position.
- **Squats on Whole Feet (12 repetitions)**
    - **Start Position:** The squat to the right angle, keeping knees in line with feet. Keep sending hips backward and keep back straight with neutral body spine. Extend arms out straight so they are parallel with the ground. Proceed from the start position to the standing position.
- **Lunges, Step Backward (by Turns, 10 Repetitions by Side)**
    - **Start Position:** Straight figure, keeping kness in line with shoulder, taut belly. The step backward phase is move back once of the legs and fold at a right angle the forward leg (the knee in line with the feet). Next step forward to the start position.
- **The Alternate Extension Arm and Leg in Supposted Kneel (10 Repetitions by Side)**
    - **Start Position:** Supported kneel, knees bent in right angle, back keeping straight, taut belly. The straight position is extended once of arms and alternate leg on the hips height. Both of the limb straight, core muscles taut.
- **Women's Pump (12 Repetitions)**
    - **Start Position:** Front support, back straight, taut belly, straight arms. Lift up and go down the body with the elbows close to the thorax, the chest as lower as you can. Next back to the start position by straighten arms.
- **Back Bows (12 Repetitions)**
    - **Start Position:** Lie prone with arms out straight, legs pushed together, all thorax contact to the ground. Next step is rising up arms and legs, thorax contact to the ground all the time.
- **Mountain Climbers (20 Repetitions)**
    - **Start Position:** Front support, back straight, arms straight in line with shoulders. Alternately pulling knees to the chest.
- **Burpees (12 Repetitions)**
    - **Start Position:** Standing position, arms loosely at your sides, taut belly, feet in line with hips. Drop into squat position with hands on the ground. Kick feet back, while keeping arms extended (front support). Immediately return feet to the squat position and jump up with extended up arms and back to the squat position.

The studied group was divided into two groups that were specified:

Figure 8. Jumping jack

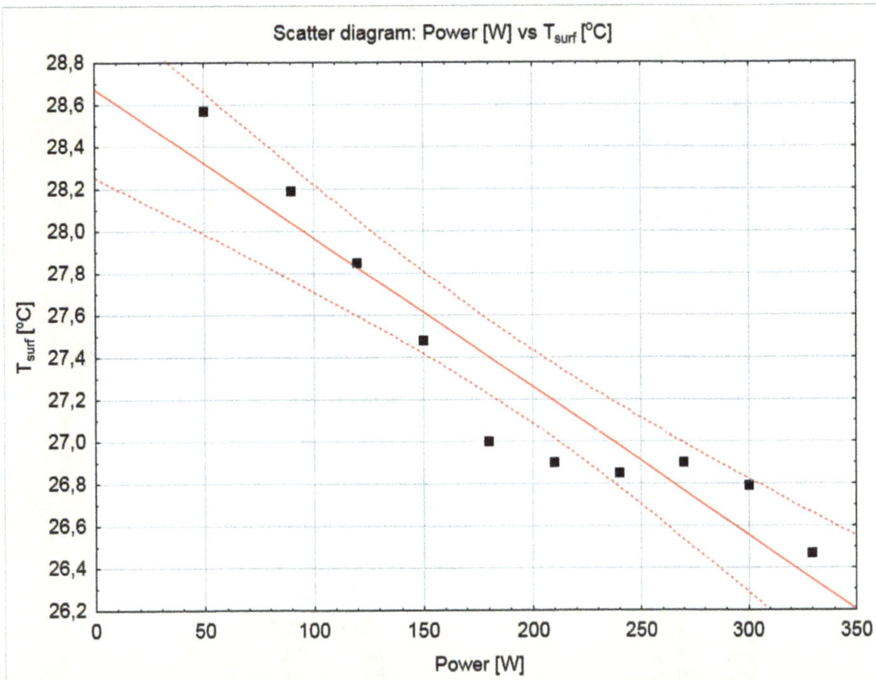

Figure 9. Squats on whole feet

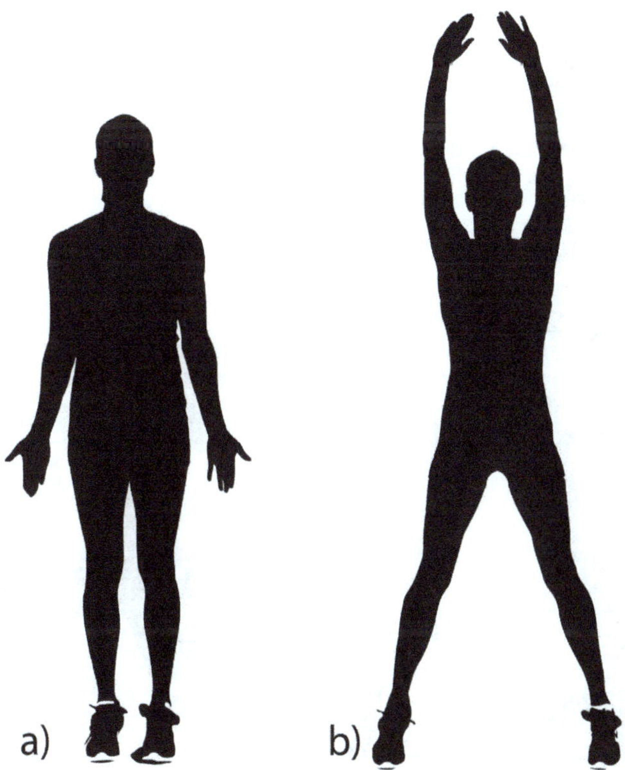

Figure 10. Lunges, step backward

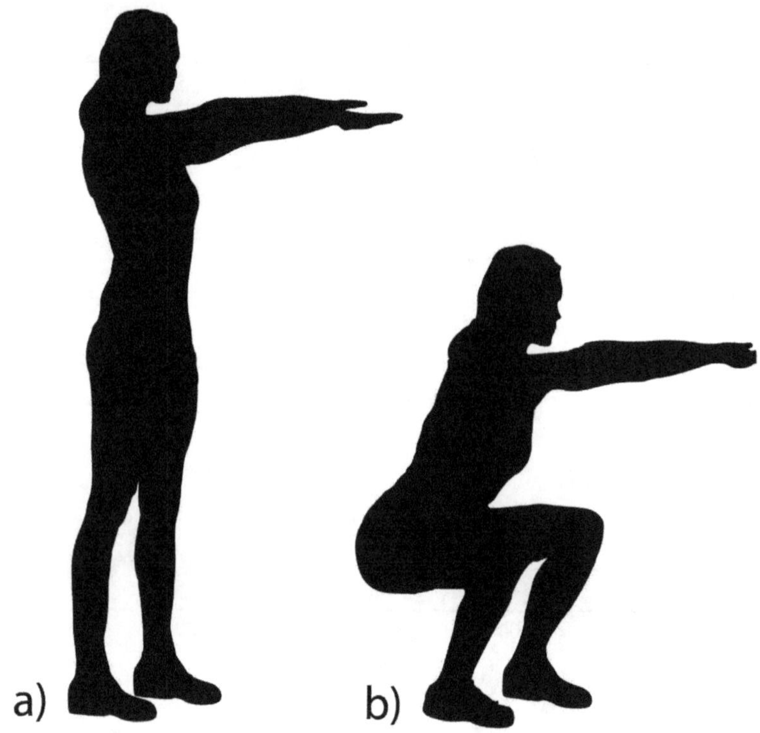

Figure 11. The alternate estension arm and leg in supposted kneel

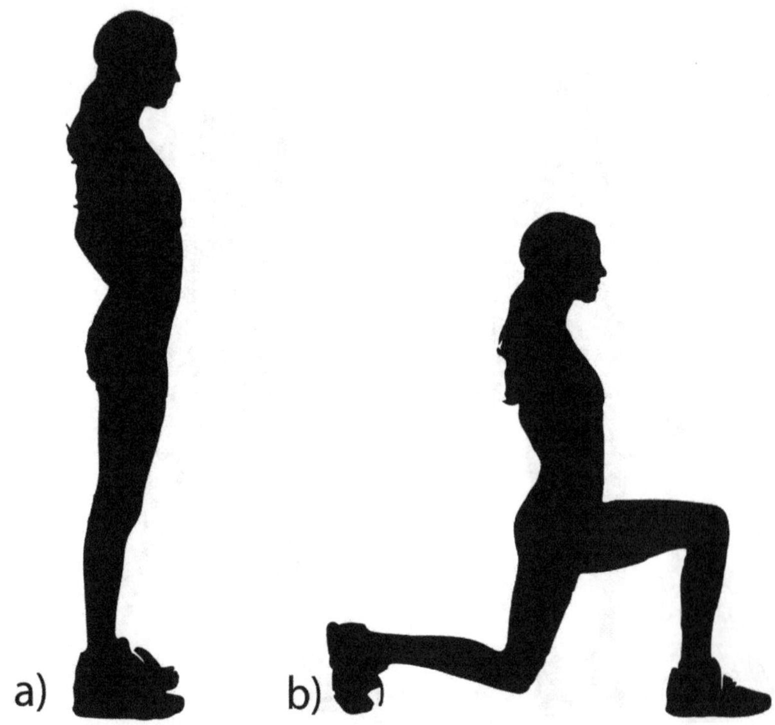

Figure 12. Women's pump

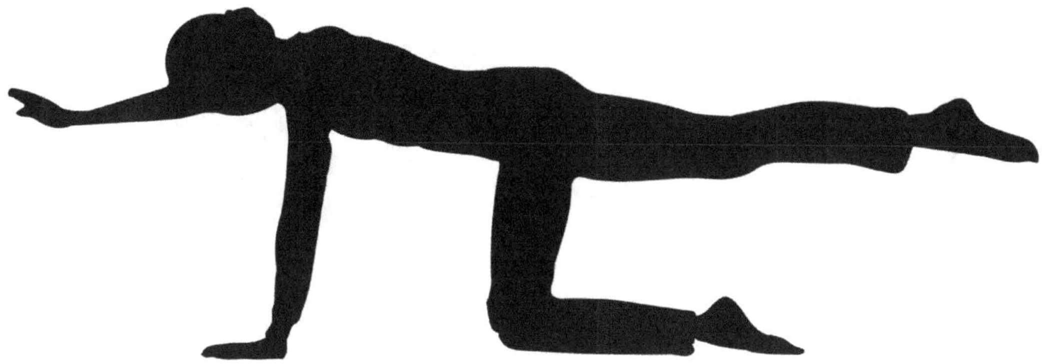

Figure 13. Back bows

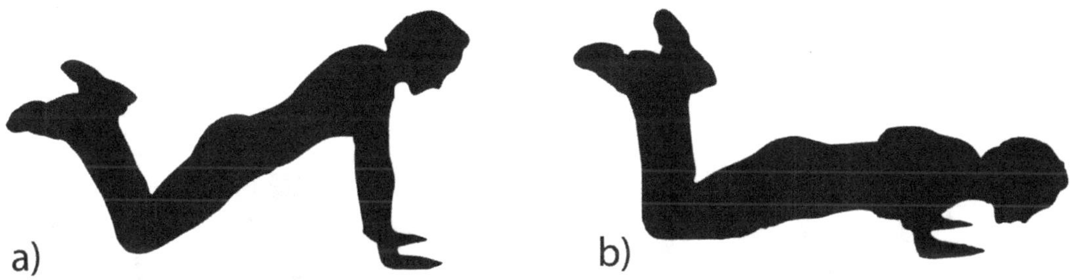

Figure 14. Mountain climbers

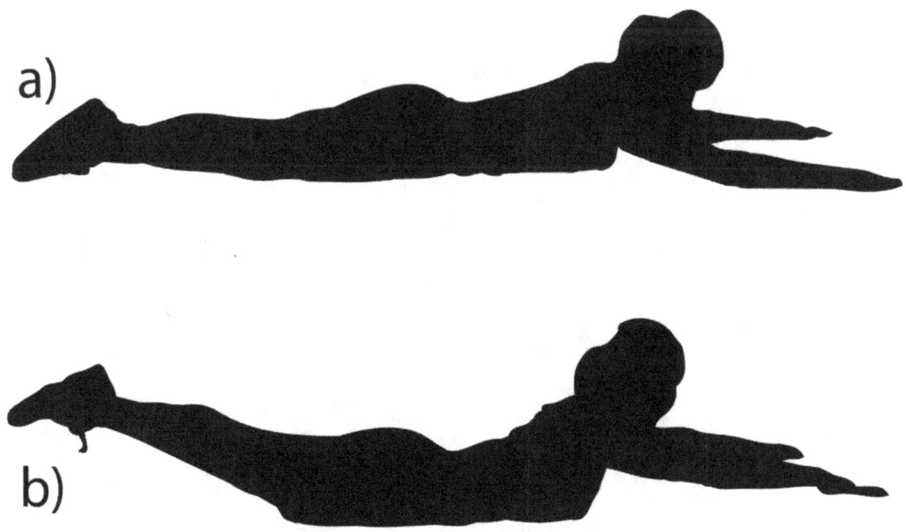

Figure 15. Burpees

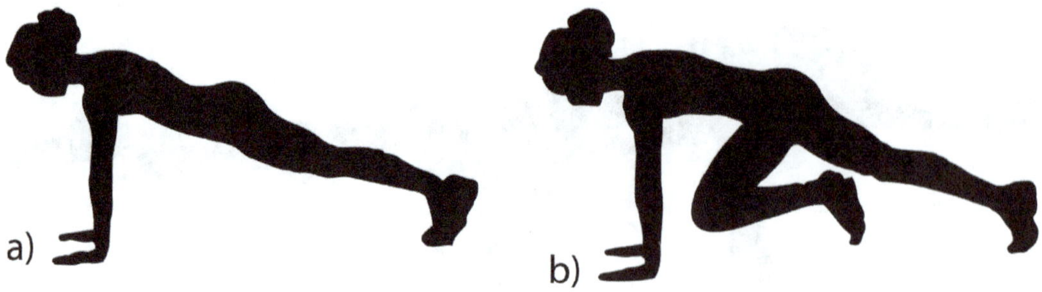

Figure 16.

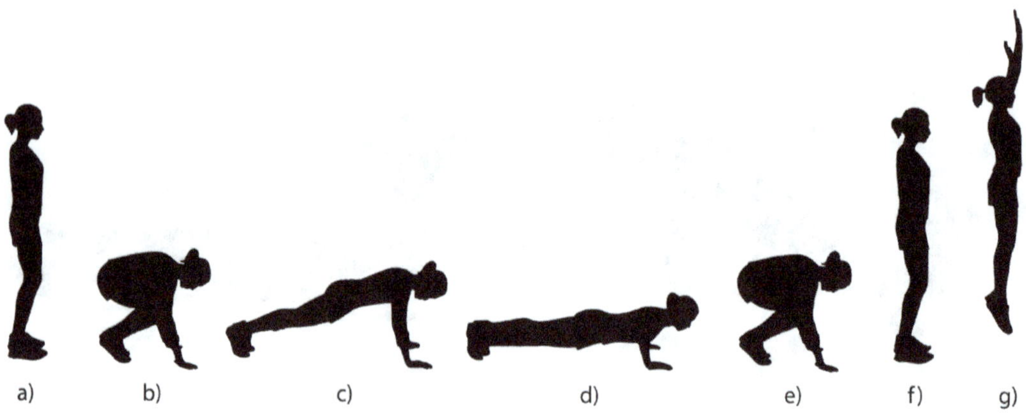

Figure 17.

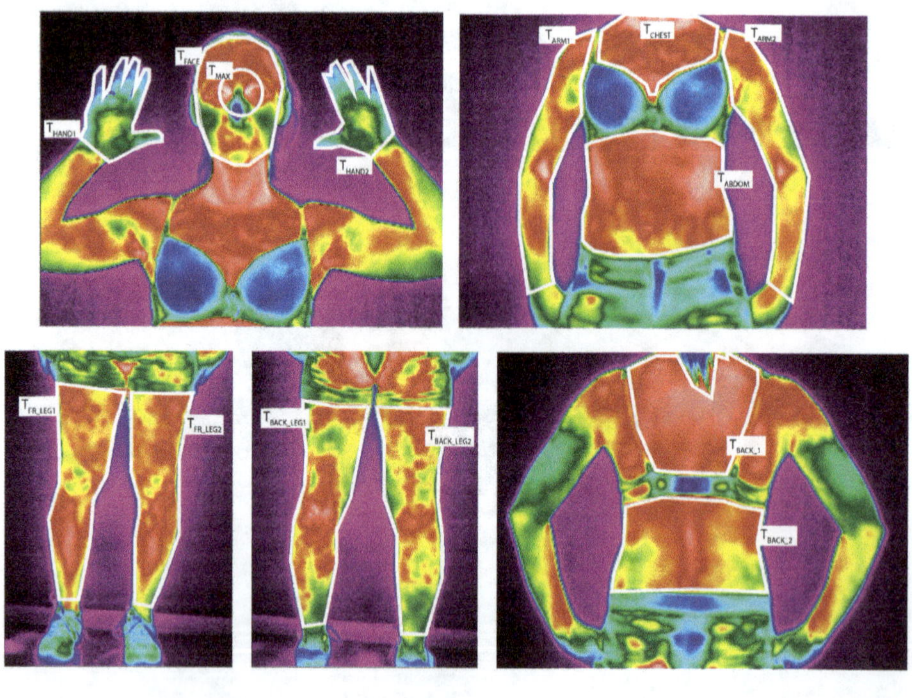

Figure 18.

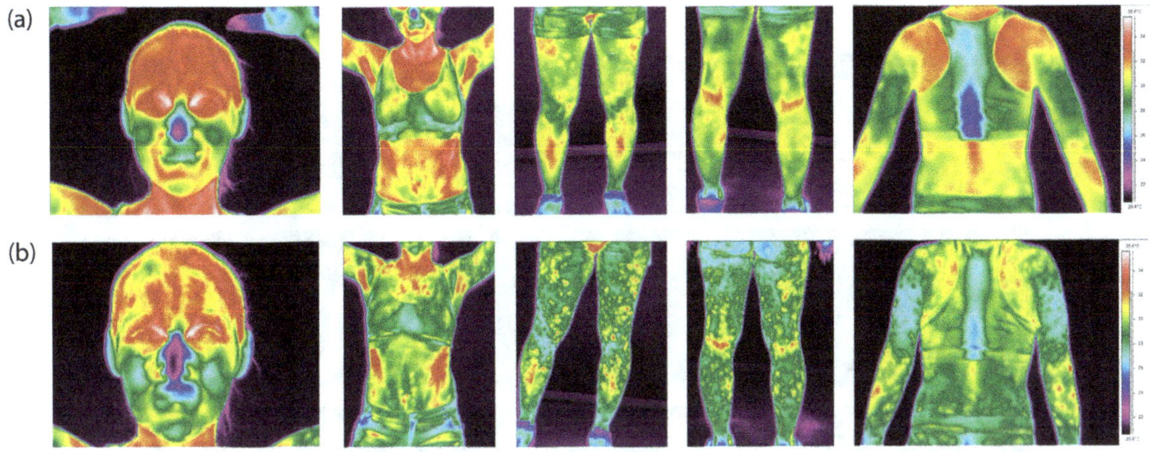

- Trainee women, which are practicing fitness regular. These women were measured before and upon 1 month of regular exercise ACT (5 times on the week, with special diet).
- Amateur women, without a daily fitness schedule.

All the measurements were performed in a similar way to *Glamorgan Protocol* which included thermal imaging in medicine standards and rules (Ammer, 2008; Ring, 2000).

The face, palm, chest, arms, back and front and back side of legs were measured during researches. The thermal imaging were done from a distance 2,0 ± 0,1 m. Researchers tried to set camera perpendicular to the measured part of the body. Also important was to kept eyes open by the imaged woman, what was needed to investigate the body core temperature from the eye corner (20). Each of the subjects had to pass the temperature adaptation process, which take about 20 minutes. The adaptation process based on uncovered the measured parts of the body. This operation purpose was to avoid the artifacts due to contact between skin and clothes. The measured parts of body had to stay uncovered till the end of researches.

Measurements were performed in closed space and the temperature was constant, kept on basic level 20 ± 2°C. There weren't any active radiation sources in the test room.

In the Figure 19 the samples of thermal images of measured body parts before one month of training for representative woman (P2, the woman which is practicing fitness regular) are shown.

It is easily to see from presented Figure 20 thermal images that forearms are characterized with higher temperature than shoulders. For body regions with larger amount of adipose tissue (e.g. lower abdomen, lower back) we can see lower surface temperature, which is appropriate to mention. It is due to worse heat conduction by the adipose tissue that muscle tissue. As it is known the adipose tissue is an insulator, which protects body from hypothermia and kept the metabolism on base level. The thermal conductivity of fat tissue is about *0,201 W/mK* and i.e. for muscles it is about *0,505 W/mK*. The more value of thermal conductivity of material indicates the better heat exchange. The percentage content of water in adipose is from 3 to 30% and for muscles it is about 75%. (Ważny, 1994; Podbielska, 2014; Valvano, 1981; Cohen, 1977). Based on this it can be conclude that adipose tissue can make the heat transfer not effective. Moreover the fat tissue vasculatore is not as good as for the muscles tissue and the blood circulation is responsible for the heat transfer (Larsen, 2010).

Figure 19. Sample thermal images of measured areas before one month of training for once woman (P2) from trainee group. Themograms were taken (a) before ACT and (b) immediately after ACT
Source: Goraj, 2015

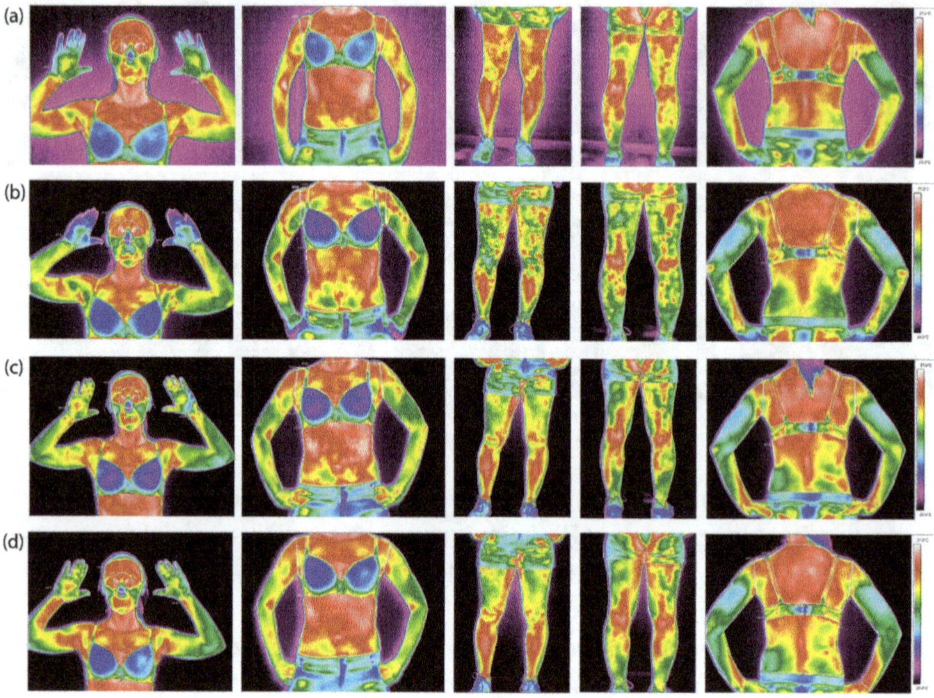

Figure 20. Samples of thermal images of measured areas after one month of training for representative woman (P2) from trainee group. Themograms were taken (a) before, (b) immediately after, (c) 15 minutes after and (d) 30 minutes after the ACT
Source: Goraj, 2015

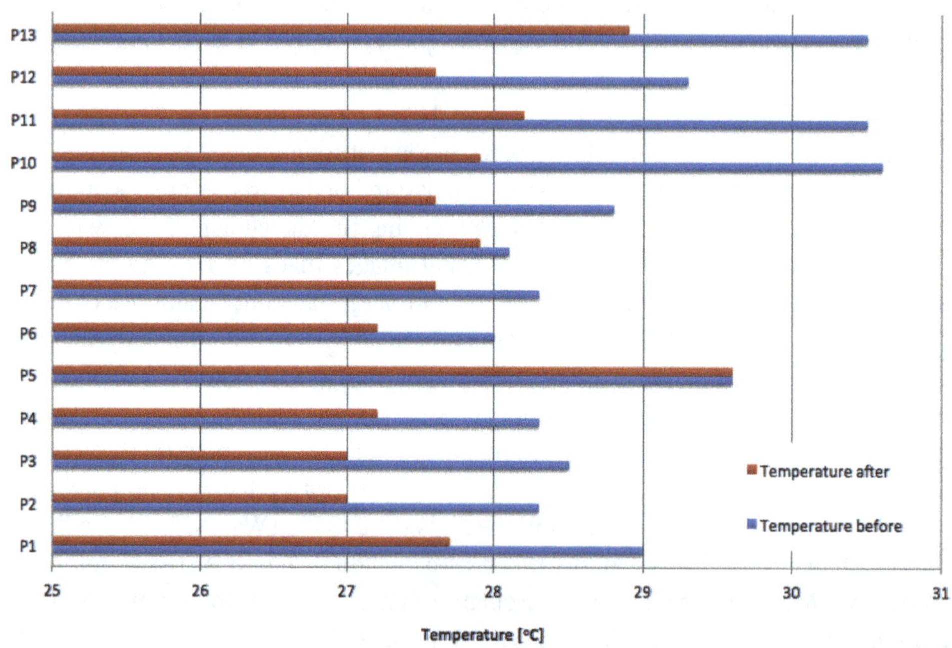

The differences between thermal images before and after 1 month of training are clearly visible (compare Figures 19 and 20). However the temperature distribution before (a) and after (b) ACT for both, before and after 1-month training, are similar. The biggest differences seem to be visible on the back thermogram – after the 1-month training the area with high temperature is greater than before training schedule.

For better analysis for patients with one month training plan (Patient 1 to 5) the average body surface temperature was calculated based on the Equation 4. The temperature of feet was skipped in calculations because of no possibility to measured feet surface. These regions had small contribution to the result. Also the chest surface was covered in part by the training top. Similar calculations were done for the group of amateur women (Patient 10 to 13).

Results are shown in Figure 21.

The Figure 21 presents the average body surface temperature for amateur group and group of trainee women after 1 month of regular exercises. The different of average body surface temperature can be easily see. For the women who did training regularly for 1 month the body surface temperature is lower than surface temperature of amateur group. The smallest temperature difference (0,2 °C) was also obtained directly after the ACT. We can also see that both of curves has got similar shape and the minimal point of average body surface temperature is just after the ACT for trainee sportsmen and for amateurs too. Then the body surface temperature is increasing a little and decreasing 30 minutes after training.

Figure 22 show the body core temperature, which was measured from the eye corner.

Based on the graph presented in Figure 22 it can be easily see that shape of body core temperature curve is more varied than for the body surface temperature (Figure 21). For women with training plan the minimal point of temperature is achieved 15 minutes after the end of ACT. Whereas for amateur

Figure 21. The relationship between average body surface temperature and the point of training for the amateur women group and group with training plan (after 1 month of regular exercising)
Source: Goraj, 2015

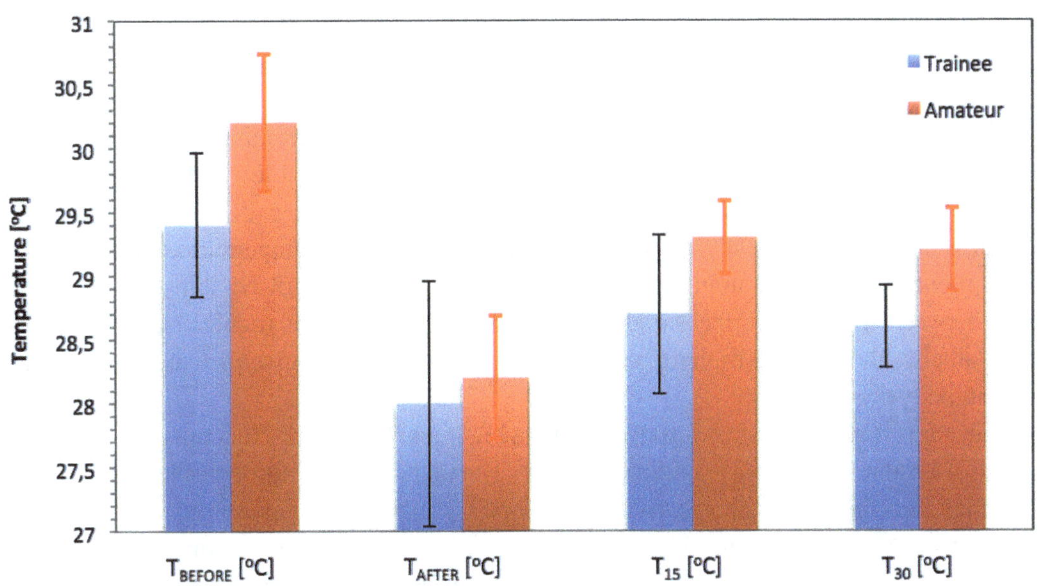

Figure 22. The relationship between average body core temperature and the point of training for the amateur women group and group with training plan (after one month of regular exercising)
Source: Goraj, 2015

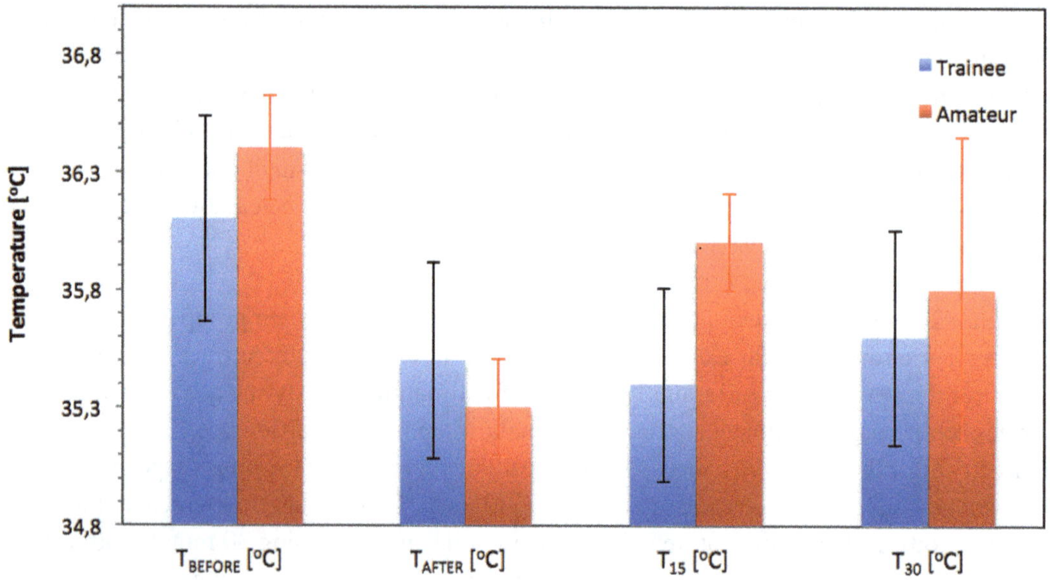

group the minimal value of body core temperature is noted directly after the ACT. Moreover is should be noted that core temperature measured for amateurs changes more dynamically during training cycle than for sportsmen with training plan. The temperature plot seems to be slightly changing against the amateurs ones. We might supposed that organism of woman with training plan has got more effective thermoregulation mechanisms. It seems that trained organism expel heat to environment better than amateur because the temperature of trained women is lower in most cases. The body of trained person is being protected from hyperthermia better.

For amateurs and trainee subjects the average surface temperature is different. However, the plots for both groups have similar shape. Moreover the values of temperature are different. For the magnitude of temperature changes between intervals: before and immediately after, as well as 15 minutes after training, the most significant shift between measured groups was obtained. Obtained results may notice that thermography may give some fresh possibilities to evaluate the physical level of sportsman. It can be also expected that this method may provide some information to planning the training cycle.

It was also interesting to check the changes between body surface temperature obtained before and after the 1-month of regular training. Obtained preliminary results showed statistically significance difference between temperature measured before and after 1 month of regular training. It might be supposed that after the 1 month training plan the thermoregulation processes are more active and more efficiency in body cooling.

It is known fact that the physical activity has got a big impact on health. It entails the positive effects for the cardiovascular system and respiratory system. The increase of erythrocytes level in blood, rising up the hemoglobin content and growth volume of blood is causing by regular physical activity. In result the body's aerobic capacity is increasing and the core and body surface temperature changes during different physical effort. This may provide to conclusion that using the thermal imaging in evaluation of fitness level of the sportsman may be useful. Presented results of the studies as well as the conclusion need further verification but they are promising.

REFERENCES

Ammer, K. (2008). The Glamorgan Protocol for recording and evaluation of thermal images of the human body. *Thermol Int.*, *18*(4), 125–144.

Baker, A. (1998). *Bicycling medicine: Cycling nutrition, Physiology, Injury prevention and treatment for riders of all levels*. Fireside.

Cholewka, A. (2005). *The influence of low temperature on organism, in vitro and in vivo studies* (Doctoral Thesis). A. Chełkowski Institute of Physics, University of Silesia Katowice Poland.

Cholewka, A., Drzazga, Z., Kajewski, B., Bogucki, R., & Wiśniowska, B. (2004). Thermal imaging of skin body surface due to whole body cryo- therapy—preliminary report. *Physica Medica*, *1*, 81–83.

Cholewka, A., Kasprzyk, T., Stanek, A., Sieroń-Stołtny, K., & Drzazga, Z. (2015). May thermal imaging be useful in cyclist endurance tests? *Journal of Thermal Analysis and Calorimetry*. doi:10.1007/s10973-015-4662-5

Cholewka, A., Stanek, A., Kasprzyk, T., Urbańczyk, P., Jagodziński, L., Sieroń, A., & Drzazga, Z. (2013). Zastosowanie termowizji w badaniach wydolności sportowców, badania pilotażowe. *PAK*, *09*, 871–874.

Clover, J. (2008). *Sports Medicine Essentials. Core Concepts in Athletic Training & Fitness Instruction*. Independence, KY: Cengage Learning.

Cohen, M. L. (1977). Measurement of the thermal properties of human skin. A review. *The Journal of Investigative Dermatology*, *69*(3), 333–338. doi:10.1111/1523-1747.ep12507965 PMID:894075

Friel, J. (2000). *The mountain biker's training bible*. VeloPress.

Goraj, M. (2015). *Applications of thermal imaging in energy cost rating during training* (Master's Thesis). A. Chełkowski Institute of Physics, University of Silesia Katowice Poland.

Górski, J. (2010). *Fizjologia Człowieka*. Warszawa: PZWL.

Kasprzyk, T. (2014). *The thermal imaging of sportsmen body surface. The influence of training cycle at organism metabolism* (Master's Thesis). A. Chełkowski Institute of Physics, University of Silesia Katowice Poland.

Larsen, R. (2010). *Anestezjologia, t. 1*. Elsevier Urban &Partner.

Mulak, J. (1982). *Lekkoatletyka – Technika Metodyka Trening*. Warszawa: Sport i Turystyka.

Olex-Zarychta, D. (2009). *Fitness: teoretyczne i metodyczne podstawy prowadzenia zajęć. Podręcznik dla studentów wychowania fizycznego i instruktorów fitness. In Wydanie III poprawione*. Gliwice: Wyd. J&D Gębka.

Pilawski, A. (1983). *Podstawy biofizyki*. New York: Springer.

Podbielska, H., & Skrzek, A. (2014). *Biomedyczne zastosowania termowizji*. Wrocław: Oficyna Wydawnicza Politechniki Wrocławskiej.

Ring, E. F. J., & Ammer, K. (2000). The technique of infrared imaging in medicine. *Thermol Int.*, *10*(1), 7–14.

Ring, J. F., & Mercer, J. (2007). Thermal Imaging for Fever Screening. *The Magazine of the International Organization for Standardization*, *4*, 33–35.

Tuszynski, J., & Dixon, J. (2002). *Biomedical applications for introductory physics*. New York: Wiley.

Usamentiaga, R., Venegas, P., Guerediaga, J., Vega, L., Molleda, J., & Bulnes, F. G. (2014). Infrared Thermography for Temperature Measurement and Non-Destructive Testing. *Sensors (Basel, Switzerland)*, *14*(7), 2305–2348. doi:10.3390/s140712305 PMID:25014096

Valvano, J.W., Allen, J.T., & Bowman, H.F. (1981). *The simultaneous measurement of thermal conductivity, thermal diffusivity, and perfusion in small volumes of tissue*. ASME 81- WA/HT-21.

Van Den Bosh, P. (2006). *Cycling: A year round plan*. Meyer & Meyer Sport.

Ważny, Z. (1994). *Leksykon treningu sportowego*. Warszawa: AWF.

Wendt, D., van Loon, L., & van Marken Lichtenbelt, W. (2007). Thermoregulation during Exercise in the heat. *Sports Medicine (Auckland, N.Z.)*, *37*(8), 669–682. doi:10.2165/00007256-200737080-00002 PMID:17645370

Wendt, D., van Loon, L., & van Marken Lichtenbelt, W. (2007). Thermoregulation during Exercise in the heat. *Sports Medicine (Auckland, N.Z.)*, *37*(8), 669–682. doi:10.2165/00007256-200737080-00002 PMID:17645370

Wiśniewski, S., & Wiśniewski, S. T. (2009). *Heat transfer* (6th ed.). Warszawa: WNT.

Zatoń, M., Herbisz, R., & Herbisz, P. (2011). *Fizjologiczne podstawy treningu w kolarstwie górskim*. Wrocław: Wydawnictwo AWF Wrocław.

Chapter 8
Infrared Thermography as a Means of Monitoring and Preventing Sports Injuries

Manuel Sillero-Quintana
Universidad Politécnica de Madrid, Spain

Pedro M. Gomez-Carmona
Universidad Politécnica de Madrid, Spain

Ismael Fernández-Cuevas
Universidad Politécnica de Madrid, Spain

ABSTRACT

Sports injuries are one of the most important problems in sports. Moreover, professional sports injuries lead to a difficult recovery process for the athletes, reduced athletic performance, and large economic costs. Infrared thermography (IRT) is a safe, non-invasive and low-cost technique that allows for the rapid and non-contact recording of Skin Temperature (Tsk). Recent research results have demonstrated new applications for this technique; among them, the monitoring and prevention of sports injuries appears to be one of the most interesting applications. Although IRT is not as objective as other methods, it may be sufficiently accurate and reliable as a complementary tool considering the theory that musculoskeletal structures should be in thermal equilibrium when in a healthy state. Therefore, the main contribution of IRT is to help identify an injury before it occurs, providing an opportunity for preventative action.

INTRODUCTION

Infrared Thermography (IRT) is a safe, non-invasive and low-cost technique that allows for the rapid and non-contact recording of the irradiated energy that is released from the body (E. Akimov & Son'kin, 2011; J. T. Costello, McInerney, Bleakley, Selfe, & Donnelly, 2012; Hildebrandt, Raschner, & Ammer, 2010; Merla, 2005; Ng, 2009).

DOI: 10.4018/978-1-5225-2072-6.ch008

Although IRT is not as objective as other methods, it may be sufficiently accurate and reliable as a complementary tool considering the theory that musculoskeletal structures should be in thermal equilibrium when in a healthy state. Regarding the practical application of thermography, thermal asymmetry in body areas can aid in the early detection of overload and skeletal muscle fatigue and may therefore help prevent injuries in individuals who practice sports.

Comparing real life with cars, sports practice maybe considered as the "Formula 1" of physical activity. Athletes are exposed to a higher injury risk because the intensity and volume of the physical activity demanded by hard training seasons (and competitions) are much higher than a normal physical activity, with the injury risk proportional to the competition level.

All the research performed on athletes, which is mainly oriented toward improving the athletes' performance, can be easily transferred to "real-life" when the physiological and psychological differences between athletes and sedentary people are considered. Consequently, when we use the term "sport" in this chapter, the term "physical activity" could also be applied in many of the contexts.

The objectives of this chapter are:

1. To review the evolution of applied thermography in the field of physical activity and sports.
2. To analyze the current applications of thermography in that field, mainly as a tool for monitoring and preventing injuries and
3. To identify the main controversies and problems of thermography application as a means to prevent sports injuries
4. To propose solutions to those issues and suggest some future research lines and approaches to improve the utility of thermography as a tool to assist in the prevention and monitoring of sports injuries.

INFRARED THERMOGRAPHY IN PHYSICAL ACTIVITY AND SPORTS

Evolution of Sports Thermography

Apart from medical research and applications, the existing studies in the field of physical activity and sports are quite scarce. The first investigations regarding thermography and high-performance sports were performed in the 1970s by a small number of research groups. Some prominent groups are the Clinical Research Centre from Middlesex UK (Clark, Goff, & Mullan, 1977; Clark, Mullan, & Pugh, 1974; Clark, Mullan, & Pugh, 1977), the University of California (Veghte, Adams, & Bernauer, 1979; Wade & Veghte, 1977), the Universitätsklinik Orthopädische München Germany (Keyl & Lenhart, 1975) and in the 1980s the research group from Addenhrooke's Hospital took over from Cambridge (Binder, Parr, Thomas, & Hazleman, 1983; Devereaux, Parr, Lachmann, Page-Thomas, & Hazleman, 1986; Devereaux, Parr, Lachmann, Page-Thomas, & Hazleman, 1984).

In addition to those primary studies, Rochcongar and Schmitt (1979) published an interesting report describing the effects of different injuries on Tsk and highlighted the potential of IRT to indicate the degree of the lesion and control its evolution. Some years later, Ring (1990) detailed the basic skin responses after an injury as identified by Rochcongar and Schmitt: normothermic, hyperthermic and hypothermic patterns, i.e., increased and decreased temperatures.

It was not until the 1990s that research groups, such as the New York Hospital Selden (BenEliyahu, 1992; BenEliyahu, 1990), the CAM Sport Monza in Italy (Garagiola & Giani, 1990; Garagiola & Giani, 1991; Giani, Rochi, Tavoni, Montanari, & Garagiola, 1989), the Research Institute for Rheumatic Diseases in Slovakia (Tauchmannova, Gabrhel, & Cibak, 1993), the Department of Physiology from the Ruhr-Universität in Bochum, Germany (Hunold, Mietzsch, & Werner, 1992), began to perform in depth investigations in populations of athletes. Therefore, most of the studies related to thermography in the field of sports are quite old, but they conclude that, even when the resolution and validity of the cameras used where not as good as modern ones, IRT could be helpful for the diagnosis of injuries and an ideal tool for monitoring the progress of lesions and the effectiveness of their treatment (Binder et al., 1983; Busoni, Romagnoli, Bagnolesi, & Gemignani, 1988; Devereaux et al., 1986; Devereaux et al., 1984; Garagiola & Giani, 1990; Giani et al., 1989; Keyl & Lenhart, 1975). It must be noted that most of the studies published by this time were conducted in the medical field to diagnose diseases or injuries.

From the mid-1990s until recently, research in the field of sports has declined considerably, potentially because they were rapidly superseded by newer and objective diagnostic methods, such as magnetic resonance and low intensity radiographic equipment; leading to the decline of research on the use of thermography in sports medicine and physical therapy in humans, remaining only in the veterinary sector, specifically in the field of equestrian competition to detect diseases in racehorses (Autio, Neste, Airaksinen, & Heiskanen, 2006; Ciutacu, Tanase, & Miclaus, 2006; Kulesza, Rzeczkowski, & Kaczorowski, 2004; Turner, 1991).

Recently, there has been a significant increase of publications regarding this topic. In 2007, a group from the University of Ljubijana (Slovenia) (Čoh & Širok, 2007) and the pemaSiP research group from the Faculty of Sciences for Physical Activity and Sport -INEF- (UPM, Spain) (Gómez Carmona & Noya Salces, 2008) began to investigate the application of IRT for non-diagnostic purposes in the field of physical activity and sports. Research groups from:

- Austria (Hildebrandt, 2009; Hildebrandt et al., 2010),
- United States (Sands, McNeal, & Stone, 2011),
- Japan (Miyamoto, Hara, Nishimura, & Yano, 2004),
- Spain (Fernández Cuevas et al., 2011; Gómez Carmona, 2012; Sillero Quintana, Gómez Carmona, Noya Salces, Núñez, & Fernández Rodríguez, 2009; Fernández-Cuevas et al., 2015; Sillero et al., 2015; Priego Quesada et al., 2016),
- Serbia (Badža, Jovančević, Fratrić, Roglić, & Sudarov, 2012),
- Australia (Costello, Stewart, Selfe, Karki, & Donnelly, 2013),
- Brasil (Bandeira, Borba Neves, Muniz de Moura, & Nohama, 2014; Bandeira, Muniz de Moura, Abreu de Souza, Nohama, & Borba Neves, 2012; Bouzas Marins et al., 2014; da Rosa Vieira et al., 2003, Barcelos et al., 2014)
- Italy (Merla, 2005; Formenti et al., 2013 and 2016) and
- Portugal (Oliveira et al., 2016).

These are some of the research groups that have published interesting works about IRT, exercise and the new applications in the last years. Nevertheless, the number of publications and international research groups are significantly increasing since 2014.

Recent Applications of Thermography in Sports

Recent research results have shown new applications for this technique in the fields of physical activity and sports such as the following:

1. The quantification of training workload. This is one of the most promising applications of IRT in the field of physical activity and more concretely for high performance sports. Several authors have concluded that skin temperature could be affected differently depending on the intensity of the exercise workload, i.e., we could rapidly determine if an athlete has assimilated the previous workout by measuring his skin temperature (Tsk) and comparing it with his thermal baseline (Gómez Carmona, 2012). Other authors have shown how Tsk varies depending on the type of training (Fernández-Cuevas et al., 2014) and intensity (Čoh & Širok, 2007; Chudecka & Lubkowska, 2012; Priego Quesada et al., 2016; Korman et al., 2016; Balci et al., 2016), even in relation to heart rate (Arfaoui, Bertucci, Letellier, & Polidori, 2014; Borba Neves et al., 2016) or lactate levels (Akimov & Son'kin, 2011). Nevertheless, this application needs further investigation to establish the Tsk responses depending on the type and intensity of exercise.
2. The detection of anatomical and biomechanical imbalances. Abate et al. (2010) noted another interesting application regarding the detection of anatomical and biomechanical imbalances using IRT. They showed how specific thermal patterns arise as a consequence of the muscle activity associated with postural alteration and how IRT is able to highlight specific functional activations (Abate et al., 2010).
3. The evaluation of fitness and performance conditions. Another important application appears to be the evaluation of fitness and performance condition (Akimov et al., 2009; Chudecka & Lubkowska, 2010b, 2012; Formenti et al., 2013). These studies have shown that thermal skin response after exercise is different depending on fitness condition. For example, untrained subjects have cooler Tsk during exercise and need more time to reach baseline Tsk after exercise (Abate, Di Carlo, Di Donato, Romani, & Merla, 2013; Formenti et al., 2013; Borba Neves et al., 2016; Adamczyk et al., 2016). It could be concluded that untrained people have less efficient thermoregulation processes than trained athletes.
4. The detection of temperature variations during exercise in pregnant women. Exercise is recommended during pregnancy, but it must be controlled to avoid the potential risk of high temperatures to the fetus and Infrared Thermography is a very useful technique for this purpose. Sillero-Quintana and his team performed a study using IRT to control skin temperature during and after yoga and swimming practice in pregnant women (Sillero Quintana, Conde Pascual, Gómez Carmona, Fernández-Cuevas, & García-Pastor, 2012).
5. The detection of delayed onset muscle soreness (DOMS). Al-Nakhli et al. (2012) published a study where they described how DOMS is related to a significant increase of skin temperature 24 hours after an exercise, where elevated skin temperature was associated with muscle damage and pain perception.
6. The prevention and monitoring of injuries. The prevention and monitoring of injuries is currently, without any doubt, the most trending application of IRT in the sports field. Several researchers published results during the 1990s showing the potential of this technique to diagnose, as well as detect overloaded areas and prevent soft tissue injuries (BenEliyahu, 1990; Tauchmannova et al., 1993). Despite a long period without any relevant study in this research line, we have observed

increased interest in the last few years, partially due to the technological improvement of IRT and the innovative initiatives of several research groups (Gómez Carmona, 2012; Hildebrandt et al., 2010; Hildebrandt, Zeilberger, Ring, & Raschner, 2012; Sillero Quintana et al., 2010). Currently, IRT is applied in professional teams as a complementary technology, with the aim of providing immediate thermal information to medical and technical staff to adapt training programs and prevent injuries or reduce the recovery periods (Badža et al., 2012; Bandeira et al., 2014; Costello et al., 2013; Sands et al., 2011; Ramos e Corte & Hernandez, 2016).

7. The evaluation of the efficiency level in the sport. Bertucci et al. (2013) concluded that for a given cycling exercise, it appeared that IR thermography was a powerful tool to appreciate different efficiency levels between cyclists (Bertucci et al., 2013). Priego Quesada and collaborators (2015) also studied the efficiency level in cyclist.
8. The detection of the lactate threshold. Akimov and Son'kin (2011) showed that, for endurance athletes, the lactate threshold approximately correspond to the beginning of the increase in skin temperature after its initial decrease as a result of sweat evaporation.
9. Clothing design and thermal comfort. Most of the IRT applications are focused on performance, fitness and health status of the subject. Nevertheless, there is a parallel research line that is equally important related to clothing design and thermal comfort (Banerjee, Chattopadhyay, & Tuli, 2013). This topic has become more important in the last years due to the improvement and sophistication of sports clothing. Additionally, the relationship between thermal comfort and performance has been proven (Gasi & Bittencourt, 2009; Mao, Luo, Li, Luo, & Wang, 2011; Mijović, Salopek Čubrić, Skenderi, & Reischl, 2012; Purvis & Cable, 2000; Purvis & Tunstall, 2004). Therefore, IRT is an ideal technique to improve the design of sports clothing (Bulut, Janta, Senner, & Kreuzer, 2013; Faulkner et al., 2013; Fournet, Ross, Voelcker, Redortier, & Havenith, 2013).

USING THERMOGRAPHY TO PREVENT AND MONITOR SPORTS INJURIES

From all the possible applications of thermography in physical activity and sports we have selected the prevention and monitoring of sports injuries due to the relevance of injuries in the sports training process. During all this section, we will mainly illustrate those applications with football/soccer players since our experience is mostly focused on this sport. Nevertheless, we can use IRT for those purposes in other sports.

The term "injury" has been deeply linked to sports since its inception and it is currently in vogue due to the significant increase in injuries, largely due to the over-competitive seasons faced by elite performance athletes (Hagglund, Walden, & Ekstrand, 2003; Lewin, 1989; Walden, Hagglund, & Ekstrand, 2005). This high injury rate is particularly accentuated in sports such as football compared with other sports (Junge, Rosch, Peterson, Graf-Baumann, & Dvorak, 2002).

A prospective study by Hoy (1992) in European soccer shows that the average absence from work caused by soccer injuries was 5 days per season, using only all the soccer injuries registered in a Danish hospital during one year. However, Fernandez Cuevas et al. (2010), after directly recording the injuries using the REINLE questionnaire (Javier Noya Salces, Benito Peinado, Calderón, & Gómez Carmona, 2008) in 16 participants in the first Spanish soccer league and 9 from the second league, obtained 14.6 injuries per season in the first division Spanish clubs players and 12,7 days in the second division clubs during the 2008 - 2009 season.

In terms of economic costs, Inklaar (1994) estimated that the direct and indirect soccer injuries cost in Holland was at least $US 65 million. The estimation of the economic costs from work absences in a Spanish study by Fernandez-Cuevas et al. (2010) was performed by relating the quantity of days that the player was injured according to the daily salary in each single case, resulting an estimated cost of more than 102 million € in the studied teams from the first Spanish league and more than 26 million € in the second league. They also estimated an average for the teams where injuries were not directly recorded, basing their estimation on variables such as the relation between the budget of each team and the amount of salaries, number of matches won or lost or final position in the national ranking. The economic cost of work absences for all Spanish soccer teams in the first and second divisions was estimated to be more than 230 million €.

It must be noted that the costs of sports injuries are not only economical for the club or the insurance companies, which have to pay the medical, surgical, physiotherapy costs (Woods, Hawkins, Hulse, & Hodson, 2003) and the payroll of the players, but also have psychological costs for the player, considering the lack of fulfilled goals and the stress that can be generated during the long recovery process. Additionally, there are personal costs accounting for all of the short and long term disturbances that the injury generates in the player's life and the interruption of the athletic career, which may never resume.

Although the preceding data refers to soccer, to understand the relevance of the sports injuries problem, we must consider injuries from the different professional sports, which have more social and even political relevance, as well as injuries that occur during amateur and the leisure sports, which are, considering the number of cases and public health costs, much more important.

The first intervention study using thermography in a professional soccer team that focused on the use of thermography as an injury prevention tool was performed by Gomez-Carmona (2012) in his doctoral dissertation and subsequent publications. He performed a longitudinal study in 35 professional players from a team competing in the Spanish first league. The injuries were recorded during the 2008 and 2009 pre-seasons using the REINLE questionnaire (Noya Salces et al., 2008). Additionally, during the 2009 pre-season, a specific injury prevention protocol supported by the technical and medical team was performed. Thermal reports obtained using IRT, including the ROI from the whole lower limb of each single player, were released daily to the technical and medical staff to support their decisions about the individual and collective contents and load of the training sessions.

The results of this study demonstrated a significant reduction in days of work absence due to injuries of the team players and a significant reduction in the probability of a player injury between both preseasons. The injury rate decreased from 10.36 injuries per 1000 hours of exposition in the 2008 preseason to 4.02 injuries per 1000 hours of exposition in 2009, which was significant data considering that the average injury rate shown by Walden et al. (2005) during the preseason was 8.2 injuries per 1000 hours of exposition. Additionally, the days of training absence due to injuries in all of the team members during the 6 week preseason was reduced from 156 days in 2008 to 14 days in 2009.

An example of IRT use for the monitoring of sport injuries can be seen in the study by Piñonosa et al. (2013), which showed the evolution of an athlete's skin temperature on the affected and not affected limb over an 8-week ACL rehabilitation program after surgical reconstruction of the ligament. The results showed apart from a reduction in the temperature of the injured knee, they registered significant temperature increases in the posterior thigh area between the first and the last week of the rehabilitation process, most likely due to a compensatory mechanism or the effects of the rehabilitation process. It is clear from this study that during the tracking process of an injury we should account for the injured areas as well as the adjacent areas and contralateral limbs. Thermal imbalances or thermal changes in the areas surrounding the injury are particularly dangerous because they can lead to injuries on theoretically "healthy" structures.

Practically, Gomez-Carmona and Sillero (2009) summarized four main applications of thermography that could be useful for the technical teams surrounding the athlete:

Evaluative Medical Examination

IRT reports may help to evaluate objectively, quickly and non-invasively the status of an athlete. This application is extremely useful for a first assessment of athletes after holiday periods, intensive training periods, and calls for participating with national teams or when clubs are contracting a new player.

Thermography is a technique that allows us to identify potential muscle, joint and even nervous disturbances or injuries. An infrared image of an athlete provides an opportunity to locate hot spots, which can be directly related to chronic or recently recovered injuries. This initial assessment helps identify risk areas where it would be necessary to verify using a more objective method to determine how harmful or limiting the risk area is to the athlete's performance in the future.

To demonstrate the applicability of thermography as an evaluative method in medical examinations, figure 1 shows the frontal and dorsal thermograms from the lower limbs of a junior soccer player who volunteered for an academic study (Iglesias-Gutierrez, 2014).

A qualitative examination of the thermogram clearly shows a heat source in the right knee (and thigh) and the quantitative analysis identified a thermal asymmetry of 4.1 °C in that area. The player had not experienced any physical disability or discomfort. As the local club lacked a medical service and he was not aware of any vascular problem in his legs, the player was recommended to public medical

Figure 1. Anterior and posterior views of the first evaluation of a young soccer player's lower limbs
Source: Iglesias-Gutierrez, 2014

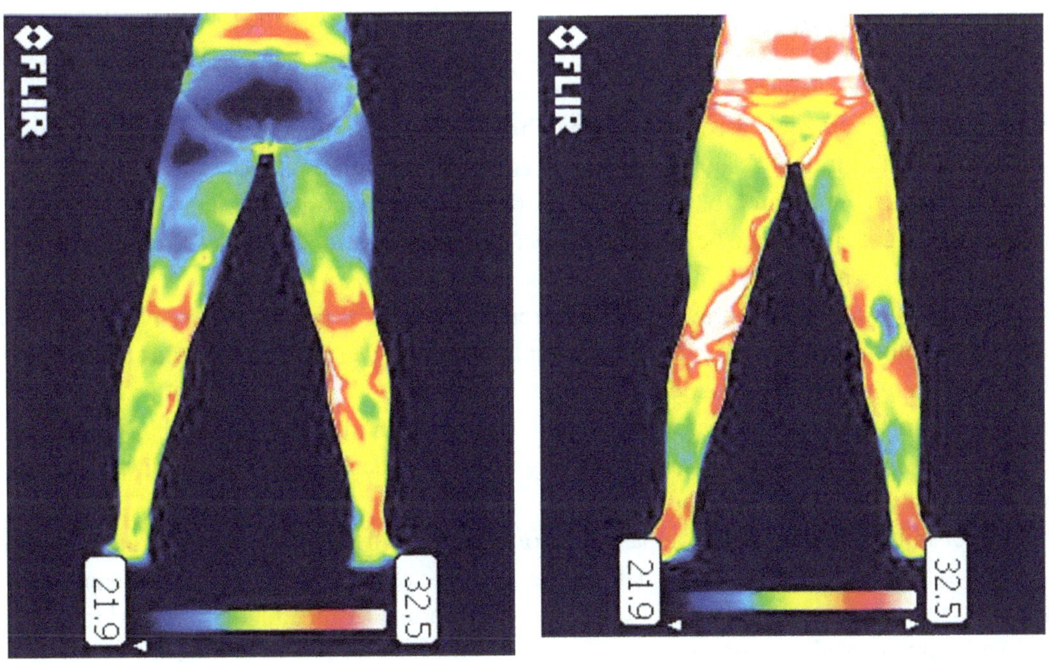

services; they automatically accepted the case for further analysis in a hospital where he was diagnosed with moderate phlebostatic syndrome and underwent an emergency vascular surgery at the hospital. Most likely, if the young player had practiced high-level physical activity for a longer time (or perhaps when he had stopped it) the vascular problem could have resulted in serious consequences for his health.

Sports Injury Prevention

Gomez Carmona et al. (2011) suggest that injury prevention is one of the most important applications of thermography in sports. Infrared thermography allows us to prevent muscle, joint or bone injuries by detecting potential overload and fatigue symptoms before they develop, almost irreparably, into an injury.

Athletes are exposed to a high risk of injury, which is directly related to their level of training. All professionals involved with physical activity sports must know and use the necessary methods to overcome this problem. IRT can be a method that will help us reduce the high "injury incidence" in athletes, a term coined by Fuller et al. (2006) to quantify the number of injuries per 1000 hours of exposure to the activity.

Consequently, we must consider the direct relationship between the increase in temperature, directly related to the emission of infrared radiation from a body area overloaded by training or competition, and harmful risk. The infrared radiation emitted by the human body depends on the flow and subcutaneous circulatory blood volume and the metabolic activity of various body systems (Thomas, Siahamis, Marion, & Boyle, 1992). Practically, both factors (i.e., increased blood flow and metabolism) could be only one factor because an area with increased metabolism also has increased blood flow.

Therefore, an increase in temperature produced by overload or fatigue after training can be due to two factors: first, a greater demand for blood from highly capillarized tissues; and second, an increase in cell metabolism of the damaged structures due to the regenerative processes following excessive muscle activation. This generates fatigue or overloading, which have been indicated as the primary cause of injury (Mair, Seaber, Glisson, & Garrett, 1996; Petibois, Cazorla, Poortmans, & Deleris, 2002).

We should analyze the evolution of the same area over time and examine the asymmetries between contralateral Regions of Interest (ROI) (i.e., left vs. right side). Figure 2 shows the reference values of asymmetry between contralateral limbs to facilitate decisions about the relevance of thermal asymmetry on injury prevention protocols based on the research by Gómez Carmona (2012).

A difference of 0.3 to 0.4ºC should lead to an intervention only if it is repeated in two different measurements and accounting for the fact that in sports with dominant sides (tennis, football, judo, etc.) the laterality of the athletes should be considered because specialization generates thermal asymmetries that are completely normal.

For differences of 0.5 to 1.0ºC preventive measurements should be performed even if the athlete does not manifest symptoms of discomfort or injury mainly when the thermal asymmetries have progressed from lower values in previous evaluations.

Values of 1.0 to 1.5ºC are, in most cases, an indication of high injury risk and when values are over 1.5ºC, the lesion will soon occur if it has not already occurred. The athlete most likely will complain of pain either in the hyperthermic or an adjacent area.

The key for injury prevention is comparing records and highlighting where there are considerable variations from the mean over time. The daily or periodic monitoring of an athlete (or team) allows us to identify the thermal response of each of the body parts worked by an athlete. In regard to preventing injuries, we need to consider two perspectives:

Figure 2. References of thermal asymmetry values for the decision making during injury prevention protocols
Source: Based on Gomez Carmona, 2012

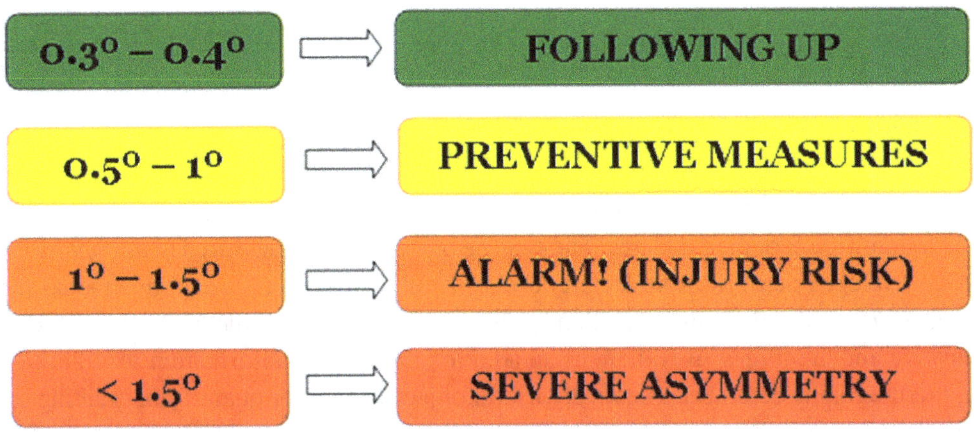

1. **Individual Comparison:** In both individual sports and team sports, injury prevention is based on the frequent comparison of the temperature recordings of each athlete over a period of training and competition. The frequency of the evaluation of the athletes and the number of considered ROI should be as high as possible to be successful. If it is not possible to perform and evaluate a high number of ROI daily, as in the work of Gomez-Carmona (2012), it would be interesting to perform the assessments close to high intensity trainings. These evaluations should occur before training when we suspect any physical problem of the athlete to consider a reduction in the intensity or volume of the training session, or the day after training when we want to assess the effects of the training and the athlete's level of recovery. Another option would be assessing the athletes after the "recovery day" of the training microcycle to estimate the level of assimilation of the training load or recovery.
2. **Group Comparison:** Comparisons between the different members of the team or the averaged values of the group can be performed if they have the same training loads and / or competitions. This analysis may help us to identify the different assimilation effects of the training load for a particular athlete of the group who will require a personalization of the training on that day, or for the whole group, which may lead to a general modification of the contents of the training season.

Tracking the Sport Injury Recovery

In the fields of physical activity and sports, it is important not only to prevent injuries but also to optimize the rehabilitation process of the athlete.

When the athletes are already injured, IRT allows us to track the injured areas, monitoring the evolution of the lesion and determining when the athlete is in good condition to initiate normal training. It is possible to do so by comparing the temperature values during rehabilitation with normal temperatures from the athlete before the injury or with data from the contralateral area in cases where bilateral comparison is possible.

Thermography is also very useful during the recovery process because it can identify the stress caused by the rehabilitation and both the physical therapist and the athlete can be aware of the effects of the work performed. Psychologically, this information should be controlled because the knowledge of the process may encourage the athletes to work harder during the rehabilitation protocol or discourage their work because the effects of the rehabilitation process does not appear to be as fast as it should be.

Quantification of the Training Load

Currently, physical activity and sports professionals have different means to measure the assimilation of the physical training loads of their athletes. They can be objective (i.e., measured in units, such as amount of kilometers, averaged heart rate and lactate levels) or subjective (i.e., based on personal feelings as the perceived exertion questionnaires fulfilled by the athlete). These parameters are not conclusive, but rather indicative and the trainer uses them as an additional source of information for training process. Therefore, thermography could become a very useful objective tool for quantifying training loads.

Through daily or periodic recording of the athlete's body temperature before starting the training session, the individual and group training thermal profile can be established and these daily records can be compared to determine the thermal behavior of the areas evaluated and how they have reacted to the training loads of the previous days.

The interpretation of the skin temperature results obtained by IRT immediately after exercise is still a challenging research topic, which will be briefly analyzed below. The acute, short- and long-term effects of the different training loads (for example, aerobic and anaerobic training, different strength training or speed training) are very complex and differentiated (Fernandes Ade et al., 2014; Fernández-Cuevas, 2012; Fernández-Cuevas et al., 2014; Korman et al., 2016) and they have to be determined in future research.

In the following section, several important points on IRT usage as an injury prevention tool or for monitoring sport injures will be developed.

Is Infrared Thermography a Diagnostic Tool?

After reviewing medical and legal journals from 1956 until 1991 related to thermography applications in musculoskeletal and neurological medicine, Awerduch (1991) concluded that little evidence existed of any thermography application that was unequivocally superior to conventional diagnostic imaging methods.

This conclusion substantially differs from Mikulska (2006), who suggested that early problems, such as low detector sensitivity and poor training of thermography technicians, was the source of error in thermography and hindered acceptance of this technique until 1990. Mikulska also stated that thermographic equipment has significantly evolved since 1990 and modern thermal imaging systems are coupled to computers with sophisticated software solutions, improving the quality of the recorded images and their further analysis to obtain more reliable information. Mikulska concluded that IRT is a reliable diagnostic method in clinical medicine and rejected the principles outlined by the European Association of Thermology, which has reduced the acceptance of this technique during medical diagnosis.

Between both extreme positions concerning the diagnostic value of IRT, there are many alternatives. It is clear that there are many tools that are more reliable and objective than IRT for medical diagnosis (i.e., radiography, MRI, ultrasound, and other imaging diagnostic tools); however, no other method is as safe, fast, portable, inexpensive and non-invasive than IRT.

We have always thought that IRT is an excellent tool for supporting medical diagnosis (Noya Salces, Sillero Quintana, Gómez Carmona, & Pastrano León, 2009). This position has also been recently defended by Bandeira and collaborators (2014) who stated that IRT can provide the practitioner with excellent additional information to identify the existence of dysfunction or thermal asymmetry in an area of the body. Most recently, the work of Sillero and collaborators (2015) showed how useful IRT could be in an Emergency Unit to help diagnosing. Nevertheless, it is important to highlight that IRT should be not use to diagnose, but helping the health professionals to get the right diagnosis thanks to the fast, non-invasive and objective information, and obviously the help of other technologies and techniques.

Apart from the example in Figure 1, we would like to refer to a non-published case of a 16 year old student who arrived at the emergency unit of a trauma clinic where a prospective study was being performed (Figure 3). He was injured when he was running during his physical education class. His diagnosis was a moderate muscle tear in the right quadriceps. The frontal image clearly shows how, even when the patient had applied an anti-inflammatory cream, the right quadriceps exhibited an altered thermogram in this area, which could benefit from a further diagnostic using ultrasound. However, the ultrasound would not have detected the vascular issue in the lateral part of the right thigh. The injury should be assessed using an appropriate methodology to determine whether the vascular problem could have influenced the injury occurrence or if it was produced by the injury.

Considering the slight vascular problems perceived in the lateral thermogram of the left (i.e., uninjured) limb and the high temperature of the feet, which was most likely promoted by poor venous return from the lower limbs, the practitioner could conclude that the injury is a result of serious vascular problems in the 16 year old patient and perform the appropriate diagnostic test. Subsequently, the physician could propose an injury prevention or intervention protocol to reduce the probability of more severe problems in the patient in the future.

Figure 3. First thermograms of a 16 year old patient diagnosed with a moderated quadriceps tear
Source: Non-published data from CEMTRO Clinic and TermoINEF

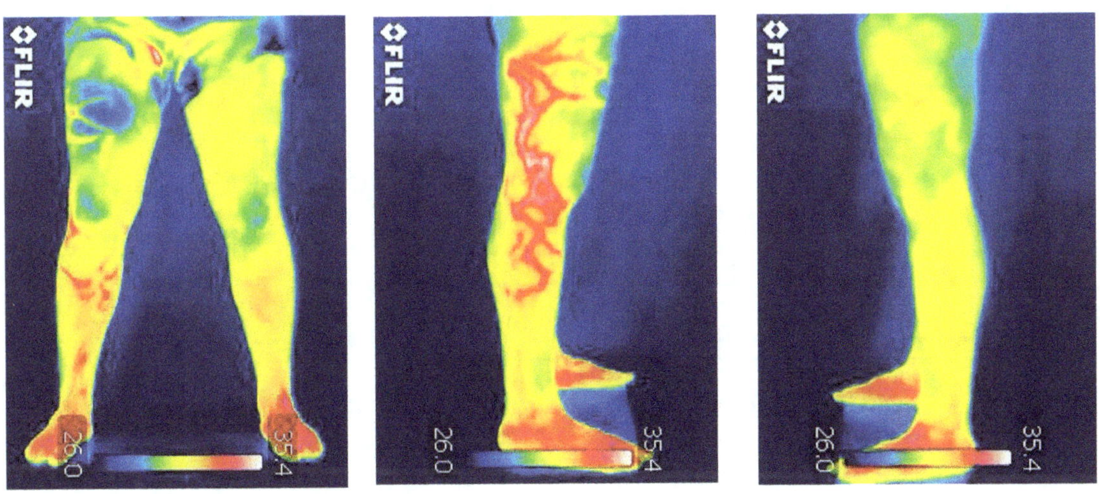

The Effects of Exercise on Skin Temperature

The possible uses of IRT for preventing and monitoring sports and physical activity injuries are clear; however, there is little knowledge and data regarding how Tsk behaves during and immediately following exercise (E. Akimov & Son'kin, 2011; Chudecka & Lubkowska, 2010b, 2012; Fernandes Ade et al., 2014; Merla, Mattei, Di Donato, & Romani, 2010).

Generally (see Figure 4), during and after exercise the hypothalamus attempts to maintain a stable body temperature. However, factors such as exercise intensity (Stannard, Brandenburg, Pitney, & Lukaszuk, 2011), increased metabolism during and after exercise (Knab et al., 2011), and the EPOC effect (LaForgia, Withers, & Gore, 2006) elevate the body temperature (and also the Tsk). On the other hand, vasoconstriction in peripheral areas (Nisha Charkoudian, 2003), blood flow redistribution (Charkoudian, 2010) and sweating (Pascoe, Mercer, & de Weerd, 2007) tend to decrease Tsk.

Many studies have been published in the previous decades that focused on the thermal effects of exercise on Tsk (Fernández-Cuevas, 2012). The first study used IRT to measure the effects of exercise in patients with deep vein thrombosis to detect vein occlusions (Cooke & Picher, 1974). Several years later, Clark et al. (Clark, Mullan et al., 1977) performed a study in which healthy subjects were assessed using IRT prior to and following running, reporting for the first time a 'dramatically' different thermal distribution following exercise, with increased Tsk over the muscles that were used in the activity. Recently, it was conclusively demonstrated that high-resolution thermal images can provide interesting information regarding the complex thermoregulation system of the body (Hildebrandt et al., 2010).

Many authors have described the use of IRT to measure the thermal response of Tsk in different body areas or ROIs under different conditions of intensity, duration, discipline, fitness level and ambient tem-

Figure 4. Factors that increase or decrease Tsk under exercise conditions

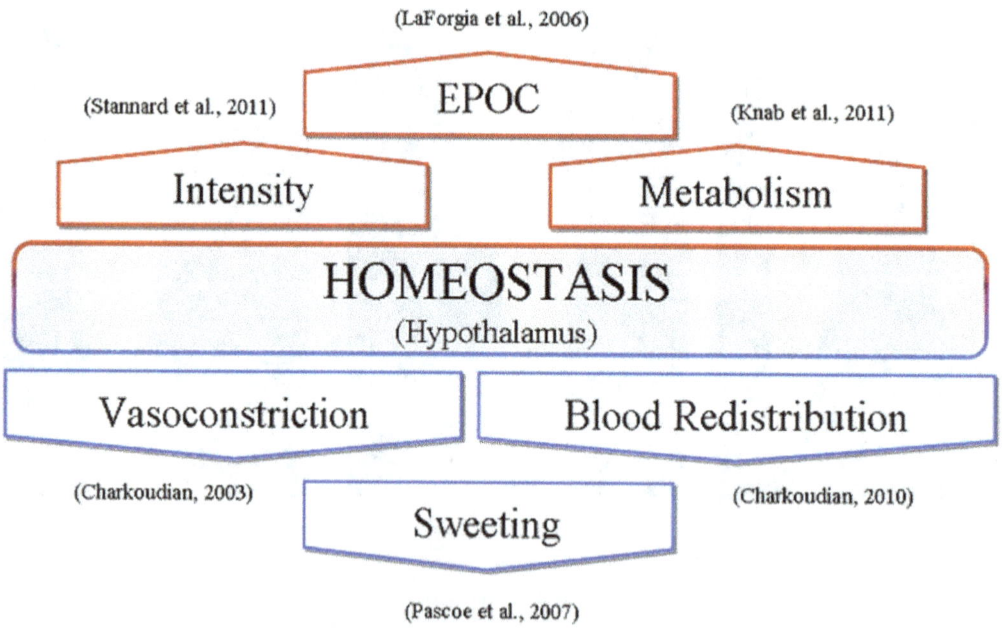

perature (Arfaoui, Polidori, Taiar, & Popa, 2012; Bonnett, Hare, Jones, Ring, & Hare, 2006; Chudecka & Lubkowska, 2010b, 2012; Chudecka, Szczepanowska, & Kempinska, 2008; Ferreira et al., 2008; Hildebrandt et al., 2012; Hirata, Nagasaka, & Noda, 1989; Hunold et al., 1992; Liu, Mimura, Wang, & Ikuda, 2003; Merla, Di Donato, & Romani, 2002; Merla et al., 2005; Merla et al., 2010; Nakayama, Ohnuki, & Kanosue, 1981; Pascoe, Skelton, Smith, Kremer, & Purohit, 1992; Torii, Yamasaki, & Sasaki, 1987; Torii, Yamasaki, Sasaki, & Nakayama, 1992; Vainer, 2005; Veghte et al., 1979; Wade & Veghte, 1977; Wang & Toh, 2001; Zaïdi, Taiar, Fohanno, & Polidori, 2007; Zontak, Sideman, Verbitsky, & Beyar, 1998)

The majority of studies in which the subjects were exposed to constant and prolonged exercise resulted in an increased Tsk (Clark, Mullan et al., 1977; Ferreira et al., 2008; Hildebrandt et al., 2012; Hirata et al., 1989; Hunold et al., 1992; Veghte et al., 1979; Wade & Veghte, 1977; Wang & Toh, 2001; Zaïdi et al., 2007). In contrast, graded, intermittent or maximal exercises, normally performed for a brief period, resulted in decreased Tsk (Akimov & Son'kin, 2011; Chudecka & Lubkowska, 2010b, 2012; Chudecka et al., 2008; Merla et al., 2005; Nakayama et al., 1981; Torii et al., 1987). Nevertheless, other factors also to the type of exercise (as the intensity), the environment (ambient temperature, outdoor-indoor activity) and the nature of the activity or sport may have also a significant influence.

It should be noted that not all studies analyze the same body areas and certain studies report opposite thermal responses during the same exercise conditions depending on the evaluated ROI (e.g., the extremities, the active musculature or the core) and its involvement in the performed exercise (Clark, Mullan et al., 1977; Vainer, 2005). There are exceptions that make this factor even more complex, with discordant results perhaps being due to inactive subjects (Bonnett et al., 2006), the special characteristics of the exercise (Zaïdi et al., 2007) or the selection of the analyzed ROI (D. D. Pascoe et al., 1992; Zontak et al., 1998).

It should also be considered that the long-term thermal behaviour of the skin after exercise may depend on the impact of physical activity on the thermoregulation system and metabolism. Certain studies monitored Tsk following exercise, reporting the tendency for Tsk to recover to the thermal baseline (Akimov & Son'kin, 2011; Merla et al., 2010). However, the normal Tsk pattern is affected for many hours following exercise, more in some areas than others depending on the activity of the structures below the considered ROI and in a different manner according to the type of exercise (Fernández-Cuevas, 2012). Further research is required to determine the duration of the thermal effects that occur following exercise in different body areas, as well as the effects of the type of exercise, its intensity, duration and the fitness level of the athlete.

Lack of Reference Patterns

The establishment of reference values for each sport and any other population group is crucial for the proper analysis of thermographic results. The normal thermal profile of healthy subjects should be considered symmetric with normal side-to-side difference values of 0.25°C ± 0.2°C in total body views and 0.2°C ± 0.15°C in regional views (Vardasca, 2008). Considering that point, side-to-side asymmetries in skin temperatures can be used to identify abnormalities, prevent injuries (Bouzas Marins et al., 2014; Gómez Carmona, 2012; Hildebrandt et al., 2012) or monitor the healing of a sports injury (Sillero Quintana et al., 2010).

Sport specialization could affect normal thermal patterns in healthy subjects (Tauchmannova et al., 1993). Athletes who participate in different sports have been assessed using IRT. These studies have been performed on athletes that participate in running (Clark, Mullan et al., 1977; Merla et al., 2010), swimming (Ludwig, Formenti, Gargano, & Alberti, 2014; Wade & Veghte, 1977; Zaïdi et al., 2007), tennis (Smith, Bandler, & Goodman, 1986), football (Bouzas Marins et al., 2014; Gómez Carmona, 2012; Tauchmannova et al., 1993), handball (Buckhout & Warner, 1980; Chudecka & Lubkowska, 2010b; Chudecka et al., 2008), cycling (Bertucci et al., 2013; Malkinson, 2002), rowing (Tauchmannova et al., 1993), basketball (Chudecka & Lubkowska, 2011; Sampedro, Piñonosa Cano, & Fernández-Cuevas, 2012), judo (Arnaiz Lastras et al., 2011), water polo (Chudecka & Lubkowska, 2010a), wrestling and weight lifting (Tauchmannova et al., 1993), volleyball (Chudecka & Lubkowska, 2012), American football (Garza et al., 2008), rugby (Bandeira et al., 2014; Selfe et al., 2014), gymnastics (Pušnik & Čuk, 2014; Sands et al., 2011), and skiing (Hildebrandt, 2009), as well as less conventional athletic disciplines, such as Taijiquan (Liu et al., 2003).

These studies are important because, as certain publications have shown, specialization can lead to sport-specific, but "normal" asymmetries. The study by Gomez-Carmona (2012) determined the normal thermal profile of elite Spanish soccer players, which was characterized, after excluding injured players, by thermally symmetric lower limbs except for the maximal and average values of the ankle in the anterior view with statistically significant differences of 0.18 and 0.30 ºC, respectively, and higher values on the dominant leg side. This asymmetry could be a result of the biomechanical or physiological specialization generated by the repetitive use of the dominant leg in soccer. Contrarily, in a study performed in junior Brazilian high-level soccer players the thermal profile was symmetric (Bouzas Marins et al., 2014); however, it should be considered that the ROI were only the legs and thighs, without considering the ankles.

Similar asymmetric results due to sport specialization have been reported in other sports such as judo (Arnaiz Lastras et al., 2011), where bilateral significant differences ($p<0.05$) were observed on the dorsal exterior forearm, with an upper 0.4-degree difference in favor of the hand-dominant side that has to perform a strong grip on the adversary's kimono. Another example is the higher dominant-hand thermal values in tennis and baseball pitchers (Smith et al., 1986).

We could generalize that in cyclic symmetric sports, such as running, rowing or cycling, the normal profile should be symmetric; however, asymmetric profiles should be observed for clear hand or foot dominance sports or physical activities, such as fencing or even in populations of supermarket cashiers. Potential asymmetry due to physiological specialization should be expected; however, properly designed research should be performed to confirm this hypothesis and to create a thermal pattern for each sport, any type of work or physical activity and even for each individual, to aid in the appropriate interpretation of acquired thermograms.

An example that illustrates perfectly the necessity of individual thermal patterns to implement injury prevention protocols appeared in the doctoral dissertation of Gomez-Carmona (2012) (Figure 5). One of the players participating in the study produced the thermogram in Figure 5 during his first evaluation. Surprisingly, the subject did not report any discomfort or injury in recent months. However, his injury history included two ACL surgical interventions, and he was the captain of the team; he was older and had been an international player at the highest level for over 10 years. His normal asymmetry in the knees was 1.5ºC, something that could be easily interpreted as a high injury risk if the personal circumstances were not considered; however, he had no injuries during the preseason. After two assessments with similar results, the team considered a 1.5ºC difference as a normal baseline instead of the symmetry for the knees and reported thermal alterations when the differences were over 1.8º-2.0ºC instead of 0.3-0.5ºC.

This is an example of how an incorrect interpretation of the player's background and influencing factors on the thermogram could lead to erroneous conclusions, which may result in a coach or doctor deciding to keep the player out of training or competition.

Figure 5. First thermogram of a player from a Spanish first division club
Source: Gómez Carmona, 2012

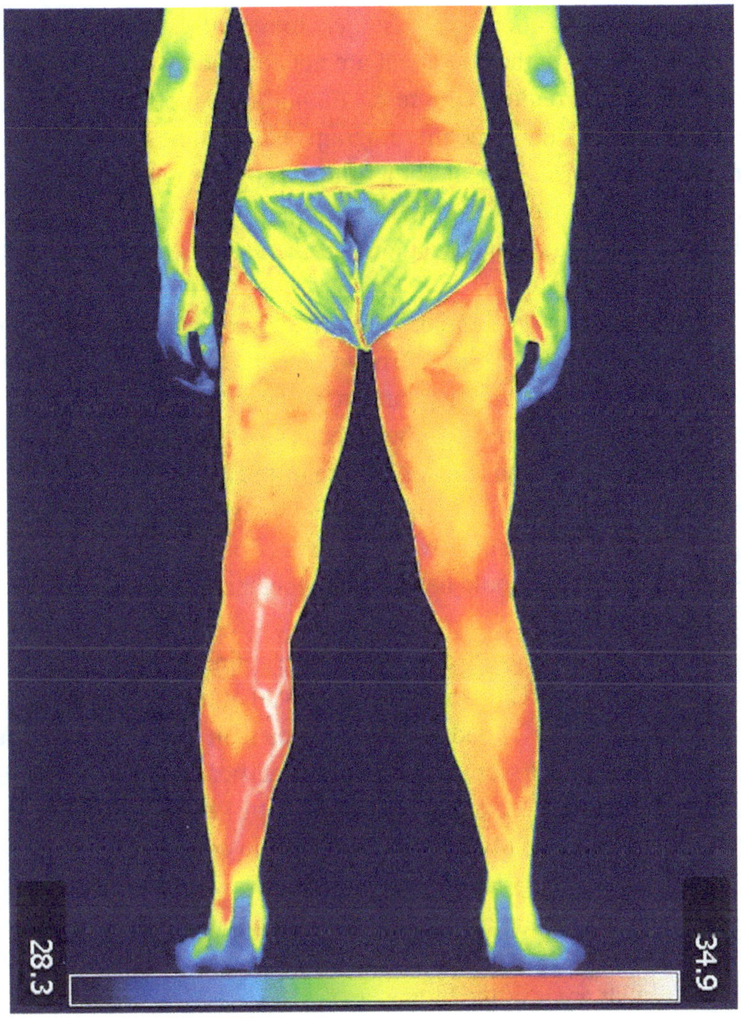

To finish the discussion of thermal patterns, it is interesting to mention an approach used to perform body mapping of different subjects to create a general thermal pattern of the group (Fournet, Redortier, & Havenith, 2012; Fournet et al., 2013). The aim of this approach is to integrate the information provided by each pixel of the thermogram included in the human shape into an ideal representation of the body while retaining the proportions of the original body. The result is an ideal human shape in which each pixels is the average of the corresponding pixels of every real person analyzed.

Delimitation of the Regions of Interest

Of the large number of academies, associations and societies, the European Association of Thermology (EAT) has been one of the most active in previous years in publishing IRT-related studies. Importantly, the EAT has contributed studies performed by the group from the University of Glamorgan, which has worked to better understand the technical factors that affect IRT measurements and to create a strict protocol for reducing errors and increasing the accuracy and the precision of temperature measurements. Their research is summarized in the Glamorgan Protocol (Ammer, 2008), which describes the conditions of data collection and positions of the subject to record the thermogram properly; however, the 90 regions of interest included in the document are not commonly used today in the field of injury prevention. Glamorgan's protocol regions of interest do not always correspond with typically injured areas, they have matching points in the same thermogram and, in some cases, the positions are difficult to reach or maintain when the subject has pain or a limited range of motion due to injury.

Generally, during thermography application in humans, particularly in the prevention and monitoring of injury, the ideal is that the delimitations of regions of interest are made based on the anatomical and functional regions of the human body.

In many studies, the delimitation of the ROI is usually achieved with rectangles (Bouzas Marins et al., 2014; Fernandes Ade et al., 2014; Marins, Fernandes et al., 2014; Marins, Moreira et al., 2014) or polygons (Piñonosa et al., 2013) edited with the standard software provided by the camera. The selection of the ROI is performed manually to ensure that the objectivity of the data collection protocol is reduced because the area selection always depends on the criteria or the researcher.

The delimitation of regions of interest in some studies is performed by locating landmarks on anatomical points to standardize the limits of the recorded area (Bouzas Marins et al., 2014). Therefore, it should be considered that the markers should never be included in the selected area because the averaged values obtained would be altered.

However, it would be ideal if the regions of interest were delineated automatically to avoid the subjectivity involved in determining the ROI manually. As a model of how the determination and collection of the data from the ROI should be performed, we will comment on some of the technical characteristics of Termotracker®, a non-commercial software that was specifically designed to analyze human IRT images by the Thermography research group of the Faculty of Physical Activity and Sport Sciences-INEF from the Technical University of Madrid (TermoINEF) in collaboration with several institutions.

The software is capable of analyzing IRT images from four views of a subject (Anterior and Posterior, Upper and Lower body) and to computationally recognize and trace 78 ROIs based on an algorithm for computer vision that can identify key anatomical points, without any external markers. The ROIs are based on articular and muscular areas of the human anatomy (as shown in Figure 6).

From the total number of pixels, Termotracker® extracts from each ROI the maximum, minimum and mean temperature with the standard deviation (SD). A comprehensive report of the validation process of the software Termotracker® can be obtained in the doctoral dissertation of Fernandez-Cuevas (2012).

Currently, there is a lack of specific software for the delimitation of areas of interest and releasing semiautomatic individual or group reports in a timely manner. The development of such software would enable the widespread application of thermography by doctors, physiotherapists and sports coaches in both the sports context as well as in the field of physical activity. Nevertheless, in the recent years, we observe and augmentation of commercial software solutions as the one proposed by the Italian company next2u or the new version of Termotracker®, known as ThermoHuman, using the same validated algorithms but with better interface and features.

Another typical problem in the delimitation of the ROIs is the concavity of the skin surface. A main factor that is likely to affect IRT recording is the angle that is subtended by the camera axis on the surface to be measured. Ammer (Kurt Ammer, 2003) described that small losses begin to occur for angles greater than 30° and that the loss of information becomes critical for 60° angles, which may lead to inaccurate temperature readings. Chen et al. (Chen, Jiang, Zheng, Liu, & Zhu, 2005) explained in their study that

Figure 6. Distribution of the 78 Regions of Interest (ROI) that are made by Termotracker® software for IRT image analysis

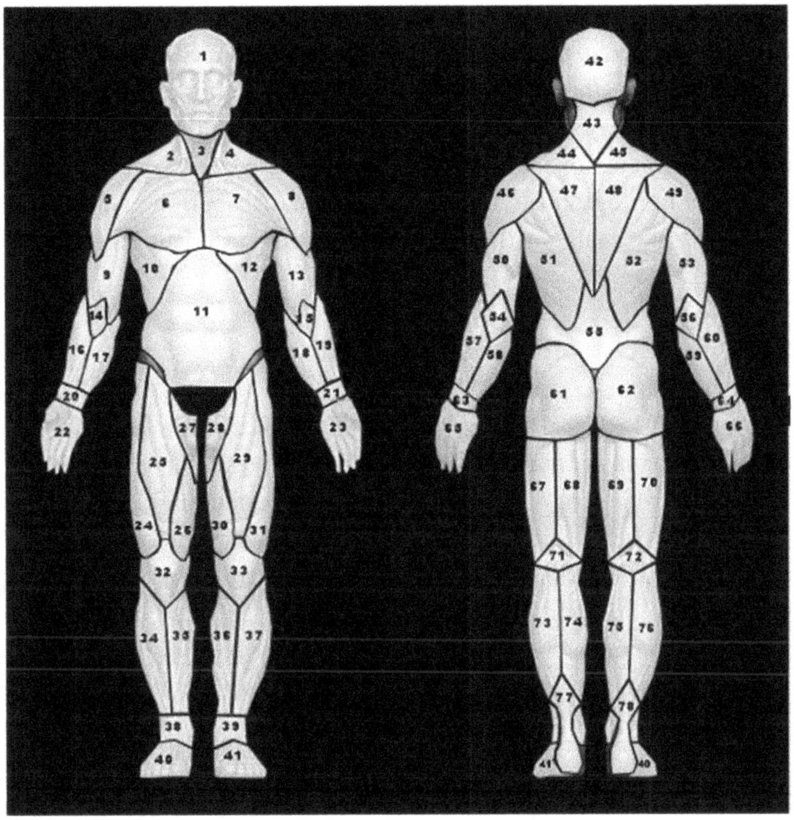

the loss of information due to the angle of view is based on Lambert's law and could be mathematically corrected. It appears that a perpendicular angle is the most desirable option for obtaining more accurate readings and an angle of more than 60° results in a critical loss of information. Considering the anatomical structure of the human body, new techniques, such as the application of Infrared in 3D, may be a solution for reducing the influence of the angle of view on thermal data (Cheng, Bai, & Chen, 2009). However, this technology is still under development and the integration of the data from different thermograms to obtain a 3D image from the body must be integrated in thermographic systems. This will be the ultimate step for the evolution of thermography use in humans.

Until 3D thermography is fully developed, to avoid the effects of the concavity of the surface, the ROI that is to be recorded should be as perpendicular as possible to the camera axis and the delimitation of the area (both in the manual or automatic selections) should exclude the limits of the human shape that have wider incidence angles with the camera axis.

Averaged Versus Maximal Values of Skin Temperatures

The majority of authors have used averaged ROI temperatures to express their results. However, averaged values may have errors because the body areas are usually traced manually. When ROIs are manually selected, they can include certain pixels from the background or from the borders of the ROI, which may exhibit lower temperature values. Therefore, the average temperature of the ROI would be lower than the actual value. In these cases, the use of maximal temperatures may be a solution.

A recent study by Ludwing and his collaborators (Ludwig et al., 2014) presented a critical comparison between the methods mainly used in the literature, i.e., average and maximal temperature. They found a high correlation between both methods, concluding that they can equally represent temperature trends in cutaneous thermographic analyses. Nevertheless, other authors continue to use both methods to better illustrate skin thermal behaviors (Bouzas Marins et al., 2014).

Other authors have used histograms to represent the data distribution and to detect possible errors (Vainer, 2005) or more complex mathematical modelling based on statistical principles for IRT analysis (Deng & Liu, 2004).

Inability to Compare Data from Different Studies

Apart from other intrinsic, extrinsic and technical factors (Fernández-Cuevas, 2012), environmental factors, such as ambient temperature or humidity, have led thermologists to obtain results that are widely variable, particularly when data from different studies are considered. For example, a comprehensive literature review has recently been published concerning the temperature of the human knee, which obtained quite variable temperature results (K Ammer, 2012). These differences complicate the comparison or discussion of the results of one study with different studies published in the literature or even with their own results obtained in another study.

Several methods can be used to standardize the temperatures to allow comparison of the results from different studies performed under different conditions.

Normalization of Temperatures

Normalization is a common technique to compare data from different sources. "Z" values from different studies are comparable because they become independent of the general averaged temperature and their standard deviation. Therefore, although the absolute data are quite different, the similarities and differences among the considered ROI in both studies can be compared.

The Phantom model was established in the 1980s after recording many anthropometric variables in a large sample of subjects (male and female). The result was an equation to convert the direct anthropometric measurements into "Z" values, which were also proportional to the height of the subject and the averaged values for this variable from the Phantom model. The result was a metaphoric and "unisex" model that could be used as a reference for any subject or group of subjects. The "Z" values were represented as a graph with "0" in the middle of the "X" axis and the results are spots in the graph with their variable names in the "Y" axis. This graph allows the identification of which variables are under- or over-normal values (Ross, Ward, Leahy, & Day, 1982).

The development of a "Thermal Phantom Model" would normalize and equalize Tsk considering average whole-body temperatures (or any other reference for Tsk or even core temperature) from both my subject and the Phantom. Therefore, any ROI with an abnormal Tsk would be detected by comparing the results obtained with those of the equivalent ROI in the model. However, the creation of this thermal Phantom model would be only possible through a coordinated multinational project to agree on the ROI to be included into the model, collect a considerable amount of data from people with different races, genders and age ranges, to finally obtain the averaged values and their standard deviations to insert in the obtained equations of the model.

Equations to Estimate Standard Conditions

Ambient temperature and humidity has a direct relationship with the Tsk measured by IRT. In a practical study (Gómez Carmona, 2012), the Tsk of different ROIs from the lower limb were tracked in professional soccer players during a 6-week training period. The training facilities used for the data collection did not allow for control of the environmental conditions for some of the 31 evaluations performed. The range of temperatures of the study was between 18.0ºC and 31.0ºC, with an average ambient temperature of 22.7ºC and a standard deviation of 3.1ºC. The variability of skin temperatures according to the background temperature suggested that the researchers should perform a correlation analysis, which showed an almost perfect direct relationship between the room temperatures (T-r) and the averaged Tsk measured (Tsk-m) in all the considered ROI (see Figure 7)

The regression equations from Figure X can be used to estimate the Tsk standardized at 21ºC (Tsk-21ºC) from Tsk-m ranging between 18 and 31ºC and the T-r as follows (Gómez Carmona, 2012):

Tsk-21ºC = Tsk-m – [0,198 * (T-r – 21ºC)] (1)

Table 1 shows a comparison of the averaged temperatures for some ROIs recorded in different studies of football players at different room temperatures, both in real data and standardized to 21ºC conditions

Figure 7. Relationship between the room temperature and averaged skin temperatures in 31 measurements. In the upper right corner is the regression equation and its determination coefficient (R^2). Source: Adapted from Gomez Carmona, 2012

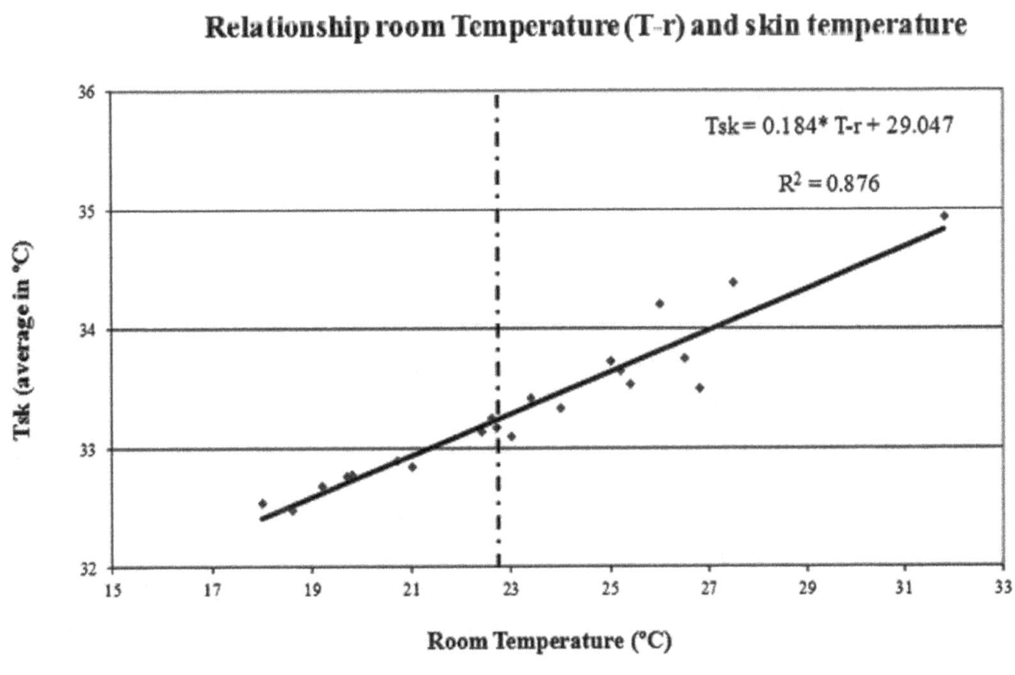

*Table 1. Comparison of middle Tsk from the same ROI in four studies using thermography on soccer players. The results are presented in real mean values (Real) and standardized by the equation: Tsk-21°C = Tsk-m – [0,198 * (T-r – 21°C)]*

	Real	Standard	Real	Standard	Real	Standard	Real	Standard
Ambient Temperature (°C)	22.7°C	21.0°C	21.1°C	21.0°C	17.1°C	21.0°C	15.2°C	21.0°C
DATA	Real	Standard	Real	Standard	Real	Standard	Real	Standard
Anterior Thigh	32.2°C	31.86°C	30.2°C	30.18°C	29.1°C	29.87°C	28.9°C	30.05°C
Posterior Thigh	32.6°C	32.26°C	30.3°C	30.28°C	29.4°C	30.17°C	29.3°C	30.45°C

with the formula 1. A direct relationship can be observed between the room temperature and the real averaged Tsk values in the anterior and posterior thigh and how, after standardizing the results to 21 °C, the differences are much closer to the original data in three of the four studies. It must be noted that the data collection in the study by Gomez-Carmona (2012) was performed daily in an intensive training season and the other three studies were performed after a resting period of at least 24 hours, which can explain the much higher values in this study compared with the other three.

The validity of the above equation can be easily criticized. A comprehensive and methodical study performed with the appropriate randomized acclimatization periods to different ambient weather conditions in a climate chamber with a large group of subjects could determine the effect of different temperatures and humidity levels on the Tsk registered by IRT and establish a more reliable set of equations to standardize the Tsk to ideal environmental conditions.

Proportions Analysis

Another possible solution for comparing our data with other data from a different camera or under different environmental conditions would be to calculate the proportions among the different ROIs. Considering that the relationship between both sets of data is linear and direct, the proportions between the Tsk values of the different ROIs of the body should remain constant independent of the environmental conditions and the camera used.

This approach can be used, as we will see below, for analyzing the temperatures of different areas of the spine, as well as the thigh, knee, leg and ankle in the lower limb or the shoulder, arm, elbow, forearm and wrist in the upper limb. The applicability of this approach depends on the establishment of an agreement on the proportions that will serve as a reference model in healthy people or in different population groups.

Consider as the Tsk reference model the cervical (32.94°C), dorsal (32.76°C) and lumbar (31.74°C) areas in a specific population and the average Tsk of the three areas (32.48°C). The percentages of these areas (or proportions coefficient dividing by 100) would be: cervical (101.4%), dorsal (100.9%) and lumbar (97.7%). If a subject has an injury in the low back, his/her Tsk would increase mainly in the lumbar area (for example, up to 33.9 °C, keeping the other two stable). In that particular case, the increment of Tsk generated by the injury cannot be quantified by comparing the contralateral area or previous data of the subject; however, it can be compared with his/her proportional data (cervical 99.2%, dorsal 98.7% and lumbar 102.1%) using the established reference data. This would allow the abnormally increased temperature on the low back area to be easily detected and quantified (97.7% being the lower of the three areas of the spine in the reference model and 102.1% being the higher in the injured person).

They are many possibilities for using our data apart from the original data and we have only discussed three of them. Only the inclusion of these proposals in the upcoming software for thermographic analysis will generalize their usage in daily thermology practice.

FUTURE RESEARCH DIRECTIONS

A considerable amount of research must still be performed to increase the knowledge and applications of IRT for injury prevention in humans, not only in professional athletes but also in any person who practices any type of physical activity. We would like to note some directions for future research in thermography applied to prevent and track the evolution sports injuries:

The establishing of protocols and methodologies that attempts to reduce the effects of the influence factors on the interpretation of IRT data to achieve a more objective application of IRT technology.

From our point of view, some of the future efforts of thermologists may be directed towards normalizing or standardizing thermal results by correcting the data for influential factors. This would make the use of IRT in humans a more objective process and allow for comparisons of different subjects (or the same subject over time) independent of environmental, individual and technical factors.

The generation of synergies among medical doctors and researchers in human thermology. When the researcher is not a medical doctor, all the protocols, data analysis, interpretation and conclusions should be supervised by medical doctors who are the effective and accredited managers of human health. Conversely, the medical doctors should be open to studying and researching new technologies that could assist them in their daily decision making processes. We strongly recommend enrolling a medical doctor in each thermography research team to ensure quality and international recognition of the results.

An extension of the knowledge about the ability of thermography to quantify the effects of workloads and assimilating them during the recovery period, describe the effects of different forms or methods of training at different volumes and intensities of work, and evaluate the effectiveness of different means of recovery after exercise as well as moderate or high physical activity.

Quantifying the effects of training load will standardize the normal response to the effort and will indirectly help the professionals working with athletes to localize overloads and non-assimilated training loads as indicators or predictors of injury risk.

Developing computer tools that are integrated with infrared devices to objectify the data collection processes and generate semiautomatic thermal reports of the athletes. This research would improve not only the work of experts in sports thermography but also the work of any thermologist who works with humans, and would generalize IRT use in the daily practice of many professionals.

Deepening the knowledge of the behavior of skin temperature depending on factors such as gender, age or type of sport, to generate "normal" or "reference" thermal profiles for different population groups (or even personal thermal profiles), including genetic research if necessary. These thermal profiles are crucial for interpreting individual data or the normal skin thermal response of an athlete in a population group to any intervention.

Applying, as soon as possible, the knowledge from research on the uses of thermography for early diagnosis, prevention of injuries and monitoring recovery processes to real practical situations, to individualize the training programs and injury prevention protocols using the information provided by the IRT.

CONCLUSION

At the moment, we must cautiously conclude that the information provided by a thermographic evaluation has been one of the aspects that helped to significantly reduce the incidence of injury during professional sport practice, contributing to the identification of an injury before it occurs, and giving us the opportunity to act preventively. IRT also appears to be an ideal tool for monitoring the progress of lesions and the effectiveness of treatment.

In the near future, when integrated systems for the analysis of the thermographic data for human applications are developed, more extensive research will be performed on issues such as incidence factors, normalization of different data collections and the effect of exercise load on skin temperature. When the medical community becomes familiar with IRT technology, IRT will most likely be considered a more reliable method for diagnosing some human diseases and injuries.

REFERENCES

Abate, M., Carlo, L. D., Romualdo, S. D., Ionta, S., Ferretti, A., Romani, G. L., & Merla, A. (2010). Postural adjustment in experimental leg length difference evaluated by means of thermal infrared imaging. *Physiological Measurement*, *31*(1), 35–43. doi:10.1088/0967-3334/31/1/003 PMID:19940346

Abate, M., Di Carlo, L., Di Donato, L., Romani, G. L., & Merla, A. (2013). Comparison of cutaneous termic response to a standardised warm up in trained and untrained individuals. *The Journal of Sports Medicine and Physical Fitness*, *53*(2), 209–215. PMID:23584330

Adamczyk, J. G., Olszewska, M., Boguszewski, D., Białoszewski, D., & Reaburn, P. (2016). Is it possible to create a thermal model of warm-up? Monitoring of the training process in athletic decathlon. *Infrared Physics & Technology*, *76*, 555–559. doi:10.1016/j.infrared.2016.04.017

Akimov, E., & Sonkin, V. (2011). Skin temperature and lactate threshold during muscle work in athletes. *Human Physiology*, *37*(5), 621–628. doi:10.1134/S0362119711050033

Akimov, E. B., Andreev, R. S., Arkov, V. V., Kirdin, A. A., Saryanc, V. V., Sonkin, V. D., & Tonevitsky, A. G. (2009). Thermal portrait of sportsmen with different aerobic capacity. *Acta Kinesiologiae Universitatis Tartuensis*, *14*, 7–16. doi:10.12697/akut.2009.14.01

Al-Nakhli, H. H., Petrofsky, J. S., Laymon, M. S., & Berk, L. S. (2012). The Use of Thermal Infra-Red Imaging to Detect Delayed Onset Muscle Soreness. *Journal of Visualized Experiments*, (59): e3551. PMID:22297829

Ammer, K. (2003). Need for standardisation of measurements in Thermal Imaging. In B. Wiecek (Ed.), *Thermography and Lasers in Medicine* (pp. 13–17). Lodz, Poland: Akademickie Centrum Graficzno-Marketigowe Lodar S.A.

Ammer, K. (2012). Temperature of the human knee – a review. *Thermology International*, *22*(4), 137–151.

Arfaoui, A., Bertucci, W. M., Letellier, T., & Polidori, G. (2014). Thermoregulation during incremental exercise in masters cycling. *Journal of Science and Cycling*, *3*(1), 32–40.

Arfaoui, A., Polidori, G., Taiar, R., & Popa, C. (2012). Infrared Thermography in Sports Activity. In R. V. Prakash (Ed.), *Infrared Thermography* (pp. 141–168). InTech. doi:10.5772/30268

Arnaiz Lastras, J., Fernández Cuevas, I., Gómez Carmona, P. M., Sillero Quintana, M., García de la Concepción, M. Á., & Piñonosa Cano, S. (2011). *Pilot study to determinate thermal asymmetries in judokas.* Paper presented at the 16th Annual Congress of the European College of Sport Sciences ECSS, Liverpool, UK.

Autio, E., Neste, R., Airaksinen, S., & Heiskanen, M. L. (2006). Measuring the heat loss in horses in different seasons by infrared thermography. *Journal of Applied Animal Welfare Science, 9*(3), 211–221. doi:10.1207/s15327604jaws0903_3 PMID:17112332

Awerbuch, M. S. (1991). Thermography--its current diagnostic status in musculoskeletal medicine. *The Medical Journal of Australia, 154*(7), 441–444. PMID:2005838

Badža, V., Jovančević, V., Fratrić, F., Roglić, G., & Sudarov, N. (2012). Possibilities of thermovision application in sport and sport rehabilitation. *Vojnosanitetski Pregled. Military-Medical and Pharmaceutical Review, 69*(10), 904–907. doi:10.2298/VSP1210904B PMID:23155613

Balci, G. A., Basaran, T., & Colakoglu, M. (2016). Analysing visual pattern of skin temperature during submaximal and maximal exercises. *Infrared Physics & Technology, 74*, 57–62. doi:10.1016/j.infrared.2015.12.002

Bandeira, F., Borba Neves, E., Muniz de Moura, M. A., & Nohama, P. (2014). A termografia no apoio ao diagnostico de lesao muscular no esporte. *Revista Brasileira de Medicina do Esporte, 20*(1), 59–64. doi:10.1590/S1517-86922014000100012

Bandeira, F., Muniz de Moura, M. A., Abreu de Souza, M., Nohama, P., & Borba Neves, E. (2012). Pode a termografia auxiliar no diagnóstico de lesoes musculares em atletas de futebol? *Revista Brasileira de Medicina do Esporte, 18*(4), 234–239. doi:10.1590/S1517-86922012000400006

Banerjee, D., Chattopadhyay, S. K., & Tuli, S. (2013). Infrared thermography in material research – A review of textile applications. *Indian Journal of Fibre & Textile Research, 38*(4), 427–437.

Barcelos, E., Caminhas, W., Ribeiro, E., Pimenta, E., & Palhares, R. (2014). A Combined Method for Segmentation and Registration for an Advanced and Progressive Evaluation of Thermal Images. *Sensors (Basel, Switzerland), 14*(11), 21950–21967. doi:10.3390/s141121950 PMID:25414972

BenEliyahu, D. (1992). Infrared thermography and the sports injury practice. *Dynamic Chiropractic, 10*(7).

BenEliyahu, D. J. (1990). Infrared thermography in the diagnosis and management of sports injuries: A clinical study and literature review. *Chiropractic Sports Medicine., 4*(2), 46–53.

Bertucci, W., Arfaoui, A., Janson, L., & Polidori, G. (2013). Relationship between the gross efficiency and muscular skin temperature of lower limb in cycling: a preliminary study. *Computer Methods in Biomechanics and Biomedical Engineering, 16*(sup1), 114-115.

Binder, A., Parr, G., Thomas, P. P., & Hazleman, B. (1983). A clinical and thermographic study of lateral epicondylitis. *British Journal of Rheumatology, 22*(2), 77–81. doi:10.1093/rheumatology/22.2.77 PMID:6682688

Bonnett, P., Hare, D. B., Jones, D. D., Ring, E. F. J., & Hare, C. J. (2006). Some preliminary observations of the effects of sports massage on heat distribution of lower limb muscles during a graded exercise test. *Thermology International*, *16*(4), 143–149.

Borba Neves, E., Martins Cunha, R., Rosa, C., Sousa Antunes, N., Vieira Felisberto, I. M., Vilaça-Alves, J., & Machado Reis, V. (2016). Correlation between skin temperature and heart rate during exercise and recovery, and the influence of body position in these variables in untrained women. *Infrared Physics & Technology*, *75*, 70–76. doi:10.1016/j.infrared.2015.12.018

Bouzas Marins, J. C., Andrade Fernandes, A., Gomes Moreira, D., Souza Silva, F., & Magno, A. (2014). Thermographic profile of soccer players lower limbs. *Revista Andaluza de Medicina del Deporte*, *7*(1), 1–6. doi:10.1016/S1888-7546(14)70053-X

Buckhout, B. C., & Warner, M. A. (1980). Digital perfusion of handball players. Effects of repeated ball impact on structures of the hand. *The American Journal of Sports Medicine*, *8*(3), 206–207. doi:10.1177/036354658000800313 PMID:7377456

Bulut, J., Janta, M., Senner, V., & Kreuzer, J. (2013). Determination of Insulation Properties of Functional Clothing Using Core Body Temperature Gradients as Quantification Parameter. *Procedia Engineering*, *60*(0), 208–213. doi:10.1016/j.proeng.2013.07.057

Busoni, F., Romagnoli, C., Bagnolesi, P., & Gemignani, G. (1988). Imaging of enthesopathies of the ligamentum patellae in athletes. Echography and computerized telethermography. *La Radiologia Medica*, *76*(1-2), 44–47. PMID:3041478

Charkoudian, N. (2003). Skin blood flow in adult human thermoregulation: How it works, when it does not, and why. *Mayo Clinic proceedings. Mayo Clinic*, *78*(5), 603–612. doi:10.4065/78.5.603

Charkoudian, N. (2010). Mechanisms and modifiers of reflex induced cutaneous vasodilation and vasoconstriction in humans. *Journal of Applied Physiology (Bethesda, Md.)*, *109*(4), 1221–1228. doi:10.1152/japplphysiol.00298.2010 PMID:20448028

Chen, Z., Jiang, G., Zheng, F., Liu, H., & Zhu, B. (2005). A Correction method of medical thermography's distortion. *Conference Proceedings; ... Annual International Conference of the IEEE Engineering in Medicine and Biology Society. IEEE Engineering in Medicine and Biology Society. Conference*, *2*, 1677–1679. PMID:17282534

Cheng, V. S., Bai, J., & Chen, Y. (2009). A high-resolution three-dimensional far-infrared thermal and true-color imaging system for medical applications. *Medical Engineering &amp. Physics*, *31*(9), 1173–1181.

Chudecka, M., & Lubkowska, A. (2010a). Evaluation of temperature changes in upper extremities of waterpolo players by thermovision [in Polish]. *Inżynieria Biomedyczna. Acta Bio-Optica et Informatica Medica*, *16*(4), 334–338.

Chudecka, M., & Lubkowska, A. (2010b). Temperature changes of selected bodys surfaces of handball players in the course of training estimated by thermovision, and the study of the impact of physiological and morphological factors on the skin temperature. *Journal of Thermal Biology*, *35*(8), 379–385. doi:10.1016/j.jtherbio.2010.08.001

Chudecka, M., & Lubkowska, A. (2011). Evaluation of the body surface temperature changes in the basketball players' after training. [in Polish]. *Inżynieria Biomedyczna. Acta Bio-Optica et Informatica Medica*, *17*(4), 271–275.

Chudecka, M., & Lubkowska, A. (2012). The use of Thermal Imaging to evaluate Body Temperature changes of athletes during training and a study on the impact of physiological and morphological factors on skin temperature. *Human Movement*, *13*(1), 33–39. doi:10.2478/v10038-012-0002-9

Chudecka, M., Szczepanowska, E., & Kempinska, A. (2008). Changes of thermoemission of upper extremities in female handball players - the preliminary study. *Medicina Sportiva*, *12*(3), 99–102. doi:10.2478/v10036-008-0019-5

Ciutacu, O., Tanase, A., & Miclaus, I. (2006). Digital infrared thermography in assessing soft tissues injuries on sport equines. *Bulletin of the University of Agricultural Sciences and Veterinary Medicine, 63*, 228-233.

Clark, R. P., Goff, M. R., & Mullan, B. J. (1977). Skin temperatures during sunbathing and some observations on the effect of hot and cold drinks on these temperatures. *The Journal of Physiology*, *267*(1), 8P–9P. PMID:874864

Clark, R. P., Mullan, B. J., & Pugh, G. C. (1974). Proceedings: Colour thermography in running. *The Journal of Physiology*, *239*(2), 81P–82P. PMID:4415246

Clark, R. P., Mullan, B. J., & Pugh, L. G. (1977). Skin temperature during running -a study using infra-red colour thermography. *The Journal of Physiology*, *267*(1), 53–62. doi:10.1113/jphysiol.1977.sp011800 PMID:874861

Čoh, M., & Širok, B. (2007). Use of the thermovision method in sport training. *Physical Education and Sport.*, *5*(1), 85–94.

Cooke, E. D., & Picher, M. F. (1974). Deep vein thrombosis: Preclinical diagnosis by thermography. *British Journal of Surgery*, *61*(12), 971–978. doi:10.1002/bjs.1800611212 PMID:4441818

Costello, J., Stewart, I. B., Selfe, J., Karki, A. I., & Donnelly, A. (2013). Use of thermal imaging in sports medicine research: A short report. *International Sportmed Journal*, *14*(2), 94–98.

Costello, J. T., McInerney, C. D., Bleakley, C. M., Selfe, J., & Donnelly, A. E. (2012). The use of thermal imaging in assessing skin temperature following cryotherapy: A review. *Journal of Thermal Biology*, *37*(2), 245–274. doi:10.1016/j.jtherbio.2011.11.008

da Rosa Vieira, L., Zaro, M. A., Cervien, A., de Lara Peres, L. H., Mendonça de Moura, A., & Corvalão de Ávila, L. (2003). *Uso da Termografia como técnica auxiliar na recuperação de atletas.* Paper presented at the X Congresso Brasileiro de Biomecânica.

Deng, Z. S., & Liu, J. (2004). Mathematical modeling of temperature mapping over skin surface and its implementation in thermal disease diagnostics. *Computers in Biology and Medicine*, *34*(6), 495–521. doi:10.1016/S0010-4825(03)00086-6 PMID:15265721

Devereaux, M., Parr, G., Lachmann, S., Page-Thomas, P., & Hazleman, B. (1986). Thermographic diagnosis in athletes with patellofemoral arthralgia. *Journal of Bone and Joint Surgery-(Br), 68*(1), 42-44.

Devereaux, M. D., Parr, G. R., Lachmann, S. M., Page-Thomas, P., & Hazleman, B. L. (1984). The diagnosis of stress fractures in athletes. *Journal of the American Medical Association*, *252*(4), 531–533. doi:10.1001/jama.1984.03350040061027 PMID:6737649

Faulkner, S. H., Ferguson, R. A., Gerrett, N., Hupperets, M., Hodder, S. G., & Havenith, G. (2013). Reducing muscle temperature drop after warm-up improves sprint cycling performance. *Medicine and Science in Sports and Exercise*, *45*(2), 359–365. doi:10.1249/MSS.0b013e31826fba7f PMID:22935735

Fernandes Ade, A., Amorim, P. R., Brito, C. J., de Moura, A. G., Moreira, D. G., & Costa, C. M. et al.. (2014). Measuring skin temperature before, during and after exercise: A comparison of thermocouples and infrared thermography. *Physiological Measurement*, *35*(2), 189–203. doi:10.1088/0967-3334/35/2/189 PMID:24398429

Fernández-Cuevas, Sillero-Quintana, Angel Garcia-Concepcion, Ribot Serrano, Gomez-Carmona, & Marins. (2014). Monitoring Skin Thermal Response to Training with Infrared Thermography. *New Studies in Athletics*, *29*(1), 57–71.

Fernández-Cuevas, I. (2012). *Effect of endurance, speed and strength training on skin temperatura measured by Infrared Thermography.* Universidad Politécnica de Madrid. Retrieved from http://oa.upm.es/14896/2/ISMAEL_FERNANDEZ_CUEVAS.pdf

Fernández-Cuevas, I., Bouzas Marins, J. C., Arnáiz Lastras, J., Gómez Carmona, P. M., Piñonosa Cano, S., García-Concepción, M. Á., & Sillero-Quintana, M. (2015). Classification of factors influencing the use of infrared thermography in humans: A review. *Infrared Physics & Technology*, *71*(0), 28–55. doi:10.1016/j.infrared.2015.02.007

Fernández Cuevas, I., Gómez Carmona, P. M., Sillero Quintana, M., Noya Salces, J., Arnaiz Lastras, J., & Pastor Barrón, A. (2010). *Economic costs estimation of soccer injuries in first and second spanish division professional teams.* Paper presented at the 15th Annual Congress of the European College of Sport Sciences ECSS, Antalya, Turkey.

Fernández-Cuevas, I., Sillero-Quintana, M., Garcia-Concepcion, M. a., Ribot Serrano, J., Gomez-Carmona, P. M., & Marins, J. C. (2014). Monitoring Skin Thermal Response to Training with Infrared Thermography. *New Studies in Athletics*, *29*(1), 57–71.

Fernández Cuevas, I., Sillero Quintana, M., Gómez Carmona, P. M., García de la Concepción, M. Á., Piñonosa Cano, S., & Arnaiz Lastras, J. (2011). *Applications of Infrared Thermography as innovative technological solution in sports injuries.* Paper presented at the Science Based Prevention, Berlin, Germany.

Ferreira, J. J., Mendonca, L. C., Nunes, L. A., Andrade Filho, A. C., Rebelatto, J. R., & Salvini, T. F. (2008). Exercise-associated thermographic changes in young and elderly subjects. *Annals of Biomedical Engineering*, *36*(8), 1420–1427. doi:10.1007/s10439-008-9512-1 PMID:18470619

Formenti, D., Ludwig, N., Gargano, M., Gondola, M., Dellerma, N., Caumo, A., & Alberti, G. (2013). Thermal imaging of exercise-associated skin temperature changes in trained and untrained female subjects. *Annals of Biomedical Engineering*, *41*(4), 863–871. doi:10.1007/s10439-012-0718-x PMID:23229282

Formenti, D., Ludwig, N., Trecroci, A., Gargano, M., Michielon, G., Caumo, A., & Alberti, G. (2016). Dynamics of thermographic skin temperature response during squat exercise at two different speeds. *Journal of Thermal Biology*, *59*, 58–63. doi:10.1016/j.jtherbio.2016.04.013 PMID:27264889

Fournet, D., Redortier, B., & Havenith, G. (2012). *A method for whole-body human skin temperature mapping*. Paper presented at the XII Congress EAT 2012, Porto, Portugal.

Fournet, D., Ross, L., Voelcker, T., Redortier, B., & Havenith, G. (2013). Body mapping of thermoregulatory and perceptual responses of males and females running in the cold. *Journal of Thermal Biology*, *38*(6), 339–344. doi:10.1016/j.jtherbio.2013.04.005

Fuller, C. W., Ekstrand, J., Junge, A., Andersen, T. E., Bahr, R., & Dvorak, J. et al.. (2006). Consensus statement on injury definitions and data collection procedures in studies of football (soccer) injuries. *Clinical Journal of Sport Medicine*, *16*(2), 97–106. doi:10.1097/00042752-200603000-00003 PMID:16603877

Garagiola, U., & Giani, E. (1990). Use of telethermography in the management of sports injuries. *Sports Medicine (Auckland, N.Z.)*, *10*(4), 267–272. doi:10.2165/00007256-199010040-00005 PMID:2247727

Garagiola, U., & Giani, E. (1991). Thermography: Description, Uses in Sports Medicine. Unpublished article by Encyclopedia of Sports Medicine and Science.

Garza, D., Rolston, B., Johnston, T., Sungar, G., Ferguson, J., & Matheson, G. (2008). *Heat-Loss Patterns in National Football League Players as Measured by Infrared Thermography*. Paper presented at the InfraMation.

Gasi, F., & Bittencourt, E. (2009). Evaluation of textile materials in physical activity. *Chemical Engineering Transactions*, *17*, 1783–1787.

Giani, E., Rochi, L., Tavoni, A., Montanari, M., & Garagiola, U. (1989). Telethermographic evaluation of NSAIDs in the treatment of sports injuries. *Medicine and Science in Sports and Exercise*, *21*(1), 1–6. doi:10.1249/00005768-198902000-00001 PMID:2648105

Gómez Carmona, P. M. (2012). *Influencia de la información termográfica infrarroja en el protocolo de prevención de lesiones de un equipo de fútbol profesional español*. Universidad Politécnica de Madrid. Retrieved from http://oa.upm.es/14694/2/PEDRO_MARIA_GOMEZ_CARMONA.pdf

Gómez Carmona, P. M., & Noya Salces, J. (2008). Prevención de lesiones en fútbol. *Training Fútbol*, (144), 36-46.

Gómez Carmona, P. M., & Sillero Quintana, M. (2009). *Termografía deportiva. I Curso básico de termografía como medio para la prevención y seguimiento de lesiones deportivas*. Madrid: pemaSIP. Facultad de Ciencias de la Actividad Física y del Deporte - INEF. Universidad Politécnica de Madrid.

Gómez Carmona, P. M., Sillero Quintana, M., Fernández Cuevas, I., Noya Salces, J., & Fernández Rodríguez, I. (2011). *Application of an injury prevention protocol based on infrared thermogrphy in professional soccer players during pre-season*. Paper presented at the 24rd Thermological Symposium of the Austrian Society of Thermography "Quantitative Thermal Imaging in Medicine", Vienna, Austria.

Hagglund, M., Walden, M., & Ekstrand, J. (2003). Exposure and injury risk in Swedish elite football: A comparison between seasons 1982 and 2001. *Scandinavian Journal of Medicine & Science in Sports, 13*(6), 364–370. doi:10.1046/j.1600-0838.2003.00327.x PMID:14617057

Hildebrandt, C. (2009). *Medical infrared thermography as a screening tool for knee injuries in professional junior alpine-ski-racers in Austria - Findings of a pilot study*. Paper presented at the 14th annual ECSS Congress.

Hildebrandt, C., Raschner, C., & Ammer, K. (2010). An overview of recent application of medical infrared thermography in sports medicine in Austria. *Sensors (Basel, Switzerland), 10*(5), 4700–4715. doi:10.3390/s100504700 PMID:22399901

Hildebrandt, C., Zeilberger, K., Ring, E. F. J., & Raschner, C. (2012). The application of medical Infrared Thermography in sports medicine. In K. R. Zaslav (Ed.), *An International Perspective on Topics in Sports Medicine and Sports Injury* (p. 534). InTech. doi:10.5772/28383

Hirata, K., Nagasaka, T., & Noda, Y. (1989). Venous return from distal regions affects heat loss from the arms and legs during exercise-induced thermal loads. *European Journal of Applied Physiology and Occupational Physiology, 58*(8), 865–872. doi:10.1007/BF02332220 PMID:2767068

Hoy, K., Lindblad, B. E., Terkelsen, C. J., Helleland, H. E., & Terkelsen, C. J. (1992). European soccer injuries. A prospective epidemiologic and socioeconomic study. *The American Journal of Sports Medicine, 20*(3), 318–322. doi:10.1177/036354659202000314 PMID:1636863

Hunold, S., Mietzsch, E., & Werner, J. (1992). Thermographic studies on patterns of skin temperature after exercise. *European Journal of Applied Physiology and Occupational Physiology, 65*(6), 550–554. doi:10.1007/BF00602364 PMID:1483445

Iglesias-Gutierrez, D. (2014). *Respuesta térmica del jugador de fútbol ante cuatro formatos diferentes de entrenamiento interválico de alta intensidad*. Trabajo Final de Master. Madrid: Facultad de Ciencias de la Actividad Física y del Deporte (INEF). Universidad Politécnica de Madrid. Retrieved from https://drive.google.com/file/d/0B7FrjSgoogHVa1FseWtXWnE3b0k/edit?usp=sharing

Inklaar, H. (1994). Soccer injuries. I: Incidence and severity. *Sports Medicine (Auckland, N.Z.), 18*(1), 55–73. doi:10.2165/00007256-199418010-00006 PMID:7939040

Junge, A., Rosch, D., Peterson, L., Graf-Baumann, T., & Dvorak, J. (2002). Prevention of soccer injuries: A prospective intervention study in youth amateur players. *The American Journal of Sports Medicine, 30*(5), 652–659. PMID:12238997

Keyl, W., & Lenhart, P. (1975). Die Thermographie bei Sportverletzungen und Sportschäden des Bewegungsapparates. *Fortschritte der Medizin, 23*(93), 124–126. PMID:1173237

Knab, A. M., Shanely, R. A., Corbin, K. D., Jin, F., Sha, W., & Nieman, D. C. (2011). A 45-minute vigorous exercise bout increases metabolic rate for 14 hours. *Medicine and Science in Sports and Exercise, 43*(9), 1643–1648. doi:10.1249/MSS.0b013e3182118891 PMID:21311363

Korman, P., Straburzyńska-Lupa, A., Kusy, K., Kantanista, A., & Zieliński, J. (2016). Changes in body surface temperature during speed endurance work-out in highly-trained male sprinters. *Infrared Physics & Technology*, *78*, 209–213. doi:10.1016/j.infrared.2016.08.003

Kulesza, O., Rzeczkowski, M., & Kaczorowski, M. (2004). Thermography and its practical use in equine diagnostics and treatment. *Medycyna Weterynaryjna*, *60*(11), 1143–1146.

LaForgia, J., Withers, R. T., & Gore, C. J. (2006). Effects of exercise intensity and duration on the excess post-exercise oxygen consumption. *Journal of Sports Sciences*, *24*(12), 1247–1264. doi:10.1080/02640410600552064 PMID:17101527

Lewin, G. (1989). The incidence of injuries in an English professional soccer club during one competitive season. *Physiotherapy*, *75*(10), 601–605. doi:10.1016/S0031-9406(10)62366-8

Liu, Y., Mimura, K., Wang, L., & Ikuda, K. (2003). Physiological benefits of 24-style Taijiquan exercise in middle-aged women. *Journal of Physiological Anthropology and Applied Human Science*, *22*(5), 219–225. doi:10.2114/jpa.22.219 PMID:14519910

Ludwig, N., Formenti, D., Gargano, M., & Alberti, G. (2014). Skin temperature evaluation by infrared thermography: Comparison of image analysis methods. *Infrared Physics & Technology*, *62*(0), 1–6. doi:10.1016/j.infrared.2013.09.011

Mair, S. D., Seaber, A. V., Glisson, R. R., & Garrett, W. E. Jr. (1996). The role of fatigue in susceptibility to acute muscle strain injury. *The American Journal of Sports Medicine*, *24*(2), 137–143. doi:10.1177/036354659602400203 PMID:8775109

Malkinson, T. J. (2002). *Skin temperature response during cycle ergometry.* Paper presented at the Electrical and Computer Engineering.

Mao, A., Luo, J., Li, Y., Luo, X., & Wang, R. (2011). A multi-disciplinary strategy for computer-aided clothing thermal engineering design. *Computer Aided Design*, *43*(12), 1854–1869. doi:10.1016/j.cad.2011.06.009

Marins, J. C. B., Fernandes, A. A., Cano, S. P., Moreira, D. G., da Silva, F. S., & Costa, C. M. A. (2014). Thermal body patterns for healthy Brazilian adults (male and female). *Journal of Thermal Biology*.

Marins, J. C. B., Moreira, D. G., Cano, S. P., Quintana, M. S., Soares, D. D., & Fernandes, A. d. A. (2014). Time required to stabilize thermographic images at rest. *Infrared Physics & Technology*.

Merla, A. (2005). Functional infrared imaging in clinical applications. In J. Bronzino (Ed.), The Biomedical Engineering Handbook. Academic Press.

Merla, A., Di Donato, L., & Romani, G. L. (2002). *Infrared functional imaging: analysis of skin temperature during exercise.* Paper presented at the Engineering in Medicine and Biology, 2002. 24th Annual Conference and the Annual Fall Meeting of the Biomedical Engineering Society EMBS/BMES Conference. doi:10.1109/IEMBS.2002.1106316

Merla, A., Iodice, P., Tangherlini, A., De Michele, G., Di Romualdo, S., & Saggini, R. (2005). Monitoring skin temperature in trained and untrained subjects throughout thermal video. *Conference Proceedings; ... Annual International Conference of the IEEE Engineering in Medicine and Biology Society. IEEE Engineering in Medicine and Biology Society. Conference*, *2*(1), 1684–1686. PMID:17282536

Merla, A., Mattei, P. A., Di Donato, L., & Romani, G. L. (2010). Thermal imaging of cutaneous temperature modifications in runners during graded exercise. *Annals of Biomedical Engineering*, *38*(1), 158–163. doi:10.1007/s10439-009-9809-8 PMID:19798579

Mijović, B., Salopek Čubrić, I., Skenderi, Z., & Reischl, U. (2012). Thermographic Assessment of Sweat Evaporation within Different Clothing Systems. *FIBRES & TEXTILES in Eastern Europe*, *20*(5 (94)), 81–86.

Mikulska, D. (2006). Contemporary applications of infrared imaging in medical diagnostics. *Annales Academiae Medicae Stetinensis*, *52*(1), 35–39, discussion 39–40. PMID:17131845

Miyamoto, T., Hara, K., Nishimura, H., & Yano, K. (2004). Thermographic evaluation in sports injury. *Journal of the Japan Society of Infrared Science and Technology*, *14*(1), 39–43.

Nakayama, T., Ohnuki, Y., & Kanosue, K. (1981). Fall in skin temperature during exercise observed by thermography. *Japanese Journal of Physiology*, *31*(5), 757–762. doi:10.2170/jjphysiol.31.757 PMID:7328924

Ng, E. Y. K. (2009). A review of thermography as promising non-invasive detection modality for breast tumor. *International Journal of Thermal Sciences*, *48*(5), 849–859. doi:10.1016/j.ijthermalsci.2008.06.015

Noya Salces, J., Benito Peinado, P. J., Calderón, J., & Gómez Carmona, P. M. (2008). *Validation of a questionnaire for the registration of injuries in the professional soccer.* Paper presented at the 13th Annual Congress of the European Collage of Sport Science ECSS Estoril, Portugal, Portugal.

Noya Salces, J., Sillero Quintana, M., Gómez Carmona, P. M., & Pastrano León, R. (2009), june 24th-27th). *Infrared Thermography as a Method for Monitoring and Preventing Injuries in Soccer.* Paper presented at the 14th Annual Congress of the European College of Sport Sciences ECSS, Oslo, Norway.

Oliveira, J., Vardasca, R., Pimenta, M., Gabriel, J., & Torres, J. (2016). Use of infrared thermography for the diagnosis and grading of sprained ankle injuries. *Infrared Physics & Technology*, *76*, 530–541. doi:10.1016/j.infrared.2016.04.014

Pascoe, D. D., Mercer, J. B., & de Weerd, L. (2007). Physiology of Thermal Signals. In N. A. Diakides & J. D. Bronzino (Eds.), Medical Infrared Imaging (pp. 6-1 - 6-20). Taylor & Francis. doi:10.1201/9781420008340.ch6

Pascoe, D. D., Skelton, M., Smith, E. W., Kremer, D., & Purohit, R. C. (1992). Infrared thermography pattern of the back of human subjects during exercise: 921. *Medicine and Science in Sports and Exercise*, *24*(5Supplement), S154. doi:10.1249/00005768-199205001-00922

Petibois, C., Cazorla, G., Poortmans, J. R., & Deleris, G. (2002). Biochemical aspects of overtraining in endurance sports: A review. *Sports Medicine (Auckland, N.Z.)*, *32*(13), 867–878. doi:10.2165/00007256-200232130-00005 PMID:12392446

Piñonosa, S., Sillero-Quintana, M., Milanović, L., Coterón, J., & Sampedro, J. (2013). Thermal evolution of lower limbs during a rehabilitation process after anterior cruciate ligament surgery. *Kinesiology*, *45*(1), 121–129.

Priego Quesada, J. I., Carpes, F. P., Bini, R. R., Salvador Palmer, R., Pérez-Soriano, P., & Cibrián Ortiz de Anda, R. M. (2015). Relationship between skin temperature and muscle activation during incremental cycle exercise. *Journal of Thermal Biology*, *48*(0), 28–35. doi:10.1016/j.jtherbio.2014.12.005 PMID:25660627

Priego Quesada, J. I., Martínez, N., Salvador Palmer, R., Psikuta, A., Annaheim, S., Rossi, R. M., & Pérez-Soriano, P. et al. (2016). Effects of the cycling workload on core and local skin temperatures. *Experimental Thermal and Fluid Science*, *77*, 91–99. doi:10.1016/j.expthermflusci.2016.04.008

Purvis, A. J., & Cable, N. T. (2000). The effects of phase control materials on hand skin temperature within gloves of soccer goalkeepers. *Ergonomics*, *43*(10), 1480–1488. doi:10.1080/001401300750003916 PMID:11083129

Purvis, A. J., & Tunstall, H. (2004). Effects of sock type on foot skin temperature and thermal demand during exercise. *Ergonomics*, *47*(15), 1657–1668. doi:10.1080/00140130412331290880 PMID:15545238

Pušnik, I., & Čuk, I. (2014). Thermal imaging of hands during simple gymnastics elements on the wooden bar with and without use of magnesium carbonate. *Science of Gymnastics Journal*, *6*(1), 67–72.

Ramos e Côrte, A. C., & Hernandez, A. J. (2016). Termografía médica infravermelha aplicada à Medicina do Esporte. *Revista Brasileira de Medicina do Esporte*, *22*(4), 315–319. doi:10.1590/1517-869220162204160783

Ring, E. F. (1990). Quantitative thermal imaging. *Clin Phys Physiol Meas*, *11*(SA), 87-95.

Rochcongar, P., & Schmitt, M. (1979). Thermographic study of muscular lesions in sport (author's transl). *Journal Belge de Medecine Physique et de Rehabilitation. Belgisch Tijdschrift voor Fysische Geneeskunde en Rehabilitatie*, 2(4), 335–342. PMID:549939

Ross, W., Ward, R., Leahy, R., & Day, J. (1982). Proportionality of Montreal Athletes. In J. Carter (Ed.), *Physical Structure of Olympic Athletes: Part 1. The Montreal Olympic Games Anthropological Project*. Basel: Karger. doi:10.1159/000406782

Sampedro, J., Piñonosa Cano, S., & Fernández-Cuevas, I. (2012). Thermography as a new assessment tool in basketball. Pilot study carried out with a professional player in the ACB. *Cuadernos de Psicología del Deporte*, *12*, 51–56. doi:10.4321/S1578-84232012000300012

Sands, W. A., McNeal, J. R., & Stone, M. (2011). Thermal imaging and gymnastics injuries: A means of screening and injury identification. *Science of Gymnastics Journal*, *3*(2), 5–12.

Selfe, J., Alexander, J., Costello, J. T., May, K., Garratt, N., Atkins, S., & Richards, J. et al. (2014). The effect of three different (-135 degrees c) whole body cryotherapy exposure durations on elite rugby league players. *PLoS ONE*, *9*(1), e86420. doi:10.1371/journal.pone.0086420 PMID:24489726

Sillero Quintana, M., Conde Pascual, E., Gómez Carmona, P. M., Fernández-Cuevas, I., & García-Pastor, T. (2012). Effect of yoga and swimming on body temperature of pregnant women. *Thermology International, 22*, 143-149.

Sillero-Quintana, M., Fernández-Jaén, T., Fernández-Cuevas, I., Gómez-Carmona, P. M., Arnaiz-Lastras, J., Pérez, M.-D., & Guillén, P. (2015). Infrared Thermography as a Support Tool for Screening and Early Diagnosis in Emergencies. *Journal of Medical Imaging and Health Informatics*, *5*(6), 1223–1228. doi:10.1166/jmihi.2015.1511

Sillero Quintana, M., Gómez Carmona, P. M., García de la Concepción, M. Á., Fernández Cuevas, I., Piñonosa Cano, S., & Cordente, C. A. (2010). *Application of thermography as injury prevention method and monitoring of the injury recovery in Athletics.* Paper presented at the World Congress on Science in Athletics, Barcelona, Spain.

Sillero Quintana, M., Gómez Carmona, P. M., Noya Salces, J., Núñez, F. J., & Fernández Rodríguez, I. (2009). Comparation of infrared thermography with tensiomyography as injury prevention method in professional soccer players. *Journal of Sports Sciences*, S174.

Smith, B. L., Bandler, M. K., & Goodman, P. H. (1986). Dominant forearm hyperthermia: A study of fifteen athletes. *Thermology*, *2*, 25–28.

Stannard, A. B., Brandenburg, J. P., Pitney, W. A., & Lukaszuk, J. M. (2011). Effects of wearing a cooling vest during the warm-up on 10-km run performance. *Journal of Strength and Conditioning Research*, *25*(7), 2018–2024. doi:10.1519/JSC.0b013e3181e07585 PMID:21448075

Tauchmannova, H., Gabrhel, J., & Cibak, M. (1993). Thermographic findings in different sports, their value in the prevention of soft tissue injuries. *Thermol Österr*, *3*, 91–95.

Thomas, D., Siahamis, G., Marion, M., & Boyle, C. (1992). Computerised infrared thermography and isotopic bone scanning in tennis elbow. *Annals of the Rheumatic Diseases*, *51*(1), 103–107. doi:10.1136/ard.51.1.103 PMID:1540012

Torii, M., Yamasaki, M., & Sasaki, T. (1987). Skin surface temperatures during submaximal cycling observed by color thermography. *Annals of Physiological Anthropology*, *6*(1), 21–24. doi:10.2114/ahs1983.6.21 PMID:3675756

Torii, M., Yamasaki, M., Sasaki, T., & Nakayama, H. (1992). Fall in skin temperature of exercising man. *British Journal of Sports Medicine*, *26*(1), 29–32. doi:10.1136/bjsm.26.1.29 PMID:1600450

Turner, T. A. (1991). Thermography as an aid to the clinical lameness evaluation. *The Veterinary Clinics of North America. Equine Practice*, *7*(2), 311–338. PMID:1933566

Vainer, B. G. (2005). FPA-based infrared thermography as applied to the study of cutaneous perspiration and stimulated vascular response in humans. *Physics in Medicine and Biology*, *50*(23), R63–R94. doi:10.1088/0031-9155/50/23/R01 PMID:16306642

Vardasca, R. (2008). Symmetry of temperature distribution in the upper and the lower extremities. *Thermology International*, *18*(4), 154.

Veghte, J. H., Adams, W. C., & Bernauer, E. M. (1979). Temperature changes during exercise measured by thermography. *Aviation, Space, and Environmental Medicine*, *50*(7), 708–713. PMID:486019

Wade, C. E., & Veghte, J. H. (1977). Thermographic evaluation of the relative heat loss by area in man after swimming. *Aviation, Space, and Environmental Medicine*, *48*(1), 16–18. PMID:831705

Walden, M., Hagglund, M., & Ekstrand, J. (2005). UEFA Champions League study: A prospective study of injuries in professional football during the 20012002 season. *British Journal of Sports Medicine*, *39*(8), 542–546. doi:10.1136/bjsm.2004.014571 PMID:16046340

Wang, J.-G., & Toh, H. L. (2001, 2001). *Visualizing skin temperature before, during and after exercise for dynamic area telethermometry.* Paper presented at the Engineering in Medicine and Biology Society.

Woods, C., Hawkins, R., Hulse, M., & Hodson, A. (2003). The Football Association Medical Research Programme: an audit of injuries in professional football: an analysis of ankle sprains. *British Journal of Sports Medicine*, *37*(3), 233–238. doi:10.1136/bjsm.37.3.233 PMID:12782548

Zaïdi, H., Taiar, R., Fohanno, S., & Polidori, G. (2007). The influence of swimming type on the skin-temperature maps of a competitive swimmer from infrared thermography. *Acta of Bioengineering and Biomechanics*, *9*(1), 47–51. PMID:17933104

Zontak, A., Sideman, S., Verbitsky, O., & Beyar, R. (1998). Dynamic thermography: Analysis of hand temperature during exercise. *Annals of Biomedical Engineering*, *26*(6), 988–993. doi:10.1114/1.33 PMID:9846937

KEY TERMS AND DEFINITIONS

Aerobic Training: Physical exercise of low to high intensity normally performed for a long period of time to increase the efficiency of energetic substrate consumption in the presence of oxygen.

Anaerobic Training: Physical exercise of high to extreme intensity performed to increase the efficiency of substrate consumption under lack of oxygen conditions. As a result, the concentration of lactic acid in the blood and the active muscles increases to extreme values that prevent the endurance of such an intense exercise for a long period of time.

Contralateral ROIs: Two symmetric ROIs. Asymmetric thermal values can be related to a dysfunction of one of them.

Influence Factor: Any condition or circumstance that may affect the values of the skin temperature of and assessed ROI.

Injury Rate: A term normally used in sports to quantify the probability of an athlete suffering an injury. It is expressed in number of injuries per 1000 hours of exposition of the sport practice or physical activity.

Microcycle: Minimal unit of the training program that includes a certain number of training sessions directed at fulfilling a training objective. Traditionally, a training program is composed of several macrocycles that consist of several mesocycles and a mesocycle is composed of several microcycles.

Region of Interest (ROI): Any region of the human skin that is delimited to obtain its thermal data. They normally correspond with anatomical regions or with a corporal structure below the skin.

Thermal Profile: The thermal values (normally mean, maximal, minimal, and standard deviation) of a collection of ROIs from an individual or from a population group that has certain characteristics such as age, gender or level of physical activity.

Training Load: The amount of exercise performed during a training activity. The training load should be of sufficient magnitude and duration to produce a physical stress and generate a physiological adaptation of the organism, which enables the athlete to perform a higher workload in later training sessions or competition.

Chapter 9
Infrared Thermography in Swimming:
Thermal Characterization of Swimming Technique

Ana Sofia Domingues
University of Porto, Portugal

Filipa Barbosa
University of Porto, Portugal

Adérito Seixas
Universidade Fernando Pessoa, Portugal

Márcio Borgonovo-Santos
University of Porto, Portugal

Eduardo M. Pereira
INESC-TEC Porto, Portugal

Ricardo Vardasca
University of Porto, Portugal

Joaquim Gabriel
University of Porto, Portugal

Ricardo J. Fernandes
University of Porto, Portugal

J. Paulo Vilas-Boas
University of Porto, Portugal

ABSTRACT

In order to verify whether there is a considerable increase in body skin temperature during different swimming techniques (crawl and backstroke) and identifying the most affected regions. The athlete's thermal symmetry was also analyzed, as well as its modification after the swimming, according to the performed technique. The accuracy of thermography as a method to identify and distinguish these different styles was also evaluated. Ten male swimmers were recruited and two different swimming techniques were assessed, crawl and backstroke. After a 10 minute acclimatization period in the pool, the swimmers were quickly dried with microfiber towels. The thermograms were taken before and after the swimming task, which consisted in a 7x200m protocol in crawl or backstroke. Infrared thermography revealed an increase of temperature after exercise and no significant differences were found between both techniques. Thermal symmetry was not affected by exercise.

DOI: 10.4018/978-1-5225-2072-6.ch009

INTRODUCTION

The study of temperature is a very comprehensive topic that applies to most contexts in science, including the study of the human body and its function. Hippocrates had already understood the importance of looking at body heat. Galilleo's thermoscope was the basis for Santorio's thermometer but it was Carl Wunderlich that introduced thermal measurements into clinical medicine later in 1868. He wrote a treatise on body temperature and health as a result of his innumerous observations that allowed him to chart the temperature variations of his patients daily (Ring, 2007).

Infrared radiation had a different development, with several milestones being achieved by several pioneers in the field contributing to the development of actual infrared thermography (IRT). In 1953, Jean Batista Della Porta made very important discoveries on the reflection of heat and, more than 200 years later, the work of William Herschell and his son – John Herschell – culminated with the first known "thermogram". JD Hardy demonstrated that the human skin behaved as a near perfect blackbody radiator and Samuel Langley contributed to the remote study of temperature with the development of the bolometer. At least, the work of Marianus Czerny on the thermal sensors and the development of an evaporograph, and the work of his former student – Bowling Barnes – resulted on the first thermal imager based on thermistors in the 1950's (Ring, 2014).

IRT is an imaging modality that has been used in medicine since the early 1960's (Ring & Ammer, 2000). Thermography is a non-invasive, non-ionizing and non-radiation emitting imaging modality that records skin temperature, providing important physiological information heat exchange processes between skin, deep tissues, local blood vessels and metabolism (Merla & Romani, 2005). The validity and reliability of technique has been widely documented in the literature (e.g. Burnham, McKinley, & Vincent, 2006).

Exercise training is known for affecting human thermoregulation, inducing changes in microvascular reactivity of the skin (Simmons, Wong, Holowatz, & Kenney, 2011). Therefore, IRT can be a powerful tool in sport medicine and research.

Early records of IRT use in sport research are available (Clark, Mullan, & Pugh, 1977; Hunold, Mietzsch, & Werner, 1992) and more recently Merla, Mattei, Di Donato, and Romani (2010) assessed skin temperature (Tsk) changes and distribution during graded treadmill exercise in trained subjects. Chudecka and Lubkowska (2012) reported a correlation between oxygen uptake and changes in the thermal profile of professional volleyball players after exercise. Evidence has also been reported suggesting that the magnitude of Tsk changes in response to localized exercise in female athletes are related to the level of physical training (Formenti et al., 2013). Bourlai, Pryor, Suyama, Reis, and Hostler (2012) reported significant correlations between skin temperature measurements of the face with IRT and measures of core temperature with ingestible core temperature capsules before, during and after treadmill exercise. Since the assessment of core temperature is vital is sport research the mass screening ability of this technique, compared to more expensive and impractical methods, can prove very useful in the future.

Swimming, as any other sport, challenges the thermal balance of the human body, increasing Tsk (Zaidi, Fohanno, Polidori, & Taiar, 2007) through a complex thermoregulation process that intends to preserve core temperature around 37.5°C (Bertucci, Arfaoui, Janson, & Polidori, 2013). Despite the study of Wade and Veghte (1977) and the increasing number of papers in sport research reporting the use of IRT, its use in swimming research is limited and few researchers have informed the use of this technology in swimming activities (Seixas, Gonjo, Vardasca, Gabriel, & Fernandes, 2014; Zaidi et al., 2007).

In the last decades the scientific community has greatly advanced in the direction of improving the quality of IRT analysis but little has been done to standardize methodologies of application of IRT in swimming research. This study aims to develop a methodology to investigate swimmers and verify whether there is a considerable increase in body temperature during different swimming techniques (crawl and backstroke) and, if confirmed, to identify the most affected regions. The athlete's thermal symmetry was also assessed before and after swimming.

BACKGROUND

Thermal Physics and Thermal Physiology

When two objects are at different temperatures heat flux, from the hotter object to the cooler object, will happen until the state of thermal equilibrium is achieved (Thomas, 1999). Heat transfer can be described by three main mechanisms, conduction, convection and radiation (Ring, 2007). Radiation is of utmost importance for IRT measurements while heat loss by other mechanisms must be avoided.

Emissivity is the most important factor in non-contact temperature measurements and can be defined as the ratio between the radiant emittance produced by an object and that of a blackbody at a specific temperature. This parameter affects the accuracy of the measurement and a perfect blackbody, as a perfect emitting surface, has an emissivity value of 1. In contrast, highly reflective materials have near 0 emissivity values (Thomas, 1999). The skin is considered a near-perfect blackbody and its emissivity value is considered to be 0.98 (Cheng & Herman, 2014).

All objects above absolute zero (-273.15ºC) radiate energy to the environment in the form of electromagnetic waves (Pidwirny & Jones, 2006). The full range of electromagnetic radiation frequencies is called electromagnetic spectrum. Biomedical utilization of this spectrum is well known as several imaging modalities capture radiation emitted by the human body at different frequencies and wavelengths (Hynes et al., 2005). Most of these imaging modalities provide anatomical information and have ionizing properties but IRT provides physiological information is noninvasive and non-ionizing, therefore totally safe to use.

The human body is homoeothermic and the thermoregulation process is mediated centrally by the hypothalamus that detects changes in temperature. The anterior hypothalamus, also known as preoptic hypothalamus, detects increments in temperature and the posterior hypothalamus detects decrements in temperature. (Charkoudian, 2003; Saxena, Marcu, & Karunasiri, 2008). Temperature homeostasis is maintained by a negative feedback mechanism (Saxena et al., 2008). The preoptic hypothalamus is sensitive to temperature changes in the hypothalamus and in the core and receives sensorial input from skin thermal receptors and the spinal cord. Looking at the processing and integration of central and peripheral thermal information occurring in the preoptic hypothalamus, it can be assumed that it influences the proper thermoregulatory responses aiming to maintain thermal balance. This homeostatic state can be affected by internal and external stressors (Boulant, 2000).

Skin temperature is influenced by peripheral blood flow (Gold, Cherniack, Hanlon, & Soller, 2010) but not exclusively. In fact, it depends on the complex interaction that characterizes heat transfer processes between the skin, internal tissues, the vascular system and metabolic activity. The skin behaves as a heat radiator or heat isolator according to the environmental conditions. Skin blood flow is regulated by the sympathetic nervous system through vasodilatation and vasonstriction mechanisms. Vasodilatation and blood flow increments are necessary to dissipate heat and, vasoconstriction and decrements in blood flow are necessary to retain heat (Charkoudian, 2003). The exposure to hot/cold environments, the presence of pathology or exercise training affects thermal balance, increasing or decreasing skin temperature. Skin blood flow is controlled by autonomic nervous system which is believed to be anatomically and histologically symmetrical (Niu et al., 2001; Ranson, 1933). Thermal symmetry has been defined as the degree of similarity between two regions of interest in different sides of the body that are identical in size and in position (Vardasca, Ring, Plassmann, & Jones, 2012) and is an indicator of normal physiological function.

Thermographic evaluation can be performed using different methodological approaches, static or dynamic methods. In a static assessment the thermogram provides information about skin temperature distribution, giving insight about hot and cold spots, and asymmetric thermal distributions. Dynamic assessments provide information about spatial temperature distribution but also about temporal behavior of skin temperature. Active thermography implies warming or cooling the area in study and the analysis of the manner and rate of thermal recovery. Passive thermography does not imply the use of thermal stressors but requires internal challenges such as exercise (Jiang et al., 2005).

Recent Use of IRT in Swimming Research

In the last two decades the technology has heavily evolved and the quality of infrared cameras has increased, as well as the knowledge about standardization techniques and physiological mechanisms of temperature distribution.

Skin temperature changes after exercise outside the water have been extensively reported in the literature but few studies addressed the skin temperature changes after exercising in the water. Studying the skin temperature changes after exercising in the water may provide important evidence on the efficiency of heat dissipation in this environment. In recent years, to our knowledge, only two investigations used IRT to assess skin temperature of swimmers or the effect of different swimming techniques in skin temperature distribution of swimmers.

Zaidi et al. (2007) published a case study aiming to demonstrate the applicability of IRT in swimming research and to understand if the skin temperature of the swimmer was affected differentially by diverse swimming techniques. The simmer's skin temperature was assessed after a 10 minute period of acclimatization in the water and after 100 meters of each swimming technique (butterfly, backstroke, breaststroke and free style). Between each swimming technique there was a 10 minute rest period to achieve thermal balance and the IRT measures after this period were the baseline for the swimming technique performed after. The authors described the changes in skin temperature after each swimming technique and concluded that each technique changed the skin temperature differently. Although this study presented a new methodology to assess skin temperature after swimming exercise some limitations can be pointed, like the fact that only one swimmer was assessed and the fact that all swimming techniques were performed in the same day since, even with a 10 minute rest period to achieve thermal balance, we may question if fatigue played a role in the observed temperature changes. Nothing was mentioned about the velocity and intensity of each swimming technique, which may have influenced the study results.

The study of Seixas et al. (2014) aimed to understand the influence of two different swimming techniques in the skin temperature distribution and analyze the relationship between IRT measurements and energy expenditure, using a respiratory snorkel AquaTrainer and valve system connected to a telemetric portable gas analyzer, in national level swimmers. Energy expenditure is commonly used in swimming research as an indicator of performance (Barbosa et al., 2006; R. Fernandes et al., 2006) but had never been related to skin temperature measurements in swimming research. Two swimmers participated in the cross-sectional study to collect energy expenditure and thermal data during 2x300m protocols (1st bout at backstroke and the 2nd at crawl). The swimming techniques were assessed in two separate days, at the same time of the day and at the same intensity and velocity. The authors concluded that higher differences between total skin temperature before exercise and after exercise were associated with lower values of energy expenditure (Seixas et al., 2014). This research findings highlight the potential use of skin temperature as an indicator of energy expenditure, however, the low number of participants advise to take this results with caution.

A study performed in Czech Republic (Novotny et al., 2015) intended to describe and assess the energetic-metabolic activity of the muscles areas in the upper limbs after backstroke swimming through IRT and electromyography. It was found that after 15 minutes after 1,000m exercise there was a significant increase in triceps brachii and in side, rear and front deltoid muscles, and a significant decrease of skin temperature in in pectoralis, rhombic and lower trapezius, erector spinae lumbalis and latissimus dorsi. The authors explain this through the influence of the swimmer's forward motion and possible cooling effect of the water.

Neuromuscular Activity in Swimming

The study of muscular involvement in human swimming has started in the 30's, however, research concerning the pattern in which muscles are activated during a rhythmical swimming movement – which provides higher insight on movement analysis – began more than 50 years ago, using electromyography (Martens, Figueiredo, & Daly, 2014). Today there is a considerable amount of research in this field but mainly presented in abstracts, congress proceedings and narrative reviews. The available evidence has recently been the subject of a systematic review focusing on the muscle activity in the four competitive strokes: crawl, breaststroke, butterfly and backstroke (Martens, Figueiredo, & Daly, 2014).

The interpretation of the eletromyographic signal allows researchers to understand the neuromuscular activation, giving insight about the force exerted as these variables are roughly proportional. The muscle force produced cannot be estimated by this analysis but the duration of muscular activation indicates if the muscle is active and it is possible to define timing and co-activation patterns of several muscles (Barbosa, Marinho, Costa, & Silva, 2011).

In crawl, according to Pink, Perry, Browne, Scovazzo, and Kerrigan (1991), the prime movers at hand entry, hand exit and recovery phases are the upper trapezius, rhomboids, supraspinatus, the middle and the anterior deltoid. During the underwater phases the main propulsive muscles are the pectoralis major and the latissimus dorsi. The rotator cuff muscles are also important because they stabilize the scapula and the humerus during all swimming phases. One of them, the teres minor, closely follows the activation of pectoralis major in all phases. Rouard and Clarys (1995) reported that at the elbow the activation of the biceps, brachioradialis, flexor carpi ulnaris and triceps was higher during the early pull-through phase, with biceps and brachioradialis as prime movers. A co-activation of the biceps and triceps is important to stabilize the elbow (Lauer, Figueiredo, Vilas-Boas, Fernandes, & Rouard, 2013; Rouard & Clarys, 1995). Caty et al. (2007), giving insight on the muscle activation at the wrist, concluded that the flexor carpi ulnaris and extensor carpi ulnaris were highly activated during the early pull-through phase to stabilize the joint.

Looking at another technique – backstroke – Pink et al. (1992), with the same equipment and protocol used in their study on crawl activation pattern, found that the deltoid muscles, supraspinatus, rhomboids, upper trapezius and serratus anterior evidenced higher activation during hand entry and exit phases. Latissimus dorsi, subscapularis and teres minor muscles were the main propulsive muscles. Compared to crawl, the activity of the pectoralis major was lower because the S-shaped movement of the upper limb is more pronounced in crawl (Martens et al., 2014).

Muscular activation during the butterfly stroke was approached by (Pink et al., 1993). The authors reported similar results to those of (Pink et al., 1991), with co-activation of all parts of the deltoid, supraspinatus, infraspinatus, trapezius and rhomboids at hand entry, hand exit and recovery phases. Pectoralis major and latissimus dorsi acted as main propulsors and close level of activation of the teres minor and subscapularis to control the humeral head and to aid in humeral medial rotation respectively.

In breaststroke, during the pull-through phase, pectoralis major and latissimus dorsi were more active and their actions was balanced by teres minor and subscapularis, correspondingly. The action of teres minor provided and eccentric external rotation force and maintained the articular congruence and the activity of the subscapularis prevented levering of the humeral head out of the glenoid joint surface. The recovery phase is characterized by activations of the deltoid portions in synchrony with the supraspinatus muscle, to lift the arm and depress the humeral head, and of the serratus anterior with the upper trapezius muscle to stabilize, protract and upward rotate the scapula (Ruwe, Pink, Jobe, Perry, & Scovazzo, 1994).

Muscle contractions during swimming produce heat that is transferred to adjacent tissues, including skin. Heat dissipation through skin can be assessed with thermal imaging, giving insight on the thermoregulatory mechanisms involved. Previous research found that, during breaststroke, skin temperature increased more importantly in the triceps area, an agonist of the swimmer forward motion (Novotny et al., 2015). Given the scarce number of reports on the skin temperature changes after swimming and its relation with muscular activity, more studies are needed to explore this application of infrared imaging.

THERMAL CHARACTERIZATION OF CRAWL AND BACKSTROKE TECHNIQUES

When trying to implement IRT in swimming several issues must be addressed to guarantee the quality of the data collected such as environmental conditions, acclimatization and skin drying protocol.

The environmental conditions of a swimming pool are different from the recommendations of previously published guidelines (Ammer, 2008; Schwartz, 2006) since the temperature and relative humidity are above the suggested values. This is a relevant issue but swimmers, as in any other sport discipline, need to be studied in the same conditions of their practice if researchers want to apply their findings to reality.

Acclimatization is important to achieve a pre-imaging equilibrium between blood pressure and skin temperature (Ring & Ammer, 2000) but the time required is not consensual and previous published literature recommend time periods of 10 minutes (Ferreira et al., 2008), 15 minutes (Zontak, Sideman, Verbitsky, & Beyar, 1998) and 20 minutes (Merla et al., 2010). Authors recommend that acclimatization should be undertaken at rest in an examination room with stable temperature to obtain baseline thermograms when using Dynamic IRT. Looking at swimming research, exercise is performed in the water and if baseline thermograms would be obtained in such conditions the analysis would be meaningless.

Water is an isotropic substance and opaque to radiation (Viskanta & Toor, 1972) therefore swimmers must be dried before thermal imaging acquisition. In this process skin friction must be avoided since it can influence local microcirculation and the skin temperature values reported by the camera.

This issues where partially addressed in the case study of Zaidi et al. (2007) but, due to the limitations of the work, further research is recommended and a cross-sectional study was conducted in 10 national level swimmers to characterize the thermal changes induced by 2 swimming techniques, crawl and backstroke.

Methodology

The local ethics committee approved the study protocol and the rules of the declaration of Helsinki were followed. The volunteers were informed about the experimental procedure, the potential risks and benefits and gave written consent to participate in the study.

Sample Characterization

The study was conducted on 10 active national level male swimmers. In order to obtain an anthropometric characterization of the dataset, age, height and mass were collected and body mass index (BMI) was estimated. The average values are presented in table 1.

The swimmers reported training 1.5-3h each session, 6-9 times per week.

Experimental Procedure

The experimental procedures took place in a covered swimming pool, with a length of 25 meters. The environmental parameters that could affect the experiment were measured during the collection period: water temperature (26.4±0.4 ºC), room temperature (29.9±0.8 ºC) and relative humidity (57.6±3.2%), with no airflow and artificial light influence.

Each participant reported for testing for two days, at the same time of the day, one for each experimental condition. During each visit, two skin temperature measurements were performed, one before and one after the swimming activity consisting of a 7x200m protocol in front crawl or backstroke.

For the capture, a FLIR A325 thermal camera was used, with spatial resolution of 320x240, sensitivity of 70mK and accuracy of ±2%. Thermogram capture and analysis was performed with FLIR® ThermaCAM Researcher v2.10 software package. Full body thermograms of different views were recorded before and after exercise: anterior, lateral (right and left) and dorsal.

In both experimental sessions the swimmers were asked to stay immersed in water up to the neck, in a static position, for 10 minutes, the minimum reported in previous literature (Ferreira et al., 2008). The acclimatization was performed in the water so that a baseline skin temperature measurement could be obtained after the same environmental conditions in which the exercise was carried out. The head was not immersed in the water for thermal comfort purposes. Subjects were in front of the swimming pool stairs, holding on to them to maintain balance during the acclimatization.

Table 1. Anthropometric characterization of the sample (mean ± standard deviation)

	Age (years)	Height (m)	Mass (kg)	BMI (Kg/m^2)
n=10	17.20±0.90	1.78±0.06	70.40±5.80	22.10±1.30

After this period the athletes were rapidly dried with a microfiber towel, a strong absorption material, without friction on the skin to avoid heating.

Thermograms were taken before and after the respective swimming exercise (crawl or backstroke 7x200m protocol).

Data Analysis

Further analyses, a total of 14 regions of interest (ROI) were selected in the anterior view (Figure 1), 16 regions for dorsal view (Figure 2) and 5 for the lateral views (Figures 3 and 4). In this selection, body extremities (hands, feet, and head) were not considered.

For each ROI, mean temperature values were extracted and average values were estimated from the results of all the 10 athletes. To analyse the changes in temperature distribution caused by exercise, a difference between the values collected before and after exercise (ΔT) was calculated for each ROI. These values were also used to compare the swimming techniques (crawl and backstroke) and their effect on skin temperature. Finally, thermal symmetry and its modification after the swimming activity was calculated as the difference between the values of symmetric ROIs (left-right) in the same view.

Figure 1. ROIs in the anterior view. Anterior Neck Right (ANR); Anterior Neck Left (ANL); Anterior Torax Right (ATXR); Anterior Torax Left (ATXL); Anterior Arm Right (AAR); Anterior Arm Left (AAL); Anterior Forearm Right (AFR); Anterior Forearm Left (AFL); Anterior Abdomen Right (AABR); Anterior Abdomen Left (AABL); Anterior Thigh Right (ATR); Anterior Thigh Left (ATL); Anterior Leg Right (ALR); Anterior Leg Left (ALL)

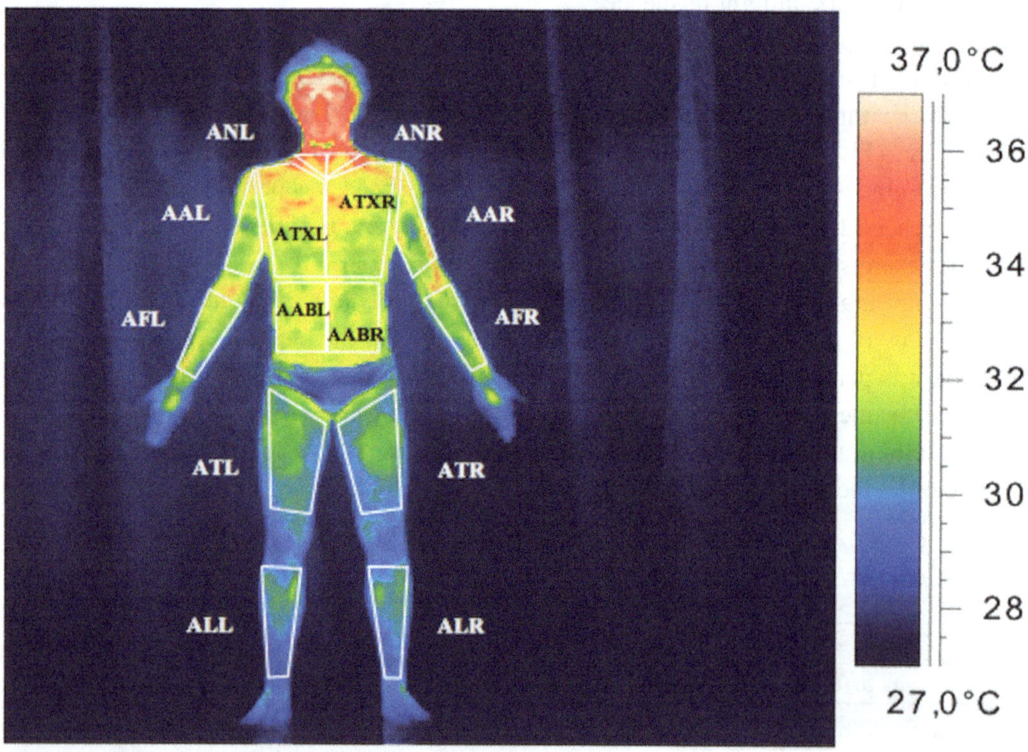

Figure 2. ROIs in the Dorsal View. Dorsal Neck Left (DNL); Dorsal Neck Right (DNR); Dorsal Upper Back Left (DUBL); Dorsal Upper Back Right (DUBR); Dorsal Arm Left (DAL); Dorsal Arm Right (DAR); Dorsal Middle Back Left (DMBL); Dorsal Middle Back Right (DMBR); Dorsal Forearm Left (DFAL); Dorsal Forearm Right (DFAR); Dorsal Lower Back Left (DLBL); Dorsal Lower Back Right (DLBR); Dorsal Thigh Left (DTL); Dorsal Thigh Right (DTR); Dorsal Leg Left (DLL); Dorsal Leg Right (DLR)

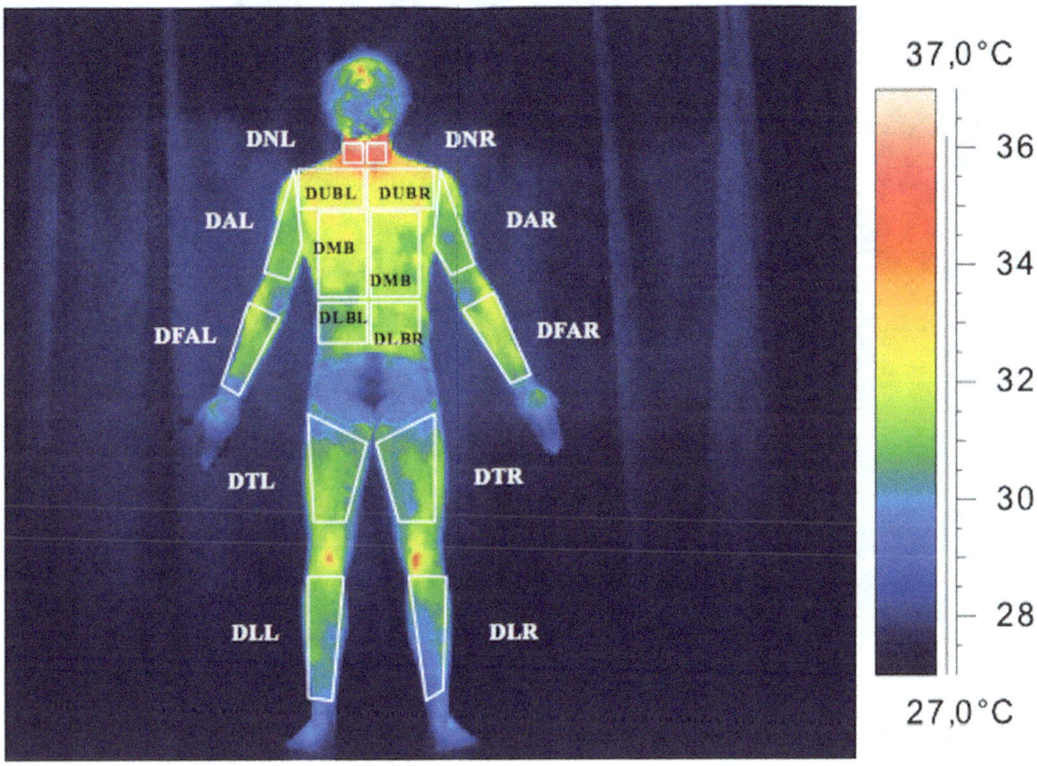

Recorded temperature values from the selected regions of interest were analysed using IBM SPSS statistics 20 for Windows. Descriptive statistics were used for anthropometric measures and ROI temperature description. Shapiro Wilk's normality test was performed and since variables did not followed normal distribution, non-parametric tests were selected (Wilcoxon Signed Ranks Test) to compare skin temperature before and after the exercise protocol and between swimming technique in each region of interest. Significance level was set at $p \leq 0.05$.

Results

The results are organized in 4 different sections:

1. Temperature differences after the swimming techniques,
2. Differences between swimming techniques,
3. Thermal symmetry and
4. Statistics.

Figure 3. ROIs in the right lateral view. Lateral Right Neck (LRN); Lateral Right Arm (LRA); Lateral Right Forearm (LRF); Lateral Right Thigh (LRT); Lateral Right Knee (LRK); Lateral Right Leg (LRL)

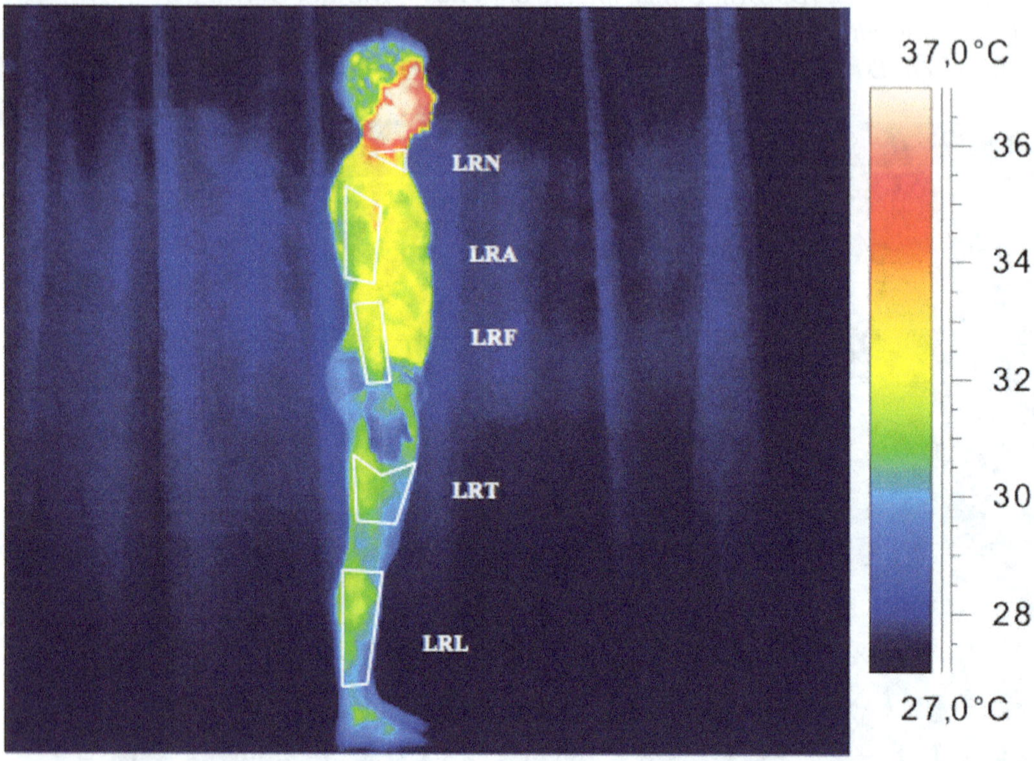

Temperature Differences After Exercise

The obtained results of temperature difference before and after the exercise for each ROI are summarized in histograms presented in Figure 5 (anterior view), Figure 6 (dorsal view), Figure 7 (lateral left view) and Figure 8 (lateral right view). The standard deviation bars were not considered because with a small sample of 10 subjects it would be of poor illustrability.

Skin temperature increased in all regions of interest after both swimming techniques. The regions with higher ΔT, for both techniques, are the upper limb (arm and forearm) and upper trunk region (thoracic, upper back and middle back).

Although the abdomen and lower back are located in the trunk, they do not indicate significant differences in temperature, as well as, in the neck and leg regions.

Differences Between Swimming Techniques

To understand whether skin temperature changes were different between the swimming techniques calculations were made subtracting the backstroke ΔT values to the front crawl ΔT values (ΔT front crawl – ΔT backstroke). The results are shown in Figure 9 (anterior view), Figure 10 (dorsal view), Figure 11 (lateral left view) and Figure 12 (lateral right view).

Figure 4. ROIs in the left lateral view. Lateral Left Neck (LLN); Lateral Left Arm (LLA); Lateral Left Forearm (LLF); Lateral Right Thigh (LRT); Lateral Left Knee (LLK); Lateral Left Leg (LLL)

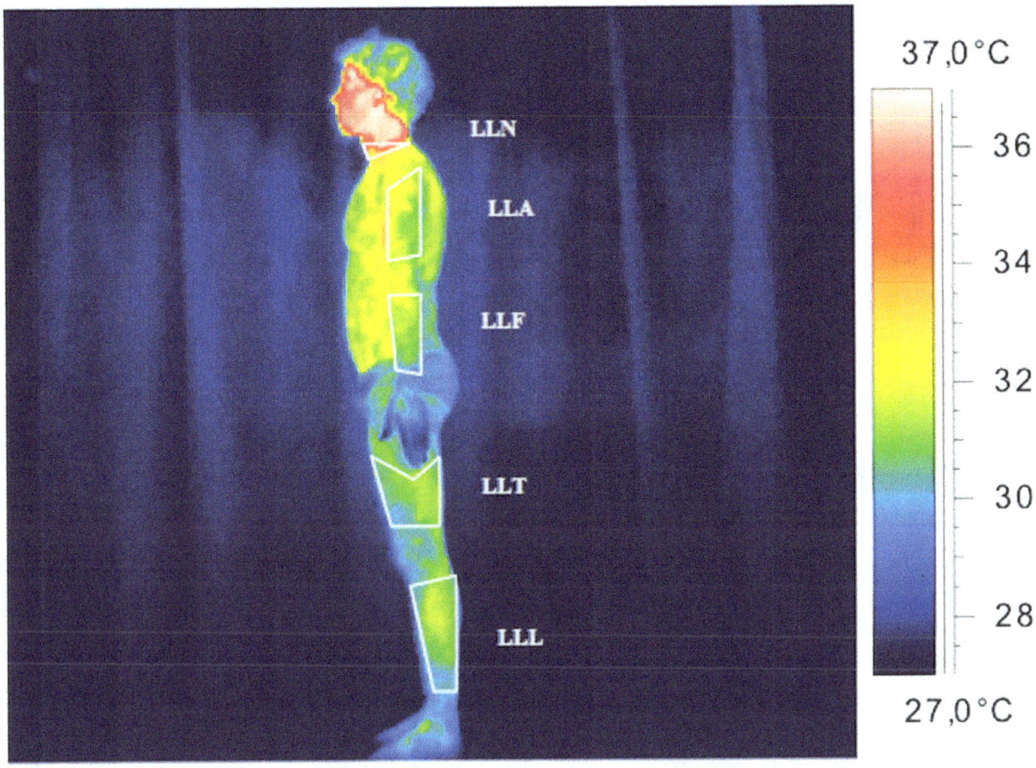

Figure 5. Temperature difference before and after exercise for Anterior ROIs (N=10)

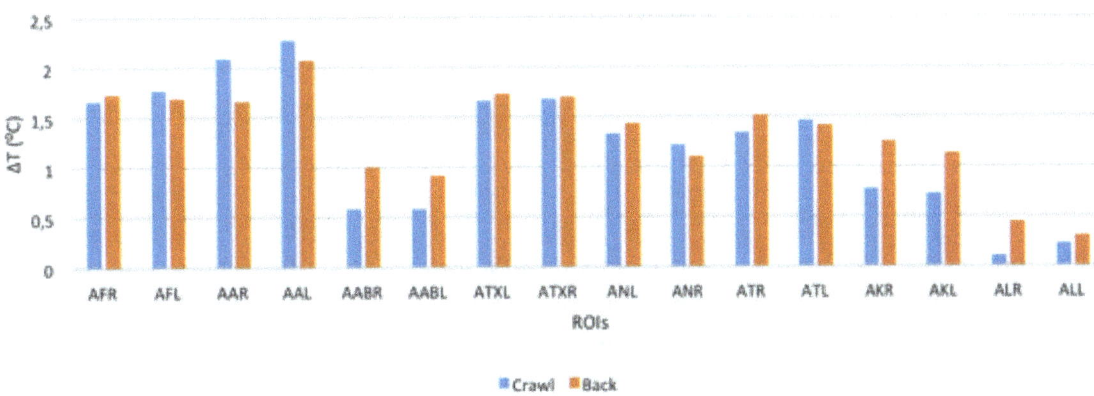

Figure 6. Temperature difference before and after exercise for Dorsal ROIs (N=10)

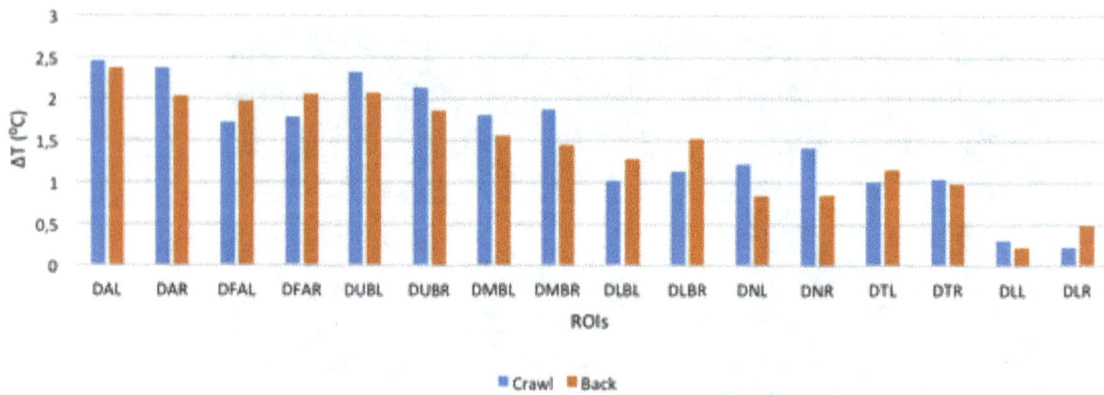

Figure 7. Temperature difference before and after exercise for Lateral Left ROIs (N=10)

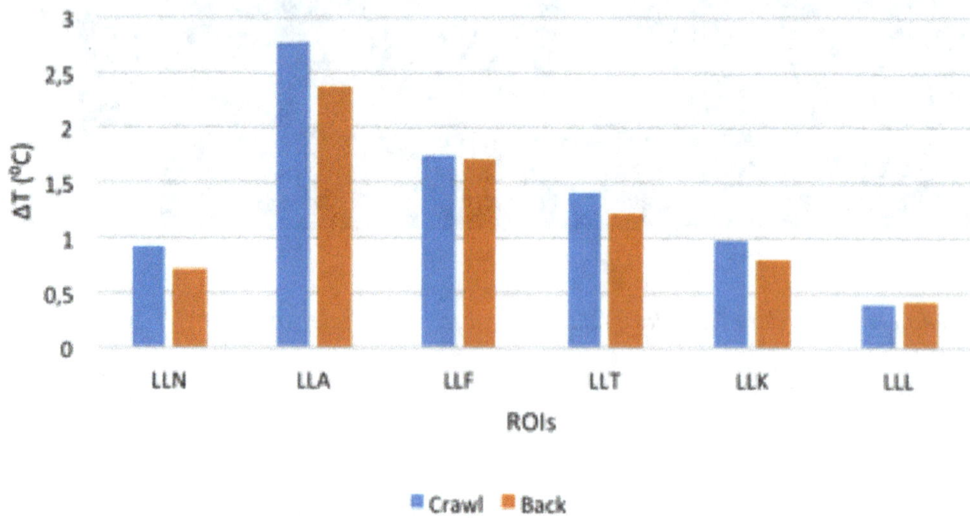

With this graphical analysis, it is possible to identify, for each ROI, the technique that induced a greater increase in temperature during the swimming activity. A negative value indicates that backstroke induced higher temperature differences whereas a positive value indicates the opposite.

Considering the presented data (anterior, posterior and both lateral views), no general tendency is observed. There is no obvious difference between each style and group of ROIs.

When comparing the skin temperature values of each ROI before exercise we found no significant differences between the values obtained in both assessment days. From the analysis through the Related-Samples Wilcoxon Signed Rank Test we can observe that there is statistical evidence ($p<0.05$), for every ROI, that skin temperature increases with both swimming techniques. However, no significant differences between the values achieved after exercise in both techniques and therefore, differentiating swimming techniques based in skin temperature values was not possible.

Figure 8. Temperature difference before and after exercise for Lateral Right ROIs (N=10)

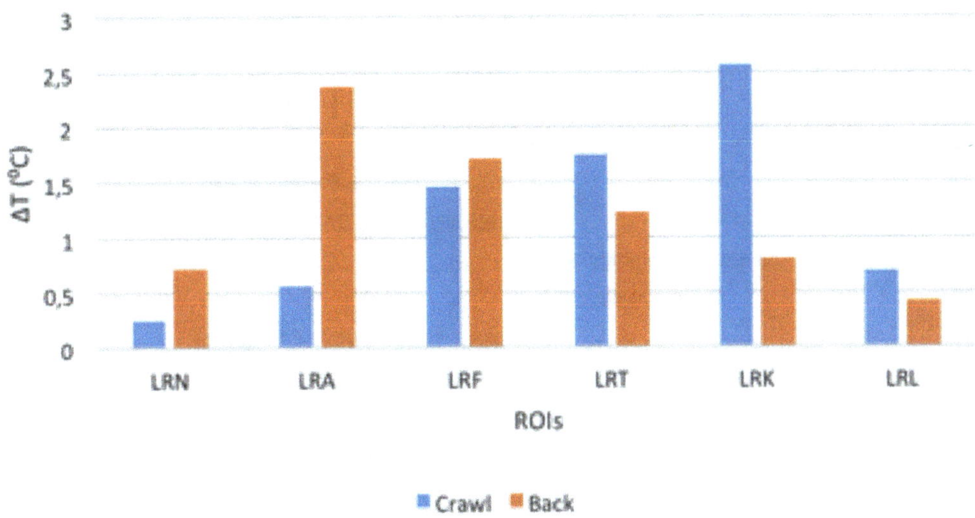

Figure 9. Temperature difference between styles (crawl – backstroke) for anterior view (N=10)

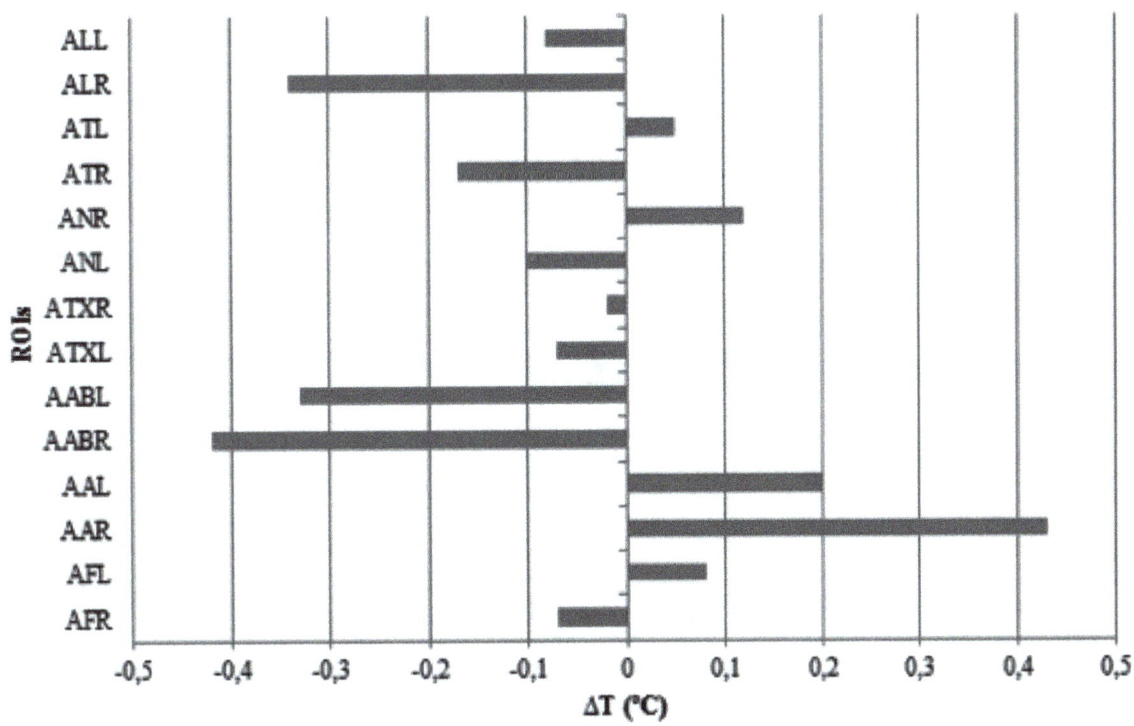

Figure 10. Temperature difference between styles (crawl – backstroke) for dorsal view (N=10)

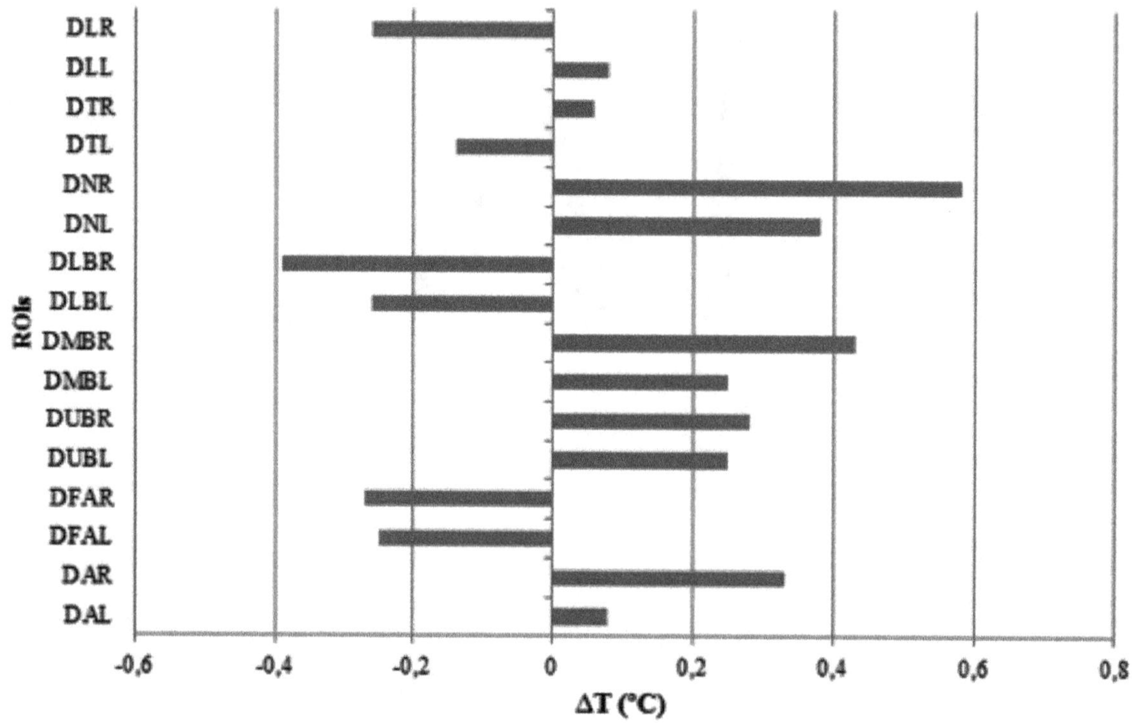

Figure 11. Temperature difference between styles (crawl – backstroke) for lateral left view (N=10)

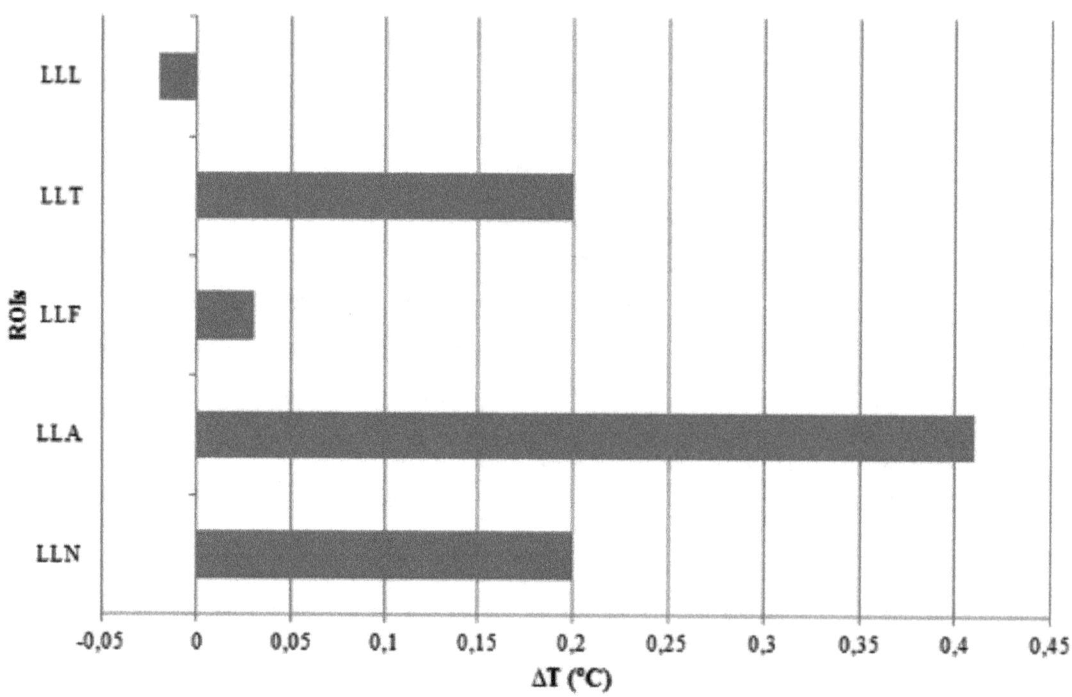

Figure 12. Temperature difference between styles (crawl – backstroke) for lateral right view (N=10)

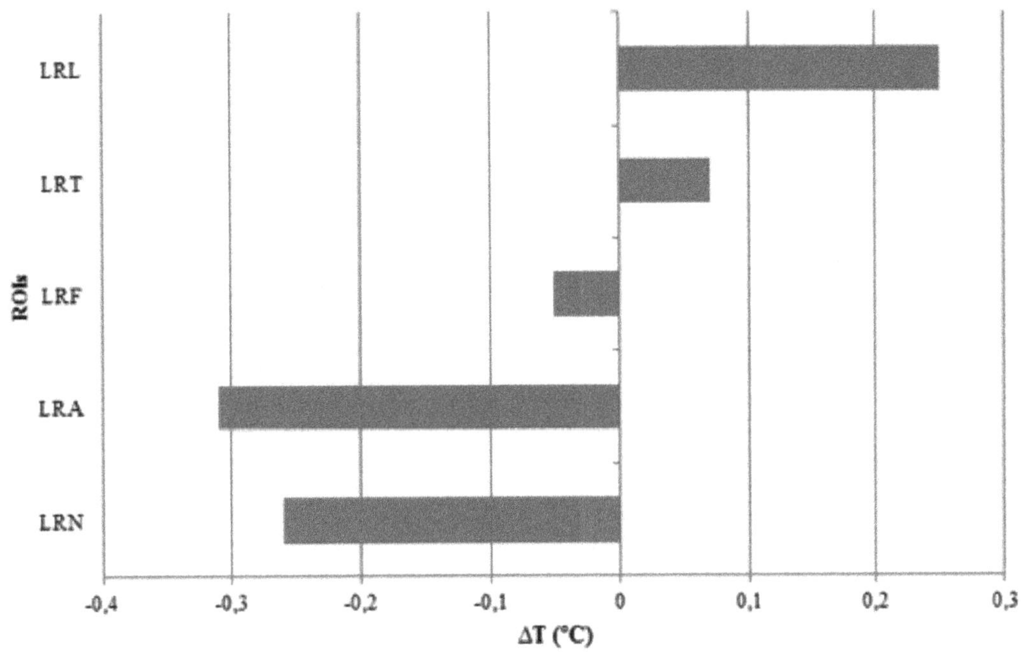

Thermal Symmetry

Thermal symmetry was assessed before and after exercise. The values obtained before the swimming protocol, allow the evaluation of the athletes health condition. With the post-exercise values, it is possible to verify if the swimming activity was equally demanding for both sides of the body.

The temperature difference between left and right regions did not exceed more than 0.5°C for all ROIs (table 2).

Thermal symmetry never exceeded 0.5°C, the value reported by Vardasca et al. (2012) as a reference in healthy subjects.

Discussion

The aim of the study was to characterize the thermal changes induced by 2 swimming techniques, crawl and backstroke.

Several issues were identified that needed to be addressed – environmental conditions, acclimatization and skin drying protocol – to increase the quality of the thermograms. In this study, different regions were evaluated in the anterior, dorsal and lateral (left and right) views, after an acclimatization period of 10 minutes, before and after two swimming techniques in two different days. The proposed methodology proved to be feasible.

It is known that exercise affects human thermoregulation (Formenti et al., 2013). Through exercise chemical energy is transformed in kinetic and thermal energy, increasing heat generation in the human body (Fernandes et al., 2014) that must be dissipated through the skin. The results obtained for the two

Table 2. Thermal symmetry values before and after the swimming techniques

ROI	ΔT Before Backstroke (°C)	ΔT After Backstroke (°C)	ΔT Before Front Crawl (°C)	ΔT After Front Crawl (°C)
Anterior Arm	0.30±0.29	0.39±0.27	0.44±0.34	0.20±0.10
Anterior Forearm	0.23±0.18	0.23±0.44	0.29±0.18	0.17±0.21
Anterior Thigh	0.20±0.14	0.20±0.12	0.29±0.30	0.21±0.16
Anterior Leg	0.20±0.14	0.30±0.13	0.30±0.18	0.30±0.12
Anterior Thorax	0.16±0.14	0.17±0.10	0.11±0.07	0.16±0.10
Anterior Abdomen	0.19±0.12	0.13±0.11	0.14±0.20	0.14±0.10
Dorsal Arm	0.31±0.20	0.26±0.41	0.23±0.11	0.16±0.17
Dorsal Forearm	0.30±0.24	0.34±0.29	0.30±0.16	0.39±0.51
Dorsal Thigh	0.20±0.17	0.16±0.10	0.16±0.08	0.09±0.09
Dorsal Leg	0.17±0.14	0.24±0.21	0.14±0.10	0.20±0.10
Dorsal Upper Back	0.14±0.10	0.16±0.08	0.19±0.12	0.09±0.07
Dorsal Mid Back	0.24±0.20	0.11±0.09	0.11±0.11	0.20±0.08
Dorsal Lower Back	0.17±0.13	0.20±0.17	0.23±0.19	0.23±0.18

swimming techniques, considering the different ROIs, corroborate this information, since an increase in temperature was verified in all regions of interest as a result of the swimming activity. The methodological approach in this study allowed to achieve this results, the acclimatization in the water prevented results similar to the results of Novotny et al. (2015), having reported a decrease in skin temperature 1 minute after swimming. In this study, the acclimatization period was outside the water and this is the most likely reason for the differences regarding our results. Drying the skin carefully, without friction, was also important being a common procedure in studies assessing thermal imaging in swimming (Novotny et al., 2015; Zaidi et al., 2007).

The thoracic region and upper limbs were the regions with higher temperature variations. The physiological processes that occur during the exercise sustain this. The upper limbs are, naturally, the key elements to the movement of the swimmer (Martens, Figueiredo, & Daly, 2014) and the thoracic region includes vital organs, which have to function more efficiently during exercise. Lower values were obtained for the lower limbs, lower back and abdomen that are also located in the trunk. However, the reduced participation of these regions in the swimming technique may be the cause of these exceptions. According to the literature (Caty et al., 2007; Lauer et al., 2013; Pink et al., 1991; Rouard & Clarys, 1995), the most active muscles in crawl, depending on the movement phase, are the upper trapezius, rhomboids, supraspinatus, middle and anterior deltoid, pectoralis major, latissimus dorsi, rotator cuff, biceps, triceps, brachioradialis, flexor carpi and extensor carpi ulnaris. In backstroke the most active muscles are the deltoid muscles, supraspinatus, rhomboids, upper trapezius, serratus anterior, latissimus dorsi, subscapularis, teres minor and pectoralis major (Pink et al., 1992). The location of these muscles corresponds to the regions of interest where higher temperatures differences were found after both swimming techniques: the upper back, mid back, the arm and the forearm in the dorsal view; the thorax, the arm and the forearm in the anterior view and the arm in the lateral view. The most active muscles reported in the literature are similar for both crawl and backstroke. This fact gives insight on the lack of differences in the thermal patterns of both swimming techniques. Total skin temperature was not calculated in this study but this might be a differentiating characteristic between the techniques as suggested by Zaidi et al. (2007) and Seixas et al. (2014).

Thermal asymmetry may indicate the presence of pathology related to the autonomic nervous system (Niu et al., 2001). In our study all thermal symmetry values were below 0.5ªC, the reference value proposed by (Vardasca et al., 2012).

Thermography has also been a useful tool to verify the symmetry of the sport modality, in this case swimming. Crawl and backstroke techniques were symmetric, requiring similar exercise intensity from both sides of the body, which was corroborated by the results, which are certainly related to the training level of the athletes. Thermal symmetry values were not affected by the swimming activity, reinforcing the idea of symmetrical activity by the swimmers. When the exercise is not symmetrically demanding, thermal symmetry is affected as reported in another study assessing the effects of vibration exercise (Seixas, Silva, Vardasca, & Gabriel, 2012).

The techniques adopted in this study are different than those reported by Zaidi et al. (2007), being difficult to compare results. The authors studied only 1 swimmer that performed 4x100 meters, 100 meters for each swimming technique, with 10-minute intervals and in our study athletes performed a 7x200 meters protocol in each of the testing days, one for each swimming technique. The intensity of the exercise is not similar and certainly this is one of the factors that can explain the differences observed. Zaidi et al. (2007) assessed the thermal response of the swimmer to four swimming techniques – butterfly, backstroke, breast stroke and free style – and we assessed the thermal response of the participants in two swimming techniques, backstroke and front crawl. We can argue if the 10 minute interval given by the authors was enough to achieve thermal balance, if the results obtained after one technique are not influenced by the thermoregulation processes that initiated after the previous technique and if the 100 meters are enough to understand the thermal pattern of the athlete. These concerns lead us to conduct a study assessing a larger distance in two different days.

It is important to notice that in this study the athletes were dried using absorbing microfiber towels avoid friction to not increase skin temperature, not taking the procedure more than 1 minute, this reduces the effect of 15 minutes waiting after the exercise (Novotny et al., 2015), that might erase the effect of the swimming challenge.

Although with a reduced sample this study reinforced the value of thermal imaging in assessing skin temperature responses after physical exertion in swimmers, and athletes in general.

FUTURE RESEARCH DIRECTIONS

Future research should clarify if the swimming technique has any influence in total skin temperature or in the temperature of individual ROIs and if the nature of thermograms plays a role in the analysis (full body or regional). The influence of the swimmer level and specialization is another issue that needs to be explored, as the influence of age and gender on the thermal response. The intensity of the swimming technique and its effect in skin temperature also needs to be addressed.

CONCLUSION

This chapter provided a literature overview on the use of thermal imaging in swimming research, on relevant background concepts and proposed a methodology to characterize the thermal changes induced by front crawl and backstroke techniques. Thermal imaging proved useful to assess the skin temperature in swimmers and the purposed methodology was reliable and repeatable. Both swimming techniques increased skin temperature but no differences were found in thermograms between swimming techniques. The regions of interest with higher temperature changes match to the locations of the most active muscles. Thermal symmetry values were not affected by exercise, suggesting a symmetrical demand to the swimmers.

REFERENCES

Ammer, K. (2008). The Glamorgan Protocol for recording and evaluation of thermal images of the human body. *Thermology International, 18*(4), 125-144.

Barbosa, T., Fernandes, R., Keskinen, K., Colaço, P., Cardoso, C., Silva, J., & Vilas-Boas, J. (2006). Evaluation of the Energy Expenditure in Competitive Swimming Strokes. *International Journal of Sports Medicine, 27*(11), 894–899. doi:10.1055/s-2006-923776 PMID:16612740

Barbosa, T., Marinho, D., Costa, M., & Silva, A. (2011). Biomechanics of competitive swimming strokes. In V. Klika (Ed.), *Biomechanics in Applications* (pp. 367–388). Intech.

Bertucci, W., Arfaoui, A., Janson, L., & Polidori, G. (2013). Relationship between the gross efficiency and muscular skin temperature of lower limb in cycling: a preliminary study. *Computer Methods in Biomechanics and Biomedical Engineering, 16*(sup1), 114-115.

Boulant, J. A. (2000). Role of the preoptic-anterior hypothalamus in thermoregulation and fever. *Clinical Infectious Diseases, 31*(Supplement 5), S157–S161. doi:10.1086/317521 PMID:11113018

Bourlai, T., Pryor, R. R., Suyama, J., Reis, S. E., & Hostler, D. (2012). Use of thermal imagery for estimation of core body temperature during precooling, exertion, and recovery in wildland firefighter protective clothing. *Prehospital Emergency Care, 16*(3), 390–399. doi:10.3109/10903127.2012.670689 PMID:22510022

Burnham, R. S., McKinley, R. S., & Vincent, D. D. (2006). Three types of skin-surface thermometers: A comparison of reliability, validity, and responsiveness. *American Journal of Physical Medicine & Rehabilitation, 85*(7), 553–558. doi:10.1097/01.phm.0000223232.32653.7f PMID:16788385

Caty, V., Aujouannet, Y., Hintzy, F., Bonifazi, M., Clarys, J., & Rouard, A. (2007). Wrist stabilisation and forearm muscle coactivation during freestyle swimming. *Journal of Electromyography and Kinesiology, 17*(3), 285–291. doi:10.1016/j.jelekin.2006.02.005 PMID:16677829

Charkoudian, N. (2003). *Skin blood flow in adult human thermoregulation: how it works, when it does not, and why.* Paper presented at the Mayo Clinic. doi:10.4065/78.5.603

Cheng, T.-Y., & Herman, C. (2014). Analysis of skin cooling for quantitative dynamic infrared imaging of near-surface lesions. *International Journal of Thermal Sciences*, *86*(0), 175–188. doi:10.1016/j.ijthermalsci.2014.06.033

Chudecka, M., & Lubkowska, A. (2012). The use of thermal imaging to evaluate body temperature changes of athletes during training and a study on the impact of physiological and morphological factors on skin temperature. *Human Movement*, *13*(1), 33–39. doi:10.2478/v10038-012-0002-9

Clark, R., Mullan, B., & Pugh, L. (1977). Skin temperature during runninga study using infra-red colour thermography. *The Journal of Physiology*, *267*(1), 53–62. doi:10.1113/jphysiol.1977.sp011800 PMID:874861

Fernandes, A. A., Amorim, P. R. S., Brito, C. J., de Moura, A. G., Moreira, D. G., Costa, C. M. A., & Marins, J. C. B. et al. (2014). Measuring skin temperature before, during and after exercise: A comparison of thermocouples and infrared thermography. *Physiological Measurement*, *35*(2), 189–203. doi:10.1088/0967-3334/35/2/189 PMID:24398429

Fernandes, R., Billat, V., Cruz, A., Colaço, P., Cardoso, C., & Vilas-Boas, J. (2006). Does net energy cost of swimming affect time to exhaustion at the individual's maximal oxygen consumption velocity? *The Journal of Sports Medicine and Physical Fitness*, *46*(3), 373. PMID:16998440

Ferreira, J. J., Mendonca, L. C., Nunes, L. A., Andrade Filho, A. C., Rebelatto, J. R., & Salvini, T. F. (2008). Exercise-associated thermographic changes in young and elderly subjects. *Annals of Biomedical Engineering*, *36*(8), 1420–1427. doi:10.1007/s10439-008-9512-1 PMID:18470619

Formenti, D., Ludwig, N., Gargano, M., Gondola, M., Dellerma, N., Caumo, A., & Alberti, G. (2013). Thermal Imaging of Exercise-Associated Skin Temperature Changes in Trained and Untrained Female Subjects. *Annals of Biomedical Engineering*, 1–9. PMID:23229282

Gold, J. E., Cherniack, M., Hanlon, A., & Soller, B. (2010). Skin temperature and muscle blood volume changes in the hand after typing. *International Journal of Industrial Ergonomics*, *40*(2), 161–164. doi:10.1016/j.ergon.2009.07.001

Hunold, S., Mietzsch, E., & Werner, J. (1992). Thermographic studies on patterns of skin temperature after exercise. *European Journal of Applied Physiology and Occupational Physiology*, *65*(6), 550–554. doi:10.1007/BF00602364 PMID:1483445

Hynes, A., Scott, D. A., Man, A., Singer, D. L., Sowa, M. G., & Liu, K. Z. (2005). Molecular mapping of periodontal tissues using infrared microspectroscopy. *BMC Medical Imaging*, *5*(1), 2. doi:10.1186/1471-2342-5-2 PMID:15890072

Jiang, L., Ng, E., Yeo, A., Wu, S., Pan, F., Yau, W., & Yang, Y. et al. (2005). A perspective on medical infrared imaging. *Journal of Medical Engineering & Technology*, *29*(6), 257–267. doi:10.1080/03091900512331333158 PMID:16287675

Lauer, J., Figueiredo, P., Vilas-Boas, J. P., Fernandes, R. J., & Rouard, A. H. (2013). Phase-dependence of elbow muscle coactivation in front crawl swimming. *Journal of Electromyography and Kinesiology*, *23*(4), 820–825. doi:10.1016/j.jelekin.2013.02.004 PMID:23489716

Martens, J., Figueiredo, P., & Daly, D. (2014). Electromyography in the four competitive swimming strokes: A systematic review. *Journal of Electromyography and Kinesiology*. PMID:25556010

Merla, A., Mattei, P. A., Di Donato, L., & Romani, G. L. (2010). Thermal imaging of cutaneous temperature modifications in runners during graded exercise. *Annals of Biomedical Engineering*, *38*(1), 158–163. doi:10.1007/s10439-009-9809-8 PMID:19798579

Merla, A., & Romani, G. L. (2005). *Biomedical applications of functional infrared imaging*. Paper presented at the 27th Annual International Conference of the Engineering in Medicine and Biology Society, Shanghai, China.

Niu, H.-H., Lui, P.-W., Hu, J. S., Ting, C.-K., Yin, Y.-C., Lo, Y.-L., & Lee, T.-Y. et al. (2001). Thermal symmetry of skin temperature: Normative data of normal subjects in Taiwan. *Chinese Medical Journal-Taipei*, *64*(8), 459–468. PMID:11720145

Novotny, J., Rybarova, S., Zacha, D., Bernacikova, M., & Ramadan, W. A. (2015). The influence of breaststroke swimming on the muscle activity of young men in thermographic imaging.Acta of bioengineering and biomechanics/Wrocław University of Technology, 17(2), 121-129.

Pidwirny, M., & Jones, S. (2006). Energy and MatterFundamentals of physical geography (2nd ed.). Retrieved from http://www.physicalgeography.net/fundamentals/6f.html

Pink, M., Jobe, F. W., Perry, J., Kerrigan, J., Browne, A., & Scovazzo, M. L. (1992). The Normal Shoulder During the Backstroke: An EMG and Cinematographic Analysis of 12 Muscles. *Clinical Journal of Sport Medicine*, *2*(1), 6–12. doi:10.1097/00042752-199201000-00002

Pink, M., Jobe, F. W., Perry, J., Kerrigan, J., Browne, A., & Scovazzo, M. L. (1993). The normal shoulder during the butterfly swim stroke. An electromyographic and cinematographic analysis of twelve muscles. *Clinical Orthopaedics and Related Research*, (288): 48–59. PMID:8458154

Pink, M., Perry, J., Browne, A., Scovazzo, M. L., & Kerrigan, J. (1991). The normal shoulder during freestyle swimming An electromyographic and cinematographic analysis of twelve muscles. *The American Journal of Sports Medicine*, *19*(6), 569–576. doi:10.1177/036354659101900603 PMID:1781492

Ranson, S. (1933). The anatomy of the autonomic nervous system with special reference to the innervation of the skeletal muscles and blood vessels. *Annals of Internal Medicine*, *6*(8), 1013–1021. doi:10.7326/0003-4819-6-8-1013

Ring, E. F. J. (2007). The historical development of temperature measurement in medicine. *Infrared Physics & Technology*, *49*(3), 297–301. doi:10.1016/j.infrared.2006.06.029

Ring, E. F. J. (2014). Pioneering progress in infrared imaging in medicine. *Quantitative InfraRed Thermography Journal*, *11*(1), 57–65. doi:10.1080/17686733.2014.892667

Ring, E. F. J., & Ammer, K. (2000). The technique of infrared imaging in medicine. *Thermology International*, *10*(1), 7-14.

Rouard, A., & Clarys, J. (1995). Cocontraction in the elbow and shoulder muscles during rapid cyclic movements in an aquatic environment. *Journal of Electromyography and Kinesiology*, *5*(3), 177–183. doi:10.1016/1050-6411(95)00008-N PMID:20719649

Ruwe, P. A., Pink, M., Jobe, F. W., Perry, J., & Scovazzo, M. L. (1994). The Normal and the Painful Shoulders During the Breaststroke Electromyographic and Cinematographic Analysis of Twelve Muscles. *The American Journal of Sports Medicine*, *22*(6), 789–796. doi:10.1177/036354659402200610 PMID:7856803

Saxena, V., Marcu, L., & Karunasiri, G. (2008). A novel noninvasive all optical technique to monitor physiology of an exercising muscle. *Physics in Medicine and Biology*, *53*(21), 6211–6225. doi:10.1088/0031-9155/53/21/021 PMID:18854609

Schwartz, R. (2006). Guidelines for neuromusculoskeletal thermography. *Thermology International, 16*(1), 5-9.

Seixas, A., Gonjo, T., Vardasca, R., Gabriel, J., & Fernandes, R. (2014). *A preliminary study on the relationship between energy expenditure and skin temperature in swimming*. Paper presented at the 12th International Conference on Quantitative InfraRed Thermography, Bordeaux. doi:10.21611/qirt.2014.097

Seixas, A., Silva, A., Vardasca, R., & Gabriel, J. (2012). The Effect of Whole-body Vibration in the Skin Temperature of Lower Extremities in Healthy Subjects. *Thermology International, 22*(3), 59-66.

Simmons, G. H., Wong, B. J., Holowatz, L. A., & Kenney, W. L. (2011). Changes in the control of skin blood flow with exercise training: Where do cutaneous vascular adaptations fit in? *Experimental Physiology*, *96*(9), 822–828. doi:10.1113/expphysiol.2010.056176 PMID:21602295

Thomas, R. A. (1999). *The thermography monitoring handbook.* Coxmoor Publ.

Vardasca, R., Ring, E. F. J., Plassmann, P., & Jones, C. D. (2012). Thermal symmetry of the upper and lower extremities in healthy subjects. *Thermology International, 22*(2), 53-60.

Viskanta, R., & Toor, J. (1972). Radiant energy transfer in waters. *Water Resources Research*, *8*(3), 595–608. doi:10.1029/WR008i003p00595

Wade, C., & Veghte, J. (1977). Thermographic evaluation of the relative heat loss by area in man after swimming. *Aviation, Space, and Environmental Medicine*, *48*(1), 16–18. PMID:831705

Zaidi, H., Fohanno, S., Polidori, G., & Taiar, R. (2007). The influence of swimming type on the skin-temperature maps of a competitive swimmer from infrared thermography. *Acta of Bioengineering and Biomechanics*, *9*(1), 47. PMID:17933104

Zontak, A., Sideman, S., Verbitsky, O., & Beyar, R. (1998). Dynamic thermography: Analysis of hand temperature during exercise. *Annals of Biomedical Engineering*, *26*(6), 988–993. doi:10.1114/1.33 PMID:9846937

Chapter 10
Thermal Imaging:
Concepts in Application to Safety Studies of Vaccines

Andreas Hoffmann
Paul-Ehrlich-Institute, Federal Institute for Vaccines and Biomedicines, Germany

Claudia Dumke
Paul-Ehrlich-Institute, Federal Institute for Sera and Vaccines, Germany

Kay-Martin Ove Hanschmann
Paul-Ehrlich-Institute, Federal Institute for Vaccines and Biomedicines, Germany

ABSTRACT

This chapter describes an approach to quantifying the local inflammatory response at the injection site after a vaccination by infrared imaging. The aim is to develop a thermographic procedure providing support to evaluate the reactivity of a vaccine. The development of the experimental design had to consider an optimum timeframe for infrared imaging, the variability of the local thermal emission, questions regarding the thermal left-right symmetry and further biometric aspects. To verify this concept, more than 80 participants of the influenza vaccination campaign were involved. Even if this study is based on a well-tolerated seasonal influenza vaccination, nearly 40% of all subjects show a pronounced thermal reaction of approximately 1°C. Apart from this, 25-30% displays no signs of any thermal response. The question of how far thermal imaging will contribute to facilitating the assessment of the reactivity of a vaccine has several aspects which are discussed in this chapter.

INTRODUCTION

Technical developments in high resolution Infrared Thermography provide further promising opportunities for their use in biomedical research. In this this chapter, a new thermographic application to support safety studies of vaccines is described. Vaccines are a heterogeneous class of medicinal products containing antigenic substances capable of inducing specific immunity against infective agents or toxins, or against other antigenic substances. In contrast to other biological and chemical medicinal products

DOI: 10.4018/978-1-5225-2072-6.ch010

used for the treatment of diseases, vaccines are a preventive measure usually given to large cohorts of healthy subjects (Lopalco et.al., 2010). A high standard of safety and low reactogenicity is generally requested. For the safety evaluation, extensive clinical studies are demanded. The whole procedure remains always in the focus of public attention and is the subject of the subsequent pharmacovigilance survey (Waldman, Luhm, Monteiro, & Freitas, 2011). The outcome of clinical studies, however, may be more or less influenced by individual subjective reports about aches and pain or other discomfort. Possibly, thermal imaging provides a non-subjective approach to supplement evaluation of the vaccine reactivity here. This chapter tries to explain the steps on the way to a standardized thermographic protocol. After a suitable procedure to characterize the thermographic response after vaccination is confirmed, at least two aspects are of peculiar interest:

- What is known about the statistical distribution?
- Is it a Gaussian one or another one?

This is a relevant issue for statistical planning in future surveys. Furthermore, a relevant question is, whether and to what extent any relation to clinical or further attributes exists. An extracurricular vaccination program by several vaccines and each with 40 or more participants will never pass an ethical review. Thus, it was decided to join the local seasonal influenza vaccination campaign, performed regularly in Germany in each autumn. This provides the opportunity to involve a relevant number of participants and to demonstrate the feasibility of the concept under practical conditions.

A separate sub-chapter is inserted, which deals with investigations of vaccines in farm animals. These vaccines must also fulfill specific requirements of safety and must comply with standards of animal welfare. In contrast to studies in human beings, there are several different aspects. Obviously, no narrative and no subjective influence by the "vaccinee" itself is possible. However, there are quite a few critical physiological properties of the skin. Significantly, they have more thermal isolation in their skin. This is either by the fur in sheep and in cattle or by a strong subcutaneous fat layer in pigs (Eckert, 2002). Moreover, the effort in fixation of the animals to take a thermal picture cannot be underestimated. Several experiences from field studies under farm conditions were presented.

BACKGROUND

The biological background of this concept is based on the interaction of cellular and humoral factors in the immune reactive network, finally leading to an efficient immune response (Pichler, 2006). This is accompanied by a more or less strong local inflammatory response at the injection site. Local clinical symptoms are the mostly expected side effects and will be neglected, if not too painful. In contrast, the frequency of unexpected and severe adverse reactions after vaccination needs much more attention. These events however, are often extremely rare and can only be observed within higher numbers of vaccinated subjects or over a longer period in post marketing studies. The idea of this thermographic approach is to develop a marker to support clinical surveys to characterize the reactivity of a vaccine. It is assumed that even a slight local inflammation causes an increased local blood flow beside pain or discomfort. This leads to a more or less higher surface temperature. In contrast to the discomfort, a higher blood flow can be well quantified by metering the increase in the surface temperature of a defined area around the injection site. In doing this, a limited amount of subjects may be sufficient to provide reliable objective information about the reactivity of a vaccine and should provide data which may serve as a surrogate marker to support the evaluation of the safety profile of a vaccine.

METHODS OF THERMAL INVESTIGATION IN INFLUENZA VACCINATION STUDIES

In this chapter, a survey is presented, that was initiated to describe the thermal reactivity at the injection site after regular seasonal influenza vaccination in human beings (Hoffmann, Dumke, Hanschmann & Wicker, 2015). This vaccination is recommended in general for those carrying a higher risk of influenza infection such as health professionals. This provides the opportunity to acquire a representative number of participants working in medical facilities in a limited local area and in a period of few weeks. Because the seasonal influenza vaccination is known as very safe and well tolerated, a low frequency of reports of adverse reactions was expected.

Subjects

In the main course of this study, 86 individuals were involved during the seasonal influenza vaccination campaign in 2013/14 (Hoffmann et.al.2015). Two pilot studies including nine and 73 vaccinees, respectively, were done in the preceding years to develop the procedure and the final protocol step by step.

The study protocol was reviewed and approved by the local ethic review committee. All participants read and signed a consent form prior to participation. To find out whether a relation between thermal response and some clinical signs or other clinical relevant information can be observed, data about pain, time of onset of the pain and its degree, local redness, swelling or any other discomfort were collected.

Infrared Imaging

Local facilities for the thermal investigations must ensure protection from direct sun light, mean temperature between 21°C and 23°C, a draft free investigation room, and low relative humidity. Only a very slow increase in the room temperature was accepted. This complies largely with the specific requirements, outlined in detail by Ammer and Ring (Ammer & Ring, 2007).

For thermal equilibration, all subjects had to remain with free arms and free shoulders for at least ten minutes. The vaccination site (V), located on the upper arm, was with an "O" by metallic Edding® -pencil. The same position at the non-vaccinated site (C) was marked by a "K". In addition, the subject identification number was notified on a transparent Tesa®-filmstrips at the forearm. The distance from the infrared- camera to the vaccinee was approximately 1-1.5 meters. To ensure a standardized position for each subject, the TFT- flat screen monitor from the infrared -camera was superimposed by a transparent template, which facilitated positioning the upper arm of the subjects always in a similar place. Further processing of infrared data was performed by thermo-analytic imaging software.

Camera, Software and Data Processing

For thermal imaging, the Jenoptic -VarioCAM® HiRes (Infratec, 2007) from Infratec Dresden, Germany was used throughout. Processing of IR-data was performed by thermo-analytic software EXAM 5.7 and

5.8 from InfraMedic®-GmbH Mörfelden-Walldorf (Germany). The region of interest was defined by an elliptic form, fixed at the upper edge of the shoulder and on the midpoint of the upper arm axis (Figure 1) The Exam software supports free positioning and selection of a metering form, offering a direct read out of the mean and the 80th or any other percentile from the metering form. For further analysis, the Exam software allows an Excel file to be exported, containing all thermopixel from the selected metering form.

Pilot Studies

Which injection site is suited and what is the optimum time frame for the infrared imaging procedure are basics, which must be clarified before the survey of the yearly seasonal influenza vaccination campaign can be started. Obviously, the expected thermal inflammatory response will be transient. The most widely preferred injection site at the upper arm or shoulder seems to be suited for the investigation. First observations revealed that a thermal response at the shoulder is indeed detectable, at least in a majority of vaccinated subjects. Free shoulders and arms are easy to arrange, even if a great number of subjects have to be investigated within a short time interval. A typical characteristic of this injection site is that the area of maximum thermal response more or less fluctuates by several foci around or below the injection site. An elliptic metering form allows the covering of all areas and foci of thermal interest. Elliptic forms are available in most of the typical software programs used to analyze thermometric images. In contrast, a vaccination site in the area of the gluteal muscle seems to be unsuited. A more or less large subcutaneous tissue layer prevents the transfer of thermal signals to the surface of the skin and no clear-cut metering field can be detected.

To evaluate the optimum time frame to describe a local thermal response in a first pilot investigation, nine subjects were monitored at intervals of several hours until the third day after vaccination (Figure 2). Remarkably, only five out of nine participants developed a significant thermal response after influenza vaccination. Among them, a maximal thermal response could be observed 24 h after the vaccination, even if the persistency of an increased thermal response varies. In a subsequent pilot survey involving

Figure 1. Female subject, 24 hrs. after vaccination with OPTAFLU®
Left: Non-vaccinated arm, mean temperature 31.4°C; Right: vaccinated arm, mean temperature 32°C; Histogram indicates frequency distribution inside of the elliptic form

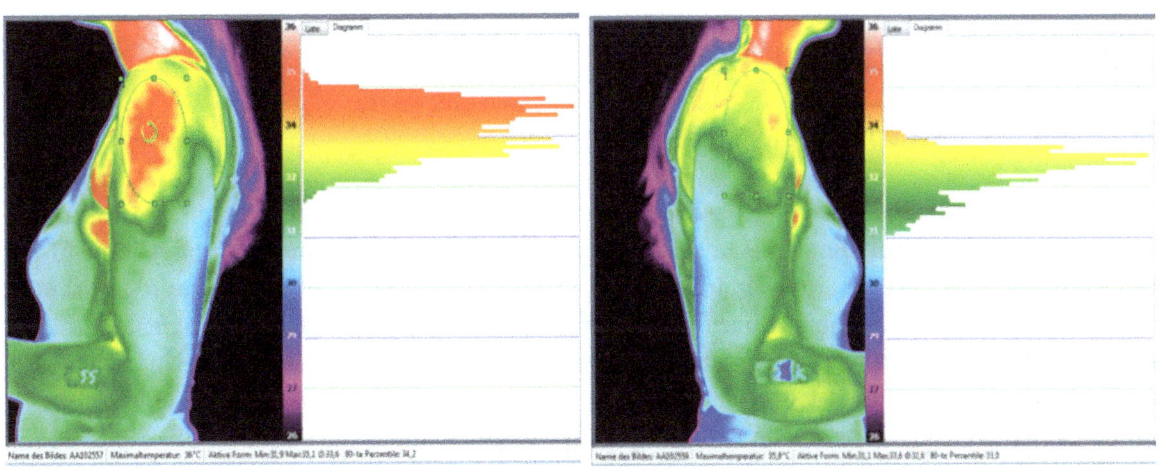

Figure 2. First monitoring of nine subjects within three days after influenza vaccination. Points indicate the difference between the vaccinated and non-vaccinated control side. Note that four of nine subjects appear as thermal non-responders at day one after

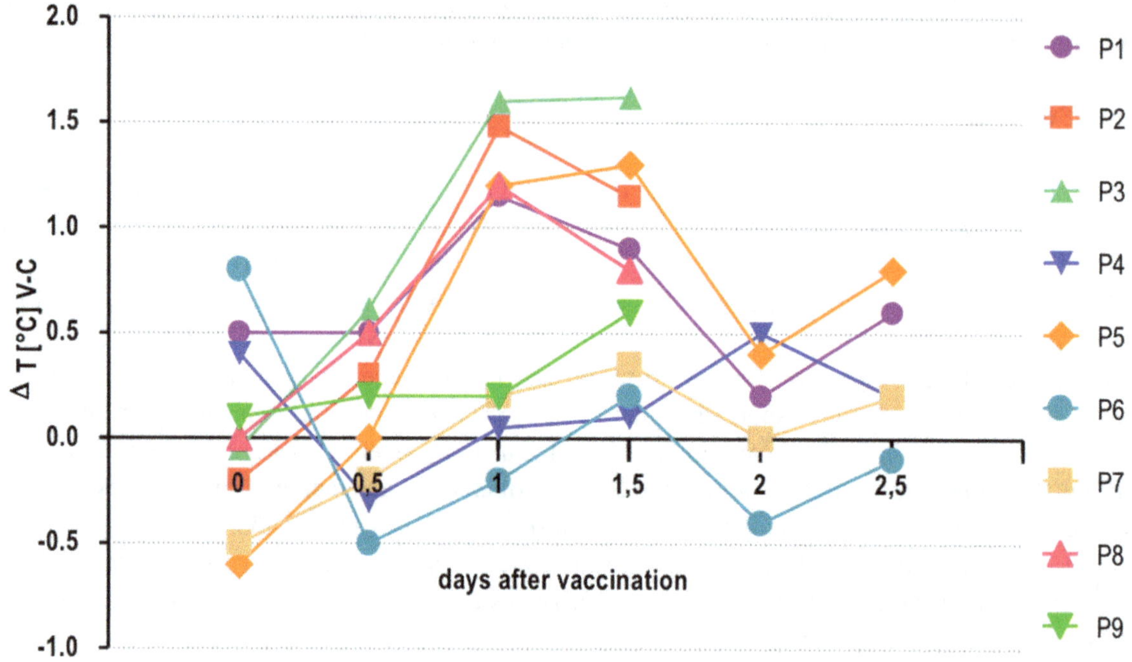

73 subjects, thermal images were recorded at a time point of 24 h after vaccination by using the non-vaccinated side as control to calculate the increase in temperature. Because approximately 15 percent of the subjects showed a decrease in temperature after vaccination, interpreting of the results was difficult. The assumption of a thermal left-right symmetry was at least in doubt. Consequently, the final protocol for the survey has to include an additional date for the infrared investigation without any influence of vaccination. This also allows an evaluation of how far individual deviations in left-right asymmetry may influence results of thermal imaging.

BIOMETRIC CONSIDERATIONS

Mean Versus Percentile

To evaluate the thermal response an ellipse seems to be the optimal form, covering the upper arm around the injection site also including an area below the injection site, because a part of the volume of the injected liquid may descend. However, the distribution of hot spots and cold areas varies to a considerable extent. The form may include one or more confluent hotspots, and sizable cold areas were also observed. Thus, the characterization of the thermal field only by the mean temperature of all included pixels can be insufficient and too much influenced by extremes. For this reason, the applicability of percentiles was considered as an alternative. To see which percentile is the optimum, all results from a

Figure 3. Box-and-whisker plot for temperature differences between vaccinated and control site, 24 hrs after vaccination. Data from 73 vaccines from the pilot survey, calculated for each from the 50th to the 100th percentile. Boxes include 50% of the vaccines' data with median (horizontal line inside the box), whiskers depict 2.5th and 97.5th percentiles, and dots mark most extreme differences. Percentiles above 90% show a slightly higher variability (wider boxes) and are therefore not suitable as target variable

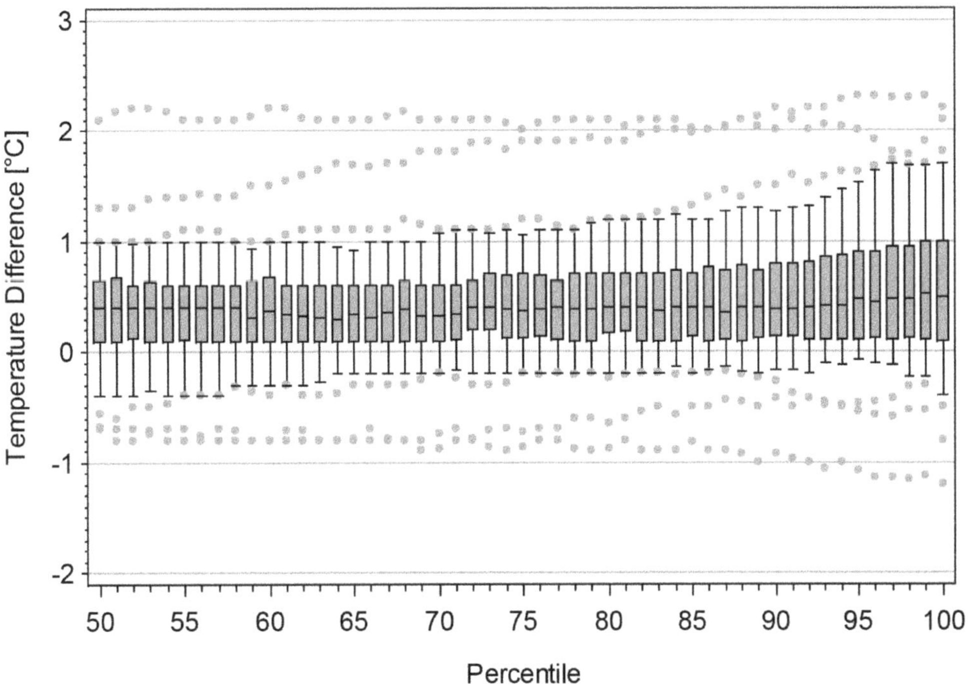

the second pilots survey, including 73 participants, were used. All percentiles both for the vaccinated and the control site, 24hrs after vaccination between the 50th (median) and the 100th (maximum) were calculated, and the difference was determined.

Different Ways to Express the Increase in Temperature After Vaccination

The simplest way to describe the increase in temperature after vaccination is to compare the vaccinated (V) with the non-vaccinated site 24 hrs. after (C). If differences (V_{24}-C_{24}) are plotted by columns, covering a range of 0.5 °C, the shape of the distribution gives some first information, shown in Figure 4A left and 4B left as an example). This simple approach is based on the assumption that the left and right upper arm show nearly the same temperature. If left-right differences cannot be neglected, an additional thermographic picture must be taken immediately before vaccination (designated points of time: V_0 and C_0 respectively). This involves a considerable effort, because all participants had to keep two subsequent appointments in the thermography station, beside the vaccination itself. In the result, four respectively eight values: V_{24}, C_{24}, V_0, C_0, both with the mean or the 80the percentile are provided for further calculation. Thus, the influence of left to right and day to day variation can be reduced.

To summarize, six ways to calculate the increase in temperature at the vaccination site are possible by three formulas applicable both for the mean and the 80th percentile:

1. Comparing temperatures on the vaccinated with the non-vaccinated side 24 hrs. after: $\mathbf{V_{24}\text{-}C_{24}}$. It is only suitable, if the left-right variation can be neglected.
2. Comparing the temperatures only at the vaccinated arm, before and 24 hrs. after vaccination: $\mathbf{V_{24} - V_0}$. For this, day to day variation must be very small.
3. Comparing temperatures on the vaccinated with the non-vaccinated side 24 hrs. after, including compensation measurement at the same sites before injection:
   $\mathbf{(V_{24}\text{-} C_{24}) \text{-} (V_0\text{-}C_0)}$. This will minimize the influence of both left- right and day to day variations.

Survey After Seasonal Influenza Vaccination by Infrared Monitoring

This survey refers to results of a study with altogether 86 subjects, participating in the seasonal influenza vaccination (Hoffmann et. al. 2014b). The infrared images were taken regularly before and 24 h after the influenza vaccination.

A typical infrared picture, indicating a thermal response 24 h after influenza vaccination was shown in Figure 1. Temperatures in the measuring form (marked ellipse) are presented both by the mean value and the 80th percentile. Infrared- data from all 86 vaccinees, taken before and 24 hrs. after vaccination, allowed us to express the thermal response by six different methods. Results are plotted in Figure 4A or 4B and summarized in Table 1. Even the simplified protocol $V_{24}\text{-}C_{24}$, shows a significant mean rise in temperature of 0.4°C after vaccination. However, around 10% of the subjects show a minor negative temperature difference. Does this means that the vaccination sometimes causes cooling by edemas or anything else? (Figure 4A, left column).

In the alternative approach ($V_{24} - V_0$), which took into account only temperature developments on the vaccinated arm before and 24 h after the vaccination, possible influences of existing asymmetry were avoided and a rise in the difference in temperature of 0.38°C to 0.47°C was shown. Since these values are obviously also influenced by day-to-day fluctuations, this leads to doubling of the variation, which is seen in the increased width of the frequency distribution as shown in Table 1 and Figure 4 (AB, medium column). As a "secondary" effect, the portion of "negative-responders" has increased to 25% caused by the higher variation.

Finally, it was examined whether the third difference formula $(V_{24}\text{-}C_{24})\text{-}(V_0\text{-}C_0)$ can be used to compensate both for a possible left-right asymmetry and for daily variations. Indeed, the mean value of the increase in temperature post vaccination rises to 0.66 and 0.76 (mean and 80th percentile respectively). In the distribution diagram (Figure 4, AB right column), the portion of subjects showing a drop in temperature post vaccination is almost entirely eliminated. Most of the variations in temperature differences lie on the right side of zero, i.e. in the direction of an increase in temperature. The distribution becomes asymmetric and reaches a skewness value of about 2 (Table 1).

Skewness $\left(\frac{1}{n}\sum_{i=1}^{n}\left(x_i - \overline{x}\right)^2\right)^3 / \sqrt{\left(\frac{1}{n}\sum_{i=1}^{n}\left(x_i - \overline{x}\right)^2\right)^3}$

Figure 4. Distribution diagram of the thermal response from 86 subjects. Comparing tree approaches for calculating the temperature increase: Left (V_{24}-C_{24}):Difference between vaccinated arm and control arm only 24 hours post vaccination. Middle: (V_{24}-V_0), Comparing values before and after vaccination, only at the vaccinated side. Right: (V_{24}-C_{24}) – (V_0-C_0) Difference between vaccinated arm and control arm 24 hrs. post vaccination including a compensation by initial values for both sides. Each for mean temperatures (line A) and 80th percentiles (line B)

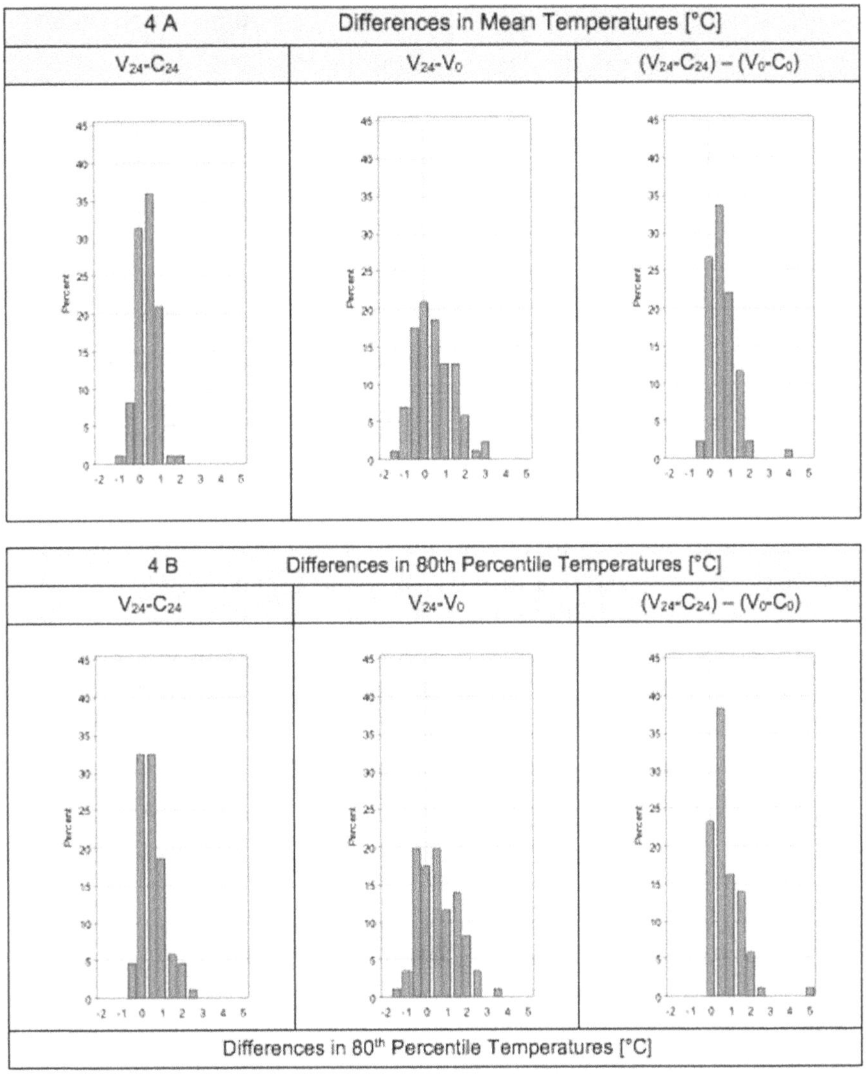

About Thermal Left Right Asymmetry

Subjects who obviously show a deviation in the functional or morphological lateral symmetry, such as partial paralysis or hypertrophies on the upper arm have been explicitly excluded from this study. The vast majority of the participants, however, did not show any abnormalities concerning this, so that, in

Table 1. Summary of results from thermal survey after influenza vaccination in 86 Subjects. Differences from six ways to express the thermal response are compared by mean, standard deviation (SD, confidence interval (CI) and the median

Calculation	Read out	N	Mean	SD	95% CI	Median	Skewness
V_{24}-C_{24}	Mean	86	0.38	0.49	0.27 – 0.49	0.30	0.47
	80th PCTL	86	0.51	0.62	0.38 – 0.64	0.50	0.79
V_{24}-C_0	Mean	86	0.47	0.93	0.27 – 0.67	0.30	0.42
	80th PCTL	86	0.57	1.00	0.36 – 0.79	0.45	0.47
(V_{24}-C_{24}) _ (V_0-C_0)	Mean	86	0.66	0.65	0.52 – 0.80	0.50	2.02
	80th PCTL	86	0.76	0.77	0.60 – 0.93	0.60	2.31

1. PCTL Percentile

general, similar thermal emissions of the skin were assumed on both sides (Uematsu,1985, Goodman, Murphy, Siltanen, Keller, & Rucker, 1986).

For the evaluation of the vaccine reaction, an appointment for an examination 24 h post vaccination should thus be sufficient, since the non-vaccinated arm serves as control. Because the result of the pilot survey in 2012 showed a portion of 15% of the subjects with a negative thermal reaction on the vaccinated side, severe doubts occurred about the general validity of this assumption. To clarify, whether deviations existed from the thermal lateral symmetry, thermographic images were taken on both arms also before the vaccination in the study in the subsequent survey in 2013. Figure 5 shows the result of the difference in temperature before the vaccination using this formula: **V_0-C_0**.

Thus, when observing the mean of all 86 subjects from 2013, there is a negative temperature value of **-0.28°C (SD=0.48).** The arm which is planned for vaccination is thus on average around 0.3°C colder before the vaccination. Finally, this is also plausible, since the subjects themselves decide that they wish the vaccination to be performed preferably on the more inactive arm. In this examination, this affected the left arm in the majority of the cases. Only 5 of 86 subjects preferred the right arm for the vaccination. This also explains why the results which were calculated according to the third method **(V_{24}-C_{24}) _ (V_0-V_0)** were about 0.3°C higher than in the simplified calculation **(V_{24}-C_{24})**, since this eliminates existing asymmetries.

Comparison of Thermal Response in Classified Responder Groups

The thermal response of the individual subjects turned out to be very different, which is also shown in the frequency presentations in Figure 4. To describe the thermal reactivity of a group beside the mean or median value, a separation in few classes of high,- low- and non- responder was also conducted. According to this, results from the survey can be described, based on the mean value of the metering form, with 37% of the subjects as high responders with more than 0.75°C increase in temperature. A slight increase of around 0.5°C (0.25 to 0.75°C) was seen in 33% (low-responders). The remaining 30% showed no reactions or reactions below 0.25°C (non-responders). On average, the rise in temperature post vaccination was about 0.66°C. The relation between high- and non-responders is 1.3.

When calculating in 80th percentiles from the metering form, 38% of the subjects showed an increase of 0.75°C or more and also 38% a slight increase of 0.5°C. 23% did not show any reactions, which is

Figure 5. Left-right variation of surface temperature from the upper arm. X-axis indicates the left-right difference of mean temperatures, recorded before vaccination. Points indicate the temperature difference from each subject. In the mean the non-vaccinated (C_0) right side was around 0.28°C warmer, compared to the vaccinated right side (V_0). Five subjects, displayed by unfilled symbols, preferred vaccination on the right side. For supplementary information, the age in years and the sex are indicated

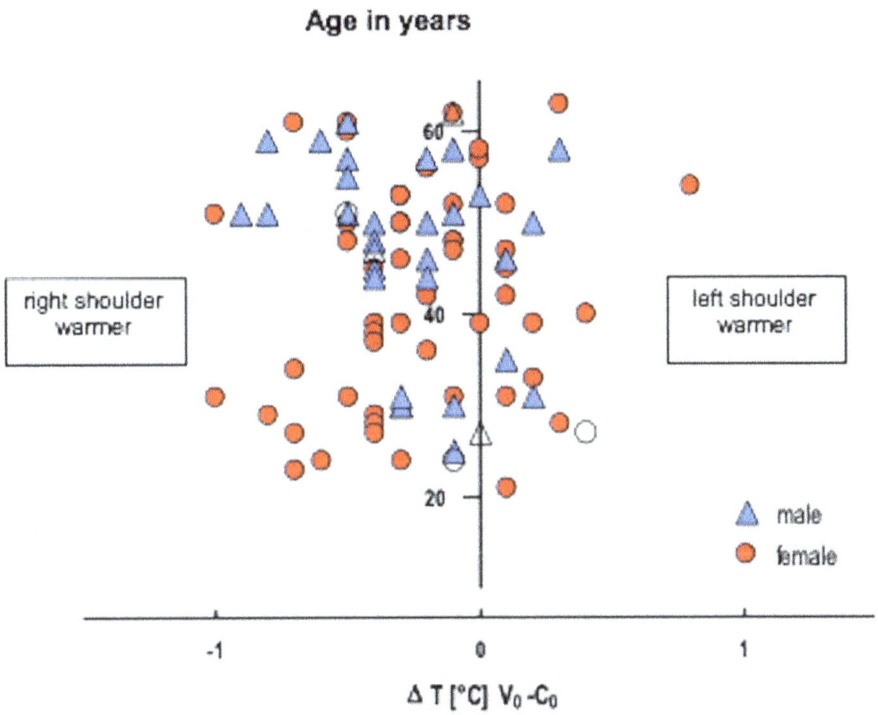

equivalent to a high- to non-responder ratio of 1.6. In addition, with 0.76°C the increase in temperatures is on average somewhat higher, as summarized in Table 2.

Association Between Thermal Response, Clinical Signs and Further Attributes

The association of thermal reactions after vaccination with clinical signs such as the subjective sensation of pain, local redness, age and gender are of special interest, since the original aim of the infrared study is to develop a surrogate parameter which facilitates the evaluation of the reactivity of vaccines.

The question as to whether there is a relation between thermal response and subjective discomfort cannot be answered in a simple manner. Data, as shown in Figure 6 reveal that a majority with 51 of 86 subjects reports only a mild pressure pain. Among them, the thermal response shows a broad variety. There are 19 high- 16 low- and 16 thermal non- responders. Furthermore 19 subjects affirmed that they had no pain. Among them were 9 high-, 8 low-, and 2 thermal non-responder. Within the group of 16 subjects suffering from higher and severe local pain after vaccination, 5 displayed a high, 9 a low and 2 no thermal response.

Table 2. Classification of thermal response after vaccination in high-, low- and non-responders, comparing the read-out by mean and 80th percentile (PCTL)

Read Out from Metering Form	High Responder (>0.75°C)	Low Responder (0.25°-0.75°C)	Non-Responder (<0.25°C)	High -to non-Responder Ratio	Mean of Temperature Differences
Mean	37%	34%	29%	1.28	0.66 (°C)
80th PCTL	38%	38%	23%	1.65	0.76 (°C)

The generally low reactivity of influenza vaccines, the not well specified subjectively determined "pain signals", as well as the marked differences in individual dispositions show that significant relations between thermal response and "pain signal" can hardly be expected here.

Local swelling on the side of the vaccination following the influenza vaccination could be detected in only eight subjects. Swelling usually originates from deeper regions of the arm and is difficult to discern and to measure on the shoulder. Redness was seen in six subjects. This always coincided with an increased thermal reaction, on average 1.4°C. Figure 7 shows typical examples.

With regard to the role of age groups and the number of previous vaccinations, there is a tendency that the 55+ age group may display an increased thermal response following the vaccination, as shown in Figure 8 This phenomenon partly also showed in pilot studies. However, these data do not allow a secured statistical interpretation. It could be possible that the 55+ age group had more frequent contacts with individual influenza strains. On the other hand, the reactivity of the blood vessel system could be

Figure 6. Association of local pain and thermal response. The mean temperature increase, 24 hrs after Vaccination [Δ T(°C)] is plotted against four degrees of subjective pain reporting

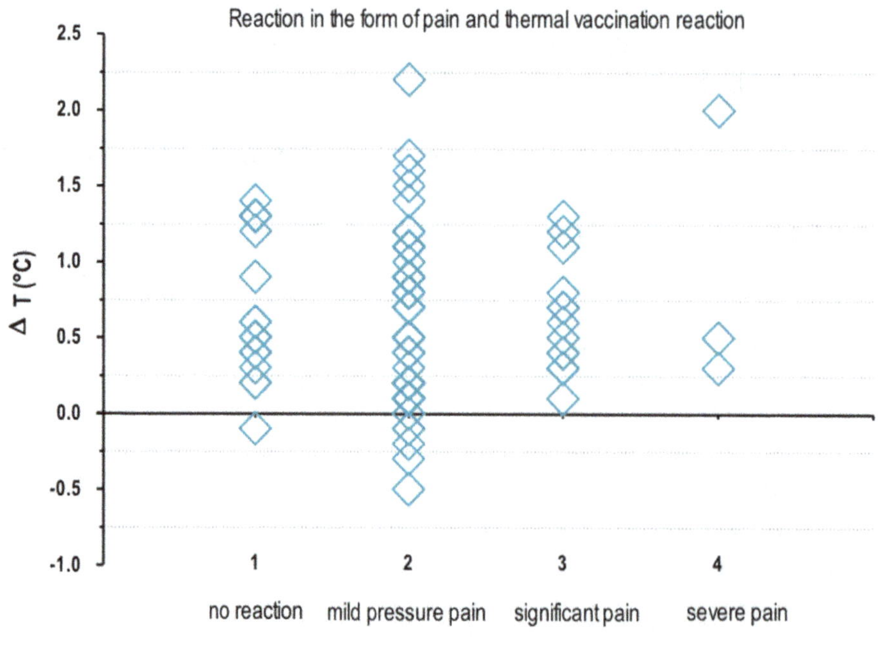

Figure 7. Local redness and thermal response. Subject, 24 hrs. post vaccination with redness of the skin on the vaccinated arm. Left: Thermogram, right photo, redness highlighted
Source: Hoffmann et al., 2015

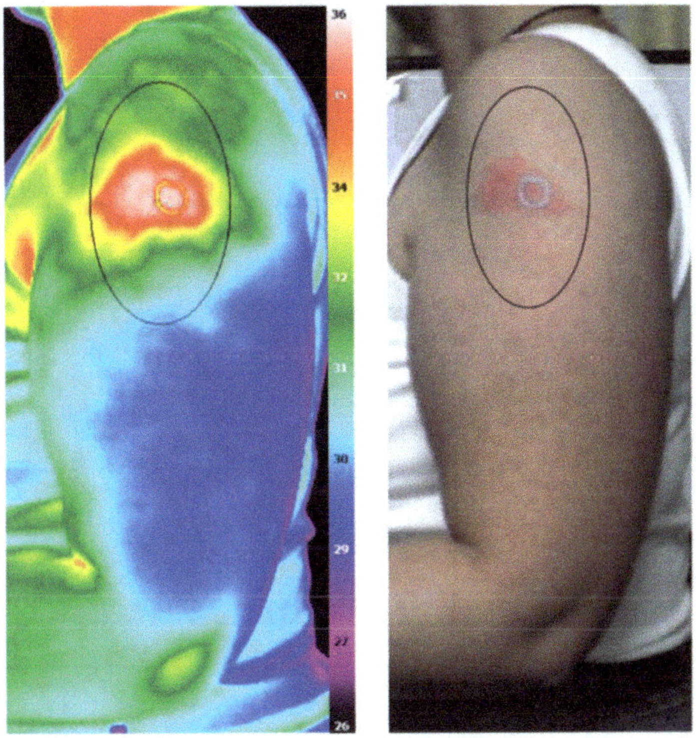

declining. In addition, the fact that there is a certain association with the number of previous vaccination is not unexpected, as displayed in Figure 9.

Any evidence pointing to a relation between gender and post vaccination thermal response could neither be found in this study nor in additional examinations

CONCLUSION

The reported survey was performed in 86 subjects following the seasonal influenza vaccinations in autumn 2013. Approximately, between 35 and 40 percent of the participants showed a mean increase in temperature of more than 0.75°C on the vaccinated arm. On the other hand, a portion of between 20 and 35 percent did not show a thermal reaction, at least until 24hrs. after vaccination. Signs of pain were low in most cases and were usually limited to minor pressure pain. Accordingly, an association to thermal response could hardly be established. Local redness occurred only in few cases in the group of thermal high responders. Its morphological manifestation by infrared or visual light was nearly identical. A certain trend towards a relationship between thermal reaction and age, especially in the 55+ group was noticeable.

Figure 8. thermal response after influenza vaccination and age cohorts
Temperature differences stratified by age groups (box-and-whisker plot shows median increase in temperature (connected with lines), interquartile range (boxes), 10th and 90th percentile (whiskers), and outlying values (blue dots)

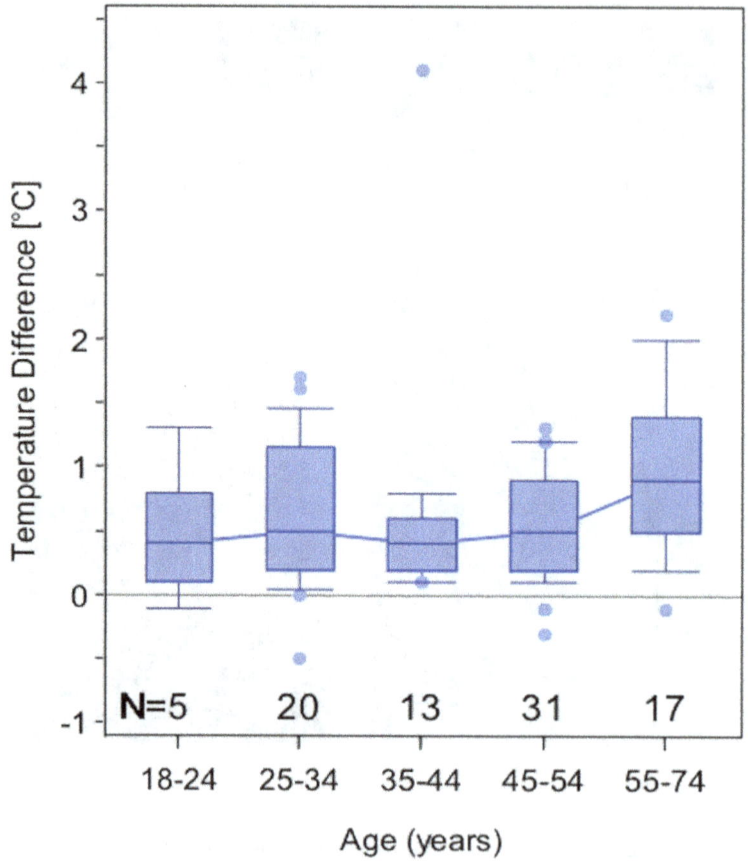

To gain more precise results, additional thermal imaging before vaccination is recommended. Especially, individual variations of the thermal lateral symmetry due to right or left handedness could be compensated for almost entirely. The parameter to describe the thermal response can be the mean increase in temperature, if the simplest method is preferred. A more informative method, however, is the analysis by indicating the distribution of high-, low- and non-responders which can be condensed to the high to non-responder ratio.

In principle, infrared thermography seems to be a promising method of demonstrating accurately the reactivity of a vaccine in a simple manner. However, the final assessment of the clinical relevance of the suggested parameters needs further comparable studies with more significant reactive vaccines. A unique value of the reported study is that, for the first time, basic data on dimension and standard deviations of the thermal response after vaccination are available, a precondition for planning further systematic surveys.

Great disparities in the thermal response after influenza vaccination, some extreme high responders or on the other hand complete non-responders, will be a challenge for succeeding advanced studies. Further

Figure 9. Thermal vaccination reaction as a variable of the number of previous influenza vaccinations (no vaccination, one vaccination or multiple vaccinations.) The mean temperature increase, 24 hrs after Vaccination [Δ T(°C)], is plotted against three categories of previous vaccinations
Source: modified from Hoffmann et al., 2015

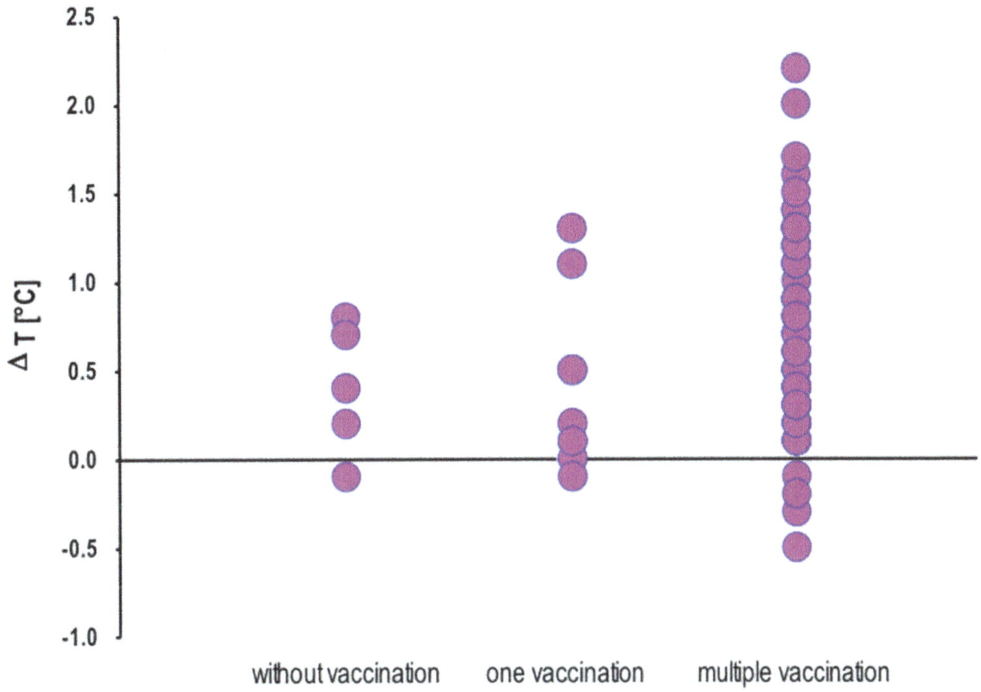

investigations, including immunoprofiling, may provide a better understanding of the local immune-inflammatory network, a special requirement, if novel synthetic adjuvants are introduced in the future.

Thermal Studies in Farm Animals

Requirements for safety of veterinary vaccines are in general not less strict than those for human beings (Martinod,1997). The procedure for licensing a vaccine includes a number of inquiries to ensure a well-tolerated vaccine without significant temporary injury or permanent damage at the injection site. For this reason, pre-authorization studies for licensing must contain several investigations including pathological studies at the injection site. To avoid multiple pathological investigations (Bernau et.al. 2013), it was proposed that possible deeper injuries at the injection site should be studied by magnet resonance tomography (MRT) and ultrasonic monitoring. This may be an alternative to multiple pathological studies and could be a way to reduce the effort and some burdens for the animals during the procedure of licensing. Parallel thermographic monitoring could also be helpful to identify a local inflammatory response which is caused by a vaccination.

In contrast to human beings, standardized studies by infrared imaging, especially in farm animals involve some problems due to certain effects: The skin of farm animals, particularly the strong subcutaneous fat layer in pigs blocks a rapid thermal transfer. Furthermore, the fur in calves and to a greater extent in sheep protects the animals very efficiently from thermal loss. For the purpose of thermal studies, this problem could be circumvented by shearing large areas. However, any unsteadiness during the shearing is visible in the thermal picture and would influence the metering. Finally, a fixation of the animal, always in the same position is needed for standardized metering of a thermal response. If fixation by the animal keeper cannot be realized in a proper manner, anesthesia will be inevitable.

Figure 10 shows an example for a local thermal response after vaccination in pigs. Vaccination with an adjuvanted Gonadotropin-releasing-factor-analogon causes a significant thermal reaction several days after second vaccination. Obviously, a considerable amount of swelling and increase in the surface temperature at the vaccinated side can be demonstrated. If the pigs were left, non fixed images were always taken from different positions. Thus, only clinical interpretation, but no comparative metering of the thermal response was possible.

In a further series, following a combined study with MRT and ultrasonic testing, the pigs were anesthetized, as described in detail by Bernau et.al.2015. This allows serial thermal investigations in pigs always in a standardized position. In general, an increase in the mean thermal response, persisting between 24 and 72 hrs., could be observed. However, the variability between the individual piglets remains high, despite the fixation of the animals.

In summary, thermal studies after vaccination in farm animals may be useful for monitoring local injuries caused by a vaccination. Strong reactions accompanied by an increased local blood flow can be documented well as shown after the second vaccination by Gonadotropin-releasing-factor-analogon. Other vaccines in pigs, containing Mycoplasma-Antigens, cause rather a local oedematization, accompanied by a slight drop down of the surface temperature. Besides, in horses, thermal response after repeated yearly vaccination against influenza- and Herpes-virus infection results in a strong thermal response. (v.d. Wense, pers .comm. Nov,10th. 2009). Problems with the proper fixation of the animals should not be underestimated. Thus, thermal studies in horses are easier to realize in contrast to other free running animals. Anesthesia can be realized only in a specific experimental set up. In addition, the thermal loss during anesthesia must be borne in mind if the investigation period is too long. Certainly, thermographic studies in animals are more complex. A comprehensive understanding of specific thermoregulation and physiology from each species is helpful.

Figure 10. Severe local swelling, accompanied by distinct increased thermal irradiadion caused several days after the second vaccination with adjuvanted Gonadotropin-releasing factor
Source: from Hoffmann et.al. 2014

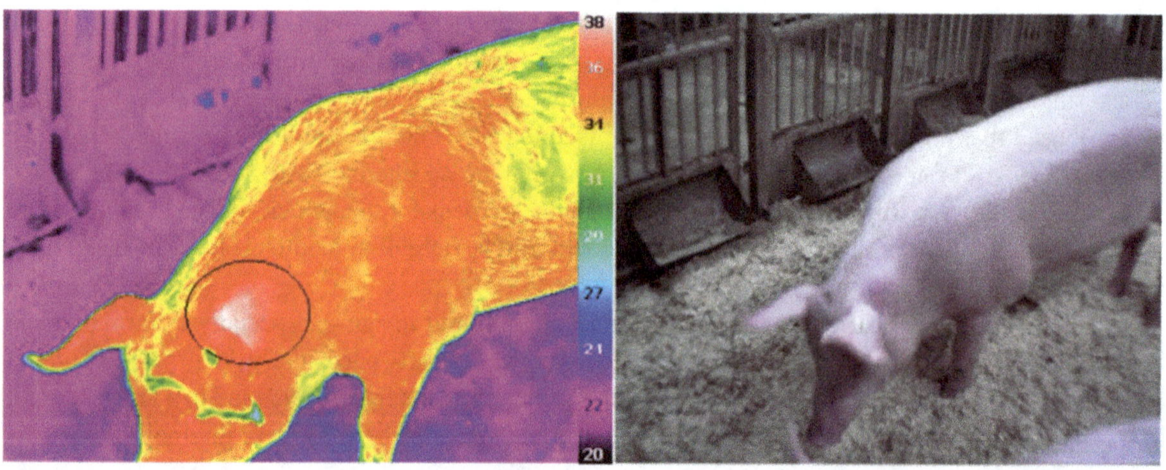

REFERENCES

Ammer, K., & Ring, F. (2007). Standard procedures in Infrared imaging. In N. A. Diakides & J. D. Bronzie (Eds.), *Medical Infrared Imaging* (p. 1). Boca Raton, FL: CRC Press. doi:10.1201/9781420008340.ch22

Bernau, M., Kremer, P., Papenberger, E., Kreuzer, L., Cussler, K., Hoffmann, A., & Scholz, A. (2015). *Safety Testing of Veterinary Vaccines Using Magnetic Resonance Imaging in Pigs Altex*. Academic Press.

Eckert, R. (2002). Energiehaushalt-Auseinandersetzung mit den Anforderungen der Umwelt. In R. Eckert (Ed.), *Tierphysiologie* (pp. 767–840). Stuttgart: Georg-Thieme.

Goodman, P. H., Murphy, M. G., Siltanen, G. L., Kelley, M. P., & Rucker, M. (1986). Norman Temperature Asymmetry of the Back and Extremities by Computer-Assisted Infrared Imaging. *Thermology*, *1*, 195–202.

Hoffmann, A., Dumke, C., Bernau, M., Krämer, P., Scholz, A., Balks, E., & Cußler, K. et al. (2014). Thermal imaging - alternative concepts for refinement and reduction of animal use for testing of biologicals. In *Proceedings of the 9th World Congress on Alternatives and Animal Use in Life Sciences.*

Lopalco, P.L, Johansen, K., Ciancio, B., De Carvalho Gomes, H., Kramarz, P., Giesecke, J. (2010). Monitoring and assessing vaccine safety: A European perspective. *Expert Rev Vaccines, 9*(4), 371-80. doi: Group10.1586/erv.10.20.EMA-Vacc-

Martinod, S. (1997). Adverse effects of vaccination. In P. P. Pastoret, J. Blancou, P. Vannier, & C. Verschuren (Eds.), *Veterinary Vaccinology* (pp. 574–580). Amsterdam: Elsevier.

Pichler, W. J. (2006). Adverse side-effects to biological agents. *Allergy*, *61*(8), 912–920. doi:10.1111/j.1398-9995.2006.01058.x PMID:16867042

Uematsu, S. (1985). Symmetry of temperatures comparing one side of the other. *Thermology*, *1*, 4–7.

Waldman, E.A., Luhm, K.R., Monteiro, S.A., Freitas, F.R. (2011). Surveillance of adverse effects following vaccination and safety of immunization programs. *Rev. Saude Publica., 45*(1), 173-84.

KEY TERMS AND DEFINITIONS

Adverse Events After Vaccination: Possible side effects that occur after administration of vaccines.

Animal Welfare Science: Scientific studies of the welfare of animals as pets, in zoos, laboratories, on farms and in the wild. The investigation of animal welfare using scientific methods is a relatively recent development.

Influenza Vaccines: Vaccines that protect against influenza.

Pharmacovigilance: Pharmacovigilance is the pharmacological science relating to the collection, detection, assessment, monitoring, and prevention of adverse effects with pharmaceutical products.

Reactogenicity of a Vaccine: The term reactogenicity was coined by the US Food and Drug Administration. It refers to the property of a vaccine of being able to produce common, "expected" adverse reactions, especially excessive immunological responses and associated signs and symptoms- fever, sore arm at injection site, etc.

Thermal Imaging: Infrared imaging science using thermographic cameras combined with digital image processing.

Vaccinovigilance: Science and activities relating to the detection, assessment, understanding and communication of adverse events following immunization.

Chapter 11
Thermography in Animal Models of Cancer:
A Tool for Studying Oncobiology in Laboratory Animals

Rui M. Gil da Costa
LEPABE, CI-IPOP,University of Porto, Portugal

António Ramos Silva
INEGI, University of Porto, Portugal

Ana Faustino Rocha
CITAB, QOPNA University of Trás-os-Montes and Alto Douro, Portugal

Paula Alexandra Oliveira
CITAB, University of Trás-os-Montes and Alto Douro, Portugal

Joaquim Gabriel
INEGI, University of Porto, Portugal

Ana Margarida Abrantes
Biophysics Institute, University of Coimbra, Portugal

Maria Filomena Botelho
CIMAGO, CNC.IBILI, University of Coimbra, Portugal

ABSTRACT

Laboratory animals provide important models for studying human diseases, including many types of cancer. Mice are among the most commonly used laboratory animals, allowing for the study of carcinogenic agents, cancer development and for testing innovative preventive and therapeutic strategies. Thus, monitoring angiogenesis in animal models is a major goal for cancer research. Among the currently available imaging techniques, thermography is a useful approach for studying the superficial vascularization of cancer, based on their heat emissions. At this chapter emphasis is placed on thermography and its applications on laboratory animals, in comparison with other available and applicable imaging techniques. In conclusion, thermography may be usefully applied to the study of cancer vascularization in animal models, particularly when using laboratory rodents such as mice. Care is needed in adapting existing approaches to the specificities of each animal species.

DOI: 10.4018/978-1-5225-2072-6.ch011

INTRODUCTION

Among the major public health problems of our time, cancer occupies a prominent place. Cancer develops through a complex, multistage process, driven by the cellular accumulation of genetic mutations and epigenetic events (Bignold, 2003; Bignold, Coghlan, Jersmann 2006; Oliveira et al., 2007; Iacobuzio-Donahue, 2009). This process of carcinogenesis often proceeds through multiple distinguishable morphological stages as shown in Figure 1. Thus, pre-cancerous lesions may develop into benign and later malignant tumors. The term cancer is reserved for malignant lesions, while the term neoplasia (used of a tissue which has become independent of normal physiological regulatory mechanisms) applies to both benign and malignant tumors. Hence, early non-tumoral lesions are often referred to as pre-neoplastic. Environmental carcinogens are biological (e.g. human papillomavirus, HPV), chemical (e.g. nitrosamines) or physical (e.g. ionizing radiations) agents that initiate carcinogenesis by inducing genetic mutations or promote it otherwise (Oliveira et al., 2007). Genetic mutations occurring in healthy cells are, most often, successfully repaired or else they trigger programmed cell death mechanisms (as a way to prevent carcinogenesis). However, unrepaired mutations that block DNA repair mechanisms (encoded by so-called tumor suppressor genes) will promote the unchecked accumulation of further mutations (genomic instability). Mutations that activate genes (so-called proto-oncogenes) that contribute to make the cell independent from its environment (e.g. by producing its own growth factors) are also important in driving carcinogenesis. Accordingly, during the early phases of carcinogenesis, cells tend to survive and proliferate in an unregulated fashion, accumulating additional mutations (Oliveira et al., 2007) that will drive carcinogenesis further on Figure 1. As already pointed out, neoplastic tissues are not necessarily malignant. While benign tumors are well-delimited and damage adjacent tissues mainly by compressing them, malignant tumors (cancers) are able to invade adjacent tissues or event to spread to distant body parts through lymphatic or blood vessels. Progression from a benign to a malignant stage is commonly observed in many epithelial tumors. The malignant phenotype requires an ability to interact with and invade the adjacent connective tissue (called the stroma). When neoplastic cells have acquired the typical traits of malignancy, they degrade the basement membrane that separates them from the stroma, and spread into the adjacent tissues. By invading blood and lymphatic vessels (a phenomenon called intravasation) in the stroma, malignant cells may gain access to distant organs, where they may establish distant tumor foci, called metastasis. The interaction between malignant or pre-malignant cells and the adjacent stroma is highly complex.

In order to study these phenomena, researchers have long resorted to employing animal models, which allow for fast and efficient experimental approaches. Thermography, as an imaging technique, is able to provide valuable additional information on the physiology and pathology of these models, namely concerning superficial inflammation and blood irrigation. The present chapter deals with laboratory animal models of cancer, followed by multiple imaging techniques available for use in these models. Special emphasis is given to the use of thermographic techniques to evaluate laboratory mice and rats.

ANGIOGENESIS IN CANCER

One key feature of the interaction between cancer cells and their adjacent stroma is the development of new, and often abundant, blood vessels, termed angiogenesis (Potente, Gerhardt, Carmeliet, 2011). Tumor-associated angiogenesis is of particular importance clinically and also from the viewpoint of thermographic analysis, as it provides the basis for temperature differences between healthy and tumoral tissues (Carmeliet & Jain, 2011).

Angiogenesis is essential to deliver nutrients to tumor cells. Tumors do not grow beyond 1 or 2 mm in diameter without developing their own blood supply. Beyond that size, oxygen and nutrients do not diffuse from adjacent blood vessels in the necessary amount, resulting in hypoxia and cell death (Potente, Gerhardt, Carmeliet, 2011). In fact, many tumors are hypoxic and necrotic areas where the blood supply is limited. A number of pro-angiogenic and anti-angiogenic factors exist, that govern the development of arrest of angiogenesis in physiological and pathological conditions. During tumor development, some tumor cells acquire the possibility of modifying the balance between pro-angiogenic and anti-angiogenic factors in favor of angiogenesis, a phenomenon known as the angiogenic switch (Shojaei, 2012). In order to achieve this, tumor cells (and, frequently, certain stromal cells) secrete a number of pro-angiogenic factors, most importantly vascular endothelial growth factor (VEGF) and basic fibroblast growth factor (bFGF). Down-regulating the expression of anti-angiogenic factors is also an important strategy, *e.g.* mutational inactivation of the p53 protein leads to decreased production of the anti-angiogenic protein thrombospondin-1 (Grossfeld, 1997). VEGF acts through its receptor (VEGFR) to attract circulating endothelial precursor cells, drive the proliferation of endothelial cells (which line the lumen of blood vessels) and their differentiation at the tumor site, as well as promoting the sprouting of new capillaries from existing blood vessels (Potente, Gerhardt, Carmeliet, 2011). The blood vessels that develop show

Figure 1. An overview of multistage cancer development in epithelial tissues. a- normal stratified epithelium (blue), with basal cells covered by differentiated cells. The epithelium lies over a basement membrane, which separates it from the underlying stroma, containing fibroblasts (yellow) and capillaries with red blood cells. b- one epithelial cell suffers DNA mutations, triggering carcinogenesis. c- loss of normal epithelial structure, and development of multiple cellular clones harboring additional different mutations. d- an aggressive, angiogenic cellular clone develops, secreting pro-angiogenic factors and re-structuring the adjacent stroma, which shows numerous capillaries, fibroblasts and leukocytes. e- malignant (cancer) cells degrade the basement membrane, invading the stroma and blood vessels. d- cancer cells migrate through the blood and lymph vessels, establishing metastasis in distant organs

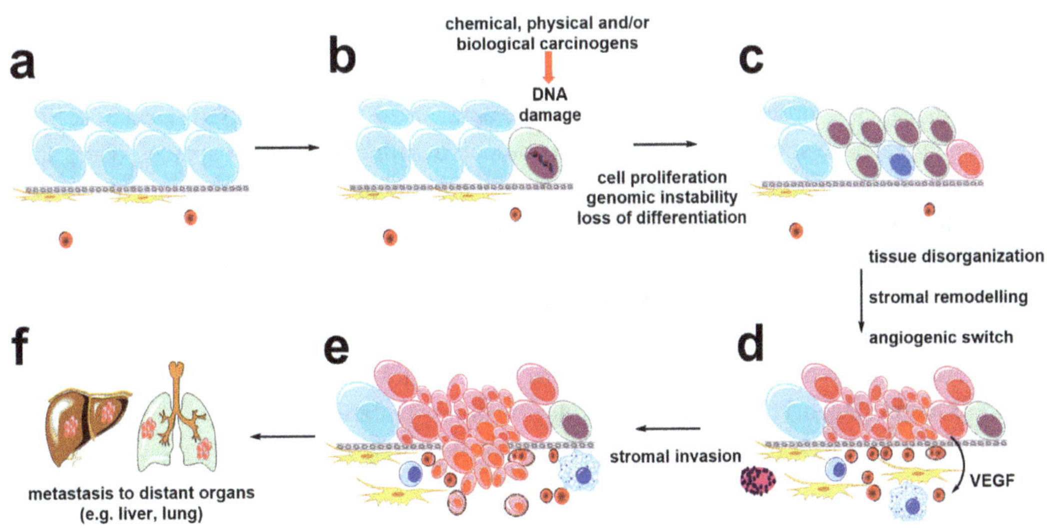

an irregular, tortuous, abnormal architecture and increased leakiness, compared with blood vessels from healthy tissues (Shojaei, 2012). In some cases, tumor cells may line structures resembling capillaries, a phenomenon known as vasculogenesis mimicry. Besides delivering oxygen and nutrients to tumor cells, endothelial cells also provide them with important polypeptide growth factors, such as insulin-like growth factor and platelet-derived growth factor. Furthermore, the development of an extensive and accessible capillary bed facilitates tumor intravasation and metastasis.

According to the most recent GLOBOCAN data, cancer incidence rates are consistently increasing, both in developed and in developing countries, with an estimated 14.1 million new cancer cases diagnosed in 2012 (Torre, 2015). The leading causes of death by cancer are lung, breast and colorectal cancers. The rising cancer incidence is believed to reflect the increasing life expectancy and changing life habits, especially the adoption of cancer-causing behaviors such as smoking. Cancer mortality tends to be higher in developing countries, due to limited access to early diagnosis and to adequate therapy (Torre, 2015). Overall, during 2012, cancer caused an estimated 8.2 million deaths worldwide (Torre, 2015). Breast cancer is now the leading cause of death by cancer among women in developed countries. Screening and vaccination programs are good examples of how understanding the biopathology of cancer were translated into effective preventive strategies. Another highly significant example, is the development of anti-angiogenic therapies, mainly based on blocking VEGF-mediated signaling (Carmeliet & Jain, 2011). The main challenges in this area are inherent or acquired resistance to angiogenesis inhibitors, a possibly increased tumor aggressiveness during anti-angiogenic treatment, and the absence of validated biomarkers to select suitable patients and monitor tumor responses (Shojaei, 2012).

Animal Models of Cancer: General Concepts

In vivo animal models of cancer are critical tools to study the biopathology of cancer and the effects of carcinogens, as well as for developing innovative preventive and therapeutic anti-cancer strategies. In the last years, with the development of genetics, sophisticated animal models have been developed that better represent specific cancer features. Nowadays, animal models of cancer come in a diversity of forms, ranging between cancer cell lines and genetically engineered animals.

Animal models provide an alternative mean to understand the causes and to evaluate new treatments for cancer, being a resource of a great potential in oncology. The use of animal cancer models has provided a better understand of cancer's biology and, more recently, its genetics (Frese & Tuveson, 2007). Several animal species, namely dogs, large animals, rabbits, fish, guinea pigs, hamsters, rats and mice have been used in experimental protocols, the rat and mouse being most frequently used (Decker & Sausville, 2011). Rats and mice have some advantages when compared with other animal species. They are mammals, small, their accommodation and maintenance are cheap, they are easy to handle and reproduce, have a high number of offspring, their physiology and genetics are well understood and are similar to humans in various aspects, namely concerning their anatomy, physiology, genetics and biochemistry. The similarities between such animal models and humans allow their use to find new diagnostic methods, as well as discovering and testing new therapies (Oliveira, Colaco, De la Cruz, Lopes, 2006).

A wide variety of animal models of cancer is currently available. *In vivo* cancer animal models can be divided into different categories: genetically engineered, transplantation (syngeneic and xenotransplant), spontaneous and carcinogen-induced models (Table 1). Researchers may select the model according their investigation's aim.

Table 1. Characteristics of animal models of cancers: some advantages and disadvantages

Animal models		Advantages	Disadvantages
Genetically engineered		Tumor arise "naturally". Tumor and stromal cells interact in their normal microenvironment. Closely mimics human cancer pathogenesis.	Mutation usually only in a single gene, failing to mimic the genetic complexity and heterogeneity of human tumors. Tumors arise at different stages. Expensive models.
Transplantation	Syngeneic	Tumor cells and the host share a common genetic background. Host immune system is not compromised (immune-competent host) Mimics the normal tumor microenvironment. Rapid development of tumors. Reproducible. Low expensive.	Tumor cells are non-human In some cases, tumors are implanted in a non-natural site.
	Xenograft	Tumor cells are from human. Wide variety of tumor cell lines available.	Host is an immune-deficient animal. Longer latency period (compared with syngeneic model). In some cases, tumors are implanted in a non-natural site. Does not mimic normal tumor microenvironment. Lack of protective immune response and tumor-promoting inflammation. Expensive models.
Spontaneous		Allow the identification of cancer susceptibility genes.	Long latency period. Difficult to obtain a sample with an adequate size.
Carcinogen-induced		Short period of latency. Easily reproducible. Allows the study of carcinogenesis (e.g. mutagenesis, oxidative stress, inflammation). Allow the identification of potential targets for cancer therapy.	Non-natural tumors. In some models, induced tumors are internal and difficult to monitor Some models simultaneously develop tumors in multiple organs.

Following the identification of many mutations responsible for the development of some human cancers, transgenic and gene targeting technology allowed the development of a large number of genetically engineered rodent strains. These genetically engineered cancer models express oncogenes or mutations in tumor suppressors found in human tumors (Hanahan, Wagner, Palmiter, 2007). In these genetically engineered animal models there is the interaction between tumor and stromal cells in their normal microenvironment, which mimics the human cancer pathogenesis better than in transplanted models. However, genetically engineered rodent strains have some limitations. Since these models usually have mutations in a single gene, they do not accurately mimic the genetic complexity and heterogeneity of human tumors. In order to overcome this limitation, mouse strains possessing combinations of oncogenic mutations have recently been developed. However, these genetically engineered animal models are expensive and not yet affordable for many research teams (Farago, Snyder, Jacks, 2012; Singh, Murriel, Johnson, 2012).

In transplantation models, tumor cell lines or a part of a human tumor, may be transplanted into immune-deficient (xenograft models) or immunocompetent (syngeneic models) animals. When tumor cells are well accepted, they result in tumor formation within a few weeks. According to the aim of the researchers, there are several ways to transplant cells: subcutaneously (heterotopically) to allow the study of tumor development, intravenously to mimic the formation of metastasis, or orthotopically when the tumor cells are transplanted to their organ of origin, mimicking tumor development in its own microenvironment (Loi et al., 2011).

In xenograft models, human tumor cells are transplanted into an immune-deficient animal. These models do not mimic the natural tumor microenvironment due to a lack of protective immune response and tumor-promoting inflammation (Dranoff, 2012).

In syngeneic models, the tumor cells and the host share an inbred genetic background. The host immune system is not compromised and transplanted tissues are not rejected by the immune system of the host. This model mimics the normal tumor microenvironment. These models are rapid, reproducible and affordable when compared with xenografts and genetically engineered models (Polin, 2011).

Decades of studies in animal models allowed researchers to discover that some animal species and strains develop cancer in a certain organ or in various organs when exposed to a specific agent, under appropriate conditions, namely age of the exposure, number of exposures/administrations, dose or time of exposure. The agents that have the capacity to induce the formation of tumors are classified as carcinogen agents. These agents can be chemicals (e.g. polycyclic aromatic hydrocarbons, nitrosoureas, nitrosamines, cadmium, arsenic, tobacco compounds), virus (e.g. mouse mammary tumor virus), radiations (e.g. ultraviolet radiation, ionizing radiation) or minerals (e.g. asbestos fibers). The tumors in carcinogen-induced models have a short period of latency and are easily reproducible (Jonkers & Berns, 2005).

Spontaneous cancer animal models are animals that naturally develop cancers, these models allow researchers to identify the genes that generate susceptibility to cancer development (Hansen & Khanna, 2004). Spontaneous tumors in dogs and cats are frequently used in cancer research, as these animals frequently develop tumors with histopathologic and biologic behavior similar to those that occurs in humans (MacEwen, 1990).

Despite the limitations of each type, *in vivo* animal models of cancer are invaluable tools to study the biopathology of cancer, understand the complexity of carcinogenesis, the effects of different carcinogens and to develop innovative preventive and therapeutic anti-cancer strategies.

Imaging Techniques in Animal Models of Cancer

Medical imaging allows the creation of visual representations of the anatomy and physiology of the interior of a body. The technology, which may or may not apply ionizing radiation, is used as diagnosis tool to identify abnormalities in comparison with normal conditions. Besides this application, it is also possible to perform imaging of removed organs and tissues using pathological techniques.

The discovery of different types of radiation and its use as a diagnostic and therapeutic methods constituted a significant advance in medicine. Small animal-dedicated scanners were produced only in the late 1990s. However, the large number of research centers interested, quickly made this equipment very popular. Therefore, nowadays there are dedicated animal cameras for all the main imaging techniques, such as microSPECT, microPET, microMRI, microCT and thermography.

X-Ray Imaging

The X-rays are electromagnetic radiation similar to visible light, but with a shorter wavelength. Considering its particular characteristics, this type of radiation allows both, to obtain images, and also to be used for therapy (radiotherapy). Thus, its use as a diagnostic tool is based on the ability of the X-radiation to propagate throughout the body. The penetrating power of X-ray is inversely proportional to its wavelength, and when a volume is exposed, some portion of the radiation energy is absorbed, while the other is scattered through the matter (Lima, 1995).

The obtained image is defined as conventional radiography, and is achieved after the X-rays pass through the object and the emerging photons are able to cause fluorescence in enhancing screens. The emitted light strikes the emulsion on a film, giving rise to a latent image. Computed radiography differs from this conventional technique because the emerging photons interact with a phosphor plate, thus creating the latent image which is automatically converted into a digital image through a scanner (Gaivão, Lima, Agostinho, Oliveira, Peres, 2001).

Concerning animal applications, the X-ray is one of the most commonly used diagnostic tools, with the possibility of obtaining 2-dimensional images which are representations of 3-dimensional objects. Due to its characteristics, this technique provides a large amount of information through non-invasive and affordable means. Besides this, X-ray do not change the disease process and does not cause pain. The results obtained with X-rays imaging depend on the combination of different parameters such as the beam voltage, the number of X-rays produced and the exposure time. Besides these instrumentation characteristics, the tissue density also influences the obtained image (Lima, 1995; Gaivão, Lima, Agostinho, Oliveira, Peres, 2001).

To perform animal imaging using X-ray (Figure 2), the animal must be adequately restrained and positioned to obtain high-quality radiographic images, whereby sedation or short-acting anesthesia is often necessary. Besides that, image acquisition parameters may also be manipulated in order to minimize the effects of animal motion. Specifically, these conditions are the decrease of exposure time and the maximization of the power (Merck Sharp, Dohme Corp, 2014).

Figure 2. Skull radiograph of the mouse in profile with changes in bone structure suggesting bone involvement by an orthotopic osteosarcoma model

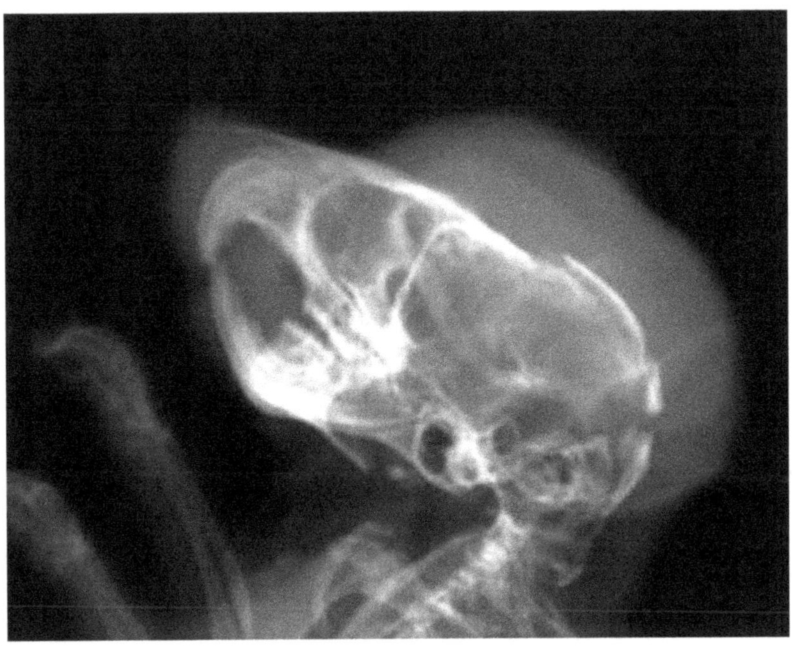

Computed Tomography (CT)

Since the 1970s, CT has been established as an imaging approach which produces axial slice images using a source of X-rays. Using this imaging technique it is possible to estimate the linear attenuation coefficient of the X-rays in each pixel of slice, which are obtained around the patient considering different angles. Whereas the final images on radiographs are obtained by the compression of a volume in a 2D level, in which the radiological projection information from a three-dimensional object is represented, with CT it is possible to get a flat image of a three-dimensional object visualized in a gray scale. This imaging methodology, allows a better temporal and spatial resolution, more anatomic imaging, improved signal/noise ratio as well as a better image processing potential and a retrospective reconstruction, especially taking into account the innovations using multi-slice imaging and newly developed contrast media (Gaivão, Lima, Agostinho, Oliveira, Peres, 2001).

For animal imaging studies, all CT scanners that provide higher spatial resolution than current scanners used in clinics are named micro-CT. The spatial resolution of these equipment is in the order of a few hundred μm. In this imaging technique, anesthesia is not required for intravenous, intraperitoneal or oral administration of contrast agents. However, mice or rats are imaged under anesthesia. To perform a CT study, animals are positioned within the scanner, and visually monitored during the scan (Bartling, Stiller, Semmler, Kiessling, 2007). Employing this imaging technique, it is possible to design *in vivo* research experiments allowing repeated measurements of the same animal. This approach reduces the variability associated with images coming from different animals (Bartling, Stiller, Semmler, Kiessling, 2007).

Nuclear Medicine (NM)

Nuclear medicine it is a diagnostic imaging and therapeutic technique also known as molecular medicine or molecular imaging, which allows in some situations, the performance of metabolic radiotherapy. This technique uses properties of radioactive isotopes and the energetic radiation emitted by them. This is always ionizing radiation and may be of different natures (particles or electromagnetic). Nuclear medicine uses both types of radiation for different purposes, the particles for therapy and the electromagnetic (gamma rays and annihilation photons) for imaging. Concerning the utilization of X-rays, radiology is more dedicated to morphological studies, whereas nuclear medicine enables the assessment of functional information. Nuclear medicine can be divided into single-photon emission computed tomography (SPECT) and positron emission tomography (PET), each technique associated with a specific and/or dedicated equipment. In nuclear medicine using SPECT, images are acquired after collimation of the photons, which are detected by a crystal that gives off a light signal. This is, in turn, amplified and converted into count data, planar or, after processing, 3D tomographic images. This imaging technique allied to a CT scanner can provide information about localization and function simultaneously. In SPECT imaging, Technetium-99m is the radionuclide most used. This isotope labels the majority of the molecules with different biodistributions (Lima, 2011) (Figure 3).

PET uses a short-lived positron-emitting isotope such as Fluor-18, which is the most commonly used (Figure 4). Modern scanners used in small animal imaging may integrate PET with CT and MRI, allowing the production of PET-CT or PET-MRI images. In small animal imaging equipment, these combinations are possible and can all be simultaneously present in the same equipment without physically moving the animal off the gantry. This possibility allows the generation of images that match information from different sources. The resultant hybrid image with functional and anatomical information is a useful tool

Figure 3. Nuclear medicine (SPECT) imaging using 99mTc-MIBI. Static image of an animal model with colostomy and colorectal cancer with 99mTc- MIBI uptake in tumor localization

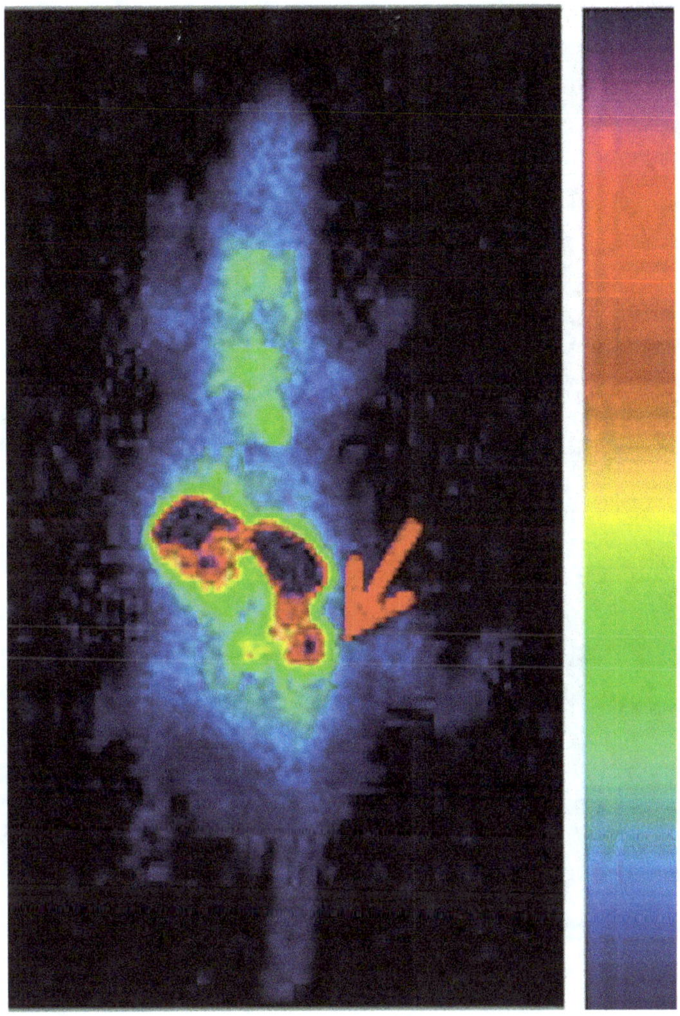

in non-invasive diagnosis and provides information over time, promoting respect for the 3Rs principles of animal research ethics (Lima, 2011; Rowland, Cherry, 2008, May).

Ultrasonography

Since the discovery of the piezoelectric properties of quartz in 1880 by Marie Curie until its current status, ultrasound imaging is the result of several decades of research. This medical imaging uses high frequency sound waves in the megahertz range that, once applied on tissues, are reflected to various degrees, being useful to produce 3D images (Gaivão, Lima, Agostinho, Oliveira, Peres, 2001).

Employing the transmission and reception of sound pressure waves it is possible to perform tissue characterization, using frequencies ranging from 20 kHz up to several GHz, which allow for a different medical image modality. The high frequency sound waves are applied on tissues and, depending on the

Figure 4. Nuclear medicine (PET) imaging using ^{18}F-FDG. Static image of an animal model with colostomy and colorectal cancer with ^{18}F-FDG uptake in tumor localization, 60 minutes after radiopharmaceutical administration

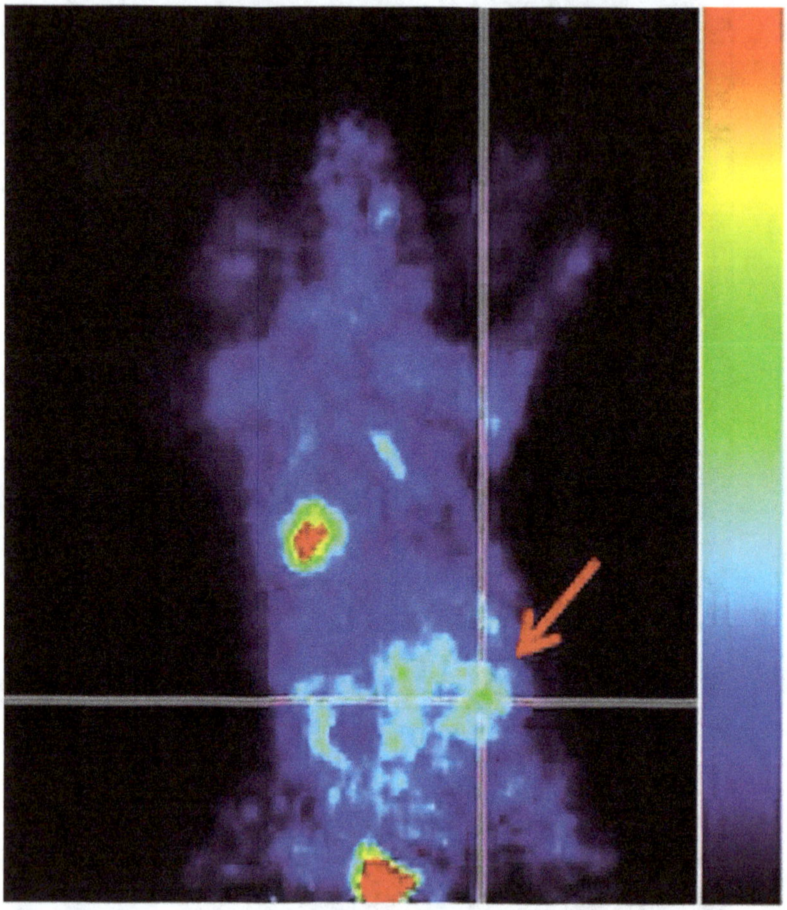

composition of the different tissues crossed, the signal is differently attenuated, and the returned echo is also separated by different intervals. This imaging approach is safe, not appear to cause any adverse effects in the body. Besides that, it is also relatively inexpensive and quick to perform and the equipment does not use ionizing radiation (Gaivão, Lima, Agostinho, Oliveira, Peres, 2001). However, the final quality of the image depends on the technician skills.

Concerning ultrasonography for animals, higher frequencies are used when compared with clinical devices used in human patients. Besides that, there is the possibility to use different contrast agents in order to study specific pathologies related with cellular receptors. This imaging approach has also the advantage of enabling real-time imaging, with the possibility of capturing about 1000 frames per second and allowing the visualization of blood flow *in vivo*, which is adequate, for instance, for cardiac studies. Considering its spatial resolution, ultrasonography is also suitable to study angiogenesis related with tumor development. However, the limited depth of penetration, influences the type of pathology in which ultrasound can be used, and should be considered as an inconvenient characteristic of this technique (Gaivão, Lima, Agostinho, Oliveira, Peres, 2001; Renault et al., 2006).

Magnetic Resonance Imaging (MRI)

A magnetic resonance imaging instrument (MRI scanner), or a nuclear magnetic resonance (NMR) imaging scanner as it was originally known, uses powerful magnets to polarize and excite hydrogen nuclei (single proton) in water molecules of biological tissues, producing a detectable signal which is spatially encoded, resulting in images of the body. The MRI machine emits a radio frequency (RF) pulse that specifically tilts the magnetic moment of the hydrogen nuclei. This pulse causes the protons in that area to absorb the energy needed to make them spin in a different direction. This is the "resonance" part of MRI. The resonance frequency is called the Larmor frequency and is calculated based on the particular tissue being imaged and the strength of the main magnetic field. MRI uses three kinds of electromagnetic fields: a very strong (in the range of a few tesla) static magnetic field to polarize the hydrogen nuclei, called the static field; one or more weaker time-varying (on the order of 1 kHz) field(s) for spatial encoding, called the gradient field(s); and a weak radio-frequency (RF) field for the manipulation of the hydrogen nuclei to produce measurable signals, collected through a RF antenna (Gaivão, Lima, Agostinho, Oliveira, Peres, 2001).

As for CT imaging, MRI traditionally creates a two dimensional image of a thin "slice" of the body and is therefore considered a tomographic imaging technique. Modern MRI instruments are able to produce images in the form of 3D blocks, which may be considered a generalization of the single-slice, maintaining the tomographic concept. However, unlike CT, MRI does not involve the use of ionizing radiation and is therefore not associated with the same health hazards. On the other hand, because MRI has only been in use since the early 1980s, there is not much confidence what are the effects of long-term exposure to strong static fields. Because of that, there is currently no limit to the number of scans to which an individual can be subjected, in contrast to what happens with radiology, CT and nuclear medicine. However, the health risks associated with tissue heating due to exposure to the RF field and to the magnetic field, are well-identified, namely if there are devices implanted in the body, such as pacemakers or other metal apparatus. These risks are strictly controlled as part of the design of the instrument and the scanning protocols used (Gaivão, Lima, Agostinho, Oliveira, Peres, 2001; Chatham, Blackband, 2001).

Because CT and MRI are sensitive to different tissue properties, the appearance of the images obtained with the two techniques differ markedly. In CT, the X-rays are more attenuated by dense tissue to create an image, whereby the image quality of soft tissues is poor. In MRI, although any nucleus with a net nuclear spin can be used, the proton of the hydrogen atom remains the most widely used, especially in the clinical setting, because it is ubiquitous and returns a large signal. This nucleus, present in water molecules, allows the excellent soft-tissue contrast achievable with MRI (Gaivão, Lima, Agostinho, Oliveira, Peres, 2001; Bartling, Stiller, Semmler, Kiessling, 2007).

Pathology

Pathological analysis is older than any of the imaging techniques already described. Using a tissue sample, it is possible to perform a morphological evaluation of tissues in search for clues concerning its histogenesis and biological behavior. Nowadays, the pathology is able not only to label diseases but also to characterize and define them morphologically as well as elucidates their underlying mechanisms (Cross, 2013; Van Middendorp, Sanchez, Burridge, 2010).

When using body tissues for pathological analysis, it is necessary first to fixate them before proceeding to histological analysis through microscopy. Fixation allows the preservation of tissues permanently in a life-like state.

Over the years, the role of pathology in medicine has benefitted from the application of specialized techniques allowing a more complete characterization of the specimen. Both, enzyme histochemistry and electron microscopy, have expanded the role of pathology from the primary microanatomical (histological) evaluation to the assessment of biochemical and subcellular structural features, exploring immunological markers and chemical signatures of cells. Over the years, advances on fixation, embedding, cutting, immunohistochemical staining, molecular methods, microscopy, as well as in image processing have improved the diagnostic ability and the research applicability of pathology (Cross, 2013; Van Middendorp, Sanchez, Burridge, 2010).

In animal research, pathological approaches have an add value, in order to obtain a complete tissue characterization in comparison with the other imaging techniques available (Figure 5). However, it is necessary to keep in mind the implications of performing a technique which involves a highly invasive procedure, i.e. removing a sample of tissue. Accordingly, pathological analysis is often performed at the end of experimental protocols or when animals are sacrificed at intermediate time points.

Figure 5. Representative images of histology specimens obtained from an orthotopic colorectal cancer animal model, stained with hematoxylin and eosin (H&E) and isolated from: colorectal cancer (A), liver (B), lung (C) and lymph node (D). Magnifications: 40x

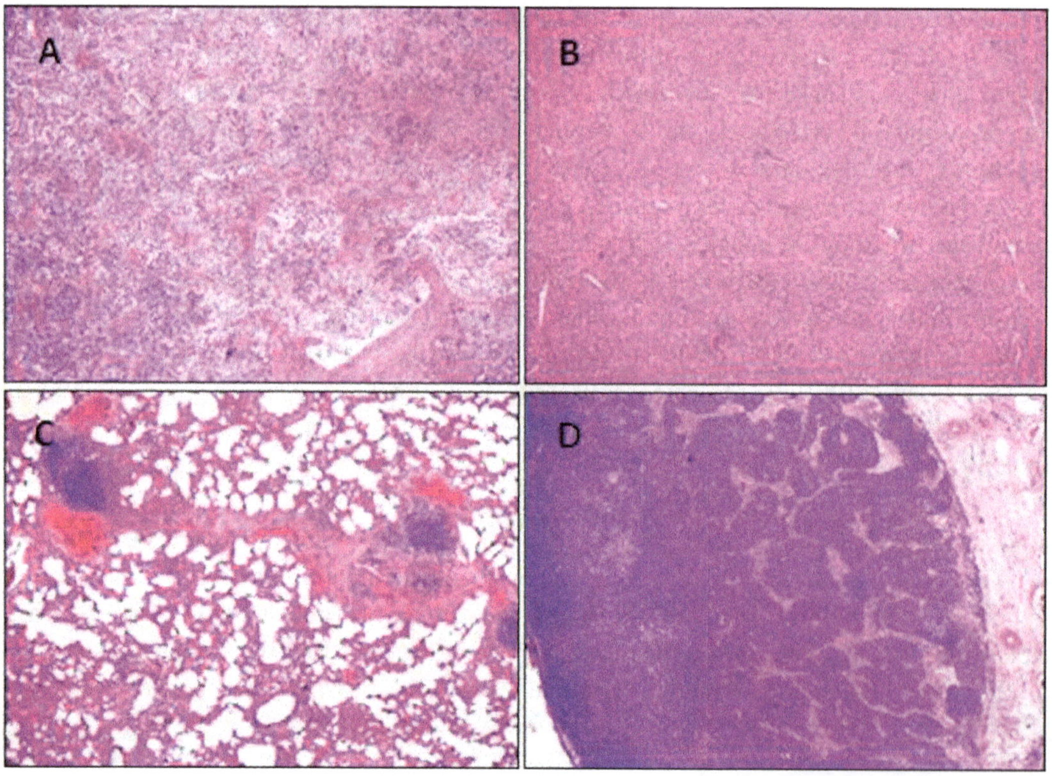

THERMOGRAPHIC TECHNOLOGY: FUNDAMENTALS FOR ANIMAL STUDIES

The image techniques seen before can be processed in order to get some useful medical information that can support the diagnosis:

- Geometry,
- Density,
- Flow,
- Size,
- Symmetry,
- Of the organ or zone of interest.

Thermography is an imaging technique that captures infrared radiation and uses it to create a temperature mapping image. Therefore, thermography not only reads the thermal patterns of a certain zone but simultaneously quantifies the temperature in each of the image picture. This adds value to the technology but requires correct equipment, conditions and protocols to perform a rigorous and useful thermographic analysis.

The majority of published thermographic studies tries to correlate a temperature variation (increase or decrease) with a certain pathology or physical disorder (Snekhalatha, Anburajan, Venkatraman, Menaka, 2013). In fact, since thermography measures radiation to create an image representing the temperature of objects, it is the most suitable method to assess the thermogenesis and thermoregulation in the majority of animals. However, the thermographic measurement of the body temperature is a challenging task as it depends on the environment, animal fur, and a precise protocol.

Infrared Measuring Principle

Measuring Temperature

Temperature is due to the kinetic movement of the molecules inside the objects. As this movement increases in amplitude and frequency, the object's temperature also increases, and thus the infrared radiation emission. The correlation between the temperature and the spectral radiation distribution can be described by the Plank law. This law states that the amount of radiation and the distribution peak frequency increases proportionally with the temperature. This way, it is possible to calculate the temperature of an object by measuring the amount of radiation in a specific waveband. A thermal camera captures infrared radiation and converts it into an electric signal that is then converted into a digital value. Through a calibration procedure, using a black body, it is possible to calculate the temperature at every pixel of the thermal image. A black body is an ideal physical object that absorbs all incident radiation, regardless of the incidence angle or radiation frequency. As an output, the emitted radiation follows the Plank law perfectly and is only modified by changing the black body's temperature (Figure 6). Another important aspect is that the radiation density is not dependent on the viewing angle. Even if the radiation is not isotropically distributed, this aspect is usually ignored since the camera's viewing angle is relatively small (less than 30º) and therefore their inherent errors are acceptable. The emissivity can then be seen has the "closeness" that an object is from being a black body, resulting in values from 1 (black body) to 0.

Figure 6. Black body radiation distribution at several temperatures, according to the Plank's law. LWIR - Long Wavelength Infrared (8-14 µm), represents the main waveband used in quantitative infrared thermography as it corresponds to the peak for environment temperatures

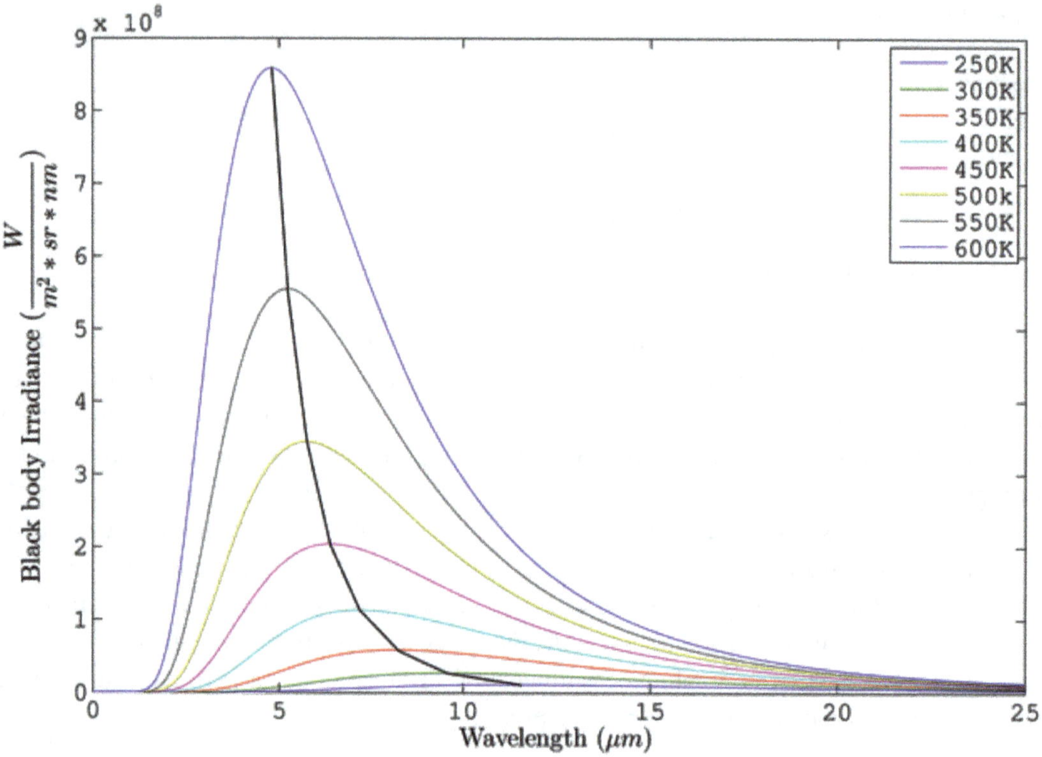

The majority of the studies take place at room temperature (approximately between 293 and 297 K). Therefore, it is necessary to use a camera that is able to capture the maximum amount of radiation in that temperature range, in order to obtain readings as precise as possible. According with the Plank law represented in Figure 6, the majority of the emitted radiation, at the ambient temperature (approximately 300K) is located between the 7 and 17 µm of wavelength. This type of radiation is known as infrared radiation (ranging from 0.77 to 1000 µm), (Ryer & Light, 1997).

Temperature Calculation

Since thermography uses and measures radiation to calculate temperature, it is influenced by some properties of the object, the environment and the camera itself. The main factors influencing thermographic measurements are:

- Objet
  - Emissivity
  - Reflected temperature and radiation
- Environment
  - Environmental temperature

- ◦ Relative humidity
- ◦ Distance

The emissivity is the balance between the emitted radiation due to the object's temperature and the radiation reflected and transmitted through the object. The skin emissivity is very high, approximately 0.98, and is the most important parameter to be set when acquiring thermal images. Another important aspect is the reflected radiation, emitted by any object in the vicinity, which interferes with temperature measurements. This effect also takes place due to background radiation emitted by the room walls, especially if the room temperature is far from the recommended. Depending on the study, and mainly the animal being studied, the ideal room temperature may vary. Although the room temperature is generally assumed to be stable during the entire image acquisition process, the reflected radiation often changes (e.g., when the hands of the researcher manipulate the animals). This aspect is far more important when working with mice compared with human patients. As mice are so small, researcher's hand occupies a considerable part of the image, thereby increasing the errors and uncertainties associated with the measurements. Ideally, animals should be pictured without any handling, which often requires sedation or a light transient anesthesia (e.g. volatile anesthesia using isoflurane). Care is needed to avoid prolonged anesthesia protocols, as these interfere with body temperature regulation.

Ideally, the lenses of the thermal camera should be completely transparent to the infrared radiation. In reality, this is impossible and the lens' transmissibility should be considered in temperature calculations. Consequentially, part of the radiation received by the sensor will derive from the lenses and not from the object. This is the reason why the thermal camera should be kept at a stable temperature.

Thermography Operating Issues

One of the most important procedures when acquiring a thermal image is the focus. An unfocused image can lead to increased uncertainty or even wrong evaluation of the thermal image. If the temperature is important for interpretation, this aspect is even more important. Figure 7, shows two thermographic images of a Wistar rat presenting chemically-induced mammary tumors in an early phase. The animal was partially shaved over the tumor area, however hair scatters the emitted infrared radiation and severely affects image quality. In Figure 7a) it is possible to observe the shaved area exhibiting three hot areas and a central colder zone. However, after adjusting the focus to the central colder area, it shows up as a clump of unshaved hair, interfering with image analysis (Figure 7b). Shaving the animal may cause light trauma to the skin, with associated inflammation, thus increasing local temperature. Care should be taken to allow sufficient time for the inflammatory phenomena to abate (usually up to 48 hours should be enough).

Another important aspect is the correct distance from the object. To achieve a perfect focus, the area to analyze is expected to be as flat as possible, which is more relevant as the camera approaches the animal. However, due to the natural round form of rats and other small animals, this situation is not usually verified. In order to minimize this problem, the object to be analyzed should be positioned as far as possible, without losing the necessary detail. An example of this situation is represented in Figure 8, representing a mouse skin tumor. The lesion was imaged using a macro lens in order to emphasize the referred effect: by focusing on the tumor basis and contour, surface and center areas become blurred. The ideal situation would be to place the camera at a 90° angle from the animal's surface, which is difficult, in this case, due to the natural shape of these animals.

Figure 7. N-methyl-N-nitrosourea-induced model of mammary cancer in a female Wistar rat. a) poorly focused thermal image of the tumor, b) correctly focused of the central area of the tumor

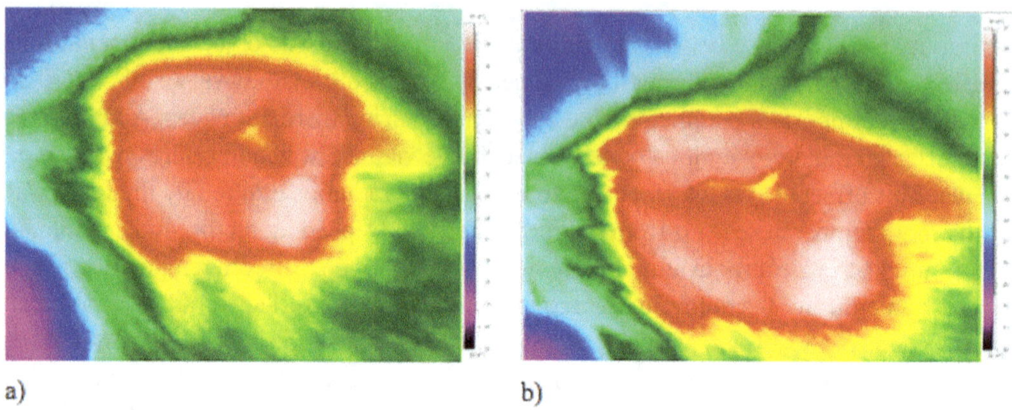

Figure 8. Two-stage skin cancer model developed with 12-O-tetradecanoylphorbol-13-acetate and 7,12-dimethylbenz(a)anthracene in a mouse. a) Poorly focused image of the tumor, b) Correctly focused image of the tumor

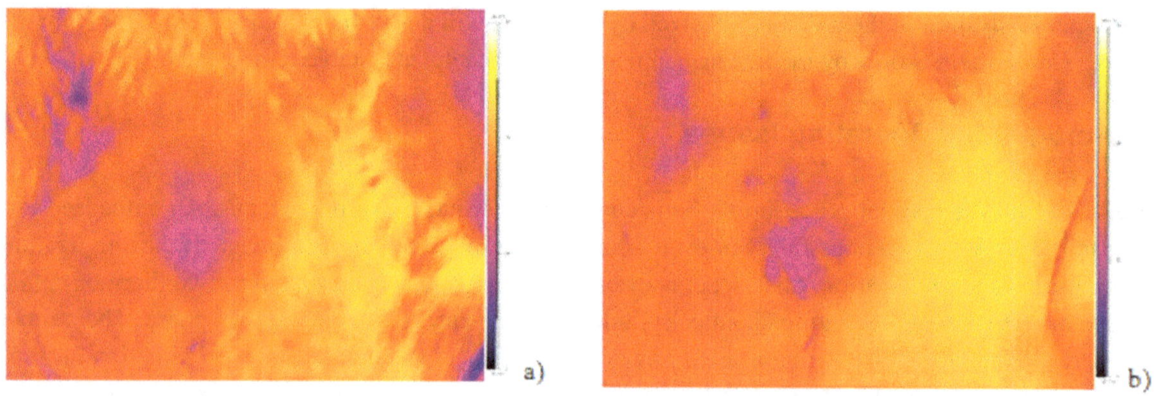

IMAGE ACQUISITION AND PROCEDURE

Image Acquisition Modalities

Thermal images may be acquired for several purposes, therefore the acquisition methodology and modality should be chosen for each case. Thermal imaging modalities can be divided into passive and active thermography (Figure 9).

In passive thermography, a single thermal image is enough to detect and characterize the object of analysis. Skin temperature changes may be detected in consequence of anomalies in the skin or in organs near the surface. For this reason, passive thermography has been the most used method in health applications, being also the easiest method to use.

Figure 9. Thermography modalities

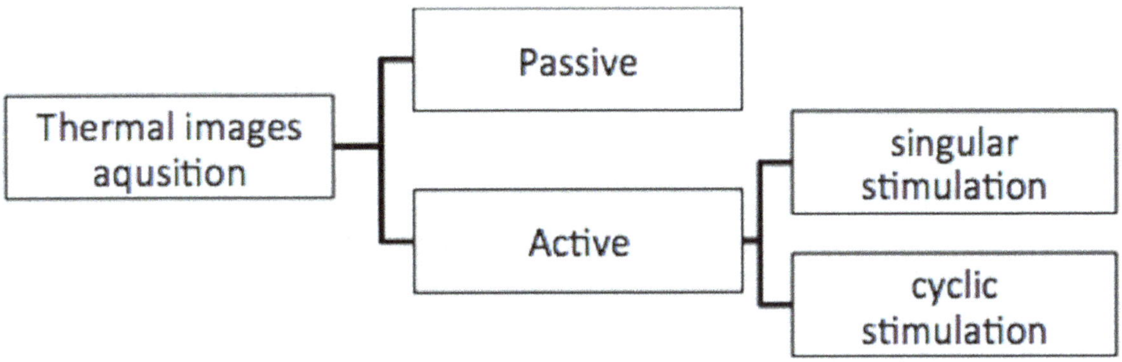

On the other hand, active thermography uses a heat flow to induce temperature changes and thus increase the accuracy of thermal readings, or to study a particular aspect e.g. thermoregulation phenomena.

Active thermography can be divided in two modalities, singular and cyclic stimulation. In the first case, the object is submitted to a single thermal stimulation; its reaction and its recovery after stimulation are then observed. Thermal transient analysis is used for example in the evaluation of the effect of physical exercise, or the response cold stress test.

Cyclic thermography is characterized by the repetition of the stimulation along the time. In this way, it is possible to achieve an accurate time-response, even if the thermal amplitudes are very small.

Preparing an Image Acquisition Setup

To perform a good thermal evaluation, it is extremely important to use not only the adequate modality but also to have a good preparation and appropriate setup. This should include a steady support for the camera, a clean table to manipulate the animal with high emissivity and low reflection and conductivity.

Firstly, a camera with the appropriate lenses should be employed. There are two types of thermal cameras (cooled and uncooled), thus the first step is to select the appropriate technology. Cooled cameras tend to be considerably more expensive but are more precise, and their sensitivity can go up to 13 mK. However, for most applications, a sensibility of 50 mK (provided by the vast majority of uncooled cameras) is sufficient. On the other hand, a very important aspect is the spatial resolution. Since the areas to observe in rats and mice are often very small, it is important to have an image with a high spatial resolution, to allow observation of small details after image acquisition. An image resolution of 320x240 pixels or higher is advisable. The lenses are also an important detail and will determine the distance to the focus area. A lens with a wide angle will be able to view a large area but not the small details and will lead to unfocussed images, as those presented in Figure 8. On the other hand, a lens with a small angle may require a far greater working space, by requiring a higher distance to view the same area. Small viewing areas also tend to create difficulties in interpreting the image and centering the object.

A relevant aspect in a thermal image is the thermal patterns, specially the natural body symmetry. Usually relative temperature (left compared to right) usually provide more information than the absolute temperature values. Another important aspect is to consider the average temperature in small areas, instead of evaluating a single point, which will necessarily conduct to wide errors.

Thermography in Animal Models of Cancer

Over the last 60 years, thermography has been used in clinical and pre-clinical (animal) studies (Ring, Hartmann, Ammer, Thomas, Land, Hand, 2010). Temperature changes at the surface of the skin may result from several biological phenomena, like: exercise (Aughey, Goodman, McKenna, 2014), articulation disorders, tumor development (Bendele, 2001; Magnan, Bondi, Pierantoni, Samaila, 2014) and drug delivery (Snekhalatha, Anburajan, Venkatraman, Menaka, 2013).

Heat and cold in a hot-blooded mammal can be either a diagnostic tool or a treatment procedure. Typically, a temperature increment or a left/right difference higher than 0.5 K is sufficient to require a more precise and complete diagnostic (Vardasca, 2012). However, for treatment purposes, a temperature variation of approximately 12 K is usually required (Portela et al., 2013, Rodrigues et al., 2013).

The thermographic evaluation of cancer patients usually takes place in hospitals, under thermoneutral temperature at approximately at 23 °C. In order to develop reliable thermographic animal cancer models, such comfort conditions must be mimicked. However, for mice the thermoneutrality should be achieved at temperatures between 30 and 32 °C (Gordon, 2012), which is far above the usual temperature in animal facilities. Other factors such the gender and the menstrual cycle of animals may also affect temperature readings (Renault et al., 2006).

The dynamics of angiogenesis in cancer have been intensively studied with recourse to animal models. Different models have allowed researchers to explore many features of cancer-associated angiogenesis, as well as to develop and test anti-angiogenic drugs. However, data from animal models must be carefully interpreted and extrapolation to human patients is not straightforward. For instance, clinical results obtained with anti-angiogenic drugs are often below what could be anticipated based on animal studies (Carmeliet & Jain, 2011). Choosing - and often, creating - adequate animal models to study specific aspects of angiogenesis is a critical step for planning translational research experiments.

Monitoring angiogenesis in animal models of cancer is also challenging. *Post-mortem* evaluations can be readily performed histologically, or by employing immunohistochemical or immunofluorescent techniques to detect and quantify blood or lymphatic vessels in tissue samples. *In vivo* monitoring of cancer-associated angiogenesis presents other difficulties. In this context, thermography offers its well-known advantages as a safe and non-invasive method. Several experiments have been performed using thermography to monitor physiological parameters and pathological changes in laboratory animals. However, only a few reports refer the use of thermography to monitor tumor growth and/or response to therapy in animal models of cancer.

From the point of view of physiology, thermographic techniques have been used to study the effects of dietary components on thermogenesis (Smriga, Murakami, Mori, Torii, 2000) and to correlate body temperature and cage behavior in rats (Bilodeau, 2011). Recently, David *et al.* (2013) used thermography to study the effects of environmental temperature in animal facilities on the metabolic status of mice. This study pointed thermography as an ideal tool for assessing husbandry practices and manage thermal stress in laboratory animals.

Thermography has also been used to study pathological phenomena, like the effects of sciatic nerve crush on the thermal status of the affected limb (Sacharuk et al., 2011). Thermography also allowed the detection of experimentally-induced pneumotorax in rats by demonstrating the presence of cooler thoracic areas Rich et al. (2004) and was shown to be useful in studying the viability of surgical skin flaps (Shejbal, Drvis, Bedekovic, 2012). In a rat model of serotonin-induced itch, thermography was used to study the local vasoregulation in response to serotonin administration, and a negative correlation between serotonin dose and local temperature was observed (Jasemian, Gazerani, Dagnaes-Hansen, 2012). In a recent study, Snekhalatha *et al.* (2013) showed that thermography may be used to monitor the development of arthritis in an experimental rat model and that thermographic findings significantly correlate with radiographic and other clinical data.

The need for adequate animal models to develop thermographic cancer research was recognized as early as 1986 (Jochimsen, Folk, Sundell, Loh, 1986). Two years later, Konerding and Steinberg (1988), reported the use of thermography to study subcutaneous (heterotopic) tumor xenografts in nude mice (Figure 10). Nude mice are particularly attractive for thermographic studies, since even a moderately thick hair coat will produce dramatic radiation scattering effects as well as change the skin temperature. Their extensive use in cancer biology for developing heterotopic (almost always subcutaneous) tumor xenografts is another reason why these models are so promising from the point of view of thermography.

An identical approach was used by Xie *et al.* (2004) to study the vascularization of breast cancer xenografts in mice. Both studies concluded that tumor xenografts showed reduced temperature, compared with the surrounding tissues. These findings were later confirmed by Song *et al.* (2007), who reported that tumor temperature progressively decreased as they developed, reaching a minimum of 3 °C when compared with adjacent tissues, at 14 days post-implantation. These reports are in accordance with our own findings, depicted in Figure 10. The reason why mouse xenografts showed reduced temperature when compared with adjacent tissues, in stark contrast with previous thermographic in human cancer patients, is not fully understood. Mouse xenografts do not develop through the usual multistep carcinogenesis process, but are a population of, often, highly malignant cells, cultured *in vitro* and then injected into the animal. As such, it is possible that some tumors do not adequately represent the histological and, especially, vascular aspects of the original human tumors. Despite these surprising findings, early studies using mouse xenografts suggested that thermography could be a useful method to monitor tumor response to anticancer drugs in animal models (Xie, McCahon, Jakobsen, Parish, 2004; Song et al. 2007). Orthotopic rat xenografts (tumors or tumor cell lines transplanted into their corresponding organ of origin) are expected to be a more realistic model than heterotopic xenografts. One such model, mimicking colon carcinoma, is depicted in Figure 11.

However, thermography has seldom been adopted for this purpose. Recently, Rodrigues *et al.* (2013), reported on the successful use of thermography to monitor the response of mouse tumor xenografts treated with hyperthermia induced by magnetic nanoparticles. The same group also reported that thermographic data significantly correlated with readings obtained by intratumoral fiber-optic thermometers. A similar approach was successfully used by Tepper *et al.* (2013), for assessing the effects of diffusing alpha-emitters radiation therapy (DaRT) wires on subcutaneous breast cancer xenografts in mice. Intratumoral temperature differences were higher in treated *versus* untreated tumors, which agrees with the hypothesis that DaRT wires induced localized tumor destruction at implantation sites. The authors also found that tumor area estimated based on thermographic images was significantly correlated with direct visual caliper measurements. In a recent study, Hashida *et al.* (2014) successfully used a thermographic approach to monitor the thermal ablation of subcutaneous colon cancer xenografts using modified carbon nanotubes. Given the importance of nude mice xenografts in developing anti-cancer therapies, and the high costs associated with other imaging technologies, it is expected that thermography, with its inherent advantages, will attract the attention of researchers working with this kind of models in the near future.

When using hirsute animals, clipping the hair that overlies the tumor area is necessary in order to obtain suitable readings (Figure 12). This problem is frequently encountered when employing common rat strains (e.g. Fischer or Wistar rats). Poljak-Blazi *et al.* (2009) studied thermographically the effects

Figure 10. Nude mouse showing subcutaneous colon cancer xenograft (circle). The tumor temperature varies between 33.1 and 33.9 ºC (33.3 ± 0.1, average ± standard deviation) For the adjacent tissue, the average temperature is 34.1 ± 0.1

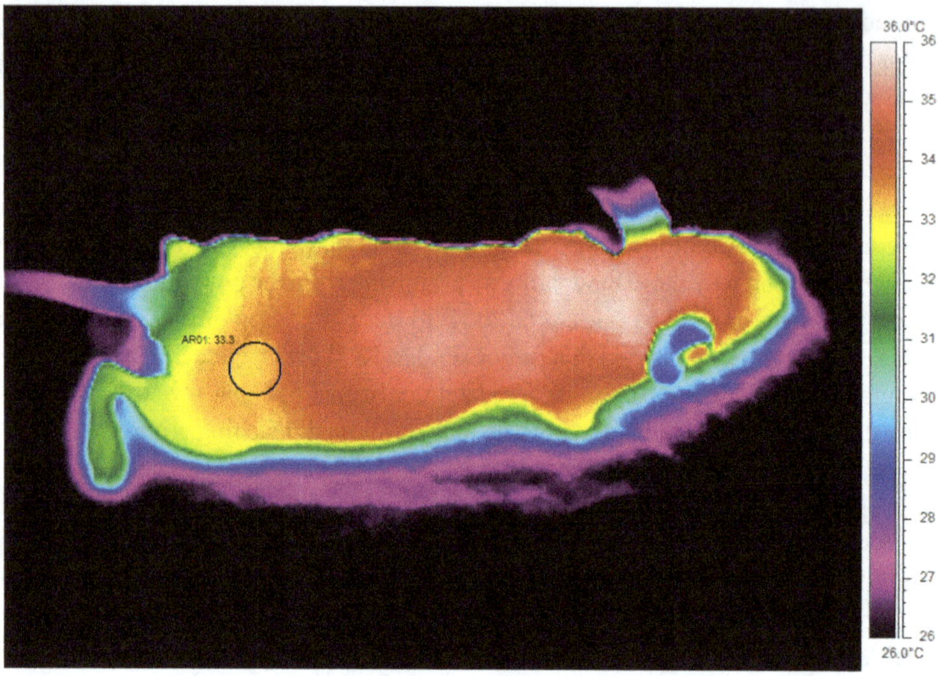

Figure 11. Nude rat with an orthotopic colon xenograft tumor. The tumor (AR01) shows an average temperature of 31.3 ºC, the subcutaneous tumor invasion area (AR02) 32.6 ºC and the adjacent tissue (AR03) 34.1 ºC

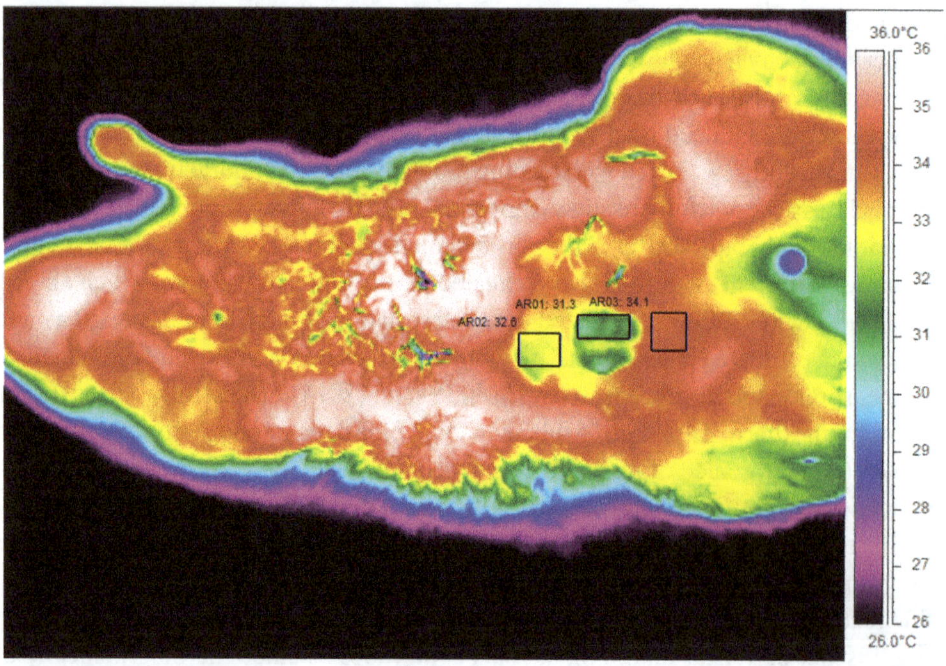

of experimental tumor transplantation, local inflammation and hematoma in Sprague-Dawley rats. As expected, the authors observed a raise in skin temperature following inflammation or hematoma induction. As observed in mouse xenografts, transplanted tumors (Walker 256 carcinoma) showed reduced temperature compared with adjacent tissues. However, contrary to what has been described for mice, this trend changed from day 10 post-transplantation onwards, when tumor temperature increased up to 1 °C over adjacent tissues. The authors reported that, histologically, the tumors showed abundant vascularization, which may, to some degree, explain these findings. A more recent study addressed the relationship between thermographic findings and tumor vascularization, as detected by ultrasonography, in nitrosamine-induced mammary cancer (Faustino-Rocha, 2013). In this study, significant intratumoral thermal heterogeneity was observed. Maximum intratumoral temperature and thermal amplitude were found to correlate positively with tumor size. This may reflect tumor heterogeneity, typically found in large lesions, which partially agrees with the findings of Poljak-Blazi *et al.* (2009), suggesting that, at least in rats, long-term tumor progression leads to increasing tumor temperatures. However, the comparison between the results of Faustino-Rocha *et al.* (2013) and of Poljak-Blazi *et al.* (2009) is necessarily limited, because the previous study does not compare tumor temperature with that of adjacent tissues. Concerning the relationship between tumor temperature and vascularization, the authors reported that maximum tumor temperature and thermal amplitude were also correlated with blood vessel density, as determined using an ultrasonographic technique (power Doppler). A more recent study came to confirm these findings, Faustino-Rocha et al. (2016) show that thermal readings may be correlated with tumor vascularization, as assessed histologically and immunohistochemically (VEGF immunoexpression).

Figure 12. N-methyl-N-nitrosourea-induced model of mammary cancer in a female Wistar rat. Visible (a) and infrared thermal images using two different temperature scales (b and c) provide complementary information regarding the tumor (circled area)

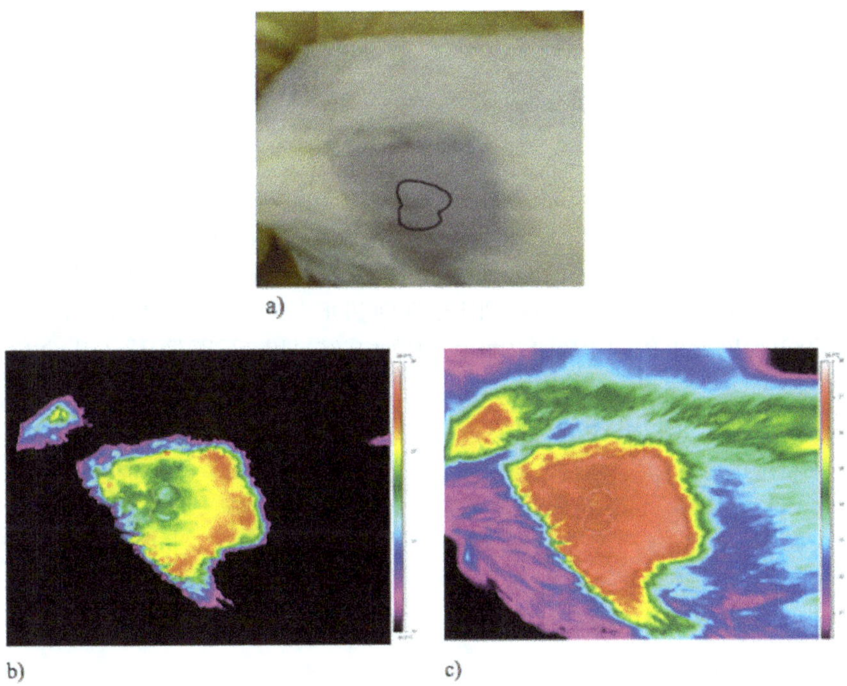

The thermal differences that have been observed between tumors in different animal models certainly reflect important differences in tumor development and biology. Over recent years, it has become evident that mouse xenografts only mimic the original human tumor to a limited extent (Eklund, Bry, Alitalo, 2013). Importantly, it has been found that anti-angiogenic agents which are highly effective in mouse xenografts show comparatively low efficacy in human patients, who present a more complex scenario. As a result, there is a search for models that recapitulate multistep carcinogenesis more accurately, including the progressive development of tumor vasculature (Eklund, Bry, Alitalo, 2013). A detailed and systematic characterization of such models is also mandatory. In this setting, thermography, with its inherent advantages over other invasive, expensive, or radiation-emitting techniques, maintains all its untapped potential to become a standard technique for monitoring tumor angiogenesis in animal models.

CONCLUSION

Thermography is a viable technique to assess the vascularization of superficial (cutaneous or subcutaneous) tumors in laboratory animals. As demonstrated by various studies, it may complement other techniques, such as ultrasound imaging and histopathology, providing relevant information on tumor biology. However, the presence of a dense haircoat on many mouse and rat strains, as well as the presence of a thick subcutaneous fat layer (e.g. in pigs), may limit the use of thermography. Other limitation of this technique when used in laboratory rodents is the frequent need for animal handling, restrainment or sedation, which may influence thermal readings. Also, it is not always possible to obtain thermal images from a 90° angle, as recommended, due to the animal's shape.

Finally, thermal cameras suppliers have recently started offering devices, which make it possible to obtain simultaneous and superimposable thermal and visible images, which will add to the potential of this technology. At the same time, the continuous development of smaller thermal cameras also offers new possibilities and applications.

ACKNOWLEDGMENT

The authors would like to acknowledge to Project POCI-01-0145-FEDER-006939, LEPABE and POCI-01-0145-FEDER-006958, funded by FEDER funds through COMPETE2020 - POCI – and by Portuguese Government and the Social European Fund through FCT, grant SFRH/BPD/85462/2012, UID/EMS/50022/2013(LAETA), UID/AGR/04033/2013, PTDC/DES/114122/2009, SFRH/BD/102099/2014, PEst-C/SAU/UI3282/2013 and IBILI-FMUC through PEst-C/SAU/UI3282/2013, UID/NEU/04539/2013 and ACIMAGO.

REFERENCES

Aughey, R. J., Goodman, C. A., & McKenna, M. J. (2014). Greater chance of high core temperatures with modified pacing strategy during team sport in the heat. *Journal of Science and Medicine in Sport, 17*(1), 113–118. doi:10.1016/j.jsams.2013.02.013 PMID:23689104

Bartling, S. H., Stiller, W., Semmler, W., & Kiessling, F. (2007). Small animal computed tomography imaging. *Current Medical Imaging Reviews, 3*(1), 45–59. doi:10.2174/157340507779940327

Bendele, A. (2001). Animal models of rheumatoid arthritis. *Journal of Musculoskeletal & Neuronal Interactions, 1*(4), 377–385. PMID:15758488

Bignold, L. P. (2003). Initiation of genetic instability and tumour formation: A review and hypothesis of a nongenotoxic mechanism. *Cellular and Molecular Life Sciences, 60*(6), 1107–1117. doi:10.1007/s00018-003-2314-6 PMID:12861379

Bignold, L. P., Coghlan, B. L. D., & Jersmann, H. P. A. (2006). Cancer morphology, carcinogenesis and genetic instability: a background. In Cancer: Cell Structures, Carcinogens and Genomic Instability (pp. 1-24). Birkhäuser Basel. doi:10.1007/3-7643-7378-4_1

Bilodeau, G. A., Ghali, R., Desgent, S., Langlois, P., Farah, R., St-Onge, P. L., . . . Carmant, L. (2011, June). Where is the rat? Tracking in low contrast thermographic images. In CVPR 2011 Workshops (pp. 55-60). IEEE. doi:10.1109/CVPRW.2011.5981685

Carmeliet, P., & Jain, R. K. (2011). Molecular mechanisms and clinical applications of angiogenesis. *Nature, 473*(7347), 298–307. doi:10.1038/nature10144 PMID:21593862

Chatham, J. C., & Blackband, S. J. (2001). Nuclear magnetic resonance spectroscopy and imaging in animal research. *ILAR Journal, 42*(3), 189–208. doi:10.1093/ilar.42.3.189 PMID:11406719

Cross, S. (2013). *Underwood's Pathology* (6th ed.). Elsevier Health Sciences.

David, J. M., Chatziioannou, A. F., Taschereau, R., Wang, H., & Stout, D. B. (2013). The hidden cost of housing practices: Using noninvasive imaging to quantify the metabolic demands of chronic cold stress of laboratory mice. *Comparative Medicine, 63*(5), 386–391. PMID:24210014

Decker, S., & Sausville, E. (2011). Perspectives on the History and Evolution of Tumor Models. In *Tumor Models in Cancer Research* (pp. 3–20). Humana Press. doi:10.1007/978-1-60761-968-0_1

Dranoff, G. (2012). Experimental mouse tumour models: What can be learnt about human cancer immunology? *Nature Reviews. Immunology, 12*(1), 61–66. PMID:22134155

Eklund, L., Bry, M., & Alitalo, K. (2013). Mouse models for studying angiogenesis and lymphangiogenesis in cancer. *Molecular Oncology, 7*(2), 259–282. doi:10.1016/j.molonc.2013.02.007 PMID:23522958

Farago, A. F., Snyder, E. L., & Jacks, T. (2012). SnapShot: Lung cancer models. *Cell, 149*(1), 246–246. doi:10.1016/j.cell.2012.03.015 PMID:22464334

Faustino-Rocha, A. I., Silva, A., Gabriel, J., da Costa, R. G., Moutinho, M., Oliveira, P. A., & Ginja, M. et al. (2016). Long-term exercise training as a modulator of mammary cancer vascularization. *Biomedicine and Pharmacotherapy*, *81*, 273–280. doi:10.1016/j.biopha.2016.04.030 PMID:27261604

Faustino-Rocha, A. I., Silva, A., Gabriel, J., Teixeira-Guedes, C. I., Lopes, C., da Costa, R. G., & Ginja, M. et al. (2013). Ultrasonographic, thermographic and histologic evaluation of MNU-induced mammary tumors in female Sprague-Dawley rats. *Biomedicine and Pharmacotherapy*, *67*(8), 771–776. doi:10.1016/j.biopha.2013.06.011 PMID:23906759

Frese, K. K., & Tuveson, D. A. (2007). Maximizing mouse cancer models. *Nature Reviews. Cancer*, *7*(9), 654–658. doi:10.1038/nrc2192 PMID:17687385

Gaivão, F. D. M., de Lima, J. P., Agostinho, A. G., Oliveira, A. S., & Peres, A. P. (2001). *Imagiologia Clínica-Princípios e Técnicas*. Academic Press.

Gordon, C. J. (2012). Thermal physiology of laboratory mice: Defining thermoneutrality. *Journal of Thermal Biology*, *37*(8), 654–685. doi:10.1016/j.jtherbio.2012.08.004

Grossfeld, G. D., Ginsberg, D. A., Stein, J. P., Bochner, B. H., Esrig, D., Nichols, P. W., & Cote, R. J. et al. (1997). Thrombospondin-1 expression in bladder cancer: Association with p53 alterations, tumor angiogenesis, and tumor progression. *Journal of the National Cancer Institute*, *89*(3), 219–227. doi:10.1093/jnci/89.3.219 PMID:9017002

Hanahan, D., Wagner, E. F., & Palmiter, R. D. (2007). The origins of oncomice: A history of the first transgenic mice genetically engineered to develop cancer. *Genes & Development*, *21*(18), 2258–2270. doi:10.1101/gad.1583307 PMID:17875663

Hansen, K., & Khanna, C. (2004). Spontaneous and genetically engineered animal models: Use in preclinical cancer drug development. *European Journal of Cancer*, *40*(6), 858–880. doi:10.1016/j.ejca.2003.11.031 PMID:15120042

Harshaw, C., Culligan, J. J., & Alberts, J. R. (2014). Sex differences in thermogenesis structure behavior and contact within huddles of infant mice. *PLoS ONE*, *9*(1), e87405. doi:10.1371/journal.pone.0087405 PMID:24498099

Hashida, Y., Tanaka, H., Zhou, S., Kawakami, S., Yamashita, F., Murakami, T., & Hashida, M. et al. (2014). Photothermal ablation of tumor cells using a single-walled carbon nanotube–peptide composite. *Journal of Controlled Release*, *173*, 59–66. doi:10.1016/j.jconrel.2013.10.039 PMID:24211651

Iacobuzio-Donahue, C. A. (2009). Epigenetic changes in cancer. *Annual Review of Pathological Mechanical Disease*, *4*(1), 229–249. doi:10.1146/annurev.pathol.3.121806.151442 PMID:18840073

Jasemian, Y., Gazerani, P., & Dagnaes-Hansen, F. (2012). Infrared thermography in serotonin-induced itch model in rats. *Open Dermatology Journal*, *6*(1), 1–7. doi:10.2174/1874372201206010001

Jochimsen, P. R., Folk, G. E., Sundell, M., & Loh, P. M. (1986). B16 melanoma in hairless mice: A model for thermographic research. *Journal of Surgical Oncology*, *33*(1), 50–52. doi:10.1002/jso.2930330114 PMID:3762175

Jonkers, J., & Berns, A. (2005). *Animal models of cancer: Introduction to the cellular and molecular biology of cancer*. Oxford University Press.

Konerding, M. A., & Steinberg, F. (1988). Computerized infrared thermography and ultrastructural studies of xenotransplanted human tumors on nude mice. *Thermology*, *3*(1), 7–14.

Lima, J. J. D. (2011). *Nuclear Medicine Physics. Series in Medical Physics and Biomedical Engineering*. Taylor and Francis.

Lima, J. J. P. D. (1995). *Física dos métodos de imagem com raios X*. Coimbra: Edições ASA.

Loi, M., Di Paolo, D., Becherini, P., Zorzoli, A., Perri, P., Carosio, R., & Ponzoni, M. et al. (2011). The use of the orthotopic model to validate antivascular therapies for cancer. *The International Journal of Developmental Biology*, *55*(4-5), 547–555. doi:10.1387/ijdb.103230ml PMID:21858775

MacEwen, E. G. (1990). Spontaneous tumors in dogs and cats: Models for the study of cancer biology and treatment. *Cancer and Metastasis Reviews*, *9*(2), 125–136. doi:10.1007/BF00046339 PMID:2253312

Magnan, B., Bondi, M., Pierantoni, S., & Samaila, E. (2014). The pathogenesis of Achilles tendinopathy: A systematic review. *Foot and Ankle Surgery*, *20*(3), 154–159. doi:10.1016/j.fas.2014.02.010 PMID:25103700

Merck Sharp & Dohme Corp. (2014). *The Merck Veterinary Manual - Diagnostic Imaging, Radiology*. Retrieved from http://www.merckmanuals.com/vet/clinical_pathology_and_procedures/diagnostic_imaging/radiography.html

Oliveira, P. A., Colaço, A., Chaves, R., Guedes-Pinto, H., De-La-Cruz, P., Luis, F., & Lopes, C. (2007). Chemical carcinogenesis. *Anais da Academia Brasileira de Ciencias*, *79*(4), 593–616. doi:10.1590/S0001-37652007000400004 PMID:18066431

Oliveira, P. A., Colaço, A., De la Cruz, P. L., & Lopes, C. (2006). Experimental bladder carcinogenesis-rodent models. *Experimental Oncology*, *28*(1), 2–11. PMID:16614700

Polin, L., Corbett, T. H., Roberts, B. J., Lawson, A. J., Leopold, W. R., III, White, K., . . . Horwitz, J. P. (2011). Transplantable Syngeneic Rodent Tumors: Solid Tumors in Mice. In Tumor Models in Cancer Research (pp. 43-78). Humana Press.

Poljak-Blazi, M., Kolaric, D., Jaganjac, M., Zarkovic, K., Skala, K., & Zarkovic, N. (2009). Specific thermographic changes during Walker 256 carcinoma development: Differential infrared imaging of tumour, inflammation and haematoma. *Cancer Detection and Prevention*, *32*(5), 431–436. doi:10.1016/j.cdp.2009.01.002 PMID:19232842

Portela, A., Vasconcelos, M., Fernandes, M. H., Garcia, M., Silva, A., Gabriel, J., & Cavalheiro, J. et al. (2013). Highly focalised thermotherapy using a ferrimagnetic cement in the treatment of a melanoma mouse model by low temperature hyperthermia. *International Journal of Hyperthermia*, *29*(2), 121–132. doi:10.3109/02656736.2013.767478 PMID:23418916

Potente, M., Gerhardt, H., & Carmeliet, P. (2011). Basic and therapeutic aspects of angiogenesis. *Cell*, *146*(6), 873–887. doi:10.1016/j.cell.2011.08.039 PMID:21925313

Renault, G., Bonnin, P., Marchiol-Fournigault, C., Gregoire, J. M., Serriere, S., Richard, B., & Fradelizi, D. (2006). High-resolution ultrasound imaging of the mouse. *Journal de Radiologie*, *87*(12 Pt 2), 1937–1945. doi:10.1016/S0221-0363(06)74179-8 PMID:17211308

Rich, P. B., Dulabon, G. R., Douillet, C. D., Listwa, T. M., Robinson, W. P., Zarzaur, B. L., & Katz, L. M. et al. (2004). Infrared thermography: A rapid, portable, and accurate technique to detect experimental pneumothorax. *The Journal of Surgical Research*, *120*(2), 163–170. doi:10.1016/j.jss.2004.02.026 PMID:15234209

Ring, E. F. J., Hartmann, J., Ammer, K., Thomas, R., Land, D., & Hand, J. W. (2010). Infrared and Microwave Medical Thermometry. *Experimental Methods in the Physical Sciences*, *43*, 393–448. doi:10.1016/S1079-4042(09)04307-0

Rodrigues, H. F., Mello, F. M., Branquinho, L. C., Zufelato, N., Silveira-Lacerda, E. P., & Bakuzis, A. F. (2013). Real-time infrared thermography detection of magnetic nanoparticle hyperthermia in a murine model under a non-uniform field configuration. *International Journal of Hyperthermia*, *29*(8), 752–767. doi:10.3109/02656736.2013.839056 PMID:24138472

Rowland, D. J., & Cherry, S. R. (2008, May). Small-animal preclinical nuclear medicine instrumentation and methodology. *Seminars in Nuclear Medicine*, *38*(3), 209–222. doi:10.1053/j.semnuclmed.2008.01.004 PMID:18396180

Ryer, A., & Light, V. (1997). *Light measurement handbook*. Academic Press.

Sacharuk, V. Z., Lovatel, G. A., Ilha, J., Marcuzzo, S., Pinho, A. S. D., Xavier, L. L., & Achaval, M. et al. (2011). Thermographic evaluation of hind paw skin temperature and functional recovery of locomotion after sciatic nerve crush in rats. *Clinics (Sao Paulo)*, *66*(7), 1259–1266. doi:10.1590/S1807-59322011000700023 PMID:21876984

Shejbal, D., Drvis, P., & Bedekovic, V. (2012). Thermography-measured effect of capsaicin, methylprednisolone and mitomycin on the survival of random skin flaps in rats. *Skin Research and Technology*, *18*(2), 157–161. doi:10.1111/j.1600-0846.2011.00547.x PMID:21545651

Shojaei, F. (2012). Anti-angiogenesis therapy in cancer: Current challenges and future perspectives. *Cancer Letters*, *320*(2), 130–137. doi:10.1016/j.canlet.2012.03.008 PMID:22425960

Singh, M., Murriel, C. L., & Johnson, L. (2012). Genetically engineered mouse models: Closing the gap between preclinical data and trial outcomes. *Cancer Research*, *72*(11), 2695–2700. doi:10.1158/0008-5472.CAN-11-2786 PMID:22593194

Smriga, M., Murakami, H., Mori, M., & Torii, K. (2000). Use of thermal photography to explore the age-dependent effect of monosodium glutamate, NaCl and glucose on brown adipose tissue thermogenesis. *Physiology & Behavior*, *71*(3), 403–407. doi:10.1016/S0031-9384(00)00350-4 PMID:11150573

Snekhalatha, U., Anburajan, M., Venkatraman, B., & Menaka, M. (2013). Evaluation of complete Freunds adjuvant-induced arthritis in a Wistar rat model. *Zeitschrift fur Rheumatologie*, *72*(4), 375–382. doi:10.1007/s00393-012-1083-8 PMID:23208192

Song, C., Appleyard, V., Murray, K., Frank, T., Sibbett, W., Cuschieri, A., & Thompson, A. (2007). Thermographic assessment of tumor growth in mouse xenografts. *International Journal of Cancer*, *121*(5), 1055–1058. doi:10.1002/ijc.22808 PMID:17487841

Tepper, M., Shoval, A., Hoffer, O., Confino, H., Schmidt, M., Kelson, I., & Gannot, I. et al. (2013). Thermographic investigation of tumor size, and its correlation to tumor relative temperature, in mice with transplantable solid breast carcinoma. *Journal of Biomedical Optics*, *18*(11), 111410–111410. doi:10.1117/1.JBO.18.11.111410 PMID:23934014

Torre, L. A., Bray, F., Siegel, R. L., Ferlay, J., Lortet-Tieulent, J., & Jemal, A. (2015). Global cancer statistics, 2012. *CA: a Cancer Journal for Clinicians*, *65*(2), 87–108. doi:10.3322/caac.21262 PMID:25651787

Van Middendorp, J. J., Sanchez, G. M., & Burridge, A. L. (2010). The Edwin Smith papyrus: A clinical reappraisal of the oldest known document on spinal injuries. *European Spine Journal*, *19*(11), 1815–1823. doi:10.1007/s00586-010-1523-6 PMID:20697750

Vardasca, R. Â. R. (2012). *The effect of work related mechanical stress on the peripheral temperature of the hand*. Academic Press.

Xie, W., McCahon, P., Jakobsen, K., & Parish, C. (2004). Evaluation of the ability of digital infrared imaging to detect vascular changes in experimental animal tumours. *International Journal of Cancer*, *108*(5), 790–794. doi:10.1002/ijc.11618 PMID:14696108

Chapter 12
Thermographic Evaluation of Racehorse Performance

Maria Soroko
Wroclaw University of Environmental and Life Sciences, Poland

ABSTRACT

Thermography has found a broad range of applications in equine sport and veterinary medicine. Thermographic diagnosis is useful in monitoring changes of horse surface temperature resulting from exercise allowing evaluation of the work of individual parts of the body in racing performance. Regular assessment of body surface temperature allows the detection of training overloads and identification of pathological conditions of the musculoskeletal system during the racing training cycle. The usefulness of thermography in veterinary medicine has been proved in detecting pathological conditions associated mainly with inflammation processes of the distal parts of the limbs and back. The main advantage of thermography is the detection of subclinical signs of inflammation before the onset of clinical signs of pathology, providing great value in veterinary medicine diagnosis. Thermography has also found application in detecting illegal performance procedures to improve horse performance and in assessing the saddle fit to the horse's back.

INTRODUCTION

Thermography in equine veterinary medicine was introduced in 1965 and since that time has been considered for use in a wide range of applications (Delahanty & Georgi, 1965).

Thermography enables abnormal patterns in skin surface temperatures (and hence vascularity and metabolic activity within and below the skin surface) due to injury to be detected (Turner, 1991). One of the clinical signs of inflammation is heat, related to metabolic activity and an elevated local circulation, recognised thermographically as a 'hotspot' (Ring, 1990). Other pathological conditions reduce blood circulation due to either vascular shunts, thrombosis or autonomic nervous system abnormalities and are recognised as 'coldspots' (Turner, 1991; von Schweinitz, 1999).

Therefore thermography has been used increasingly in equine veterinary practice as an efficient tool for detection of injuries of the musculoskeletal system in sport horses (Turner et al., 2001). It has been

DOI: 10.4018/978-1-5225-2072-6.ch012

employed especially in the racing industry, where the physical demands put on racing horses are extreme (Figure 1). Constant overload of the musculoskeletal system due to regular training and racing can cause abnormalities associated with painful conditions or diseases, leading to loss of performance (Jeffcott et al., 1982; Rossdale et al., 1985). Injuries are mainly associated with soft tissue or bone fractures of the distal parts of limbs (Jeffcott, 1999; Parkin et al., 2004; Head, 2009). They are often variably clinically manifested, ranging from overt lameness but also pain on palpation or gait alterations (Jeffcott, 1999; Denoix, 1999; Haussler et al., 1999).

Lameness is a significant disorder for racehorses, recognized as an abnormality associated with painful conditions or mechanical injuries, which affect the horse's way of movement. Numerous reports describing lameness incidence in racehorses have been recorded in the United Kingdom. Investigations presented by Buchner et al. (1996), Ramdy (1997), Oliver et al. (1997), Jeffcott (1999), Kane et al. (2000), and Keegan et al. (2000) indicated that lameness is the main reason for training days being lost and wastage in the horse industry. In the study presented by Jeffcott et al. (1982), out of 163 Thoroughbred racehorses 53% suffered from lameness, which was the main cause of elimination of the horses from performance. A more recent study involving Thoroughbred racehorses recorded an 81% incidence of lameness (Williams et al., 2001).

One of the main problems with injuries is the long period of rehabilitation. Additionally, the reduced tissue functionality decreases the chance of the horse returning to its previous performance and soundness. It was reported that 70% of Thoroughbred horses failed to return to regular training after injury (Oikawa & Kasashima, 2002). Monitoring the impact of racehorse exercise programmes through the measurement of body surface temperature can help to detect potential injuries, maintain horse health and condition, and extend a horse's career in sport.

Figure 1. Thermogram of a racehorse with the rider from the lateral aspect

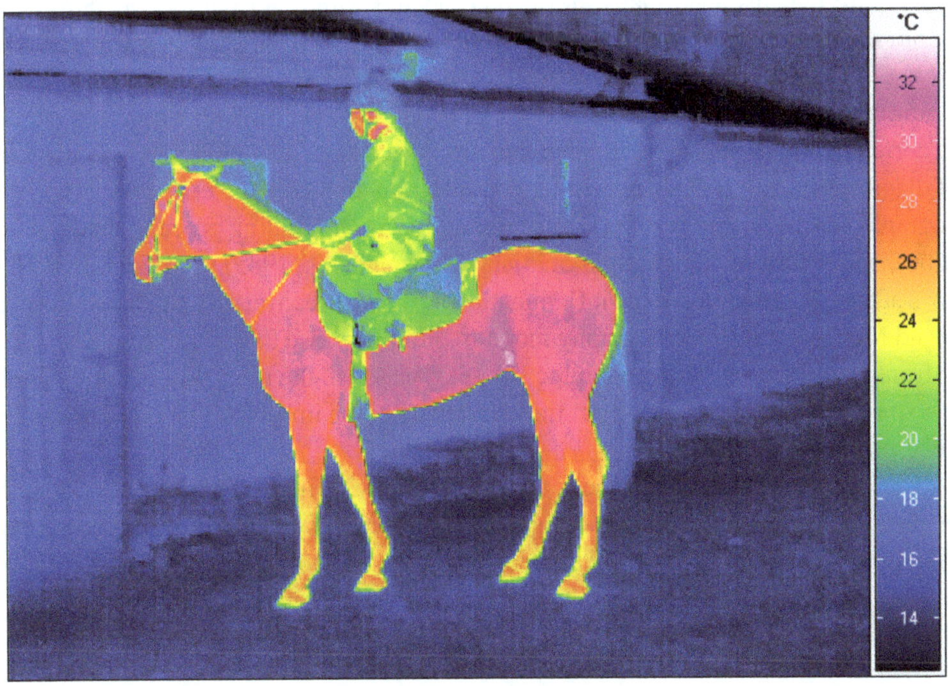

APPLICATION OF THERMOGRAPHY IN VETERINARY MEDICINE

Potential equine veterinary applications of thermography in identifying areas of pathology have been described (Purohit & McCoy, 1980; Bowman et al., 1983; Turner et al., 1983; Turner, 1991). These reports mostly address the detection of injuries, especially at the back and the distal parts of the limbs (Vaden et al., 1980; von Schweinitz, 1999; Turner et al., 2001; Turner, 2003; Soroko et al., 2013).

Clinical diseases of the distal limbs including tendonitis, carpal and tarsal joint inflammation and bucked shins have been recognized and characterized by thermography (Purohit & McCoy, 1980; Bowman et al., 1983; Turner et al., 1983; Turner, 1991; Soroko, 2011a). Thermography is also useful in recognizing abnormal conditions of the hoof including navicular syndrome, laminitis, sole abscesses, corns and other hoof-related structural pathologies (Purohit & McCoy, 1980; Turner et al., 1983; Turner, 1991). Thermography not only provides additional information about localizing the problem but also evaluates the degree of associated inflammation.

Thermography and radiography are complementary diagnostic tools for the study of inflammation diseases of distal parts of the limbs (Collins et al., 1976). They cooperate together in diagnosis of joint diseases, as radiography recognizes osseous changes, while thermography indicates changes associated with capsulitis and synovitis in joints. Cooperation between those two methods was successfully applied for diagnosis of osteoarthritis. The study presented by Vaden et al. (1980) indicated that thermography can be a useful tool for chronic tarsal joint arthritis diagnosis together with radiography, and also in the early stages of joint disorders, when no changes are detected in radiography examinations. Similar conclusions were indicated in the case of carpal inflammatory joint disease (Bowman et al., 1983).

Thermography and ultrasonography are also used as complementary tools for the examination of tendons in the distal parts of the limbs. While ultrasonography evaluates morphology of the tendonitis (the size and the shape of the injury), thermography localizes the injury. Moreover thermography can be useful to follow the healing process. As the tendon heals the thermal pattern becomes more uniform, but the temperature remains abnormally elevated compared with a normal tendon (Stromberg, 1972; 1974). Later in the recovery process, as the scar tissue is deposited, the skin over the injured area may actually show a decrease in temperature. According to Hall et al. (1987), ultrasonographic assessment of the structural reorganization of the tendon during healing did not correlate with the thermal changes. However a correlation between thermography and ultrasonography examinations was demonstrated at the time of diagnosis of the clinical signs of tendon inflammation (Soroko et al., 2012a).

Thermography has been shown to be useful in monitoring the healing process, being able to detect inflammation in cases with no clinical signs of injury (Bowman et al., 1983). Additionally, thermography was used to grade the significance of the inflammation during the recovery phase. In the study presented by Purohit and McCoy (1980) thermography monitored the response to anti-inflammatory drugs in the area of the front splints bones. Thermographic images confirmed the reduction of inflammation, however when no heat was detected manually at the affected area, the image continued to suggest increased blood circulation.

Other studies indicated the effectiveness of thermography in monitoring the development of cast sores in the distal parts of the limb. Thermographic evaluations of sored limbs were performed between 18-31 days after the cast. It was found that the technique was able to detect superficial and deep dermal sores. The results indicate that thermography can be useful in monitoring casts and the complications associated with them (Levet et al., 2009).

In the case of back abnormalities, thermography can diagnose muscular and spinous process inflammation of the thoracic vertebrae (Turner et al., 1996; Kold & Chappel, 1998). It has also been used to diagnose clinical cases of lumbosacral muscle tension (Turner, 1991; Turner et al., 1996). In another study thermography diagnosed the clinical signs of neuromuscular disease as caused by nerve dysfunction of the thoracolumbar region (von Schweintiz, 1999). Thermography has been compared with radiographic examination to detect an area of subluxation of the third lumbar vertebrae. The large mass of soft tissue meant that radiographic images did not detect the site of injury, whereas thermography was effective in identification of the exact site of the pathology (Purohit & McCoy, 1980). Thermography was shown to be an effective diagnostic tool in finding active or degenerative places of lesion. Another study presented by Kold and Chappel (1998), investigated the effectiveness of thermography in detecting inflammation along the spine in acute stages. Diagnoses were successful in identification of increased activity of the superficial soft tissue of the thoracic spine and symmetrically over the sacroiliac area. It has been suggested that additional thermography diagnosis can help to locate the site of pain allowing other diagnosis to work more effectively (Turner, 2003). In another study, thermography (along with ultrasonography) was efficient at detecting supraspinous and interspinous ligament inflammation, dorsal intervertebral osteoarthritis and kissing spines of the thoracolumbar spine (Fonseca et al., 2006). Thermography has also been used as a first examination tool for the detection of subclinical inflammation, before the onset of clinical signs of injury. It diagnosed subclinical signs of tendonitis and joint arthritis prior to the appearance of clinical signs of inflammation (Stromberg, 1974; Vaden et al., 1980; Bowman et al., 1983). Recent studies also report possible detection of subclinical inflammation in racehorses (Turner, 1991; Turner et al., 2001; Soroko, 2011a; Soroko et al., 2013). In the study presented by Turner et al. (2001), out of 127 specific limb problems in racehorses, 120 abnormalities were predicted 2 weeks before they became evident clinically. Thermography may therefore help to avoid future loss of soundness by applying treatment or by changing the training program.

PROCEDURES FOR THERMOGRAPHIC EXAMINATION

Internal and external factors have a significant effect on body surface temperature distribution. The proper use of thermography to evaluate surface thermal patterns therefore requires a controlled environment, and the physiological state of the horse must be considered in order to reduce variability and eliminate errors of interpretation (Head & Dyson, 2001; American Academy of Thermology, 2013; Soroko & Davies – Morel 2016).

Indoor thermography measurement standards have been established in equine veterinary practice (Purohit, 2009). To enhance the diagnostic value of thermography, the thermographic examination should be performed in an area sheltered from the sunlight, in the absence of air drafts (Palmer, 1981; Turner, 2001; Westermann et al. 2013). The ambient temperature of the examination room should be maintained between 21°C to 26°C. Slight variation in some cases may be acceptable, but room temperature should always be cooler than the animal's body temperature and free from bright lights. It is also recommended to acclimatise the horse for 15-20 minutes prior to imaging in the room where thermography will take place. A longer period of equilibration may be required in cases where the animal is transported from an extreme cold or hot environment. According to Tunley and Henson (2004), the thermographic pattern does not change significantly during acclimatization, but the time taken for stabilisation of the absolute temperature of the body surface is between 39 and 60 minutes. The major factor affecting this equilibration time is the temperature difference between the original environment and that in which the images are to be obtained. Therefore a stabilisation period of one hour is suggested after exposure to a different ambient temperature (Palmer, 1983). Another factor affecting the quality of thermograms is sweating. Therefore imaging should be performed prior to exercise (Purohit, 2009). The examimed horse must have a clean, dry hair coat and should be groomed at least one hour before the examination. Artifacts can be produced by any material on the body surface such as dirt, thick coat, scars and bands (Stromberg, 1974; Palmer, 1981). The feet should be brushed to remove external contamination. Anti – inflammatory medications, vasoactive drugs, regional and local blocks, sedation and tranquilisation should be avoided because of their effect on superficial perfusion (Purohit, 2009). Blankets should be removed at least 30 minutes before thermographic examination, and any bandages should be removed at least two hours before imaging (Palmer, 1981).

Emissivity of the hair coat is generally assumed to be 1, but a lack of precise knowledge of this value will have a small impact on accuracy of perhaps a few tenths of a degree Celsius (Soroko & Davies-Morel, 2016).

Hair coat has been shown to be an effective insulator by blocking heat emission from the skin (Turner, 1991). It has been found that clipping does not cause any change in the thermal distribution but does result in an increase in overall thermal emission. This indicates that clipping is not necessary for a reliable thermogram, however it is necessary that the hair coat be short, of uniform length, and lay flat against the skin to permit thermal conduction (Turner et al., 1983). This is important in the feet area, where some horses can have long “feathers”.

The effect of the coat on thermal distribution has many considerations, because its emission presents a rough surface causing an error in reading the surface temperature. The coated animal surface seen by the camera includes some layers within the coat. Its equilibrium temperature in air is determined by the balance between the loss of heat by radiation and convection to the surrounding environment, and heat conduction through the coat, (Cena, 1974). Clark and Cena (1973) described the transmission of thermal radiation through animal coats of various colours and the related effects of environmental factors. The influence of radiant solar energy on pigmented and non-pigmented areas of the coat was also examined. There was a significant difference in coat surface temperature, up to 8°C between hotter black pigments compared to white areas. It was concluded that skin temperature differences are clearly expressed on the thermal image, but the effect of environmental factors can disturb a reliable thermal image of the animal. In a later study, it was confirmed that under direct sun exposure, black areas of the skin are significantly warmer compared to unpigmented areas. However, indoor examination did not present a significant difference between pigmented and non-pigmented areas (Palmer, 1981). It was also suggested that solar energy absorption depended on the shape and posture of exposed areas to sun (Clark & Cena, 1973). Errors of reading can also be influenced by curvature of the anatomical surface, variations in coat thickness, or pigmentation differences (Clark & Cena, 1977; Turner et al., 1983).

Notes of the thermographic examination should include age, gender and breed of the horse, type of performance and training intensity, and also information about saddle fit. A medical history is also required, including results of other veterinary examinations like radiography, ultrasonography and palpation. This is crucial because many musculoskeletal injuries can be detected by thermography not only in the acute or chronic but also the subclinical stage of inflammation (Soroko & Davies-Morel, 2016).

Thermographic examination of the horse for veterinary diagnosis should include a lateral aspect of the whole body from both sides (Eddy et al., 2001). In these views there should be equal loading of four all limbs with the lateral and medial aspects of the limbs visible. Imaging distance should be about 7

m. The distal parts of the forelimbs and hindlimbs can be imaged from a distance of approximately 2 m (Van Hoogmoed & Snyder, 2002) and should include dorsal, palmar/plantar, lateral and medial aspects. Symmetrical limbs imaged together for palmar or dorsal aspects in one thermographic image should be positioned next to each other; the horse should stand straight without lateral and medial rotation, and the limbs should be evenly loaded.

It is also important to include both lateral aspects of the head, neck, thoracic and pelvic areas, imaged from a distance of around 3 m. The thoracolumbar and sacral parts of the spine should be imaged in the dorsal aspect (von Schweinitz, 1999) from a height of approximately 1.2 m and at a distance of 1.5 m.

SURFACE TEMPERATURE DISTRIBUTION

Thermographic patterns of the healthy horse have been described, enabling improved diagnostic interpretation of equine thermography (Soroko & Davies-Morel, 2016). It was found that every horse has its own individual and reproducible thermographic pattern, which is related to the vasculature and tissue metabolism and is influenced by ambient air temperature (Purohit & McCoy, 1980; Waldsmith & Oltmann, 1994). However, a number of studies have demonstrated repeatability of body surface temperature distribution on the same areas in different horses (Vaden et al., 1980; Purohit & McCoy, 1980; Palmer, 1981). The skin overlying major vessels will appear warm, whereas areas distal to a major blood supply will appear cooler. Normally veins are warmer compared to arteries because they are in metabolically active areas and closer to the skin surface. Venous drainage from tissue with a high metabolic rate is warmer than venous drainage from normal tissue. The temperature of skin overlying a muscle mass depends on muscle activity.

Based on the above findings, some generalisations can be made regarding the thermal pattern of the horse. The midline of the horse is warm, including the back, chest, and the area between the hindlimbs along the ventral midline (Turner, 1991). Temperature over the limbs decreases from the proximal to the distal part.

Studies by Purohit et al. (1977), Purohit and McCoy (1980), Turner (1991) and Tunley and Henson (2004) has established normal thermographic patterns of the distal parts of the limbs and the back for clinical use.

The patterns obtained in the distal parts of the limbs are characterised by right and left temperature symmetry. Also the thermal symmetry was found to be identical between distal parts of forelimbs and hindlimbs (Purohit & McCoy, 1980). Variations in local blood supply determine the thermal pattern. Areas of increased temperature follow the vascular patterns, including the 3rd metacarpal/metatarsal from the medial and lateral aspects, and coronary band arteries in the dorsal aspect (Vaden et al., 1980; Turner, 1991). In the dorsal aspect joints are cooler compared to the surrounding structures, except the tarsal joint which has a vertical area of increased temperature medially corresponding to the saphenous vein. The route of the median palmar vein in the forelimb and the metatarsal vein in the hindlimb produces a warm region between the 3rd metacarpal/metatarsal and the flexor tendons (Figure 2). Therefore the medial metacarpal/metatarsal region is warmer than the lateral. In contrast, areas distant from major blood vessels appear cooler, including the 3rd metacarpal/metatarsal bone, fetlock, and pastern from the dorsal and palmar/plantar aspects (Turner et al., 1996) (Figure 3, 4).

Figure 2. Thermogram of lateral aspect of the distal part of right forelimb and medial aspect of distal part of left forelimb. Areas of increased temperature follow the vascular patterns in 3rd metacarpal region

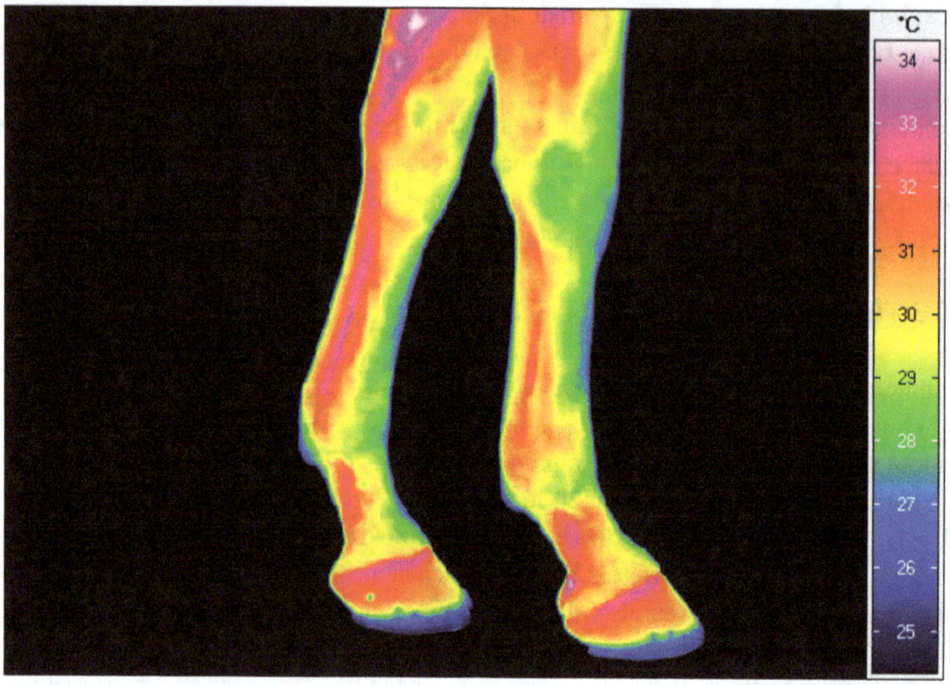

Figure 3. Thermogram of dorsal aspect of the distal part of forelimbs. The highest temperature is in the coronary band. Lower temperatures follow the tendons

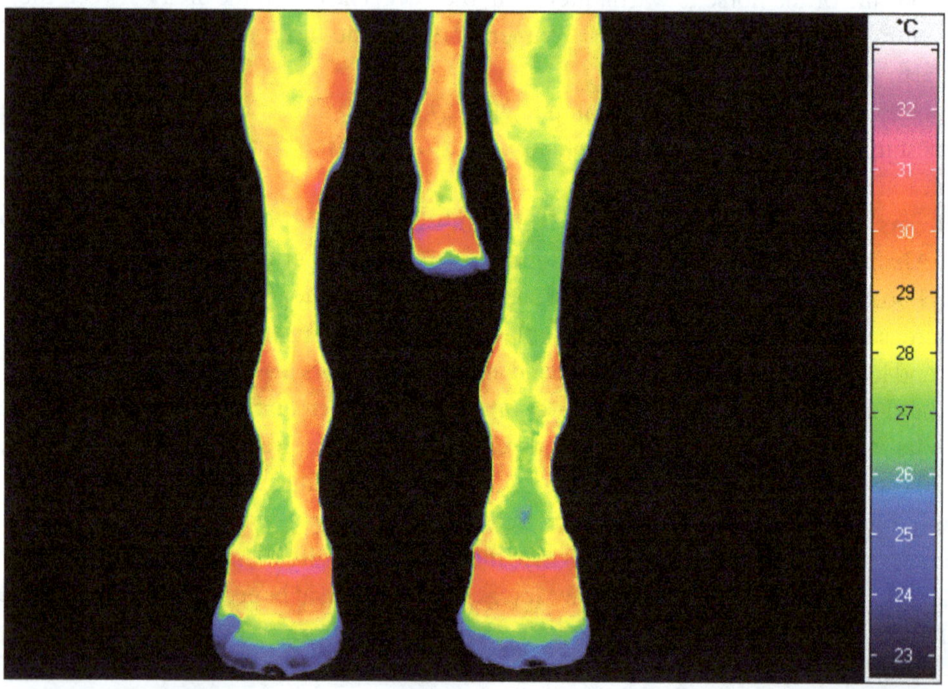

Figure 4. Thermogram of palmar aspect of the distal part of forelimbs. Increase in the heat between the heel bulbs. Lower temperatures follow the tendons

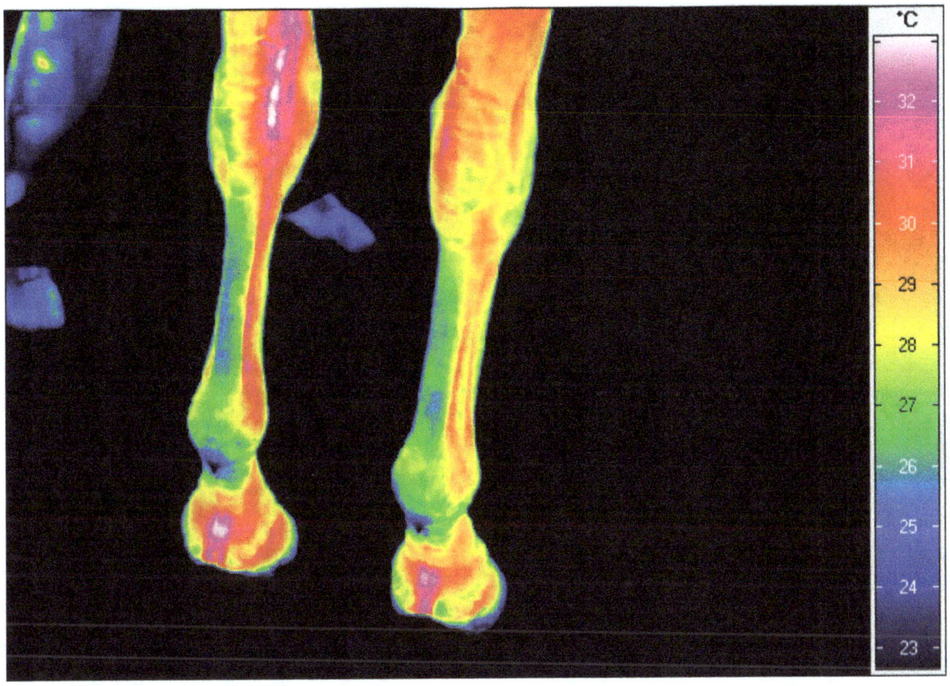

The highest temperature is in the coronary band, as it is situated close to the major arterio-venous plexus (Kold & Chappell, 1998; Turner, 2001) (Figure 3). The coronary band is 1-2°C warmer than the remainder of the hoof. The surface temperature of the hoof becomes gradually cooler towards the ground, because of the specific anatomic build of the hoof (Verschooten et al., 1997). Tendons have a low blood supply and will appear cold in the dorsal and palmar/plantar aspects because of their location far from superficial vessels. From palmar/plantar aspects, a high surface temperature is indicated in the area between the bulbs of the heels (Turner, 1991) (Figure 4).

Lateral and medial aspects of the distal part of the limb are more reliable than the palmar/plantar aspects for detecting and monitoring abnormalities in increased blood flow.

The thermographic image of a clinically healthy back presents with left and right temperature distribution symmetry along the midline of the spine (Kold & Chappell, 1998). Similar conclusions were found in another study where the thoracolumbar spine was divided into 6 horizontal lines along which the temperatures were measured. All thermograms indicated increased temperature along the midline of the spine, with a temperature 3°C higher at the midline at the thoracic and lumbar vertebrae (Tunley & Henson, 2004). A possible explanation is a high number of superficial subcutaneus blood vessels in that area (von Schweinitz, 1999) (Figure 5).

Any thermal asymmetry between compared bilateral surfaces can indicate abnormalities (Verschooten et al., 1997). However, not every asymmetry should be defined as an abnormal condition (Kold & Chappell, 1998). Temperature variations up to 1°C between the compared limbs represents normal variation. Where there is a temperature difference of more than 1°C over 25% of the compared body area, it is considered to be abnormal (Turner, 1991). Temperature differences of 1.25°C between the

Figure 5. Thermogram of dorsal aspect of back. Increased temperatures follow the midline of the spine in the thoracic and lumbar vertebrae with temperature symmetry between right and left side of the back

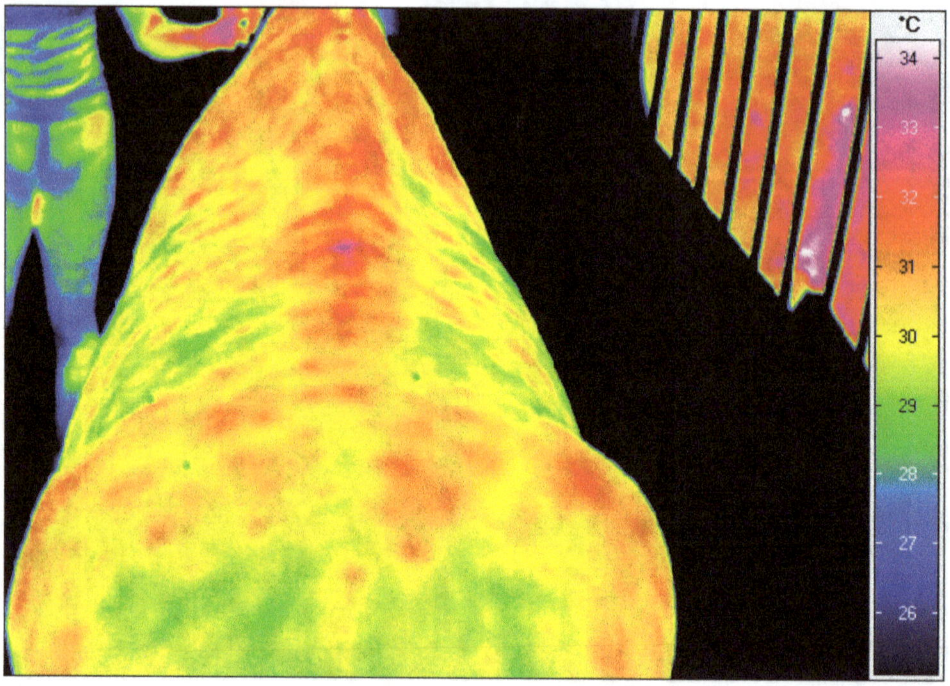

right and left distal parts of limbs indicated subclinical inflammation of the superficial digital flexor tendon and bucked shins in racehorses (Soroko et al., 2013). In another study, the early stages of bucked shins (Figure 6) were diagnosed when local temperatures over the dorsal 3rd metacarpal bone were 1°C to 2°C higher compared to the surrounding distal limb areas (Turner, 1991) .

In the early phase of laminitis, the coronary band had significantly increased surface temperature compared to the distal hoof wall and soles of the hooves (Noeck, 1997). In navicular disease, there was a reduction of the blood flow, especially in the heel region, because of vascular constriction. Affected horses presented with a lack of temperature increase in the suspected limb after exercise. The results were correlated with radiography findings, which showed an increased vascular foramina of the affected navicular bone (Turner et al., 1983). Therefore navicular disease can be recognized by thermography in the early stages, with the decreased blood flow appearing as a cooler area (Waldsmith & Oltmann, 1994).

Not every temperature asymmetry may lead to pathological conditions (Kold & Chappell, 1998). In the distal parts of the limbs, local skin temperature variations may be associated with the horse's homeostatic response to ambient temperature extremes. At low ambient temperature there is a maximal temperature gradient between the skin and the environment, because of vasoconstriction of the local vasculature in the extremities to conserve metabolic energy. At high ambient temperatures, vasodilation causes warming of the extremities, encouraging heat loss to the environment. Bilateral symmetry of the limbs is clinically valid throughout the range of ambient temperature (Palmer, 1983).

Figure 6. Thermogram of dorsal aspect of distal part of forelimbs. Subclinical inflammation of the right and left 3rd metacarpal bone

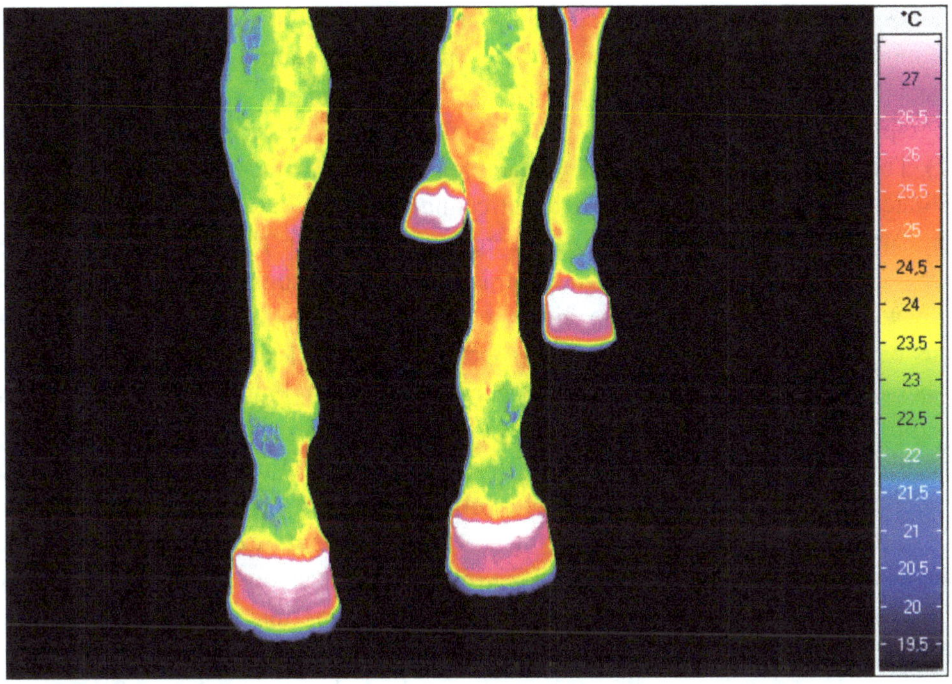

APPLICATIONS OF THERMOGRAPHY IN RACEHORSE TRAINING

Body surface temperature distribution depends on movement, and the type of physical exercise performed, as the skin overlying muscle is subjected to an increase in temperature during muscular activity (Turner et al., 1996). Thermograms documenting the changes of horse surface temperature resulting from exercise could be useful in the evaluation of the work of individual parts of the body in racing performance (Purohit & McCoy, 1980; Waldsmith & Oltmann, 1994; Jodkowska et al., 2001; Jodkowska, 2005).

The study presented by Simon et al. (2006) highlighted the influence of exercise on body surface temperature changes in the forelimbs and hindlimbs. Thermal images of examined horses were taken before and after exercise on a treadmill. The skin temperature overlying muscle surfaces after exercise was increased by 6°C, whereas areas of distal parts of the limbs were increased by 8°C. There was a significant temperature difference during the first 15 minutes after exercise, whereas thermographic examinations performed 45 minutes after exercise were not influenced by the mechanism of thermoregulation. It was also found that muscular areas in the upper part of the body returned more quickly to the basal temperature compared to the dorsal parts of the limbs. In the study by Turner et al. (2001), racehorses had an increased hoof surface temperature for almost 24 hours after an intensive gallop.

Symmetrical temperature distribution on both sides from the front and from the back aspect should be present at rest, and also after exercise (Jodkowska et al., 2001). Any temperature asymmetry after training could be useful in the evaluation of the work of individual parts of the body in sport performance. Jodkowska (2005) determined a model of horse temperature before and after exercise. During the study the rectal temperature, pulse rate and blood parameters, as well as environmental factors were correlated with changing temperature patterns. It was concluded that body surface temperature patterns depend on exercise performance. Surface temperature examination of the distal limbs and back was helpful in assessing the quality of exercises and preparation of a horse for training. It was also found that the optimum period for measurements of body surface temperature was the time before exercise, or on the day after exercise.

Thermography was also confirmed as a valuable aid in regular assessment of racehorses by Turner et al. (2001). Thermographic imaging of the distal parts of the limbs and back at rest during the training season facilitated identification of inflammation affecting performance (Soroko at al., 2013). In the study presented by Turner et al. (2001) there was a high correlation between Thoroughbred racehorse trainers' and veterinary diagnosis supported by thermographic assessment. Additionally, in most cases subclinical inflammation was detected 2 weeks before clinical problems were noted. This finding confirmed reports in a previous paper that indicated injury of the superficial digital flexor tendon of racehorses prior to the appearance of clinical signs of inflammation (Stromberg, 1974) (Figure 7). The injured area showed increased temperature on the thermographic image even though radiogram did not show any changes. Stromberg (1974) concluded that thermography can predict tendon injures up to 14 days before clinical signs appear and can play an essential role in preventing lameness in racehorses.

The type of training has an influence on changes of body temperature distribution. Horses in training put more strain on the forelimbs, especially on the digital flexor tendons and bones (Nilson & Bjorck, 1969). Regular thermographic examination of racehorses found thermal abnormalities of forelimbs associated with strains and overloads (Soroko, 2011b; Soroko et al., 2014). This confirms that racehorses are more likely to develop injury associated with the forelimb than the hindlimb (Peloso et al., 1994).

Figure 7. Thermogram of lateral aspect of the distal part of left forelimb and medial aspect of distal part of right forelimb. Subclinical inflammation of superficial digital flexor tendon of right forelimb

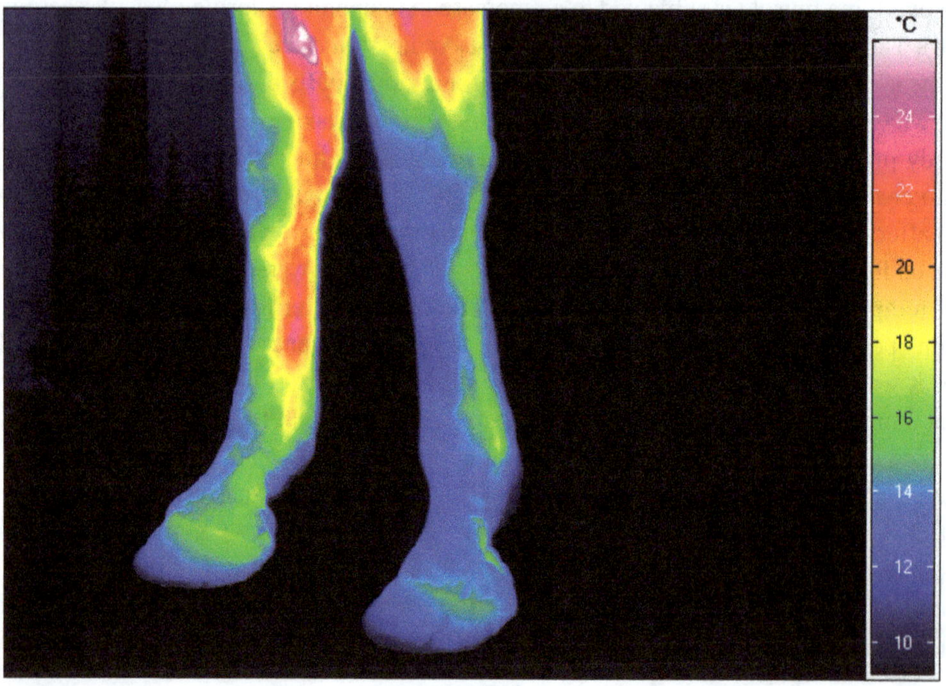

The same conclusions have been presented in another study, where more signs of injuries in 4-year-old Standardbreed Trotters were recorded in the left forelimb compared to the right one (Magnusson, 1985). Possibly, as horses during racing and exercise were loaded on the right forelimb due to the clockwise race track, when resting they were overloading the opposite side.

Increased body surface temperature in the back area may indicate pathological conditions caused by intensive performance of a horse, the rider's imbalance, or an incorrectly fitted saddle (Harman, 1999; De Cocq et al., 2004; Arruda at al., 2011). The study by Jeffcott et al. (1985) proved that injuries of the paraspinal muscles and the ligaments were diagnosed in 25% of horses in intensive training. Other research indicated body temperature surface variations in the sacroiliac joint region, which were found to be typical injuries for show jumping horses with indicated abnormalities of hind limb movement patterns (Haussler et al., 1999). Racehorse back surface temperature distribution changes were characterised in response to increasing training intensity in long-term training by Soroko et al. (2012b). The study found that the spine had the highest temperature in the thoracic vertebrae compared to the lumbar vertebrae and sacroiliac joint area. Higher temperatures in the thoracic vertebrae could be associated with riding techniques in trot. Peham et al. (2010) detected the highest load on the horse's back at the sitting trot (2112 N), followed by the rising trot (2056 N) and the two-point seat (1688 N). Saddles, analysed for the pressure distribution over the thoracic vertebrae during movement, indicated the highest pressure at trot (Latif et al., 2010).

Gradual increments of training intensity in long - term training caused a decrease of average temperature differences between thoracic vertebrae compared to the lumbar vertebrae and sacroiliac joint areas in racehorses at rest (Soroko et al., 2012b). Regular thermographic examination of racehorse performance indicated an increment of the temperature at the back and the distal parts of the forelimbs at rest (Soroko, at al., 2015). In another study, the best performing racehorses were warmer than their poorer performing peers at all body sites. Differences in temperature between the groups were significantly higher at the carpal joint, 3rd metacarpal bone, fetlock joint, the short pastern bone, the tarsus joint, (although only on the left side) and also the thoracic vertebrae (Soroko et al., 2014). This temperature difference may reflect an increased physiological training impact on the best performing horses. According to Evans et al. (1992), strains and overloading of the musculoskeletal system due to physical work under demanding exercise results in increased blood circulation in a defensive adaptation process, predisposing the animal to future lameness injuries. This agrees with Estberg et al. (1995) who confirmed that training intensity and regular exercise predispose horses to fatal skeletal injures. According to Soroko et al. (2014) identification of the most reliable body regions recommended for monitoring the impact of training should facilitate the detection of pathological conditions during the training cycle. This is particularly important in racehorses, where immediate diagnosis might help to maintain their health and condition, positively influencing their further career in sport.

Thermography is able to diagnose an area of inflammation associated with superficial muscles or muscle groups. Muscle inflammation is usually identified as an area of increased temperature directly overlying the affected muscle. Although thermography measures only skin surface temperature it also reflects alterations in the circulation of deeper tissue. The most common cause of muscle inflammation is muscle strain, which can be detected by thermography, however it has not been well documented in studies. Turner (1998) detected by thermography inflammation of muscles in forelimbs including the pectoralis muscles and biceps brachialis muscles. In the upper hindlimb, the gluteal muscles and the biceps femoris muscles appeared warmer when the croup region was injured (Turner et al., 1996). In another study horses with croup and caudal thigh myopathy were diagnosed. Thermography was recommended as a tool for detecting upper limb lameness, by confirming inflammation of sore areas requiring further diagnostics (Turner, 1998). Figures 8-10 present examples of thermographically detected muscle inflammation processes in four cases of sport horses. Thermography was able to detect upper limb problems associated with: gluteus muscles inflammation (Figure 8), tensor fasciae latae muscle inflammation (Figure 9) inflammation of the semitendinosus (Figure 10) and biceps femoris muscles (Figure 11). Once abnormalities have been detected, thermography can determine the effectiveness of different types of therapeutic and rehabilitation applications (Turner, 1991; Turner, 1998).

In racing performance horses intensively trained for high level racing, musculoskeletal injures can impair the horse's ability to perform and can lead to dismissal from competition. Common areas which are frequently a source of lameness in racing horses are the distal parts of limbs and back. Therefore regular thermographic analysis will enable horseback overloads to be monitored and facilitate identification of pathological conditions during the training cycle. With the veterinarians and breeders working together, new heights in performance can be reached when training and conditional diagnosis are combined.

ILLEGALLY ENHANCING PERFORMANCE

Thermography has also found application in detecting abnormal temperature caused by chemical and mechanical abrasion of performance horses. In equestrian events intense competition promotes the use of procedures designed to illegally enhance performance including application of counterirritants, subdermal injections, irritants or use of regional nerve block via chemical or surgical neurectomies. The majority of these methods are an attempt either to mask lameness from veterinarians or enhance a horse's natural

Figure 8. Thermogram of dorsal aspect of hindlimb. Inflammation of left and right gluteus muscles

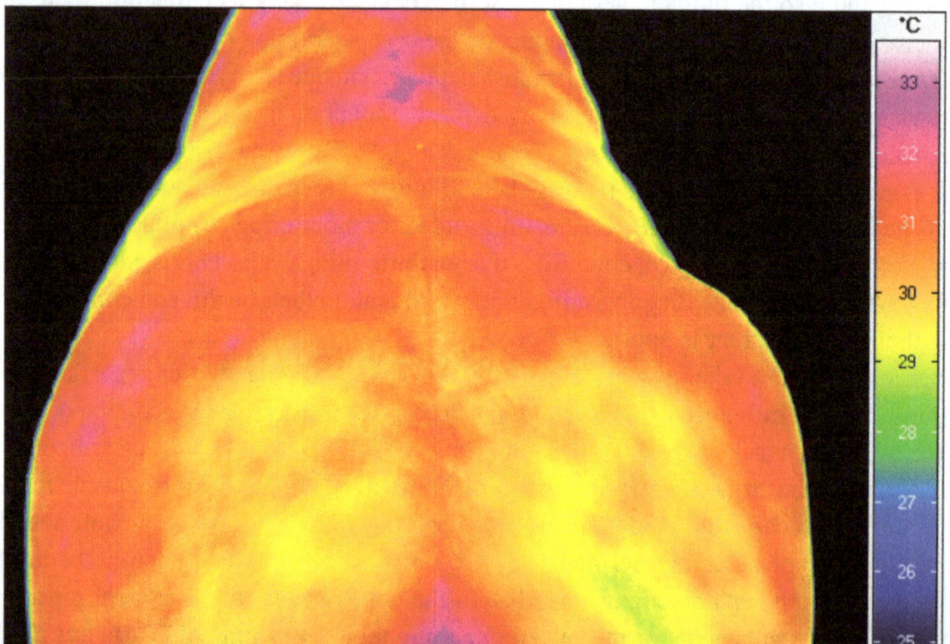

Figure 9. Thermogram of lateral aspect of left hindlimb. Inflammation of tensor fasciae latae muscle

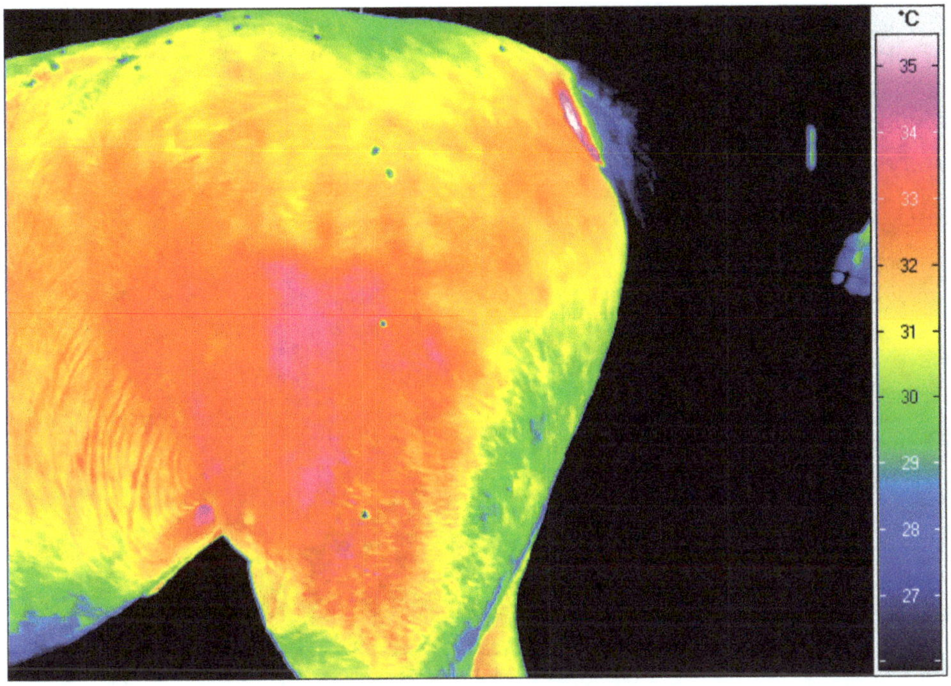

Figure 10. Thermogram of caudal aspect of hindlimb. Inflammation of left semitendinosus muscle

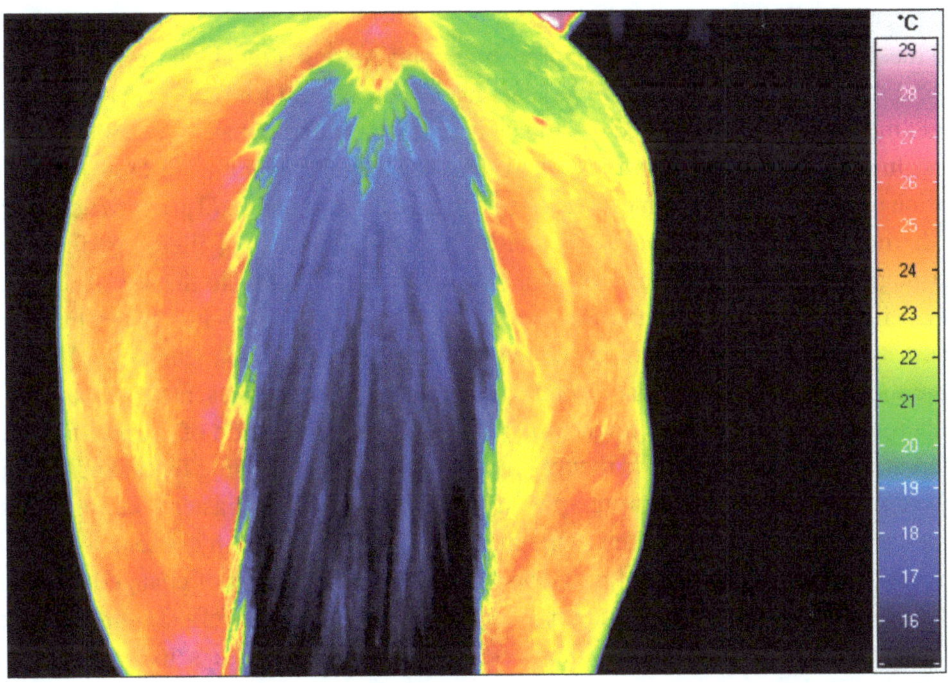

Figure 11. Thermogram of lateral aspect of right hindlimb. Inflammation of biceps femoris muscle

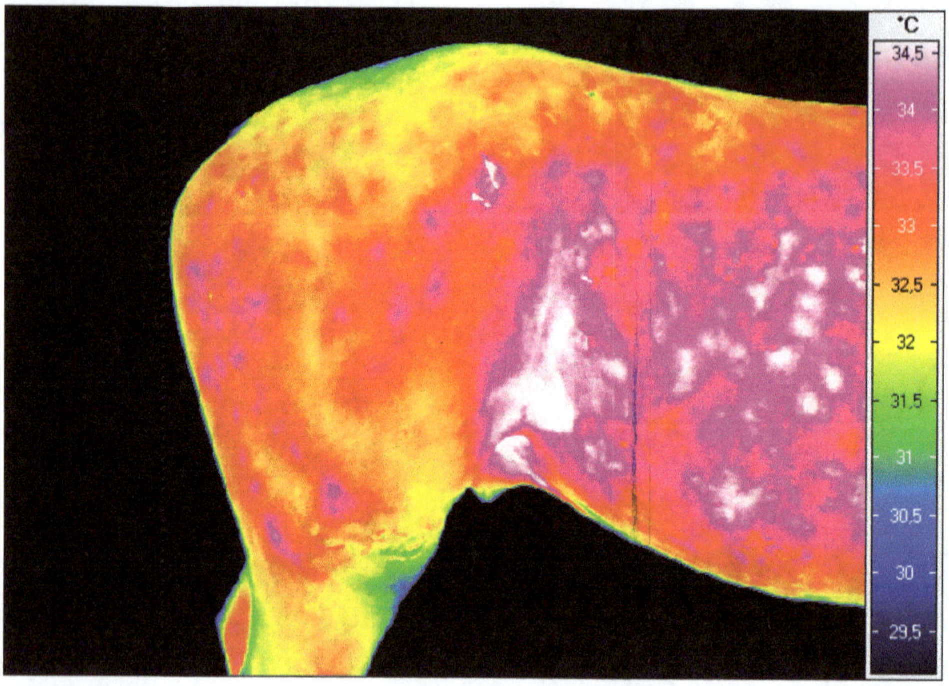

gait by artificially producing more action or suspension. Some techniques are not detectable, and may be difficult to prove, using conventional methods.

In 1970 the passage of the US federal Horse Protection Act put a legal ban on the use of chemical or mechanical means of soring horses. Five years later Nelson and Osheim (1975) demonstrated that chemical and mechanical soring caused definite abnormalities in the radiation emission patterns of the horse's digit. In a later publication, thermography detected illegal procedures in show horses, detecting the application of irritants to the perineal region to enhance rail evaluation (Turner & Scroggins, 1989). Therefore thermography became an appropriate tool for the detection of illegal performance procedures. Thermography successfully detected limb sensitivity, which refers to the sensation perceived by horses in their limbs. When the sensation is increased above normal limits it is called hypersensitivity, as from traumatic or surgical cutting of the nerves in that area of the limb (neurectomy). It is practiced to encourage sport horses to jump more carefully and higher. In a study presented by Van Hoogmoed et al. (2000) thermography was used to investigate the detection and duration of counter-irritants applied topically and injected subdermally, and induction of hypersensitisation using limb bandages containing metallic objects. Counter-irritations were applied to the dorsum of the pastern, and metallic irritants contained in limb bandages were applied to the metacarpal area to induce hypersensitivity of that area. Thermography images were found useful to detect and monitor the effect of changed thermal patterns after a single application of an irritant: mercuric iodine for 6 days, and the effect of metallic bottle caps within the leg wraps for 24h after application, presenting thermography as a sensitive tool for detecting hypersensitisations in horses.

Another study evaluated the ability of thermography to detect procedures used to obscure lameness, ranging from local injections of various pharmaceuticals. The injection of analgesic agents was applied to horses' limbs and backs. Thermographic images were recorded before, and 30, 60, 90 and 120 min. after the experimental procedures, until temperature differences from the opposite non-treated site were no longer significant. A single injection of neurolitic agents in the area of lumbar vertebrae and in the suspensory ligament caused an increase of temperature which persisted for 2 days. The highest temperature differences peaked at 60 min. and later declined. The study identified thermography as potential tool for detecting temperature changes in heat patterns compared to control regions. In the same study, the application of thermography was investigated for detecting and monitoring palmar digital neurectomy. Horses with palmar digital neurectomy did not show a persistent increase in temperature compared to the control limb. The significantly increased temperature was present on the first day of treatment in the limb with neurectomy compared to opposite control limb. However, no temperature differences between limbs were detected by day 6. It is suspected that nervous interruption causes a vasodilator effect, persistent for a short period of time until the vascular system compensates, influencing a return to normal circulation (Van Hoogmoed & Synder, 2002). It has been concluded that thermography is sensitive enough to detect changes in heat patterns from innervated regions, however it is not specific enough to discriminate between procedures and injury inducing an inflammatory response.

Since 2002 thermography has been recommended as a potential screening technique for illegal limb sensitivity of competition horses by the International Federation for Equestrian Sports. If the examining veterinarians observe excessively sensitive, or insensitive limbs together with abnormal thermal patterns detected by thermography, a horse can be disqualified from competition on the basis of horse welfare and fair play.

Thermography was also used for examination of the correct fit of the saddle to the horse's back (Turner, 1991). Tack related problems can be identified by the thermal patterns caused by the tack while the horse is being ridden. Thermal image assessment of the dynamic interaction between the saddle and the back of the horse showed not only the heat generated in areas of greater interaction with the saddle, but also the physiological effects of riding on the back of the horse (Turner et al., 2004; Arruda et al., 2011)

CONCLUSION

Thermography is becoming increasingly popular as an aid to assist the diagnosis of musculoskeletal and neurological injuries in racehorses. It can detect subclinical problems at least 2 weeks before they are visually detectable. It helps veterinarians to diagnose the exact site of injury and follow the response to treatment. Thermography detects training overloads and muscle strains which can lead to injury, allowing the trainer to make decisions about the horse's training programme and management. It is more sensitive than palpitation for detecting subtle temperature variations (Turner, 2001). This high sensitivity makes it useful in conjunction with other veterinary diagnostic tools that provide more specific information. Thermography, as a non-invasive tool, allows the horses to be examined without being touched, thus causing no stress or discomfort to the animal.

Infrared imaging technology has improved extraordinarily in recent years. New generations of thermographic imagers are user-friendly, portable and have a high temperature sensitivity. Current thermographic equipment is sensitive enough to detect skin temperature differences of 0.1°C.

The development of infra-red technology and better availability of this type of equipment should contribute to more extensive use of this diagnostic method, applicable not only to horses, but also to other animals.

REFERENCES

American Academy of Thermology. (2013). *Veterinary guidelines for infrared thermography*. Available from: http://www.aathermology.org/organization/guidelines/veterinary-guidelines-for-infrared-thermography

Arruda, T. Z., Brass, K. E., & De La Corte, F. D. (2011). Thermographic assessment of saddles used on jumping horses. *Journal of Equine Veterinary Science*, *31*(11), 625–629. doi:10.1016/j.jevs.2011.05.011

Bowman, K. F., Purohit, R. C., Ganjam, V. K., Pechman, R. D. Jr, & Vaughan, J. T. (1983). Thermographic evaluation of corticosteroid efficacy in amphotericin B – induced arthiritis in ponies. *American Journal of Veterinary Research*, *44*(1), 51–56. PMID:6824225

Buchner, H. H. F., Savelbergh, H. H., Schamhardt, H. C., & Barneveld, A. (1996). Head and trunk movement adaptations in horses with experimentally induced fore or hind limb lameness. *Equine Veterinary Journal*, *28*(1), 71–76. doi:10.1111/j.2042-3306.1996.tb01592.x PMID:8565958

Cena, K. (1974). Radiative heat loss from Animal and Man. In J. L. Monteih & L. E. Mount (Eds.), *Heat loss from animals and man* (pp. 34–57). London: Butterworths. doi:10.1016/B978-0-408-70652-0.50009-3

Clark, J. A., & Cena, K. (1973). Thermographic measurements of the surface temperatures of animals. *Journal of Mammalogy*, *54*(4), 1003–1007. doi:10.2307/1379105 PMID:4761360

Clark, J. A., & Cena, K. (1977). The potential of infra-red thermography in veterinary diagnosis. *The Veterinary Record*, *100*(19), 402–404. doi:10.1136/vr.100.19.402 PMID:325877

Collins, A. J., Ring, E. F., Bacon, P. A., & Brookshaw, J. D. (1976). Thermography and radiology: Complementary methods for the study of inflammatory diseases. *Clinical Radiology*, *27*(2), 237–243. doi:10.1016/S0009-9260(76)80153-5 PMID:1277739

De Cocq, P., Van Weeren, P. R., & Back, W. (2004). Effects of girth, saddle and weight on movements of the horse. *Equine Veterinary Journal*, *36*(8), 758–763. doi:10.2746/0425164044848000 PMID:15656511

Delahanty, D. D., & Georgi, J. R. (1965). Thermography in equine medicine. *Journal of the American Veterinary Medical Association*, *147*, 235–238. PMID:14325456

Denoix, J. M. (1999). Spinal biomechanics and functional anatomy. *The Veterinary Clinics of North America. Equine Practice*, *15*, 27–60. PMID:10218240

Eddy, A. L., van Hoogmoed, L. M., & Snyder, J. R. (2001). The role of thermography in the management of equine lameness. *Veterinary Journal (London, England)*, *162*(3), 172–181. doi:10.1053/tvjl.2001.0618 PMID:11681868

Estberg, L., Gardner, I. A., Stover, S. M., Johnson, B. J., Case, J. T., & Ardans, A. (1995). Cumulative racing – seed distance cluster as a risk factor for fatal musculoskeletal injury in Thoroughbred racehorses in California. *Preventive Veterinary Medicine*, *24*(4), 253–263. doi:10.1016/0167-5877(95)00489-J

Evans, G. P., Behiri, J. C., Vaughan, L. C., Vaughan, L. C., & Bonfield, W. (1992). The response of equine cortical bone to loading at strains rates experienced in vivo by the galloping horse. *Equine Veterinary Journal*, *24*(2), 125–128. doi:10.1111/j.2042-3306.1992.tb02796.x PMID:1582390

Fonseca, B. P. A., Alves, A. L. G., Nicoletti, J. L. M., Thomassian, A., Hussini, C. A., & Mikaik, S. (2006). Thermography and ultrasonography in back pain diagnosis of equine athletes. *Journal of Equine Veterinary Science*, *26*(11), 507–516. doi:10.1016/j.jevs.2006.09.007

Hall, J., Bramlage, L. R., Kantrwitz, B. M., Page, L., & Simpson, B. (1987). Correlation between contact thermography and ultrasonography in the evaluation of experimentally – induced superficial flexor tendonitis.*Proceedings of the American Association of Equine Practitioners*, *38*, 429-431.

Harman, J. C. (1999). Tack and saddle fit. In S. Turner & K. K. Haussler (Eds.), *Veterinary Clinics of North American Equine Practice: Back Problems* (pp. 247–261). Philadelphia: W.B. Saunders Company.

Haussler, K. K., Stover, S. M., & Willits, N. H. (1999). Pathology of the lumbosacral spine and pelvis in Thoroughbred racehorses. *American Journal of Veterinary Research*, *60*(2), 143–153. PMID:10048543

Head, J., & Dyson, S. (2001). Taking the temperature of equine thermography. *Veterinary Journal (London, England)*, *162*(3), 166–167. doi:10.1053/tvjl.2001.0639 PMID:11681865

Head, M. J. (2009). Back pathology in racehorses. In F. M. D. Henson (Ed.), *Equine back pathology* (pp. 213–222). Wiley-Blackwell.

Jeffcott, L. B. (1999). Historical perspective and clinical indications. *The Veterinary Clinics of North America. Equine Practice*, *15*(1), 1–12. PMID:10218238

Jeffcott, L. B., Dalin, G., Ekman, S., & Olsson, S.-E. (1985). Sacroiliac lesions as a cause of chronic poor performance in competitive horses. *Equine Veterinary Journal*, *17*(2), 111–118. doi:10.1111/j.2042-3306.1985.tb02063.x PMID:3987658

Jeffcott, L. B., Rossdale, P. D., Freestone, J., Frank, C. J., & Towers-Clark, P. F. (1982). An assessment of wastage in Thoroughbred racing from conception to 4 years of age. *Equine Veterinary*, *14*(3), 185–198. doi:10.1111/j.2042-3306.1982.tb02389.x PMID:7106081

Jodkowska, E. (2005). Temperatura powierzchni ciała jako kryterium predyspozycji wysiłkowych konia. Zeszyty Naukowe Akademii Rolniczej nr 511, Wroclaw.

Jodkowska, E., Dudek, K., & Bek-Kaczkowska, I. (2001). Wpływ treningu wyścigowego na temperaturę powierzchni ciała koni różnych ras. *Roczniki Naukowe Zootechniki*, *14*, 63–72.

Kane, A. J., Trau, J., Dargatz, B., Losinger, W. C., & Carber, L. P. (2000). The occurrence and causes of lameness and laminitis in the US horse population. *Procedure of the Annual Convention of the American Association of Equine Practitioners, 46*, 277-280.

Keegan, K. G., Wilson, D. A., Smith, B. K., & Wilson, D. J. (2000). Changes in kinematic variables observed during pressure induced forelimb lameness in adult horses trotting on a treadmill. *American Journal of Veterinary Research, 61*(6), 612–619. doi:10.2460/ajvr.2000.61.612 PMID:10850834

Kold, S. E., & Chappell, K. A. (1998). Use of computerized thermographic image analysis (CTIA) in equine orthopedics: Review and presentation of clinical cases. *Equine Veterinary Education, 10*(4), 198–204. doi:10.1111/j.2042-3292.1998.tb00877.x

Latif, S. N., Von Peinen, K., Wiestner, T., Bitschnau, C., Renk, B., & Weishaupt, M. A. (2010). Saddle pressure patterns of three different training saddles (normal tree, flexible tree, treeless) in Thoroughbred racehorses at trot and gallop. *Equine Veterinary Journal, 42*(38), 630–636. doi:10.1111/j.2042-3306.2010.00237.x PMID:21059072

Levet, A., Martens, L., Devisscher, L., Duchateur, L., Bogaert, L., & Vlamink, L. (2009). Distal limb cast sores in horses: Risk factors and early detection using thermography. *Equine Veterinary Journal, 41*(1), 18–23. doi:10.2746/042516408X343046 PMID:19301577

Magnusson, L. E. (1985). *Studies on the conformation and related traits of the Standardbred Trotters in Sweden. Relationship between conformation and soundness in four year old Standardbred Trotters. Swedish University of Agricultural Sciences*. Skara.

Nelson, H. A., & Osheim, D. L. (1975). Soring in tennessee walking horses: detection by thermography. United States Department of Agriculture - APHIS, Veterinary Services Laboratories, Ames, IA.

Nilson, G., & Bjorck, G. (1969). Surgical treatment of chronic tendinitis in the horse. *Journal of the American Veterinary Medical Association, 155*(5), 920–926. PMID:5817732

Nocek, E. (1997). Bovine acidosis: Implications on laminitis. *Journal of Dairy Science, 80*(5), 1005–1008. doi:10.3168/jds.S0022-0302(97)76026-0 PMID:9178142

Oikawa, M., & Kasashima, Y. (2002). The Japanese experience with tendonitis in racehorses. *Journal of Equine Science, 13*(2), 41–56. doi:10.1294/jes.13.41

Oliver, A., Nurton, J. P., & Guthrie, A. J. (1997). An epizoological study in wastage in Thoroughbred racehorses in Gauteng, South Africa. *Journal of the South African Veterinary Association, 68*, 125–129. PMID:9561496

Palmer, S. E. (1981). Use of portable infrared thermometer as a means of means of measuring limb surface temperature in the horse. *American Journal of Veterinary Research, 42*(1), 105–108. PMID:7224303

Palmer, S. E. (1983). Effect of ambient temperature upon the surface temperature of equine limb. *American Journal of Veterinary Research, 44*(6), 1098–1101. PMID:6870013

Parkin, T. D. H., Clegg, P. D., French, N. P., Proudman, C. J., Riggs, C. M., Singer, E. R., & Morgan, K. L. et al. (2004). Horse-level risk factors for fatal distal limb fracture in racing Thoroughbreds in the UK. *Equine Veterinary Journal, 36*(6), 513–519. doi:10.2746/0425164044877387 PMID:15460076

Peham, C., Kotschwar, A. B., Borkenhagen, B., Kuhnke, S., Molsner, J., & Baltacis, A. (2010). Comparison of forces acting on the horses back and the stability of the riders seat in different positions at the trot. *Veterinary Journal (London, England)*, *184*(1), 56–59. doi:10.1016/j.tvjl.2009.04.007 PMID:19428275

Peloso, J. G., Mundy, G. D., & Cohen, N. D. (1994). Prevalence of, and factors associated with, musculoskeletal racing injuries of Thoroughbreds. *Journal of the American Medical Association*, *204*(4), 620–626. PMID:8163419

Purohit, R. (2009). Standards for thermal imaging in veterinary medicine.*Proceedings of the XIth European Congress of Thermology. Mannheim, Germany. Thermology International, 19*, 99.

Purohit, R. C., Bergfeld, W. A., McCoy, M. D., Thomson, W. M., & Sharman, R. S. (1977). Value of clinical thermography in veterinary medicine. *Auburn Veterinarian*, *33*(3), 104–108.

Purohit, R. C., & McCoy, M. D. (1980). Thermography in the diagnosis of inflammatory processes in the horse. *American Journal of Veterinary Research*, *41*(8), 1167–1174. PMID:7447110

Ramdy, D. W. (1997). Prospective evaluation of fore limb flexion tests in practice: clinical response, radiographic correlation and predictive value for future lameness.*Proceedings of the Annual Convention American Association of Equine Practitioners*, *43*, 116-120.

Ring, F. J. (1990). Quantitative thermal imaging. *Clinical Physics and Physiological Measurement*, *11*(4A), 87–97. doi:10.1088/0143-0815/11/4A/310 PMID:2286052

Rossdale, P. D., Hopes, R., Wingfield-Digby, N. J., & Offord, K. (1985). Epidemiological study of wastage among racehorses 1982 and 1983. *The Veterinary Record*, *116*(3), 66–69. doi:10.1136/vr.116.3.66 PMID:3976145

Simon, E. L., Gaughan, E. M., Epp, T., & Spire, M. (2006). Influence of exercise on thermographically determined surface temperatures of thoracic and pelvic limbs in horses. *Journal of the American Veterinary Medical Association*, *229*(12), 1940–1944. doi:10.2460/javma.229.12.1940 PMID:17173534

Soroko, M. (2011a). Analyses of superficial temperature distribution of lower part of the limbs in young racing horses. *Measurement. Automation and Monitoring*, *57*(10), 1157–1160.

Soroko, M. (2011b). Thermographic diagnosis of sport horses' limbs. *Biomedical Engineering*, *17*(2), 104–109.

Soroko, M., & Davies - Morel, M.C.G. (2016). Equine Thermography in Practice, CABI, UK and US. doi:10.1079/9781780647876.0000

Soroko, M., Dudek, K., Howell, K., Henklewski, R., & Jodkowska, E. (2014). Thermographic evaluation of racehorse performance. *Journal of Equine Veterinary Science*, *34*(9), 1076–1083. doi:10.1016/j.jevs.2014.06.009

Soroko, M., Henklewski, R., Filipowski, H., & Jodkowska, E. (2013). The effectiveness of thermographic analysis in equine orthopedics. *Journal of Equine Veterinary Science*, *33*(9), 760–762. doi:10.1016/j.jevs.2012.11.009

Soroko, M., Henklewski, R., & Jodkowska, E. (2012a). Analiza wyników badań termograficznych, ultrasonograficznych i rentgenowskich w diagnozowaniu chorób ortopedycznych u koni wyścigowych[Comparison of thermographic, radiographic and ultrasonographic results in diagnosing racehorses orthopedic diseases]. *Medycyna Weterynaryjna*, *68*(11), 693–696.

Soroko, M., Jodkowska, E., & Dudek, K. (2015). Diagnoza termograficzna w monitorowaniu rocznego treningu koni wyścigowych[Thermography diagnosis in monitoring annual racehorses' training cycle]. *Medycyna Weterynaryjna*, *71*(01), 52–58.

Soroko, M., Jodkowska, E., & Zabłocka, M. (2012b). The use of thermography to evaluate back musculoskeletal responses of young racehorses to training. *Thermology International*, *22*(3), 152–156.

Stromberg, B. (1972). Thermography of the superficial flexor tendon in race horses. *Acta Radiologica*, *319*(319 Suppl), 295–297. doi:10.1177/0284185172013S31954 PMID:4531198

Stromberg, B. (1974). The use of thermography in equine orthopedics. *Journal of the American Veterinary Radiology*, *15*(1), 94–97. doi:10.1111/j.1740-8261.1974.tb00676.x

Tunley, B. V., & Henson, F. M. (2004). Reliability and repeatability of thermographic examination and the normal thermographic image of the thoracolumbar region in the horse. *Equine Veterinary Journal*, *36*(4), 306–312. doi:10.2746/0425164044890652 PMID:15163036

Turner, T. A. (1991). Thermography as an aid to the clinical lameness evaluation. *The Veterinary Clinics of North America. Equine Practice*, *7*(2), 311–338. PMID:1933566

Turner, T. A. (1998). The use of thermography in lameness evaluation.*Proceeding of the American Association of Equine Practitioners*, *44*, 224-226.

Turner, T. A. (2001). Diagnostic thermography. *The Veterinary Clinics of North America. Equine Practice*, *17*(1), 95–113. PMID:11488048

Turner, T. A. (2003). Back problems in horses.*49th Annual Convention of the American Association of Equine Practitioners*, New Orleans, LA.

Turner, T. A., Fessler, J. F., Lamp, M., Pearce, J. A., & Geddes, L. A. (1983). Thermographic evaluation of horses with podotrochlosis. *American Journal of Veterinary Research*, *44*(4), 535–539. PMID:6869948

Turner, T. A., Pansch, J., & Wilson, J. H. (2001). Thermographic assessment of racing Thoroughbreds. *Proceeding of the American Association of Equine Practitioners*, *47*, 344-346.

Turner, T. A., Rantanen, N. W., & Hauser, M. L. (1996). Alternate methods of soft tissue imaging.*1st Proceedings Dubai International Equine Symposium*, (pp. 165–176).

Turner, T. A., & Scroggins, R. D. (1989). Thermographic detection of gingering in horses. *Journal of Equine Veterinary Science*, *5*(1), 8–10. doi:10.1016/S0737-0806(85)80077-0

Turner, T. A., Waldsmith, J. K., & Wilson, J. H. (2004). How to assess saddle fit in horses. *Proceedings American Association of Equine Practice*, *50*, 196–201.

Vaden, M. F., Purohit, R. C., McCoy, D., & Vaughan, J. T. (1980). Thermography: A technique for subclinical diagnosis of osteoarthritis. *American Journal of Veterinary Research*, *41*(8), 1175–1180. PMID:7447111

Van Hoogmoed, L. M., & Snyder, J. R. (2002). Use of infrared thermography to detect injections and palmar digital neurectomy in horses. *Veterinary Journal (London, England)*, *164*(2), 129–141. doi:10.1053/tvjl.2002.0719 PMID:12359467

Van Hoogmoed, L. M., Snyder, J. R., Allen, A. K., & Waldsmith, J. D. (2000). Use of infrared thermography to detect performance - enhancing techniques in horses. *Equine Veterinary Education*, *12*(2), 102–107. doi:10.1111/j.2042-3292.2000.tb01772.x

Verschooten, F., Desmet, P., & Verbeeck, J. (1997). Skin surface temperature measurements in horses by electronic thermometry. *Equine Practice*, *19*(4), 16–23.

von Schweinitz, D. G. (1999). Thermographic diagnosis in equine back pain. *The Veterinary Clinics of North America. Equine Practice*, *15*, 161–177. PMID:10218248

Waldsmith, J. K., & Oltman, J. I. (1994). Thermography: Subclinical inflammation, diagnosis, rehabilitation, and athletic evaluation. *Journal of Equine Veterinary Science*, *14*(1), 8–10. doi:10.1016/S0737-0806(07)80302-9

Westermann, S., Stanek, C., Schramel, J. P., Ion, A., & Buchner, H. H. (2013). The effect of airflow on thermographically determined temperature of the distal forelimb of the horse. *Equine Veterinary Journal*, *45*(5), 637–641. doi:10.1111/evj.12019 PMID:23294196

Williams, R. B., Harkins, L. S., Hammond, C. J., & Wood, J. L. (2001). Racehorses injuries, clinical problems and fatalities recorded on British racecourses from flat racing and National Hint racing during 1996, 1997 and 1998. *Equine Veterinary Journal*, *33*(5), 478–486. doi:10.2746/042516401776254808 PMID:11558743

KEY TERMS AND DEFINITIONS

Bucked Shines: A repetitive loading injury of the third metacarpal bone. It occurs when the periosteum tears away from the front of the cannon bone. As the result of this this tear, there is bleeding with the formation of a hematoma, where new bone if forming.

Distal Parts of the Limbs: Limb from carpal joint do hoof in forelimb and from tarsal joint to hoof in hindlimb.

Laminitis: Laminitis is a crippling disease in which there is a failure of attachment of the epidermal laminae connected to the hoof wall from the dermal laminae attached to the distal phalanx.

Long Term Training: One racing training season which lasts 10 months from January till October, during which horses are regularly trained and raced.

Navicular Disease: Is an arthrosis developing on the surfaces of the navicular bone and the deep flexor tendon.

Subclinical Sign of Inflammations: Very early stage of inflammation when no clinical signs of inflammation: pain, heat, lameness, swelling and concerns of trainers are present.

Tendonitis: Inflammation of a tendon.

Compilation of References

Abate, M., Carlo, L. D., Romualdo, S. D., Ionta, S., Ferretti, A., Romani, G. L., & Merla, A. (2010). Postural adjustment in experimental leg length difference evaluated by means of thermal infrared imaging. *Physiological Measurement*, *31*(1), 35–43. doi:10.1088/0967-3334/31/1/003 PMID:19940346

Abate, M., Di Carlo, L., Di Donato, L., Romani, G. L., & Merla, A. (2013). Comparison of cutaneous termic response to a standardised warm up in trained and untrained individuals. *The Journal of Sports Medicine and Physical Fitness*, *53*(2), 209–215. PMID:23584330

Abel, G., Allen, J., & Drinnan, M. (2014). A pilot study of a new spectrophotometry device to measure tissue oxygen saturation. *Physiological Measurement*, *35*(9), 1769–1780. doi:10.1088/0967-3334/35/9/1769 PMID:25119876

Abramowit, Queral, Finn, Nora, & Peterson, Bergan, & Yao. (1979). The use of photoplethsmography in the assessment of venous insufficiency: A comparison to venous pressure measurements. *Surgery*, *86*, 434–441. PMID:473029

Adamczyk, J. G., Olszewska, M., Boguszewski, D., Białoszewski, D., & Reaburn, P. (2016). Is it possible to create a thermal model of warm-up? Monitoring of the training process in athletic decathlon. *Infrared Physics & Technology*, *76*, 555–559. doi:10.1016/j.infrared.2016.04.017

Agarwal, S. C., Allen, J., Murray, J., & Purcell, I. F. (2012). Laser Doppler assessment of dermal circulatory changes in people with coronary artery disease. *Microvascular Research*, *84*(1), 55–59. doi:10.1016/j.mvr.2012.02.002 PMID:22366028

Airaksinen, O. V., Kyrklund, N., Latvala, K., Kouri, J. P., Grönblad, M., & Kolari, P. (2003). Efficacy of cold gel for soft tissue injuries a prospective randomized double-blinded trial. *The American Journal of Sports Medicine*, *31*(5), 680–684. PMID:12975186

Akimov, E. B., Andreev, R. S., Arkov, V. V., Kirdin, A. A., Saryanc, V. V., Sonkin, V. D., & Tonevitsky, A. G. (2009). Thermal portrait of sportsmen with different aerobic capacity. *Acta Kinesiologiae Universitatis Tartuensis*, *14*, 7–16. doi:10.12697/akut.2009.14.01

Akimov, E., & Sonkin, V. (2011). Skin temperature and lactate threshold during muscle work in athletes. *Human Physiology*, *37*(5), 621–628. doi:10.1134/S0362119711050033

Allen, J. (2007). Topical Review: Photoplethysmography and its application in clinical physiological measurement. *Physiological Measurement*, *28*(3), R1–R39. doi:10.1088/0967-3334/28/3/R01 PMID:17322588

Allen, J. (2012). *Development of a clinical vascular optics measurement facility – the Newcastle upon Tyne experience. XII European Congress of Thermology*, Porto, Portugal.

Allen, J., Di Maria, C., Burnett, S., Forrest, I., & Griffiths, B. (2015a). *Imaging assessments of patients with suspected systemic sclerosis and associated inflammatory lung disease. In Infrared imaging: A casebook in clinical medicine.* Institute of Physics Publishing.

Allen, J., & Gorman, G. (2015d). *Thermographic assessment of the presence of fatty tumours in myoclonic epilepsy with ragged red fibres. In Infrared imaging: A casebook in clinical medicine*. Institute of Physics Publishing.

Allen, J., & Howell, K. J. (2014). Topical Review: Clinical Microvascular Imaging: Techniques and opportunities for clinical physiological measurements. *Physiological Measurement*, *35*(7), R91–R141. doi:10.1088/0967-3334/35/7/R91 PMID:24910968

Allen, J., Murray, A., Di Maria, C., & Newton, J. L. (2012). Chronic fatigue syndrome and impaired peripheral pulse characteristics on orthostasis - a new potential diagnostic biomarker. *Physiological Measurement*, *33*(2), 231–241. doi:10.1088/0967-3334/33/2/231 PMID:22273713

Allen, J., Oates, C. P., Chishti, A. D., Ahmed, I. A. M., Talbot, D., & Murray, A. (2006). Thermography and colour duplex ultrasound assessments of arterio-venous fistula function in renal patients. *Physiological Measurement*, *27*(1), 51–60. doi:10.1088/0967-3334/27/1/005 PMID:16365510

Allen, J., Oates, C., & Talbot, D. (2015c). *Thermal imaging and its potential for arterio-venous fistula function assessment. In Infrared imaging: A casebook in clinical medicine*. Institute of Physics Publishing.

Allen, J., Perros, P., Dickinson, J., & Murray, A. (2011). An exploratory look at the thermal characteristics of the eyes in patients with thyroid eye disease. International Consensus Guidelines on Medical Thermography. Iguazu Falls, Brazil 23-26 Nov 2011. *Thermology International*, *21*, 148.

Allen, J., Robertshaw, D., & Leech, N. (2015b). *Thermal imaging potential for assessing diabetic Charcot foot syndrome. In Infrared imaging: A casebook in clinical medicine*. Institute of Physics Publishing.

Allen, J., Young, A. L., & Griffiths, B. (2014). Subject preparation and thermal acclimatization prior to mild cold challenge testing using dynamic thermal imaging. *Pan American Journal of Medical Thermology*, *1*(1), 51–54. doi:10.18073/2358-4696/pajmt.v1n1p51-54

Al-Nakhli, H. H., Petrofsky, J. S., Laymon, M. S., & Berk, L. S. (2012). The Use of Thermal Infra-Red Imaging to Detect Delayed Onset Muscle Soreness. *Journal of Visualized Experiments*, (59): e3551. PMID:22297829

Altman, D. G., & Bland, J. M. (1994). Diagnostic tests. 1: Sensitivity and specificity. *British Medical Journal*, *308*(6943), 1552. doi:10.1136/bmj.308.6943.1552 PMID:8019315

American Academy of Thermology. (2013). *Veterinary guidelines for infrared thermography*. Available from: http://www.aathermology.org/organization/guidelines/veterinary-guidelines-for-infrared-thermography

Ammer K. (2008). The Glamorgan Protocol for recording and evaluation of thermal images of the human body. *Thermology International, 18*, 125–44.

Ammer, K. (2008). The Glamorgan Protocol for recording and evaluation of thermal images of the human body. *Thermology International, 18*(4), 125-144.

Ammer. (2004). Temperature effects of thermotherapy determined by infrared measurements. *Phys Med, 20*(S1), 64-66.

Ammer. (2004). Temperature effects of thermotherapy determined by infrared measurements. *Physica Medica, 20*(S1), 64-66.

Ammer. (2008). The Glamorgan Protocol for recording and evaluation of thermal images of the human body. *Thermology International.*

Ammer, K. (2003). Need for standardisation of measurements in Thermal Imaging. In B. Wiecek (Ed.), *Thermography and Lasers in Medicine* (pp. 13–17). Lodz, Poland: Akademickie Centrum Graficzno-Marketigowe Lodar S.A.

Ammer, K. (2004). Temperature effects of thermotherapy determined by infrared measurements. *Physica Medica, 20*, 64–66.

Ammer, K. (2008). The Glamorgan Protocol for recording and evaluation of thermal images of the human body. *Thermol Int., 18*(4), 125–144.

Ammer, K. (2008). The Glamorgan Protocol for recording and evaluation of thermal images of the human body. *Thermology International, 18*(4), 125–129.

Ammer, K. (2012). Temperature of the human knee – a review. *Thermology International, 22*(4), 137–151.

Ammer, K., & Ring, F. E. (2007). Standard procedures for infrared imaging in medicine. In N. A. Diakides & J. D. Bronzino (Eds.), *Medical infrared imaging. Principles and Practice* (pp. 32.1–32.14). Boca Raton, FL: Taylor & Francis. doi:10.1201/9781420008340.ch22

Anbar, M. (2008). Dynamic Thermal Assessment. In N. A. Diakides & J. D. Bronzino (Eds.), *Medical infrared imaging* (pp. 8.1–8.17). Boca Raton, FL: CRC Press.

Anbar, M., Gratt, B. M., & Hong, D. (1998). Thermology and facial telethermography. Part I: History and technical review. *Dento Maxillo Facial Radiology, 27*(2), 61–67. doi:10.1038/sj.dmfr.4600314 PMID:9656868

Anderson, K., Di Maria, C., & Allen, J. (2013). Novel assessment of microvascular changes in idiopathic restless legs syndrome (Willis-Ekbom disease). *Journal of Sleep Research, 22*(3), 315–321. doi:10.1111/jsr.12025 PMID:23397977

Anderson, M. E., Moore, T. L., Lunt, M., & Herrick, A. L. (2004). Digital iontophoresis of vasoactive substances as measured by laser Doppler imaging - a non-invasive technique by which to measure microvascular dysfunction in Raynauds phenomenon. *Rheumatology (Oxford, England), 43*(8), 986–991. doi:10.1093/rheumatology/keh244 PMID:15199217

Arfaoui, A., Bertucci, W. M., Letellier, T., & Polidori, G. (2014). Thermoregulation during incremental exercise in masters cycling. *Journal of Science and Cycling, 3*(1), 32–40.

Arfaoui, A., Polidori, G., Taiar, R., & Popa, C. (2012). Infrared Thermography in Sports Activity. In R. V. Prakash (Ed.), *Infrared Thermography* (pp. 141–168). InTech. doi:10.5772/30268

Arnaiz Lastras, J., Fernández Cuevas, I., Gómez Carmona, P. M., Sillero Quintana, M., García de la Concepción, M. Á., & Piñonosa Cano, S. (2011). *Pilot study to determinate thermal asymmetries in judokas.* Paper presented at the 16th Annual Congress of the European College of Sport Sciences ECSS, Liverpool, UK.

Arora, N., Martins, D., Ruggerio, D., Tousimis, E., Swistel, A. J., Osborne, M. P., & Simmons, R. M. (2008). Effectiveness of a noninvasive digital infrared thermal imaging system in the detection of breast cancer. *American Journal of Surgery, 196*(4), 523–526. doi:10.1016/j.amjsurg.2008.06.015 PMID:18809055

Arruda, T. Z., Brass, K. E., & De La Corte, F. D. (2011). Thermographic assessment of saddles used on jumping horses. *Journal of Equine Veterinary Science, 31*(11), 625–629. doi:10.1016/j.jevs.2011.05.011

Arthur, D. T., Khan, M. M., & Barclay, L. C. (2011). Thermographic investigation of osseous stress pathology. In *Engineering in Medicine and Biology Society, EMBC, 2011 Annual International Conference of the IEEE* (pp. 6250 - 6253). doi:10.1109/IEMBS.2011.6091543

Aughey, R. J., Goodman, C. A., & McKenna, M. J. (2014). Greater chance of high core temperatures with modified pacing strategy during team sport in the heat. *Journal of Science and Medicine in Sport, 17*(1), 113–118. doi:10.1016/j.jsams.2013.02.013 PMID:23689104

Autio, E., Neste, R., Airaksinen, S., & Heiskanen, M. L. (2006). Measuring the heat loss in horses in different seasons by infrared thermography. *Journal of Applied Animal Welfare Science*, *9*(3), 211–221. doi:10.1207/s15327604jaws0903_3 PMID:17112332

Awerbuch, M. S. (1991). Thermography--its current diagnostic status in musculoskeletal medicine. *The Medical Journal of Australia*, *154*(7), 441–444. PMID:2005838

Badža, V., Jovančević, V., Fratrić, F., Roglić, G., & Sudarov, N. (2012). Possibilities of thermovision application in sport and sport rehabilitation. *Vojnosanitetski Pregled. Military-Medical and Pharmaceutical Review*, *69*(10), 904–907. doi:10.2298/VSP1210904B PMID:23155613

Bagavathiappan, S., Philip, J., Raj, K., & Panicker, K. (2009). Infrared thermal imaging for detection of peripheral vascular disorders. *Journal of Medical Physics*, *34*(1), 43–47. doi:10.4103/0971-6203.48720 PMID:20126565

Baker, A. (1998). *Bicycling medicine: Cycling nutrition, Physiology, Injury prevention and treatment for riders of all levels*. Fireside.

Balci, G. A., Basaran, T., & Colakoglu, M. (2016). Analysing visual pattern of skin temperature during submaximal and maximal exercises. *Infrared Physics & Technology*, *74*, 57–62. doi:10.1016/j.infrared.2015.12.002

Bandeira, F., Borba Neves, E., Muniz de Moura, M. A., & Nohama, P. (2014). A termografia no apoio ao diagnostico de lesao muscular no esporte. *Revista Brasileira de Medicina do Esporte*, *20*(1), 59–64. doi:10.1590/S1517-86922014000100012

Bandeira, F., Muniz de Moura, M. A., Abreu de Souza, M., Nohama, P., & Borba Neves, E. (2012). Pode a termografia auxiliar no diagnóstico de lesoes musculares em atletas de futebol? *Revista Brasileira de Medicina do Esporte*, *18*(4), 234–239. doi:10.1590/S1517-86922012000400006

Banerjee, D., Chattopadhyay, S. K., & Tuli, S. (2013). Infrared thermography in material research – A review of textile applications. *Indian Journal of Fibre & Textile Research*, *38*(4), 427–437.

Banfi, L., Lombardi, G., Colombini, A., & Melegati, G. (2010). Whole-body cryotherapy in athletes. *Sports Medicine (Auckland, N.Z.)*, *40*(6), 509–517. doi:10.2165/11531940-000000000-00000 PMID:20524715

Barbosa, T., Fernandes, R., Keskinen, K., Colaço, P., Cardoso, C., Silva, J., & Vilas-Boas, J. (2006). Evaluation of the Energy Expenditure in Competitive Swimming Strokes. *International Journal of Sports Medicine*, *27*(11), 894–899. doi:10.1055/s-2006-923776 PMID:16612740

Barbosa, T., Marinho, D., Costa, M., & Silva, A. (2011). Biomechanics of competitive swimming strokes. In V. Klika (Ed.), *Biomechanics in Applications* (pp. 367–388). Intech.

Barcelos, E., Caminhas, W., Ribeiro, E., Pimenta, E., & Palhares, R. (2014). A Combined Method for Segmentation and Registration for an Advanced and Progressive Evaluation of Thermal Images. *Sensors (Basel, Switzerland)*, *14*(11), 21950–21967. doi:10.3390/s141121950 PMID:25414972

Barnes, R. B. (1964). Thermography. (Thermography & its clinical applications). *Annals of the New York Academy of Sciences*, *121*(1), 34–48. doi:10.1111/j.1749-6632.1964.tb13683.x PMID:14237524

Bartling, S. H., Stiller, W., Semmler, W., & Kiessling, F. (2007). Small animal computed tomography imaging. *Current Medical Imaging Reviews*, *3*(1), 45–59. doi:10.2174/157340507779940327

Bauer & Skrzek. (1997). Physiological basis of cryotherapy. *Acta Bio-Optica et Informatica Medica*, *3*(2-4), 115–120.

Bauer & Skrzek. (1999). Fizjologiczne podstawy krioterapii. *Medycyna sportowa*, *94*, 3-7. (in Polish)

Bauer, Hurnik, & Zdziarski, Mielczarek, & Podbielska. (1997). Thermovision and its applications in medicine. *Acta Bio-Optica et Informatica Medica*, *3*(2-4), 121–131.

Bauer, Hurnik, Zdziarski, Mielczarek, & Skrzek, Podbielska, & Zagrobelny. (1997). Thermovison evaluation of cryotherapy effects. *Acta Bio-Optica et Informatica Medica*, *3*(2-4), 133–140.

Belcaro, Dugall, Luzzi, Ippolito, & Cesarone. (2014). Postpartum Varicose Veins: Supplementation with Pycnogenol or Elastic Compression—A 12-Month Follow-Up. *International Journal of Angiology*. Available at http://santurel.net/_library/_files/Pycnogenol-studie-spataders.pdf

Benbow, C., & Bowsher, W. (1994). The prediction of diabetic neuropathic plantar foot ulceration by liquid-crystal contact thermography. *Diabetes Care*, *17*(8), 835–839. doi:10.2337/diacare.17.8.835 PMID:7956627

Bendele, A. (2001). Animal models of rheumatoid arthritis. *Journal of Musculoskeletal & Neuronal Interactions*, *1*(4), 377–385. PMID:15758488

BenEliyahu, D. (1992). Infrared thermography and the sports injury practice. *Dynamic Chiropractic, 10*(7).

BenEliyahu, D. J. (1990). Infrared thermography in the diagnosis and management of sports injuries: A clinical study and literature review. *Chiropractic Sports Medicine.*, *4*(2), 46–53.

Benson, E., & Allen, J. (2015). *Illuminating light in medical diagnostics and treatment.* British Science Week seminar on light. Portcullis House.

Bernau, M., Kremer, P., Papenberger, E., Kreuzer, L., Cussler, K., Hoffmann, A., & Scholz, A. (2015). *Safety Testing of Veterinary Vaccines Using Magnetic Resonance Imaging in Pigs Altex.* Academic Press.

Berry, D. C., & Yemm, R. (1971). Variations in skin temperature of the face in normal subjects and in patients with temporomandibular dysfunction. *The British Journal of Oral Surgery*, *8*(3), 242–247. doi:10.1016/S0007-117X(70)80086-5 PMID:5282910

Berry, D. C., & Yemm, R. (1974). A further study of facial skin temperature in patients withmandibular dysfunction. *Journal of Oral Rehabilitation*, *1*(3), 255–264. doi:10.1111/j.1365-2842.1974.tb01437.x PMID:4530064

Bertucci, W., Arfaoui, A., Janson, L., & Polidori, G. (2013). Relationship between the gross efficiency and muscular skin temperature of lower limb in cycling: a preliminary study. *Computer Methods in Biomechanics and Biomedical Engineering, 16*(sup1), 114-115.

Biagioni, P. A., Longmore, R. B., McGimpsey, J. G., & Lamey, P. J. (1996). Its role in dental research with particular reference to craniomandibular disorders. *Dento Maxillo Facial Radiology*, *25*(3), 119–124. doi:10.1259/dmfr.25.3.9084259 PMID:9084259

Biały, Zimer, & Zagrobelny. (1999) Acta Bio-Optica et Informatica Medica. *Inżynieria Biomedyczna Wpływ ogólnoustrojowej krioterapii na parametry krwi obwodowej zawodników kadry narodowej lekkoatletów,* *5*(1-2), 7-10. (in Polish)

Biały, Zimmer, Skrzek, & Zagrobelny. (1998). Cryogenic Chamber – Possibilities Of Use In Rehabilitation. *Baln. Pol*, *40*(3-4), 44–47.

Bignold, L. P., Coghlan, B. L. D., & Jersmann, H. P. A. (2006). Cancer morphology, carcinogenesis and genetic instability: a background. In Cancer: Cell Structures, Carcinogens and Genomic Instability (pp. 1-24). Birkhäuser Basel. doi:10.1007/3-7643-7378-4_1

Bignold, L. P. (2003). Initiation of genetic instability and tumour formation: A review and hypothesis of a nongenotoxic mechanism. *Cellular and Molecular Life Sciences*, *60*(6), 1107–1117. doi:10.1007/s00018-003-2314-6 PMID:12861379

Bilodeau, G. A., Ghali, R., Desgent, S., Langlois, P., Farah, R., St-Onge, P. L., . . . Carmant, L. (2011, June). Where is the rat? Tracking in low contrast thermographic images. In CVPR 2011 Workshops (pp. 55-60). IEEE. doi:10.1109/CVPRW.2011.5981685

Binder, A., Parr, G., Thomas, P. P., & Hazleman, B. (1983). A clinical and thermographic study of lateral epicondylitis. *British Journal of Rheumatology*, *22*(2), 77–81. doi:10.1093/rheumatology/22.2.77 PMID:6682688

Birkner, Sieroń, Beck, Jagodziński, & Romuk, Skrzep-Poloczek, & Stanek. (2003). Application of cryogenic temperatures in medicine. *Wiadomosci Lekarskie (Warsaw, Poland)*, *56*(1-2), 53–56. PMID:12901269

Bollinger, A., & Fagrell, B. (1990). *Clinical capillaroscopy: a guide to its use in clinical research and practice*. Toronto: Hogrefe & Huber Publishers.

Bollinger, Isenring, & Franzeck. (1982). U.K.: Lymphatic microangiopathy: a complication of severe chronic venous incompetence (CVI). *Lymphology*, *15*(2), 60–65. PMID:7109680

Bollinger, L., Leu, A. J., Hoffmann, U., & Franzeck, U. K. (1997). Microvascular changes in venous disease: An update. *Angiology*, *48*(1), 27–32. doi:10.1177/000331979704800105 PMID:8995340

Bonnett, P., Hare, D. B., Jones, D. D., Ring, E. F. J., & Hare, C. J. (2006). Some preliminary observations of the effects of sports massage on heat distribution of lower limb muscles during a graded exercise test. *Thermology International*, *16*(4), 143–149.

Borba Neves, E., Martins Cunha, R., Rosa, C., Sousa Antunes, N., Vieira Felisberto, I. M., Vilaça-Alves, J., & Machado Reis, V. (2016). Correlation between skin temperature and heart rate during exercise and recovery, and the influence of body position in these variables in untrained women. *Infrared Physics & Technology*, *75*, 70–76. doi:10.1016/j.infrared.2015.12.018

Boulant, J. A. (2000). Role of the preoptic-anterior hypothalamus in thermoregulation and fever. *Clinical Infectious Diseases*, *31*(Supplement 5), S157–S161. doi:10.1086/317521 PMID:11113018

Bourlai, T., Pryor, R. R., Suyama, J., Reis, S. E., & Hostler, D. (2012). Use of thermal imagery for estimation of core body temperature during precooling, exertion, and recovery in wildland firefighter protective clothing. *Prehospital Emergency Care*, *16*(3), 390–399. doi:10.3109/10903127.2012.670689 PMID:22510022

Bouzas Marins, J. C., Andrade Fernandes, A., Gomes Moreira, D., Souza Silva, F., & Magno, A. (2014). Thermographic profile of soccer players lower limbs. *Revista Andaluza de Medicina del Deporte*, *7*(1), 1–6. doi:10.1016/S1888-7546(14)70053-X

Bowman, K. F., Purohit, R. C., Ganjam, V. K., Pechman, R. D. Jr, & Vaughan, J. T. (1983). Thermographic evaluation of corticosteroid efficacy in amphotericin B – induced arthiritis in ponies. *American Journal of Veterinary Research*, *44*(1), 51–56. PMID:6824225

Bradbury, M., Murie, J. A., & Ruckley, C. V. (1993). Role of leucocyte in the pathogenesis of vascular disease. *British Journal of Surgery*, *80*(12), 1503–1512. doi:10.1002/bjs.1800801204 PMID:8298912

Breiman, L., Friedman, J. H., Olshen, R., & Stone, C. J. (1984). *Classification and regression trees*. Monterey, CA: Wadsworth.

Brengelmann. (1989). Body temperature regulation In H. D. Patron, A. F. Fuchs, B. Hill, A. M. Scher, & R. Steiner (Eds.), *Textbook of Physiology*. Academic Press.

Briain, L., & Takano, F. (2003). Intravascular Modalities for Detection of Vulnerable Plaque. *Arteriosclerosis, Thrombosis, and Vascular Biology*, *23*(8), 1333–1342. doi:10.1161/01.ATV.0000080948.08888.BF PMID:12805071

Briers, J. D. (2001). Laser Doppler, speckle and related techniques for blood perfusion mapping and imaging. *Physiological Measurement*, *22*(4), R35–R66. doi:10.1088/0967-3334/22/4/201 PMID:11761081

Brioschi, M. L., Teixeira, M. J., Silva, F. M., & Colman, D. (2010). *Princípios e Indicações da Termografia Médica*. São Paulo: Andreoli.

Brooks, Bogduk, & Bellamy. (2003). *Evidence based – Management of acute muscosceletal pain*. Australian Academic Press.

Browne, S., Sivananthan, U. M., Sabroe, I., & Rees, M. R. (1992). Use of thermal imaging to monitor crural thrombolysis. *Blood Coagulation & Fibrinolysis*, *3*(4), 489–492. doi:10.1097/00001721-199208000-00019 PMID:1420827

Buchner, H. H. F., Savelbergh, H. H., Schamhardt, H. C., & Barneveld, A. (1996). Head and trunk movement adaptations in horses with experimentally induced fore or hind limb lameness. *Equine Veterinary Journal*, *28*(1), 71–76. doi:10.1111/j.2042-3306.1996.tb01592.x PMID:8565958

Buckhout, B. C., & Warner, M. A. (1980). Digital perfusion of handball players. Effects of repeated ball impact on structures of the hand. *The American Journal of Sports Medicine*, *8*(3), 206–207. doi:10.1177/036354658000800313 PMID:7377456

Bulut, J., Janta, M., Senner, V., & Kreuzer, J. (2013). Determination of Insulation Properties of Functional Clothing Using Core Body Temperature Gradients as Quantification Parameter. *Procedia Engineering*, *60*(0), 208–213. doi:10.1016/j.proeng.2013.07.057

Burnham, R. S., McKinley, R. S., & Vincent, D. D. (2006). Three types of skin-surface thermometers: A comparison of reliability, validity, and responsiveness. *American Journal of Physical Medicine & Rehabilitation*, *85*(7), 553–558. doi:10.1097/01.phm.0000223232.32653.7f PMID:16788385

Busoni, F., Romagnoli, C., Bagnolesi, P., & Gemignani, G. (1988). Imaging of enthesopathies of the ligamentum patellae in athletes. Echography and computerized telethermography. *La Radiologia Medica*, *76*(1-2), 44–47. PMID:3041478

Caggiati, B., & Gloviczki, J. (2002). International Interdisciplinary Consensus Committee on Venous Anatomical Terminology. Nomenclature of the veins of the lower limbs: An international interdisciplinary consensus statement. *Journal of Vascular Surgery*, *36*(2), 416–422. doi:10.1067/mva.2002.125847 PMID:12170230

Cameron, S., Sachdev, D., Gishen, P., & Martin, J. F. (1991). Liquid crystal thermography as a screening test for deep vein thrombosis in patients with cerebral infarction. *European Journal of Clinical Investigation*, *21*(5), 548–550. doi:10.1111/j.1365-2362.1991.tb01408.x PMID:1752294

Canavan, D., & Gratt, B. M. (1995). Electronic thermography for the assessment of mild and moderate temporomandibular joint dysfunction. *Oral Surgery, Oral Medicine, Oral Pathology, Oral Radiology, and Endodontics*, *79*(6), 778–786. doi:10.1016/S1079-2104(05)80316-6 PMID:7621039

Carmeliet, P., & Jain, R. K. (2011). Molecular mechanisms and clinical applications of angiogenesis. *Nature*, *473*(7347), 298–307. doi:10.1038/nature10144 PMID:21593862

Caty, V., Aujouannet, Y., Hintzy, F., Bonifazi, M., Clarys, J., & Rouard, A. (2007). Wrist stabilisation and forearm muscle coactivation during freestyle swimming. *Journal of Electromyography and Kinesiology*, *17*(3), 285–291. doi:10.1016/j.jelekin.2006.02.005 PMID:16677829

Cena, K. (1974). Radiative heat loss from Animal and Man. In J. L. Monteih & L. E. Mount (Eds.), *Heat loss from animals and man* (pp. 34–57). London: Butterworths. doi:10.1016/B978-0-408-70652-0.50009-3

Charkoudian, N. (2003). Skin blood flow in adult human thermoregulation: How it works, when it does not, and why. *Mayo Clinic proceedings. Mayo Clinic, 78*(5), 603–612. doi:10.4065/78.5.603

Charkoudian, N. (2010). Mechanisms and modifiers of reflex induced cutaneous vasodilation and vasoconstriction in humans. *Journal of Applied Physiology (Bethesda, Md.), 109*(4), 1221–1228. doi:10.1152/japplphysiol.00298.2010 PMID:20448028

Chatham, J. C., & Blackband, S. J. (2001). Nuclear magnetic resonance spectroscopy and imaging in animal research. *ILAR Journal, 42*(3), 189–208. doi:10.1093/ilar.42.3.189 PMID:11406719

Cheng, H., Luo, Q., Liu, Q., Lu, Q., Gong, H., & Zeng, S. (2004). Laser speckle imaging of blood flow in microcirculation. *Physics in Medicine and Biology, 49*(7), 1347–1357. doi:10.1088/0031-9155/49/7/020 PMID:15128210

Cheng, T.-Y., & Herman, C. (2014). Analysis of skin cooling for quantitative dynamic infrared imaging of near-surface lesions. *International Journal of Thermal Sciences, 86*(0), 175–188. doi:10.1016/j.ijthermalsci.2014.06.033

Cheng, V. S., Bai, J., & Chen, Y. (2009). A high-resolution three-dimensional far-infrared thermal and true-color imaging system for medical applications. *Medical Engineering &amp. Physics, 31*(9), 1173–1181.

Chen, Z., Jiang, G., Zheng, F., Liu, H., & Zhu, B. (2005). A Correction method of medical thermography's distortion. *Conference Proceedings; ... Annual International Conference of the IEEE Engineering in Medicine and Biology Society. IEEE Engineering in Medicine and Biology Society. Conference, 2*, 1677–1679. PMID:17282534

Chiesa, M., & Limoni, V. (2005). Demographic factors and their relationship with the presence of CVI signs in Italy: The 24-cities cohort study. *European Journal of Vascular and Endovascular Surgery, 30*(6), 674–680. doi:10.1016/j.ejvs.2005.06.016 PMID:16055355

Cholewka & Drzazga. (2005a). Diagnostic value of thermal imaging due to whole body cryotherapy. *IFMBE Proceedings of 3rd EMBEC.*

Cholewka & Drzazga. (2005b). Krioterapia ogólnoustrojowa w kriokomorze dwu-stopniowej oraz kriokomorze z zaleganiem zimna. *Acta Bio-Optica et Informatica Medica*, 57-63. (in Polish)

Cholewka & Drzazga. (2006). Comparison Of Some Parameters Of Two-Stepped Cryogenic Chamber And Chamber With Lingering Cold. *Biomedical Engineering Acta Indygo, 11*, 103–110.

Cholewka, A. (2005). *The influence of low temperature on organism, in vitro and in vivo studies* (Doctoral Thesis). A. Chełkowski Institute of Physics, University of Silesia Katowice Poland.

Cholewka, Ciszek, & Drzazga. (2012). Cryogenic chamber used in physical medicine and their comparison. *W: Zastosowanie niskich temperatur w medycynie, redakcja: Anna Skrzek i Halina Podbielska 2012.* Oficyna Wydawnicza Politechniki Wrocławskiej, Wrocław.

Cholewka, Drzazga, Borgieł, & Kurpas. (2005). Cold penetration of the fourth layer tissue model in the whole body cryotherapy conditions. *IFMBE Proceedings of 3rd EMBEC.*

Cholewka, Drzazga, Kajewski, Sieroń, & Wiśniowska. (2004). Thermographic assessment of cryotherapy effects. *VI Konferencja Krajowa TTP2004 Ustroń-Jaszowiec, Proceedings*, (pp. 143 – 148).

Cholewka, Drzazga, Knefel, Kawecki, & Nowak. (2010). Thermal Imaging In Hyperbaric Oxygen Therapy (HBO). *Inżynieria Biomedyczna.*

Cholewka, Drzazga, Michalik, & Sieroń. (2006). Whole Body Cryotherapy and Magnetotherapy Influence on Some Cardiac Parameters. *Pol J of Environ Stud, 15*(4A), 19-21.

Cholewka, Drzazga, Sieroń, & Stanek. (2010). Thermovision diagnostics in chosen spine diseases treated by whole body cryotherapy. *Journal of Thermal Analysis and Calorymetry.*

Cholewka, Drzazga, Sieroń, & Wiśniowska. (2004). Temperature effect of whole body cryotherapy determined by thermography. *Thermology International*, 57-63.

Cholewka, Drzazga, Sieroń, Stanek, Knefel, Kawecki, & Nowak. (2010). Some Applications Of Thermal Imaging In Medicine. *Monographs of Polish Journal of Environmental Studies.*

Cholewka, Drzazga, Wiśniowska, & Sieroń. (2002). The temperature changes of the skin surface during whole body cryotherapy. *IFMBE Proceedings of 2nd EMBEC, 2*, 1330-31.

Cholewka, Sieroń, & Drzazga. (2014). Application thermal imaging in diseases of the blood vessels. W: Biomedyczne zastosowania termowizji, pod redakcją H. Podbielska i A. Skrzek, Biomedyczne zastosowania termowizji. Oficyna Wydawnicza Politechniki Wrocławskiej.

Cholewka, Stanek, Kasprzyk, Urbańczyk, Jagodziński, Sieroń, & Drzazga. (2013). The application of thermography in research efficiency athletes, pilot studies. *PAK, 9*, 871-874.

Cholewka, Stanek, Kwiatek, Sieroń, & Drzazga. (2011). The use of thermography in the diagnosis of selected changes to skin cancer - preliminary study. *Application of thermovision to diagnosis of chosen skin cancer changes – preliminary studies*. PAK.

Cholewka. (2005). *The impact of low temperatures on the body - in vivo and in vitro studies*. Rozprawa doktorska Uniwersyetet Śląski w Katowicach, Katowice.

Cholewka. (2012). Meaning of thermal diagnostic analysis of the whole body cryotherapy. *W: Zastosowanie niskich temperatur w medycynie*. Redakcja: Anna Skrzek i Halina Podbielska.

Cholewka, A., Drzazga, Z., Kajewski, B., Bogucki, R., & Wiśniowska, B. (2004). Thermal imaging of skin body surface due to whole body cryo- therapy—preliminary report. *Physica Medica, 1*, 81–83.

Cholewka, A., Stanek, A., Kasprzyk, T., Urbańczyk, P., Jagodziński, L., Sieroń, A., & Drzazga, Z. (2013). Zastosowanie termowizji w badaniach wydolności sportowców, badania pilotażowe. *PAK, 09*, 871–874.

Cholewka, D., Drzazga, Z., & Sieroń, A. (2006). Monitoring of whole body cryotherapy effects by thermal imaging – preliminary report. *Physica Medica, 22*(2), 57–62. doi:10.1016/S1120-1797(06)80054-2 PMID:17643893

Cholewka, D., Drzazga, Z., Sieroń, A., & Stanek, A. (2010). Thermovision diagnostics in chosen spine diseases treated by whole body cryotherapy. *Journal of Thermal Analysis and Calorimetry, 102*(1), 113–119. doi:10.1007/s10973-010-0873-y

Cholewka, Drzazga, & Kajewski, Bogucki, & Wiśniowska. (2004). The thermal imaging of skin body surface due to whole body cryotherapy – preliminary report. *Physica Medica, 20*(Suppl. I), 70–72.

Cholewka, K., & Stanek, K. (2012). Thermal imaging and TC oximetry measurements of hyperbaric oxygen therapy (HBO) effects on trophic ulceration of the crura. *Journal of Thermal Analysis and Calorimetry, 108*(1), 25–31. doi:10.1007/s10973-011-1934-6

Cholewka, Kasprzyk, & Stanek, Sieroń-Stołtny, & Drzazga. (2015). May thermal imaging be useful in cyclist endurance tests? *Journal of Thermal Analysis and Calorimetry*. doi:10.1007/s10973-015-4662-5

Cholewka, S., & Klimas, S. (2014). Thermal imaging application in chronic venous disease: Pilot study. *Journal of Thermal Analysis and Calorimetry*, *115*(2), 1609–1618. doi:10.1007/s10973-013-3356-0

Cholewka, Stanek, Sieroń, & Drzazga. (2011). Thermography study of skin response due to whole-body cryotherapy. *Skin Research and Technology*. PMID:21507075

Cholewka, Stanek, & Klimas, Sieroń, & Drzazga. (2014). Thermal Imaging Application In Chronic Venous Disease. *Pilot Study*, *115*, 1609–1618.

Cholewka, Stanek, & Kwiatek, Sieroń, & Drzazga. (2013). Does the temperature gradient correlate with photodynamic diagnosis parameter NCV? *Photodiagnosis and Photodynamic Therapy*, *10*, 33–38. doi:10.1016/j.pdpdt.2012.07.001 PMID:23465370

Christensen, J., Vaeth, M., & Wenzel, A. (2012). Thermographic imaging of facial skin-gender differences and temperature changes over time in healthy subjects. *Dento Maxillo Facial Radiology*, *41*(8), 662–667. doi:10.1259/dmfr/55922484 PMID:22554986

Christopoulos, N., Nicolaides, A. N., & Szendro, G. (1988). Venous reflux: Quantification and correlation with clinical severity. *British Journal of Surgery*, *75*(4), 352–356. doi:10.1002/bjs.1800750419 PMID:3359149

Chudecka, M., & Lubkowska, A. (2010a). Evaluation of temperature changes in upper extremities of waterpolo players by thermovision [in Polish]. *Inżynieria Biomedyczna. Acta Bio-Optica et Informatica Medica*, *16*(4), 334–338.

Chudecka, M., & Lubkowska, A. (2010b). Temperature changes of selected bodys surfaces of handball players in the course of training estimated by thermovision, and the study of the impact of physiological and morphological factors on the skin temperature. *Journal of Thermal Biology*, *35*(8), 379–385. doi:10.1016/j.jtherbio.2010.08.001

Chudecka, M., & Lubkowska, A. (2011). Evaluation of the body surface temperature changes in the basketball players' after training. [in Polish]. *Inżynieria Biomedyczna. Acta Bio-Optica et Informatica Medica*, *17*(4), 271–275.

Chudecka, M., & Lubkowska, A. (2012). The use of Thermal Imaging to evaluate Body Temperature changes of athletes during training and a study on the impact of physiological and morphological factors on skin temperature. *Human Movement*, *13*(1), 33–39. doi:10.2478/v10038-012-0002-9

Chudecka, M., Szczepanowska, E., & Kempinska, A. (2008). Changes of thermoemission of upper extremities in female handball players - the preliminary study. *Medicina Sportiva*, *12*(3), 99–102. doi:10.2478/v10036-008-0019-5

Chwalbińska-Moneta. (2003). Wpływ kriostymulacji ogólnoustrojowej na niektóre reakcje wysiłkowe u sportowców. *Sport Wyczynowy*, *5/6*, 50-54. (in Polish)

Ciutacu, O., Tanase, A., & Miclaus, I. (2006). Digital infrared thermography in assessing soft tissues injuries on sport equines. *Bulletin of the University of Agricultural Sciences and Veterinary Medicine*, *63*, 228-233.

Clark, J. A., & Cena, K. (1973). Thermographic measurements of the surface temperatures of animals. *Journal of Mammalogy*, *54*(4), 1003–1007. doi:10.2307/1379105 PMID:4761360

Clark, J. A., & Cena, K. (1977). The potential of infra-red thermography in veterinary diagnosis. *The Veterinary Record*, *100*(19), 402–404. doi:10.1136/vr.100.19.402 PMID:325877

Clark, R. P., Goff, M. R., & Mullan, B. J. (1977). Skin temperatures during sunbathing and some observations on the effect of hot and cold drinks on these temperatures. *The Journal of Physiology*, *267*(1), 8P–9P. PMID:874864

Clark, R. P., Mullan, B. J., & Pugh, G. C. (1974). Proceedings: Colour thermography in running. *The Journal of Physiology*, *239*(2), 81P–82P. PMID:4415246

Clark, R. P., Mullan, B. J., & Pugh, L. G. (1977). Skin temperature during running -a study using infra-red colour thermography. *The Journal of Physiology*, *267*(1), 53–62. doi:10.1113/jphysiol.1977.sp011800 PMID:874861

Clover, J. (2008). *Sports Medicine Essentials. Core Concepts in Athletic Training & Fitness Instruction*. Independence, KY: Cengage Learning.

Cohen, M. L. (1977). Measurement of the thermal properties of human skin. A review. *The Journal of Investigative Dermatology*, *69*(3), 333–338. doi:10.1111/1523-1747.ep12507965 PMID:894075

Čoh, M., & Širok, B. (2007). Use of the thermovision method in sport training. *Physical Education and Sport.*, *5*(1), 85–94.

Collard, D. C., Verhagen, E. A., Van Mechelen, W., Heymans, M. W., & Chinapaw, M. J. (2011). Economic burden of physical activity–related injuries in Dutch children aged 10–12. *British Journal of Sports Medicine*, *45*(13), 1058–1063. doi:10.1136/bjsm.2010.082545 PMID:21685503

Collins, A. J., Ring, E. F., Bacon, P. A., & Brookshaw, J. D. (1976). Thermography and radiology: Complementary methods for the study of inflammatory diseases. *Clinical Radiology*, *27*(2), 237–243. doi:10.1016/S0009-9260(76)80153-5 PMID:1277739

Cooke, E. D., & Picher, M. F. (1974). Deep vein thrombosis: Preclinical diagnosis by thermography. *British Journal of Surgery*, *61*(12), 971–978. doi:10.1002/bjs.1800611212 PMID:4441818

Costello, J. T., McInerney, C. D., Bleakley, C. M., Selfe, J., & Donnelly, A. E. (2012). The use of thermal imaging in assessing skin temperature following cryotherapy: A review. *Journal of Thermal Biology*, *37*(2), 245–274. doi:10.1016/j.jtherbio.2011.11.008

Costello, J., Stewart, I. B., Selfe, J., Karki, A. I., & Donnelly, A. (2013). Use of thermal imaging in sports medicine research: A short report. *International Sportmed Journal*, *14*(2), 94–98.

Crandell, C. E., & Hill, R. P. (1966). Thermography in dentistry: A pilot study. *Oral Surgery, Oral Medicine, and Oral Pathology*, *21*(3), 316–320. doi:10.1016/0030-4220(66)90064 8 PMID:5216735

Criado, D., & Marston, M. (1995). Physiologic variation in lower extremity venous valvular function. *Annals of Vascular Surgery*, *9*(1), 102–108. doi:10.1007/BF02015323 PMID:7703053

Criado, F., & Marston, D. (1998). The role of air plethysmography in the diagnosis of chronic venous insufficiency. *Journal of Vascular Surgery*, *27*(4), 660–670. doi:10.1016/S0741-5214(98)70231-9 PMID:9576079

Cross, S. (2013). *Underwood's Pathology* (6th ed.). Elsevier Health Sciences.

Cutolo, M. (2010). *Atlas of capillaroscopy in rheumatic diseases*. Milan: Elsevier.

Cutolo, M., Sulli, A., & Smith, V. (2010). Assessing microvascular changes in systemic sclerosis diagnosis and management. *Nature Reviews. Rheumatology*, *6*(10), 578–587. doi:10.1038/nrrheum.2010.104 PMID:20703220

da Rosa Vieira, L., Zaro, M. A., Cervien, A., de Lara Peres, L. H., Mendonça de Moura, A., & Corvalão de Ávila, L. (2003). *Uso da Termografia como técnica auxiliar na recuperação de atletas*. Paper presented at the X Congresso Brasileiro de Biomecânica.

Da Silva, Navarro, & Batalheiro. (1992). The importance of chronic venous insufficiency: Various preliminary data on its medico-social consequences. *Phlebologie*, *45*, 439–443. PMID:1302319

David, J. M., Chatziioannou, A. F., Taschereau, R., Wang, H., & Stout, D. B. (2013). The hidden cost of housing practices: Using noninvasive imaging to quantify the metabolic demands of chronic cold stress of laboratory mice. *Comparative Medicine*, *63*(5), 386–391. PMID:24210014

Davison, Ewing, & Fergason. (1972). Detection of breast cancer by liquid crystal thermography: A preliminary report. *Cancer, 29*, 1123-1132.

De Cocq, P., Van Weeren, P. R., & Back, W. (2004). Effects of girth, saddle and weight on movements of the horse. *Equine Veterinary Journal, 36*(8), 758–763. doi:10.2746/0425164044848000 PMID:15656511

de Leeuw, R. (2008). *Orofacial pain: guidelines for assessment, diagnosis and management. The American Academy of Orofacial Pain* (4th ed.). Chicago, IL: Quintessence.

de Weerd, L., Mercer, J. B., & Setså, L. B. (2006). Intraoperative dynamic infrared thermography and free-flap surgery. *Annals of Plastic Surgery, 57*(3), 279–284. doi:10.1097/01.sap.0000218579.17185.c9 PMID:16929195

Decker, S., & Sausville, E. (2011). Perspectives on the History and Evolution of Tumor Models. In *Tumor Models in Cancer Research* (pp. 3–20). Humana Press. doi:10.1007/978-1-60761-968-0_1

Delahanty, D. D., & Georgi, J. R. (1965). Thermography in equine medicine. *Journal of the American Veterinary Medical Association, 147*, 235–238. PMID:14325456

Deng, Z. S., & Liu, J. (2004). Mathematical modeling of temperature mapping over skin surface and its implementation in thermal disease diagnostics. *Computers in Biology and Medicine, 34*(6), 495–521. doi:10.1016/S0010-4825(03)00086-6 PMID:15265721

Denoix, J. M. (1999). Spinal biomechanics and functional anatomy. *The Veterinary Clinics of North America. Equine Practice, 15*, 27–60. PMID:10218240

Devereaux, M., Parr, G., Lachmann, S., Page-Thomas, P., & Hazleman, B. (1986). Thermographic diagnosis in athletes with patellofemoral arthralgia. *Journal of Bone and Joint Surgery-(Br), 68*(1), 42-44.

Devereaux, M. D., Parr, G. R., Lachmann, S. M., Page-Thomas, P., & Hazleman, B. L. (1984). The diagnosis of stress fractures in athletes. *Journal of the American Medical Association, 252*(4), 531–533. doi:10.1001/jama.1984.03350040061027 PMID:6737649

Di Benedetto, M., Huston, C. W., Sharp, M. W., & Jones, B. (1996). Regional Hypothermia in Response to Minor Injury1. *American Journal of Physical Medicine & Rehabilitation, 75*(4), 270–277. doi:10.1097/00002060-199607000-00006 PMID:8777022

Di Maria, C., Allen, J., Dickinson, J., Neoh, C., & Perros, P. (2014). 2014 Novel thermal imaging analysis technique for detecting inflammation in thyroid eye disease. *The Journal of Clinical Endocrinology, 99*(12), 4600–4606. doi:10.1210/jc.2014-1957 PMID:25238202

Di Maria, C., Perros, P., Dickinson, J., & Allen, J. (2015). *Exploratory thermal and laser speckle contrast imaging measurements of eye inflammation in a case of thyroid eye disease. In Infrared imaging: A casebook in clinical medicine.* Institute of Physics Publishing.

Diakides, N. A., Diakides, M., Lupo, I., Paul, J., & Balcerak, R. (2013). Advances in Medical Infrared Imaging: An Update. In N. A. Diakides, M. Diakides, & J. D. Bronzino (Eds.), *Medical Infrared Imaging. Principles and practice. Boca Ratón* (pp. 1.1–1.14). CRC Press.

Diakow, P. R. (1992). Differentiation of active and latent trigger points by thermography. *Journal of Manipulative and Physiological Therapeutics, 15*(7), 439–441. PMID:1431631

Dibai-Filho, A. V., Packer, A. C., Costa, A. C., & Rodrigues-Bigaton, D. (2014). The chronicity of myogenous temporomandibular disorder changes the skin temperature over the anterior temporalis muscle. *Journal of Bodywork and Movement Therapies, 18*(3), 430–434. doi:10.1016/j.jbmt.2013.11.001 PMID:25042314

Dibai-Filho, A. V., Packer, A. C., Costa, A. C., & Rodrigues-Bigaton, D. (2015). Women with more severe degrees of temporomandibular disorder exhibit an increase in temperature over the temporomandibular joint. *The Saudi Dental Journal*, *27*(1), 44–49. doi:10.1016/j.sdentj.2014.10.002 PMID:25544814

Dragan & MILIC. (2011). Prevalence and socioeconomic data in chronic venous disease: How useful are they in planning appropriate management? *Medicographia*, *33*, 253.

Dranoff, G. (2012). Experimental mouse tumour models: What can be learnt about human cancer immunology? *Nature Reviews. Immunology*, *12*(1), 61–66. PMID:22134155

Dworkin, S. F., Huggins, K. H., LeResche, L., Von Korff, M., Howard, J., Truelove, E., & Sommers, E. (1990). Epidemiology of signs and symptoms in temporomandibular disorders: Clinical signs in cases and controls. *The Journal of the American Dental Association*, *120*(3), 273–281. doi:10.14219/jada.archive.1990.0043 PMID:2312947

Dworkin, S. F., & LeResche, L. (1992). Research diagnostic criteria for temporomandibular disorders: Review, criteria, examinations and specifications, critique. *Journal of Craniomandibular Disorders*, *6*(4), 301–355. PMID:1298767

Eberhardt, R. T. (2005). Chronic Venous Insufficiency. *Circulation*, *111*(18), 2398–2409. doi:10.1161/01.CIR.0000164199.72440.08 PMID:15883226

Eckert, R. (2002). Energiehaushalt-Auseinandersetzung mit den Anforderungen der Umwelt. In R. Eckert (Ed.), *Tierphysiologie* (pp. 767–840). Stuttgart: Georg-Thieme.

Eddy, A. L., van Hoogmoed, L. M., & Snyder, J. R. (2001). The role of thermography in the management of equine lameness. *Veterinary Journal (London, England)*, *162*(3), 172–181. doi:10.1053/tvjl.2001.0618 PMID:11681868

Einspahr, T., & Saboda, N. (2007). Expression of vascular endothelial growth factor in early cutaneous melanocytic lesion progression. *Cancer*, *110*(11), 2519–2527. doi:10.1002/cncr.23076 PMID:17932890

Eklund, L., Bry, M., & Alitalo, K. (2013). Mouse models for studying angiogenesis and lymphangiogenesis in cancer. *Molecular Oncology*, *7*(2), 259–282. doi:10.1016/j.molonc.2013.02.007 PMID:23522958

Estberg, L., Gardner, I. A., Stover, S. M., Johnson, B. J., Case, J. T., & Ardans, A. (1995). Cumulative racing – seed distance cluster as a risk factor for fatal musculoskeletal injury in Thoroughbred racehorses in California. *Preventive Veterinary Medicine*, *24*(4), 253–263. doi:10.1016/0167-5877(95)00489-J

Evans, G. P., Behiri, J. C., Vaughan, L. C., Vaughan, L. C., & Bonfield, W. (1992). The response of equine cortical bone to loading at strains rates experienced in vivo by the galloping horse. *Equine Veterinary Journal*, *24*(2), 125–128. doi:10.1111/j.2042-3306.1992.tb02796.x PMID:1582390

Farago, A. F., Snyder, E. L., & Jacks, T. (2012). SnapShot: Lung cancer models. *Cell*, *149*(1), 246–246. doi:10.1016/j.cell.2012.03.015 PMID:22464334

Farella, M., Michelotti, A., Steenks, M. H., Romeo, R., Cimino, R., & Bosman, F. (2000). The diagnostic value of pressure algometry in myofascial pain of the jaw muscles. *Journal of Oral Rehabilitation*, *27*(1), 9–14. doi:10.1046/j.1365-2842.2000.00526.x PMID:10632838

Faulkner, S. H., Ferguson, R. A., Gerrett, N., Hupperets, M., Hodder, S. G., & Havenith, G. (2013). Reducing muscle temperature drop after warm-up improves sprint cycling performance. *Medicine and Science in Sports and Exercise*, *45*(2), 359–365. doi:10.1249/MSS.0b013e31826fba7f PMID:22935735

Faustino-Rocha, A. I., Silva, A., Gabriel, J., da Costa, R. G., Moutinho, M., Oliveira, P. A., & Ginja, M. et al. (2016). Long-term exercise training as a modulator of mammary cancer vascularization. *Biomedicine and Pharmacotherapy*, *81*, 273–280. doi:10.1016/j.biopha.2016.04.030 PMID:27261604

Faustino-Rocha, A. I., Silva, A., Gabriel, J., Teixeira-Guedes, C. I., Lopes, C., da Costa, R. G., & Ginja, M. et al. (2013). Ultrasonographic, thermographic and histologic evaluation of MNU-induced mammary tumors in female Sprague-Dawley rats. *Biomedicine and Pharmacotherapy*, *67*(8), 771–776. doi:10.1016/j.biopha.2013.06.011 PMID:23906759

Fawcett, T. (2006). An introduction to ROC analysis. *Pattern Recognition Letters*, *27*(8), 861–874. doi:10.1016/j.patrec.2005.10.010

Fegan, W. G., & Beesley, W. H. (1970). An investigation into the localisation of incompetent perforating veins. *British Journal of Surgery*, *57*(1), 30–32. doi:10.1002/bjs.1800570106 PMID:5411584

Fernandes Ade, A., Amorim, P. R., Brito, C. J., de Moura, A. G., Moreira, D. G., & Costa, C. M. et al.. (2014). Measuring skin temperature before, during and after exercise: A comparison of thermocouples and infrared thermography. *Physiological Measurement*, *35*(2), 189–203. doi:10.1088/0967-3334/35/2/189 PMID:24398429

Fernandes, R., Billat, V., Cruz, A., Colaço, P., Cardoso, C., & Vilas-Boas, J. (2006). Does net energy cost of swimming affect time to exhaustion at the individual's maximal oxygen consumption velocity? *The Journal of Sports Medicine and Physical Fitness*, *46*(3), 373. PMID:16998440

Fernández Cuevas, I., Gómez Carmona, P. M., Sillero Quintana, M., Noya Salces, J., Arnaiz Lastras, J., & Pastor Barrón, A. (2010). *Economic costs estimation of soccer injuries in first and second spanish division professional teams.* Paper presented at the 15th Annual Congress of the European College of Sport Sciences ECSS, Antalya, Turkey.

Fernández Cuevas, I., Sillero Quintana, M., Gómez Carmona, P. M., García de la Concepción, M. Á., Piñonosa Cano, S., & Arnaiz Lastras, J. (2011). *Applications of Infrared Thermography as innovative technological solution in sports injuries.* Paper presented at the Science Based Prevention, Berlin, Germany.

Fernández-Cuevas, I. (2012). *Effect of endurance, speed and strength training on skin temperatura measured by Infrared Thermography.* Universidad Politécnica de Madrid. Retrieved from http://oa.upm.es/14896/2/ISMAEL_FERNANDEZ_CUEVAS.pdf

Fernández-Cuevas, Sillero-Quintana, Angel Garcia-Concepcion, Ribot Serrano, Gomez-Carmona, & Marins. (2014). Monitoring Skin Thermal Response to Training with Infrared Thermography. *New Studies in Athletics*, *29*(1), 57–71.

Fernández-Cuevas, I., Bouzas Marins, J. C., Arnáiz Lastras, J., Gómez Carmona, P. M., Piñonosa Cano, S., García-Concepción, M. Á., & Sillero-Quintana, M. (2015). Classification of factors influencing the use of infrared thermography in humans: A review. *Infrared Physics & Technology*, *71*(0), 28–55. doi:10.1016/j.infrared.2015.02.007

Ferreira, J. J., Mendonca, L. C., Nunes, L. A., Andrade Filho, A. C., Rebelatto, J. R., & Salvini, T. F. (2008). Exercise-associated thermographic changes in young and elderly subjects. *Annals of Biomedical Engineering*, *36*(8), 1420–1427. doi:10.1007/s10439-008-9512-1 PMID:18470619

Fillingim, R. B., Maixner, W., Kincaid, S., Sigurdsson, A., & Harris, M. B. (1996). Pain sensitivity in patients with temporomandibular disorders: Relationship to clinical and psychosocial factors. *The Clinical Journal of Pain*, *12*(4), 260–269. doi:10.1097/00002508-199612000-00005 PMID:8969871

Fischer, A.A. (1983). Advances in documentation of pain and soft tissue pathology. *J Fam Med*, 24–31.

Fischer, A. A. (1987). Pressure algometry over normal muscles. Standard values, validity and reproducibility of pressure threshold. *Pain*, *30*(1), 115–126. doi:10.1016/0304-3959(87)90089-3 PMID:3614975

Fischer, A. A. (1988). Documentation of myofascial trigger points. *Archives of Physical Medicine and Rehabilitation*, *69*(4), 286–291. PMID:3281631

Fischer, A. A. (1991). Muscle spasm: Documentation by thermography and by clinical methods. *Thermology*, *3*, 276.

Fischer, A. A. (1991a). Trigger points: Visualization by thermography. *Thermology*, *3*, 276.

Fischer, A. A., & Chang, C. H. (1986). Temperature and pressure threshold measurements in trigger points. *Thermology*, *1*, 212–215.

Fonseca, B. P. A., Alves, A. L. G., Nicoletti, J. L. M., Thomassian, A., Hussini, C. A., & Mikaik, S. (2006). Thermography and ultrasonography in back pain diagnosis of equine athletes. *Journal of Equine Veterinary Science*, *26*(11), 507–516. doi:10.1016/j.jevs.2006.09.007

Formenti, D., Ludwig, N., Gargano, M., Gondola, M., Dellerma, N., Caumo, A., & Alberti, G. (2013). Thermal Imaging of Exercise-Associated Skin Temperature Changes in Trained and Untrained Female Subjects. *Annals of Biomedical Engineering*, 1–9. PMID:23229282

Formenti, D., Ludwig, N., Gargano, M., Gondola, M., Dellerma, N., Caumo, A., & Alberti, G. (2013). Thermal imaging of exercise-associated skin temperature changes in trained and untrained female subjects. *Annals of Biomedical Engineering*, *41*(4), 863–871. doi:10.1007/s10439-012-0718-x PMID:23229282

Formenti, D., Ludwig, N., Trecroci, A., Gargano, M., Michielon, G., Caumo, A., & Alberti, G. (2016). Dynamics of thermographic skin temperature response during squat exercise at two different speeds. *Journal of Thermal Biology*, *59*, 58–63. doi:10.1016/j.jtherbio.2016.04.013 PMID:27264889

Fournet, D., Redortier, B., & Havenith, G. (2012). *A method for whole-body human skin temperature mapping.* Paper presented at the XII Congress EAT 2012, Porto, Portugal.

Fournet, D., Ross, L., Voelcker, T., Redortier, B., & Havenith, G. (2013). Body mapping of thermoregulatory and perceptual responses of males and females running in the cold. *Journal of Thermal Biology*, *38*(6), 339–344. doi:10.1016/j.jtherbio.2013.04.005

Fowkes, L., & Evans, A. (2001). Lifestyle risk factors for lower limb venous reflux in the general population: Edinburgh Vein Study. *International Journal of Epidemiology*, *30*(4), 846–852. doi:10.1093/ije/30.4.846 PMID:11511615

Frese, K. K., & Tuveson, D. A. (2007). Maximizing mouse cancer models. *Nature Reviews. Cancer*, *7*(9), 654–658. doi:10.1038/nrc2192 PMID:17687385

Friel, J. (2000). *The mountain biker's training bible.* VeloPress.

Fuller, C. W., Ekstrand, J., Junge, A., Andersen, T. E., Bahr, R., & Dvorak, J. et al.. (2006). Consensus statement on injury definitions and data collection procedures in studies of football (soccer) injuries. *Clinical Journal of Sport Medicine*, *16*(2), 97–106. doi:10.1097/00042752-200603000-00003 PMID:16603877

Fullerton, A., Stücker, M., Wilhelm, K. P., Wårdell, K., Anderson, C., Fischer, T., & Serup, J. et al. (2002). Guidelines for visualization of cutaneous blood flow by laser Doppler perfusion imaging. A report from the Standardization Group of the European Society of Contact Dermatitis based upon the HIRELADO European community project. *Contact Dermatitis*, *46*(3), 129–140. doi:10.1034/j.1600-0536.2002.460301.x PMID:12000320

Gage & Baust. (2002). Cryosurgery – a review of recent advances and current issues. *Cryo Letters*, *23*(2), 30–32. PMID:12050774

Gaivão, F. D. M., de Lima, J. P., Agostinho, A. G., Oliveira, A. S., & Peres, A. P. (2001). *Imagiologia Clínica-Princípios e Técnicas*. Academic Press.

Ganong. (2009). FizjologiaPZWL.

Garagiola, U., & Giani, E. (1991). Thermography: Description, Uses in Sports Medicine. Unpublished article by Encyclopedia of Sports Medicine and Science.

Garagiola, U., & Giani, E. (1990). Use of telethermography in the management of sports injuries. *Sports Medicine (Auckland, N.Z.)*, *10*(4), 267–272. doi:10.2165/00007256-199010040-00005 PMID:2247727

Garza, D., Rolston, B., Johnston, T., Sungar, G., Ferguson, J., & Matheson, G. (2008). *Heat-Loss Patterns in National Football League Players as Measured by Infrared Thermography.* Paper presented at the InfraMation.

Gascó-Gómez de Membrillera, J., Gascó-Adrien, J., & Barra-Pla, A. (2002). Conceptos básicos en Traumatología infantil. Epidemiología. Tratamiento cerrado de las fracturas. Tratamiento abierto de las fracturas. Remodelamiento de fracturas mal consolidadas. *Pediatría Integral*, *6*(6), 535–546.

Gasi, F., & Bittencourt, E. (2009). Evaluation of textile materials in physical activity. *Chemical Engineering Transactions*, *17*, 1783–1787.

Gelfand, S. B., Ravishankar, C. S., & Delp, E. J. (1991). An Iterative Growing and Pruning Algorithm for Classification Tree Design. *IEEE Transactions on Pattern Analysis and Machine Intelligence*, *13*(2), 163–174. doi:10.1109/34.67645

Gerwin, R. D., Dommerholt, J., & Shah, J. P. (2004). An expansion of Simons integrated hypothesis of trigger point formation. *Current Pain and Headache Reports*, *8*(6), 468–475. doi:10.1007/s11916-004-0069-x PMID:15509461

Giani, E., Rochi, L., Tavoni, A., Montanari, M., & Garagiola, U. (1989). Telethermographic evaluation of NSAIDs in the treatment of sports injuries. *Medicine and Science in Sports and Exercise*, *21*(1), 1–6. doi:10.1249/00005768-198902000-00001 PMID:2648105

Gloviczki, Comerota, Dalsing, Eklof, & Gillespie. (2011). The care of patients with varicose veins and associated chronic venous diseases: Clinical practice guidelines of the Society for Vascular Surgery and the American Venous Forum. *J Vasc Surg, 5*, 1S-48S.

Gold, J. E., Cherniack, M., Hanlon, A., & Soller, B. (2010). Skin temperature and muscle blood volume changes in the hand after typing. *International Journal of Industrial Ergonomics*, *40*(2), 161–164. doi:10.1016/j.ergon.2009.07.001

Gómez Carmona, P. M. (2012). *Influencia de la información termográfica infrarroja en el protocolo de prevención de lesiones de un equipo de fútbol profesional español.* Universidad Politécnica de Madrid. Retrieved from http://oa.upm.es/14694/2/PEDRO_MARIA_GOMEZ_CARMONA.pdf

Gómez Carmona, P. M., & Noya Salces, J. (2008). Prevención de lesiones en fútbol. *Training Fútbol,* (144), 36-46.

Gómez Carmona, P. M., & Sillero Quintana, M. (2009). *Termografía deportiva. I Curso básico de termografía como medio para la prevención y seguimiento de lesiones deportivas*. Madrid: pemaSIP. Facultad de Ciencias de la Actividad Física y del Deporte - INEF. Universidad Politécnica de Madrid.

Gómez Carmona, P. M., Sillero Quintana, M., Fernández Cuevas, I., Noya Salces, J., & Fernández Rodríguez, I. (2011). *Application of an injury prevention protocol based on infrared thermogrphy in professional soccer players during preseason.* Paper presented at the 24rd Thermological Symposium of the Austrian Society of Thermography "Quantitative Thermal Imaging in Medicine", Vienna, Austria.

Goodman, Murphy, Siltanen, Kelley, & Rucker. (1986). Normal temperature asymmetry of the back and extremities by computer-assisted infrared imaging. *Thermology, 1*, 195-202.

Goodman, P. H., Heaslet, M. W., Pagliano, J. W., & Rubin, B. D. (1985). Stress-fracture diagnosis by computer-assisted thermography. *The Physician and Sportsmedicine*, *13*(4), 114–132. doi:10.1080/00913847.1985.11708772 PMID:27421377

Goodman, P. H., Murphy, M. G., Siltanen, G. L., Kelley, M. P., & Rucker, M. (1986). Norman Temperature Asymmetry of the Back and Extremities by Computer-Assisted Infrared Imaging. *Thermology*, *1*, 195–202.

Goraj, M. (2015). *Applications of thermal imaging in energy cost rating during training* (Master's Thesis). A. Chełkowski Institute of Physics, University of Silesia Katowice Poland.

Góralczyk, Mikuła, & Jagodzińska. (2002). Osteoarthritis. Choroba zwyrodnieniowa stawów. *Medycyna Rodzinna*, *10*, 2.

Gordon, C. J. (2012). Thermal physiology of laboratory mice: Defining thermoneutrality. *Journal of Thermal Biology*, *37*(8), 654–685. doi:10.1016/j.jtherbio.2012.08.004

Gorodkin, R., Moore, T., & Herrick, A. (2004). Assessment of endothelial function in complex regional pain syndrome type I using iontophoresis and laser Doppler imaging. *Rheumatology (Oxford, England)*, *43*(6), 727–730. doi:10.1093/rheumatology/keh158 PMID:15026582

Górski, J. (2010). *Fizjologia Człowieka*. Warszawa: PZWL.

Gratt, B. M., & Anbar, M. (1998). Thermology and facial telethermography: Part II. Current and future clinical applications in dentistry. *Dento Maxillo Facial Radiology*, *27*(2), 68–74. doi:10.1038/sj.dmfr.4600324 PMID:9656869

Gratt, B. M., Graff-Radford, S. B., Shetty, V., Solberg, W. K., & Sickles, E. A. (1996). A 6-year clinical assessment of electronic facial thermography. *Dento Maxillo Facial Radiology*, *25*(5), 247–255. doi:10.1259/dmfr.25.5.9161178 PMID:9161178

Gratt, B. M., Pullinger, A., Sickles, E. A., & Lee, J. J. (1989). Electronic thermography of normal facial structures: A pilot study. *Oral Surgery, Oral Medicine, and Oral Pathology*, *68*(3), 346–351. doi:10.1016/0030-4220(89)90222-3 PMID:2771378

Gratt, B. M., & Sickles, E. A. (1993). Thermographic characterization of the asymptomatic temporomandibular joint. *Journal of Orofacial Pain*, *7*(1), 7–14. PMID:8467300

Gratt, B. M., & Sickles, E. A. (1995). Electronic facial thermography: An analysis of asymptomatic adult subjects. *Journal of Orofacial Pain*, *9*(3), 255–265. PMID:8995925

Gratt, B. M., Sickles, E. A., Ross, J. B., Wexler, C. E., & Gornbein, J. A. (1994). Thermographic assessment of craniomandibular disorders: Diagnostic interpretation versus temperature measurement analysis. *Journal of Orofacial Pain*, *8*(3), 278–288. PMID:7812225

Green, R. J., Endersby, S., Allen, J., & Adams, J. (2014). Role of medical thermography in treatment of Freys syndrome with botulinum toxin A. Short Communication. *The British Journal of Oral & Maxillofacial Surgery*, *52*(1), 90–92. doi:10.1016/j.bjoms.2013.09.013 PMID:24238875

Gregorowicz & Dalidowski. (1998). Cryotherapy In Sclerosis Multiplex (Sm) Treatment Acta Bio-Opt. *Inform. Med.*, *4*(4), 173 – 174.

Gregorowicz. (1992). *The influence of whole body cryotherapy on chosen haemodynamic and lungs ventilation markers in rheumatoid diseases*. Praca Doktorska AM.

Gregorowiczv & Zagrobelny. (1998). Whole body cryotherapy, indications and contraindications, treatment and its physiological and clinical effects. Acta Bio-Optica et Informatica Media, 4, 120-131.

Grossfeld, G. D., Ginsberg, D. A., Stein, J. P., Bochner, B. H., Esrig, D., Nichols, P. W., & Cote, R. J. et al. (1997). Thrombospondin-1 expression in bladder cancer: Association with p53 alterations, tumor angiogenesis, and tumor progression. *Journal of the National Cancer Institute*, *89*(3), 219–227. doi:10.1093/jnci/89.3.219 PMID:9017002

Guex, Myon, & Didier, Nguyen Le, & Taieb. (2005). Chronic venous disease: Health status of a population and care impact on this health status through quality of life questionnaires. *International Angiology*, *24*, 258–264. PMID:16158036

Guex, Z., & Boussetta, N. L. (2007). Construction and validation of a patient reported outcome dedicated to chronic venous disorder: SQOR-V (Specific Quality of Life and Outcome Response-Venous). *Journal des Maladies Vasculaires*, *32*(3), 135–137. doi:10.1016/j.jmv.2007.05.004 PMID:17616292

Guyton, A. C. (2006). *Body temperature, temperature regulation and fever. In Textbook of medical physiology* (11th ed.; pp. 822–833). W.B. Saunders Company.

Haddad, D. S. (2001). *Correlação clínica e termográfica do ponto-gatilho miofascial nos músculos da mastigação* (dissertação). São Paulo: Universidade de São Paulo, Faculdade de Odontologia.

Haddad, D. S., Brioschi, M. L., & Arita, E. S. (2012). Thermographic and clinical correlation of myofascial trigger points in the masticatory muscles. *Dento Maxillo Facial Radiology*, *41*(8), 621–629. doi:10.1259/dmfr/98504520 PMID:23166359

Haddad, D. S., Brioschi, M. L., Vardasca, R., Weber, M., Crosato, E. M., & Arita, E. S. (2014). Thermographic characterization of masticatory muscle regions in volunteers with and without myogenous temporomandibular disorder: Preliminary results. *Dento Maxillo Facial Radiology*, *43*(8), 20130440. doi:10.1259/dmfr.20130440 PMID:25144605

Hagglund, M., Walden, M., & Ekstrand, J. (2003). Exposure and injury risk in Swedish elite football: A comparison between seasons 1982 and 2001. *Scandinavian Journal of Medicine & Science in Sports*, *13*(6), 364–370. doi:10.1046/j.1600-0838.2003.00327.x PMID:14617057

Hall, J., Bramlage, L. R., Kantrwitz, B. M., Page, L., & Simpson, B. (1987). Correlation between contact thermography and ultrasonography in the evaluation of experimentally – induced superficial flexor tendonitis.*Proceedings of the American Association of Equine Practitioners*, *38*, 429-431.

Hanahan, D., Wagner, E. F., & Palmiter, R. D. (2007). The origins of oncomice: A history of the first transgenic mice genetically engineered to develop cancer. *Genes & Development*, *21*(18), 2258–2270. doi:10.1101/gad.1583307 PMID:17875663

Hansen, K., & Khanna, C. (2004). Spontaneous and genetically engineered animal models: Use in preclinical cancer drug development. *European Journal of Cancer*, *40*(6), 858–880. doi:10.1016/j.ejca.2003.11.031 PMID:15120042

Harada, K., Katz, M. L., & Comerota, A. (1995). A non-invasive screening test to detect critical deep venous reflux. *Journal of Vascular Surgery*, *22*(5), 532–537. doi:10.1016/S0741-5214(95)70033-1 PMID:7494351

Harding. (1995). Liquid crystal thermography in the investigation of deep venous thrombosis: A prospective study of 800 patients. In *The Thermal Image in Medicine and Biology*. Uhlen Verlag.

Harding. (1995). Thermal imaging in the investigation of deep venous thrombosis. *Proceedings of the 1995 IEEE Engineering in Medicine and Biology conference and 21st Canadian Medica/and Biological Engineering Conference.*

Harman, J. C. (1999). Tack and saddle fit. In S. Turner & K. K. Haussler (Eds.), *Veterinary Clinics of North American Equine Practice: Back Problems* (pp. 247–261). Philadelphia: W.B. Saunders Company.

Harshaw, C., Culligan, J. J., & Alberts, J. R. (2014). Sex differences in thermogenesis structure behavior and contact within huddles of infant mice. *PLoS ONE*, *9*(1), e87405. doi:10.1371/journal.pone.0087405 PMID:24498099

Hashida, Y., Tanaka, H., Zhou, S., Kawakami, S., Yamashita, F., Murakami, T., & Hashida, M. et al. (2014). Photothermal ablation of tumor cells using a single-walled carbon nanotube–peptide composite. *Journal of Controlled Release*, *173*, 59–66. doi:10.1016/j.jconrel.2013.10.039 PMID:24211651

Hassan, M., Chernomordik, V., Vogel, A., Hattery, D., Gannot, I., Little, R., & Yarchoan, R. (2007). Infrared imaging for functional monitoring of disease processes. In N. A. Diakides & J. D. Bronzino (Eds.), *Medical Infrared Imaging. Principles and practice* (pp. 14.11–14.28). Taylor & Francis.

Haussler, K. K., Stover, S. M., & Willits, N. H. (1999). Pathology of the lumbosacral spine and pelvis in Thoroughbred racehorses. *American Journal of Veterinary Research*, *60*(2), 143–153. PMID:10048543

Head, J. F., & Elliott, R. L. (2002). Infrared imaging: Making progress in fulfilling its medical promise. *Engineering in Medicine and Biology Magazine, IEEE*, *21*(6), 80–85. doi:10.1109/MEMB.2002.1175142 PMID:12613215

Head, J., & Dyson, S. (2001). Taking the temperature of equine thermography. *Veterinary Journal (London, England)*, *162*(3), 166–167. doi:10.1053/tvjl.2001.0639 PMID:11681865

Head, M. J. (2009). Back pathology in racehorses. In F. M. D. Henson (Ed.), *Equine back pathology* (pp. 213–222). Wiley-Blackwell.

Herrick, A. (2008). Diagnosis and management of scleroderma peripheral vascular disease. *Rheumatic Disease Clinics of North America, 34*, 89-114.

Herrick, A. L., & Clark, S. (1998). Quantifying digital vascular disease in patients with primary Raynauds phenomenon and systemic sclerosis. *Annals of the Rheumatic Diseases*, *57*(2), 70–78. doi:10.1136/ard.57.2.70 PMID:9613334

Hess. (2005). Identifying and managing venous dermatitis. *Adv Skin Wound Care., 18*(5), 42-3.

Hildebrandt, C. (2009). *Medical infrared thermography as a screening tool for knee injuries in professional junior alpine-ski-racers in Austria - Findings of a pilot study*. Paper presented at the 14th annual ECSS Congress.

Hildebrandt, C., Zeilberger, K., Ring, E. F. J., & Raschner, C. (2012). The Application of Medical Infrared Thermography in Sports Medicine. In An International Perspective on Topics in Sports Medicine and Sports Injury. doi:10.5772/28383

Hildebrandt, C., Raschner, C., & Ammer, K. (2010). An overview of recent application of medical infrared thermography in sports medicine in Austria. *Sensors (Basel, Switzerland)*, *10*(5), 4700–4715. doi:10.3390/s100504700 PMID:22399901

Hirata, K., Nagasaka, T., & Noda, Y. (1989). Venous return from distal regions affects heat loss from the arms and legs during exercise-induced thermal loads. *European Journal of Applied Physiology and Occupational Physiology*, *58*(8), 865–872. doi:10.1007/BF02332220 PMID:2767068

Hoffman & Bischo. (2002). The cryobiology of cryosurgical injury. *Urology, 60*(2), 40-49.

Hoffmann, A., Dumke, C., Bernau, M., Krämer, P., Scholz, A., Balks, E., & Cußler, K. et al. (2014). Thermal imaging - alternative concepts for refinement and reduction of animal use for testing of biologicals. In *Proceedings of the 9th World Congress on Alternatives and Animal Use in Life Sciences.*

Howell, K. J., & Smith, R. E. (2009). Guidelines for specifying and testing a thermal camera for medical applications. *Thermology International, 19*, 5-12.

Howell, K. J., Lavorato, A., Visentin, M. T., Smith, R. E., Schaefer, G., Jones, C. D., & Woo, P. et al. (2009). Validation of a protocol for the assessment of skin temperature and blood flow in childhood localised scleroderma. *Skin Research and Technology*, *15*(3), 346–356. doi:10.1111/j.1600-0846.2009.00371.x PMID:19624432

Hoy, K., Lindblad, B. E., Terkelsen, C. J., Helleland, H. E., & Terkelsen, C. J. (1992). European soccer injuries. A prospective epidemiologic and socioeconomic study. *The American Journal of Sports Medicine*, *20*(3), 318–322. doi:10.1177/036354659202000314 PMID:1636863

Hrycaj & Łącki. (2002). Od zwyrodnienia do zapalenia – współczesne poglądy na patogenezę choroby zwyrodnieniowej stawów. *Nowa Medycyna*, (2), 115.

Hug, A. M., Schmidts, T., Kuhlmann, J., Segger, D., Fotopoulos, G., & Heinzerling, J. (2012). Skin hydration and cooling effect produced by the Voltaren® vehicle gel. *Skin Research and Technology*, *18*(2), 199–206. doi:10.1111/j.1600-0846.2011.00554.x PMID:22092669

Hulbert & Else. (2004). Basal Metabolic Rate: History, Composition, Regulation and Usefulness. *Physiol Biochem Zool.*, *77*(6), 869-76.

Hunold, S., Mietzsch, E., & Werner, J. (1992). Thermographic studies on patterns of skin temperature after exercise. *European Journal of Applied Physiology and Occupational Physiology*, *65*(6), 550–554. doi:10.1007/BF00602364 PMID:1483445

Hynes, A., Scott, D. A., Man, A., Singer, D. L., Sowa, M. G., & Liu, K. Z. (2005). Molecular mapping of periodontal tissues using infrared microspectroscopy. *BMC Medical Imaging*, *5*(1), 2. doi:10.1186/1471-2342-5-2 PMID:15890072

Iacobuzio-Donahue, C. A. (2009). Epigenetic changes in cancer. *Annual Review of Pathological Mechanical Disease*, *4*(1), 229–249. doi:10.1146/annurev.pathol.3.121806.151442 PMID:18840073

Iglesias-Gutierrez, D. (2014). *Respuesta térmica del jugador de fútbol ante cuatro formatos diferentes de entrenamiento interválico de alta intensidad.* Trabajo Final de Master. Madrid: Facultad de Ciencias de la Actividad Física y del Deporte (INEF). Universidad Politécnica de Madrid. Retrieved from https://drive.google.com/file/d/0B7FrjSgoogHVa1FseWtXWnE3b0k/edit?usp=sharing

Inklaar, H. (1994). Soccer injuries. I: Incidence and severity. *Sports Medicine (Auckland, N.Z.)*, *18*(1), 55–73. doi:10.2165/00007256-199418010-00006 PMID:7939040

Jaeger, B., & Reeves, J. L. (1986). Quantification of changes in myofascial trigger point sensitivity with the pressure algometer following passive stretch. *Pain*, *27*(2), 203–210. doi:10.1016/0304-3959(86)90211-3 PMID:3797015

Jagodziński, Kubacka, & Wiśniowska, Puszer, & Stanek. (2001). Whole Body Cryotherapy Part 1 Priv.[In Polish]. *Cab*, *4*(92), 10–11.

Jagodziński, S., & Gmyrek, C. (2007). Evaluation of whole - body cryotherapy on the circulatory system in patients with ankylosing spondylitis by analysis of duration and QT interval dispertion. *Fizjoterapia Polska*, *7*(3), 362–369.

Jasemian, Y., Gazerani, P., & Dagnaes-Hansen, F. (2012). Infrared thermography in serotonin-induced itch model in rats. *Open Dermatology Journal*, *6*(1), 1–7. doi:10.2174/1874372201206010001

Jazienicka, Pietrzak, & Toruniowi. (1991). New indications for cryotherapy. *Przeglad Dermatologiczny*, *78*(3), 190–194.

Jeffcott, L. B. (1999). Historical perspective and clinical indications. *The Veterinary Clinics of North America. Equine Practice*, *15*(1), 1–12. PMID:10218238

Jeffcott, L. B., Dalin, G., Ekman, S., & Olsson, S.-E. (1985). Sacroiliac lesions as a cause of chronic poor performance in competitive horses. *Equine Veterinary Journal*, *17*(2), 111–118. doi:10.1111/j.2042-3306.1985.tb02063.x PMID:3987658

Jeffcott, L. B., Rossdale, P. D., Freestone, J., Frank, C. J., & Towers-Clark, P. F. (1982). An assessment of wastage in Thoroughbred racing from conception to 4 years of age. *Equine Veterinary*, *14*(3), 185–198. doi:10.1111/j.2042-3306.1982.tb02389.x PMID:7106081

Jiang, L. J., Ng, E. Y. K., Yeo, A. C. B., Wu, S., Pan, F., Yau, W. Y., & Yang, Y. et al. (2005). A perspective on medical infrared imaging. *Journal of Medical Engineering & Technology*, *29*(6), 257–267. doi:10.1080/03091900512331333158 PMID:16287675

Jiménez-Balderas & Mintz. (1993). Ankylosing Spondylitis: Clinical Course In Women And Men. *J Rheumatol, 20*(12), 2069–72.

Jochimsen, P. R., Folk, G. E., Sundell, M., & Loh, P. M. (1986). B16 melanoma in hairless mice: A model for thermographic research. *Journal of Surgical Oncology*, *33*(1), 50–52. doi:10.1002/jso.2930330114 PMID:3762175

Jodkowska, E. (2005). Temperatura powierzchni ciała jako kryterium predyspozycji wysiłkowych konia. Zeszyty Naukowe Akademii Rolniczej nr 511, Wroclaw.

Jodkowska, E., Dudek, K., & Bek-Kaczkowska, I. (2001). Wpływ treningu wyścigowego na temperaturę powierzchni ciała koni różnych ras. *Roczniki Naukowe Zootechniki*, *14*, 63–72.

Johansson, A., Kopp, S., & Haraldson, T. (1985). Reproducibility and variation of skin surface temperature over the temporomandibular joint and masseter muscle in normal individuals. *Acta Odontologica Scandinavica*, *43*(5), 309–313. doi:10.3109/00016358509046513 PMID:3866482

John, M. T., Dworkin, S. F., & Mancl, L. A. (2005). Reliability of clinical temporomandibular disorder diagnoses. *Pain*, *118*(1-2), 61–69. doi:10.1016/j.pain.2005.07.018 PMID:16154702

Johnston, S., Schoenfeld, P., Mysore, J. V., & Dubois, A. (1999, July). Endoscopic spray cryotherapy: a new technique for mucosal ablation in the esophagus. *Gastrointestinal Endoscopy*, *50*(1), 86–92. doi:10.1016/S0016-5107(99)70352-4 PMID:10385730

Jonderko. (1990). Current state of knowledge about the application of cryotherapy for treatment of musculoskeletal diseases. *Chir Narzadow Ruchu Ortop Pol, 55*, 31-5.

Jones, B. F. (1998). A reappraisal of the use of infrared thermal image analysis in medicine. *Medical Imaging. IEEE Transactions on*, *17*(6), 1019–1027. doi:10.1109/42.746635

Jones, B. F., & Plassmann, P. (2002). Digital infrared thermal imaging of human skin. *IEEE Engineering in Medicine and Biology Magazine*, *21*(6), 41–48. doi:10.1109/MEMB.2002.1175137 PMID:12613210

Jonkers, J., & Berns, A. (2005). *Animal models of cancer: Introduction to the cellular and molecular biology of cancer*. Oxford University Press.

Jung, Z., & Kalicki, M. (2015). Thermal imaging in the screening diagnosis of crural varices in adolescents. In F. Ring, A. Jung, & J. Zuber (Eds.), Infrared Imaging. A casebook in clinical medicine. IOP Publishing.

Junge, A., Rosch, D., Peterson, L., Graf-Baumann, T., & Dvorak, J. (2002). Prevention of soccer injuries: A prospective intervention study in youth amateur players. *The American Journal of Sports Medicine*, *30*(5), 652–659. PMID:12238997

Kalodiki, Calahoras, & Geroulakos. (1995). Liquid crystal thermography and duplex in the preoperative marking of varicose veins. *Phlebology*, *10*, 110–114.

Kamida, Eklof, & Masuda. (2001). Lower extremity ascending and descending venography. In Handbook of Venous Disorders (2nd ed.). New York, NY: Arnold.

Kane, A. J., Trau, J., Dargatz, B., Losinger, W. C., & Carber, L. P. (2000). The occurrence and causes of lameness and laminitis in the US horse population. *Procedure of the Annual Convention of the American Association of Equine Practitioners, 46*, 277-280.

Kaplan, C., & Denenberg, B. (2003). Quality of life in patients with chronic venous disease: San Diego population study. *Journal of Vascular Surgery*, *37*(5), 1047–1053. doi:10.1067/mva.2003.168 PMID:12756353

Kasprzyk, T. (2014). *The thermal imaging of sportsmen body surface. The influence of training cycle at organism metabolism* (Master's Thesis). A. Chełkowski Institute of Physics, University of Silesia Katowice Poland.

Kasprzyk, Wójcik, Cholewka, Sieroń-Stołtny, Piętka, Drzazga, & Stanek. (2015). *The applications of thermal imaging in energy cost rating during Aerobic Circuit Training*. QIRT.

Kass, G. V. (1980). An Exploratory Technique for Investigating Large Quantities of Categorical Data. *Journal of Applied Statistics*, *29*(2), 119–127. doi:10.2307/2986296

Katz, L. M., Nauriyal, V., Nagaraj, S., Finch, A., Pearlstein, K., Szymanowski, A., & Pearlstein, R. D. et al. (2008). Infrared imaging of trauma patients for detection of acute compartment syndrome of the leg. *Critical Care Medicine*, *36*(6), 1756–1761. doi:10.1097/CCM.0b013e318174d800 PMID:18496371

Kawano, W., Kawazoe, T., Tanaka, M., & Hikida, Y. (1993). Deep thermometry of temporomandibular joint and masticatory muscle regions. *The Journal of Prosthetic Dentistry*, *69*(2), 216–221. doi:10.1016/0022-3913(93)90143-C PMID:8429516

Keegan, K. G., Wilson, D. A., Smith, B. K., & Wilson, D. J. (2000). Changes in kinematic variables observed during pressure induced forelimb lameness in adult horses trotting on a treadmill. *American Journal of Veterinary Research*, *61*(6), 612–619. doi:10.2460/ajvr.2000.61.612 PMID:10850834

Keith, L. E., Thomas, W. D., & Ferganson, J. L. (1973). Effects of activity, alcohol, smoking, and the menstrual cycle on liquid crystal breast thermography. *The Ohio Journal of Science*, *73*, 55–58.

Kerschan-Schindl, Uher, Zauner-Dungl, & Fialka-Moser. (1998). V Cold And Cryotherapy. A Review Of The Literature On General Principles And Practical Applications Acta Med. *Austriaca, 25*(3), 73 – 8.

Keyl, W., & Lenhart, P. (1975). Die Thermographie bei Sportverletzungen und Sportschäden des Bewegungsapparates. *Fortschritte der Medizin*, *23*(93), 124–126. PMID:1173237

Knab, A. M., Shanely, R. A., Corbin, K. D., Jin, F., Sha, W., & Nieman, D. C. (2011). A 45-minute vigorous exercise bout increases metabolic rate for 14 hours. *Medicine and Science in Sports and Exercise*, *43*(9), 1643–1648. doi:10.1249/MSS.0b013e3182118891 PMID:21311363

Knight. (1995). *Cryotherapy in sport injury management*. Human Kinetics.

Kold, S. E., & Chappell, K. A. (1998). Use of computerized thermographic image analysis (CTIA) in equine orthopedics: Review and presentation of clinical cases. *Equine Veterinary Education*, *10*(4), 198–204. doi:10.1111/j.2042-3292.1998.tb00877.x

Kolosovas-Machuca, E. S., & González, F. J. (2011). Distribution of skin temperature in Mexican children. *Skin Research and Technology*, *17*(3), 326–331. doi:10.1111/j.1600-0846.2011.00501.x PMID:21338404

Konerding, M. A., & Steinberg, F. (1988). Computerized infrared thermography and ultrastructural studies of xenotransplanted human tumors on nude mice. *Thermology*, *3*(1), 7–14.

Kontos, M., Wilson, R., & Fentiman, I. (2011). Digital infrared thermal imaging (DITI) of breast lesions: Sensitivity and specificity of detection of primary breast cancers. *Clinical Radiology*, *66*(6), 536–539. doi:10.1016/j.crad.2011.01.009 PMID:21377664

Korman, P., Straburzyńska-Lupa, A., Kusy, K., Kantanista, A., & Zieliński, J. (2016). Changes in body surface temperature during speed endurance work-out in highly-trained male sprinters. *Infrared Physics & Technology*, *78*, 209–213. doi:10.1016/j.infrared.2016.08.003

Korzonek-Szlacheta, Wielkoszynski, & Stanek. (2007). Influence of whole - body cryotherapy on the levels of some hormones in professional footballers. *Endokrynologia Polska*, *58*(1), 27–32. PMID:17354202

Kozielski & Ziora. (1997). Bronchoscopic cryotherapy. *Pneumonologia i Alergologia Polska*, *65*(5-6), 411–416. PMID:9340073

Kruse, R. A., & Christiansen, J. A. (1992). Thermographic imaging of myofascial trigger points: A follow-up study. *Archives of Physical Medicine and Rehabilitation*, *73*(9), 819–823. PMID:1514891

Księżpolska-Pietrzak. (1998). Krioterapia W Osteoporozie: Polski Merkuriusz Lekarski, D.[In Polish]. *Polski Tygodnik Lekarski*, *28*, 222–224.

Księżpolska-Pietrzak, Cygler, Lesiak, & Noniewicz. (1993). The Influence Of Low Temperature Treatment On Reumatoid Arm. *Reumatologia*, *31*(2), 179–183.

Kulesza, O., Rzeczkowski, M., & Kaczorowski, M. (2004). Thermography and its practical use in equine diagnostics and treatment. *Medycyna Weterynaryjna*, *60*(11), 1143–1146.

Kumar, N., Allen, J., Murray, A., & Griffiths, B. (2006). The assessment of single dose Sildenafil Citrate (Viagra) in the treatment of Raynaud's phenomenon in patients with systemic sclerosis. *The Journal of Rheumatology*, *33*, 1918–1919. PMID:16960964

Kurz, Kahn, & Abenhaim. (1999). Chronic venous disorders of the leg: epidemiology, outcomes, diagnosis and management: summary of an evidence-based report of the VEINES task force. *International Angiology*, *18*, 83–102. PMID:10424364

Labropolous, T. (2003). Definition of venous reflux in lower extremity veins. *Journal of Vascular Surgery*, *38*(4), 793–798. doi:10.1016/S0741-5214(03)00424-5 PMID:14560232

LaForgia, J., Withers, R. T., & Gore, C. J. (2006). Effects of exercise intensity and duration on the excess post-exercise oxygen consumption. *Journal of Sports Sciences*, *24*(12), 1247–1264. doi:10.1080/02640410600552064 PMID:17101527

Lafuma, Fagnani, Peltier-Pujol, & Rauss. (1994). Venous disease in France: An unrecognized public health problem[in French]. *Journal des Maladies Vasculaires*, *19*, 185–189. PMID:7798803

Lahiri, B. B., Bagavathiappan, S., Jayakumar, T., & Philip, J. (2012). Medical applications of infrared thermography: A review. *Infrared Physics & Technology*, *55*(4), 221–235. doi:10.1016/j.infrared.2012.03.007

Landin, L. A. (1997). Epidemiology of childrens fractures. *Journal of Pediatric Orthopaedics. Part B*, *6*(2), 79–83. doi:10.1097/01202412-199704000-00002 PMID:9165435

Larsen, R. (2010). *Anestezjologia, t. 1*. Elsevier Urban &Partner.

Lasanen, R., Julkunen, P., Airaksinen, O., & Töyräs, J. (2016). Menthol concentration in topical cold gel does not have significant effect on skin cooling. *Skin Research and Technology*, *22*(1), 40–45. doi:10.1111/srt.12226 PMID:25773465

Latif, S. N., Von Peinen, K., Wiestner, T., Bitschnau, C., Renk, B., & Weishaupt, M. A. (2010). Saddle pressure patterns of three different training saddles (normal tree, flexible tree, treeless) in Thoroughbred racehorses at trot and gallop. *Equine Veterinary Journal*, *42*(38), 630–636. doi:10.1111/j.2042-3306.2010.00237.x PMID:21059072

Lauer, J., Figueiredo, P., Vilas-Boas, J. P., Fernandes, R. J., & Rouard, A. H. (2013). Phase-dependence of elbow muscle coactivation in front crawl swimming. *Journal of Electromyography and Kinesiology*, *23*(4), 820–825. doi:10.1016/j.jelekin.2013.02.004 PMID:23489716

Laurikka, S., & Tarkka, A. (2002). Risk indicators for varicose veins in forty to sixty-year-olds in the Tampere varicose vein study. *World Journal of Surgery*, *26*(6), 648–651. doi:10.1007/s00268-001-0283-1 PMID:12053212

Lawson, R. N. (1956). Implications of surface temperatures in the diagnosis of breast cancer. *Canadian Medical Association Journal*, *75*(4), 309–311. PMID:13343098

Leonardi, R., Zaborra, G., Li Pera, A. M., & Tripi, T. R. (1991). Comparison of telethermography and electromyography in instrumental symptomologic evaluation of the anterior temporalis and the masseter.[In Italian.]. *Stomatologia Mediterranea*, *11*(1), 5–10. PMID:1871658

Leppaluto, W. (2008). Effect of long-term whole-body cold exposures on plasma concentrations of ACTH, beta-endorphin, cortisol, catecholamines and cytokines in healthy females. *Scandinavian Journal of Clinical and Labolatory Investstigation*, *68*(2), 145–153. doi:10.1080/00365510701516350

Levet, A., Martens, L., Devisscher, L., Duchateur, L., Bogaert, L., & Vlamink, L. (2009). Distal limb cast sores in horses: Risk factors and early detection using thermography. *Equine Veterinary Journal*, *41*(1), 18–23. doi:10.2746/042516408X343046 PMID:19301577

Lewin, G. (1989). The incidence of injuries in an English professional soccer club during one competitive season. *Physiotherapy*, *75*(10), 601–605. doi:10.1016/S0031-9406(10)62366-8

Lima, J. J. D. (2011). *Nuclear Medicine Physics. Series in Medical Physics and Biomedical Engineering*. Taylor and Francis.

Lima, J. J. P. D. (1995). *Física dos métodos de imagem com raios X*. Coimbra: Edições ASA.

Liu, Y., Mimura, K., Wang, L., & Ikuda, K. (2003). Physiological benefits of 24-style Taijiquan exercise in middle-aged women. *Journal of Physiological Anthropology and Applied Human Science*, *22*(5), 219–225. doi:10.2114/jpa.22.219 PMID:14519910

Loi, M., Di Paolo, D., Becherini, P., Zorzoli, A., Perri, P., Carosio, R., & Ponzoni, M. et al. (2011). The use of the orthotopic model to validate antivascular therapies for cancer. *The International Journal of Developmental Biology*, *55*(4-5), 547–555. doi:10.1387/ijdb.103230ml PMID:21858775

Lopalco, P.L, Johansen, K., Ciancio, B., De Carvalho Gomes, H., Kramarz, P., Giesecke, J. (2010). Monitoring and assessing vaccine safety: A European perspective. *Expert Rev Vaccines, 9*(4), 371-80. doi: Group10.1586/erv.10.20.EMA-Vacc-

Ludwig, N., Formenti, D., Gargano, M., & Alberti, G. (2014). Skin temperature evaluation by infrared thermography: Comparison of image analysis methods. *Infrared Physics & Technology*, *62*(0), 1–6. doi:10.1016/j.infrared.2013.09.011

MacEwen, E. G. (1990). Spontaneous tumors in dogs and cats: Models for the study of cancer biology and treatment. *Cancer and Metastasis Reviews*, *9*(2), 125–136. doi:10.1007/BF00046339 PMID:2253312

Magnan, B., Bondi, M., Pierantoni, S., & Samaila, E. (2014). The pathogenesis of Achilles tendinopathy: A systematic review. *Foot and Ankle Surgery*, *20*(3), 154–159. doi:10.1016/j.fas.2014.02.010 PMID:25103700

Magnusson, L. E. (1985). *Studies on the conformation and related traits of the Standardbred Trotters in Sweden. Relationship between conformation and soundness in four year old Standardbred Trotters. Swedish University of Agricultural Sciences*. Skara.

Mair, S. D., Seaber, A. V., Glisson, R. R., & Garrett, W. E. Jr. (1996). The role of fatigue in susceptibility to acute muscle strain injury. *The American Journal of Sports Medicine*, *24*(2), 137–143. doi:10.1177/036354659602400203 PMID:8775109

Maksymowicz, Dudek, & Bauer, Jurek, & Drozd. (2007). Assessment of the possibilities of applications of the thermovision technique in medico-legal diagnosis. *Annales Academiae Medicae Stetinensis*, *53*(suppl. 2), 102–106. PMID:20143690

Malkinson, T. J. (2002). *Skin temperature response during cycle ergometry.* Paper presented at the Electrical and Computer Engineering.

Mao, A., Luo, J., Li, Y., Luo, X., & Wang, R. (2011). A multi-disciplinary strategy for computer-aided clothing thermal engineering design. *Computer Aided Design*, *43*(12), 1854–1869. doi:10.1016/j.cad.2011.06.009

Maraso, B., Gai, G., & Massaglia, O. (1998). Radiofrequency resection of bronchial tumours in combination with cryotherapy: Evaluation of a new technique. *Thorax*, *53*(2), 106–109. doi:10.1136/thx.53.2.106 PMID:9624294

Marins, J. C. B., Fernandes, A. A., Cano, S. P., Moreira, D. G., da Silva, F. S., & Costa, C. M. A. (2014). Thermal body patterns for healthy Brazilian adults (male and female). *Journal of Thermal Biology*.

Marins, J. C. B., Moreira, D. G., Cano, S. P., Quintana, M. S., Soares, D. D., & Fernandes, A. d. A. (2014). Time required to stabilize thermographic images at rest. *Infrared Physics & Technology*.

Markel, M., & Manzo, B. (1994). A comparison of the cuff deflation method with Valsavas maneuver and limb compression in detecting venous valvular reflux. *Archives of Surgery (Chicago, Ill.)*, *129*(7), 701–705. doi:10.1001/archsurg.1994.01420310033005 PMID:8024449

Martens, J., Figueiredo, P., & Daly, D. (2014). Electromyography in the four competitive swimming strokes: A systematic review. *Journal of Electromyography and Kinesiology*. PMID:25556010

Martinod, S. (1997). Adverse effects of vaccination. In P. P. Pastoret, J. Blancou, P. Vannier, & C. Verschuren (Eds.), *Veterinary Vaccinology* (pp. 574–580). Amsterdam: Elsevier.

Martins, Ribeiro, & Cury. (2012). Diagnostic Evaluation of Chronic Venous Insufficiency Cases Using Thermal Imaging. *Thermology International*, *22*(3), 169-176.

Masuda, Eklof, & Kistner. (2001). Direct venous pressure: Role in the assessment of venous disease. In Handbook of Venous Disorders (2nd ed.). New York, NY: Arnold.

McKay, N., Griffiths, B., di Maria, C., Hedley, S., Murray, A., & Allen, J. (2014). Novel photoplethysmography cardiovascular assessments in patients with Raynauds phenomenon and systemic sclerosis: A pilot study. *Rheumatology*, *53*(10), 1855–1863. doi:10.1093/rheumatology/keu196 PMID:24850874

Meeusen & Lievens. (1986). The use of cryotherapy in sports injuries. *Sports Med.*, *3*(6), 398-414.

Mercer & Ring. (2009). Fever screening and infrared thermal imaging: Concerns and guidelines. *Thermology International*, *19*, 67–69.

Mercer, Nielsen, & Hoffmann. (2008). Improvement of wound healing by water-filtered infrared-A (wIRA) in patients with chronic venous stasis ulcers of the lower legs including evaluation using infrared thermography. *GMS German Medical Science*, *6*, 1-26.

Merck Sharp & Dohme Corp. (2014). *The Merck Veterinary Manual - Diagnostic Imaging, Radiology.* Retrieved from http://www.merckmanuals.com/vet/clinical_pathology_and_procedures/diagnostic_imaging/radiography.html

Merla, A. (2005). Functional infrared imaging in clinical applications. In J. Bronzino (Ed.), The Biomedical Engineering Handbook. Academic Press.

Merla, A., & Romani, G. L. (2005). *Biomedical applications of functional infrared imaging*. Paper presented at the 27th Annual International Conference of the Engineering in Medicine and Biology Society, Shanghai, China.

Merla, A., Di Donato, L., & Romani, G. L. (2002). *Infrared functional imaging: analysis of skin temperature during exercise*. Paper presented at the Engineering in Medicine and Biology, 2002. 24th Annual Conference and the Annual Fall Meeting of the Biomedical Engineering Society EMBS/BMES Conference. doi:10.1109/IEMBS.2002.1106316

Merla, A., Iodice, P., Tangherlini, A., De Michele, G., Di Romualdo, S., & Saggini, R. (2005). Monitoring skin temperature in trained and untrained subjects throughout thermal video. *Conference Proceedings; ... Annual International Conference of the IEEE Engineering in Medicine and Biology Society. IEEE Engineering in Medicine and Biology Society. Conference*, *2*(1), 1684–1686. PMID:17282536

Merla, A., Mattei, P. A., Di Donato, L., & Romani, G. L. (2010). Thermal imaging of cutaneous temperature modifications in runners during graded exercise. *Annals of Biomedical Engineering*, *38*(1), 158–163. doi:10.1007/s10439-009-9809-8 PMID:19798579

Merla, A., & Romani, G. L. (2008). Biomedical appplications of functional infrared imaging. In N. A. Diakides & J. D. Bronzino (Eds.), *Medical infrared imaging* (pp. 15.1–15.20). Boca Raton, FL: CRC Press.

Mettler, F. A. Jr, Bhargavan, M., Faulkner, K., Gilley, D. B., Gray, J. E., Ibbott, G. S., & Yoshizumi, T. T. et al. (2009). Radiologic and Nuclear Medicine Studies in the United States and Worldwide: Frequency, Radiation Dose, and Comparison with Other Radiation Sources—1950–2007 1. *Radiology*, *253*(2), 520–531. doi:10.1148/radiol.2532082010 PMID:19789227

Metzger, Zwingmann, Protz, & Jackel. (2000). Die Bedeutung Der Ganzkorperkaltetherapie Im Rahmen Der Rehabilitation Bei Patienten Mit Rheumatishen. *Erkrank. Rehabil.*, *39*, 93–100. doi:10.1055/s-2000-14442

Meurman, K., Somer, K., & Sjovall, J. (1980). Thermography of stress fractures in military personnel. *Acta Thermographica*, *5*, 132–136.

Mijović, B., Salopek Čubrić, I., Skenderi, Z., & Reischl, U. (2012). Thermographic Assessment of Sweat Evaporation within Different Clothing Systems. *FIBRES & TEXTILES in Eastern Europe*, *20*(5 (94)), 81–86.

Mikulska, D. (2006). Contemporary applications of infrared imaging in medical diagnostics. *Annales Academiae Medicae Stetinensis*, *52*(1), 35–39, discussion 39–40. PMID:17131845

Milic. (2011). Prevalence and socioeconomic data in chronic venous disease: How useful are they in planning appropriate management? *Medicographia, 33*, 253-258.

Misztela, Kuliński, & Rybak. (1995). Ocena Krioterapii Miejscowej W Reumatoidalnym Zapaleniu Stawów Baln.[In Polish]. *Pol*, *37*(3-4), 38–41.

Miyamoto, T., Hara, K., Nishimura, H., & Yano, K. (2004). Thermographic evaluation in sports injury. *Journal of the Japan Society of Infrared Science and Technology*, *14*(1), 39–43.

Mongini, F., Caselli, C., Macri, V., & Tetti, C. (1990). Thermographic findings in cranio-facial pain. *Headache*, *30*(8), 497–504. doi:10.1111/j.1526-4610.1990.hed3008497.x PMID:2228600

Mraz, Skrzek, & Gruszka, Chamela-Bilińska, Drak-Wojakiewicz, & Dutkiewicz. (2001). The influence of physiotherapy and whole body cryotherapy on standing position balance of patients with sclerosis multiplex. *Physiotherapy*, *9*(1), 26–29.

Mulak, J. (1982). *Lekkoatletyka – Technika Metodyka Trening*. Warszawa: Sport i Turystyka.

Nakayama, T., Ohnuki, Y., & Kanosue, K. (1981). Fall in skin temperature during exercise observed by thermography. *Japanese Journal of Physiology*, *31*(5), 757–762. doi:10.2170/jjphysiol.31.757 PMID:7328924

Neglen, E., Egger, J. F. III, Olivier, J., & Raju, S. (2004). Hemodynamic and clinical impact of ultrasound-derived venous reflux parameters. *Journal of Vascular Surgery*, *40*(2), 303–310. doi:10.1016/j.jvs.2004.05.009 PMID:15297826

Neglen, P., & Raju, S. (2000). Ambulatory venous pressure revisited. *Journal of Vascular Surgery*, *31*(6), 1206–1213. doi:10.1067/mva.2000.105669 PMID:10842158

Nelson, H. A., & Osheim, D. L. (1975). Soring in tennessee walking horses: detection by thermography. United States Department of Agriculture - APHIS, Veterinary Services Laboratories, Ames, IA.

Nelzen, B., Bergqvist, D., & Lindhagen, A. (1991). Leg ulcer etiology–a cross-sectional population study. *Journal of Vascular Surgery*, *14*(4), 557–564. doi:10.1016/0741-5214(91)90251-O PMID:1920653

Ng, E. Y.-K. (2009). A review of thermography as promising noninvasive detection modality for breast tumor. *International Journal of Thermal Sciences*, *48*(5), 849–859. doi:10.1016/j.ijthermalsci.2008.06.015

Nicolaides. (2000). Investigation of chronic venous insufficiency: A consensus statement. *Circulation*, *102*, e126-e163.

Nicolaides, A. N., & Miles, C. (1987). Photoplethysmography in the assessment of venous insufficiency. *Journal of Vascular Surgery*, *5*(3), 405–412. doi:10.1016/0741-5214(87)90047-4 PMID:3334678

Nicolaides, A. N., & Zukowski, A. J. (1986). The value of dynamic venous pressure measurements. *World Journal of Surgery*, *10*(6), 919–924. doi:10.1007/BF01658640 PMID:3798938

Nilson, G., & Bjorck, G. (1969). Surgical treatment of chronic tendinitis in the horse. *Journal of the American Veterinary Medical Association*, *155*(5), 920–926. PMID:5817732

Niu, H.-H., Lui, P.-W., Hu, J. S., Ting, C.-K., Yin, Y.-C., Lo, Y.-L., & Lee, T.-Y. et al. (2001). Thermal symmetry of skin temperature: Normative data of normal subjects in Taiwan. *Chinese Medical Journal-Taipei*, *64*(8), 459–468. PMID:11720145

Nocck, E. (1997). Bovine acidosis: Implications on laminitis. *Journal of Dairy Science*, *80*(5), 1005–1008. doi:10.3168/jds.S0022-0302(97)76026-0 PMID:9178142

Novotny, J., Rybarova, S., Zacha, D., Bernacikova, M., & Ramadan, W. A. (2015). The influence of breaststroke swimming on the muscle activity of young men in thermographic imaging.Acta of bioengineering and biomechanics/Wrocław University of Technology, 17(2), 121-129.

Nowakowski. (2001). *Postępy termografii – aplikacje medyczne*. Gdańsk: Academic Press.

Noya Salces, J., Benito Peinado, P. J., Calderón, J., & Gómez Carmona, P. M. (2008). *Validation of a questionnaire for the registration of injuries in the professional soccer.* Paper presented at the 13th Annual Congress of the European Collage of Sport Science ECSS Estoril, Portugal, Portugal.

Noya Salces, J., Sillero Quintana, M., Gómez Carmona, P. M., & Pastrano León, R. (2009), june 24th-27th). *Infrared Thermography as a Method for Monitoring and Preventing Injuries in Soccer.* Paper presented at the 14th Annual Congress of the European College of Sport Sciences ECSS, Oslo, Norway.

O'Keefe, M., OReilly, J., & Lanigan, B. (1998). Longer term visual outcome of eyes with retinopathy of prematurity treated with cryotherapy or diode laser. *The British Journal of Ophthalmology*, *82*(11), 1246–1248. doi:10.1136/bjo.82.11.1246 PMID:9924326

Oikawa, M., & Kasashima, Y. (2002). The Japanese experience with tendonitis in racehorses. *Journal of Equine Science, 13*(2), 41–56. doi:10.1294/jes.13.41

Olex-Zarychta, D. (2009). *Fitness: teoretyczne i metodyczne podstawy prowadzenia zajęć. Podręcznik dla studentów wychowania fizycznego i instruktorów fitness. In Wydanie III poprawione*. Gliwice: Wyd. J&D Gębka.

Oliveira, J., Vardasca, R., Pimenta, M., Gabriel, J., & Torres, J. (2016). Use of infrared thermography for the diagnosis and grading of sprained ankle injuries. *Infrared Physics & Technology, 76*, 530–541. doi:10.1016/j.infrared.2016.04.014

Oliveira, P. A., Colaço, A., Chaves, R., Guedes-Pinto, H., De-La-Cruz, P., Luis, F., & Lopes, C. (2007). Chemical carcinogenesis. *Anais da Academia Brasileira de Ciencias, 79*(4), 593–616. doi:10.1590/S0001-37652007000400004 PMID:18066431

Oliveira, P. A., Colaço, A., De la Cruz, P. L., & Lopes, C. (2006). Experimental bladder carcinogenesis-rodent models. *Experimental Oncology, 28*(1), 2–11. PMID:16614700

Oliver, A., Nurton, J. P., & Guthrie, A. J. (1997). An epizoological study in wastage in Thoroughbred racehorses in Gauteng, South Africa. *Journal of the South African Veterinary Association, 68*, 125–129. PMID:9561496

Palmer, S. E. (1981). Use of portable infrared thermometer as a means of means of measuring limb surface temperature in the horse. *American Journal of Veterinary Research, 42*(1), 105–108. PMID:7224303

Palmer, S. E. (1983). Effect of ambient temperature upon the surface temperature of equine limb. *American Journal of Veterinary Research, 44*(6), 1098–1101. PMID:6870013

Parkin, T. D. H., Clegg, P. D., French, N. P., Proudman, C. J., Riggs, C. M., Singer, E. R., & Morgan, K. L. et al. (2004). Horse-level risk factors for fatal distal limb fracture in racing Thoroughbreds in the UK. *Equine Veterinary Journal, 36*(6), 513–519. doi:10.2746/0425164044877387 PMID:15460076

Pascoe, D. D., Mercer, J. B., & de Weerd, L. (2007). Physiology of Thermal Signals. In N. A. Diakides & J. D. Bronzino (Eds.), Medical Infrared Imaging (pp. 6-1 - 6-20). Taylor & Francis. doi:10.1201/9781420008340.ch6

Pascoe, D. D., Mercer, J. B., & De Weerd, L. (2006). Physiology of thermal signals. In J. D. Bronzino (Ed.), *Medical devices and systems* (pp. 21.1–21.20). doi:10.1201/9781420003864.ch21

Pascoe, D. D., Skelton, M., Smith, E. W., Kremer, D., & Purohit, R. C. (1992). Infrared thermography pattern of the back of human subjects during exercise: 921. *Medicine and Science in Sports and Exercise, 24*(5Supplement), S154. doi:10.1249/00005768-199205001-00922

Pasricha, Hill, Wadwa, Gislason, & Okolo. (1999). Endoscopic cryotherapy: experimental results and first clinical use. *Gastrointest. Endosc., 49*(5), 627-631.

Patil, W., Williams, L., & Williams, K. L. (1970). Thermographic localisation of incompetent perforating veins in the leg. *British Medical Journal, 1*(5690), 195–197. doi:10.1136/bmj.1.5690.195 PMID:4904934

Peham, C., Kotschwar, A. B., Borkenhagen, B., Kuhnke, S., Molsner, J., & Baltacis, A. (2010). Comparison of forces acting on the horses back and the stability of the riders seat in different positions at the trot. *Veterinary Journal (London, England), 184*(1), 56–59. doi:10.1016/j.tvjl.2009.04.007 PMID:19428275

Peloso, J. G., Mundy, G. D., & Cohen, N. D. (1994). Prevalence of, and factors associated with, musculoskeletal racing injuries of Thoroughbreds. *Journal of the American Medical Association, 204*(4), 620–626. PMID:8163419

Perros, P., Di Maria, C., Dickinson, J., & Allen, J. (2012). Thermal imaging and characteristics in Graves' Orbitopathy. European Thyroid Journal, 1(S1), 123-65.

Petibois, C., Cazorla, G., Poortmans, J. R., & Deleris, G. (2002). Biochemical aspects of overtraining in endurance sports: A review. *Sports Medicine (Auckland, N.Z.)*, *32*(13), 867–878. doi:10.2165/00007256-200232130-00005 PMID:12392446

Petrova, N., MacDonald, A., Ainarkar, S., Plassmann, P., Ring, F., Simpson, R., & Edmonds, M. et al. (2016). Infrared thermometry reveals no differences of the skin temperatures at the plantar, dorsal, medial and lateral sites between the right foot and left foot in healthy volunteers. *Diabetic Medicine*, *33*(Suppl. 1), 35–196.

Pichler, W. J. (2006). Adverse side-effects to biological agents. *Allergy*, *61*(8), 912–920. doi:10.1111/j.1398-9995.2006.01058.x PMID:16867042

Pidwirny, M., & Jones, S. (2006). Energy and MatterFundamentals of physical geography (2nd ed.). Retrieved from http://www.physicalgeography.net/fundamentals/6f.html

Pilawski. (1983). *Podstawy biofizyki*. PZWL. (in Polish)

Pilawski, A. (1983). *Podstawy biofizyki*. New York: Springer.

Pink, M., Jobe, F. W., Perry, J., Kerrigan, J., Browne, A., & Scovazzo, M. L. (1992). The Normal Shoulder During the Backstroke: An EMG and Cinematographic Analysis of 12 Muscles. *Clinical Journal of Sport Medicine*, *2*(1), 6–12. doi:10.1097/00042752-199201000-00002

Pink, M., Jobe, F. W., Perry, J., Kerrigan, J., Browne, A., & Scovazzo, M. L. (1993). The normal shoulder during the butterfly swim stroke. An electromyographic and cinematographic analysis of twelve muscles. *Clinical Orthopaedics and Related Research*, (288): 48–59. PMID:8458154

Pink, M., Perry, J., Browne, A., Scovazzo, M. L., & Kerrigan, J. (1991). The normal shoulder during freestyle swimming An electromyographic and cinematographic analysis of twelve muscles. *The American Journal of Sports Medicine*, *19*(6), 569–576. doi:10.1177/036354659101900603 PMID:1781492

Piñonosa, S., Sillero-Quintana, M., Milanović, L., Coterón, J., & Sampedro, J. (2013). Thermal evolution of lower limbs during a rehabilitation process after anterior cruciate ligament surgery. *Kinesiology*, *45*(1), 121–129.

Plassmann, P., Ring, E. F. J., & Jones, C. D. (2006). Quality assurance of thermal imaging systems in medicine. *Thermology International, 16*, 10-5.

Podbielska & Skrzek. (2014). *Biomedical application of thermography, Biomedyczne zastosowania termowizji, praca zbiorowa*. Wrocław: Oficyna Wydawnicza Politechniki Wrocławskiej.

Podbielska & Skrzek. (Eds.). (2012). The application of low temperatures in biomedicine. Oficyna Wydawnicza Politechniki Wrocławskiej, Wrocław.

Podbielska, H., & Skrzek, A. (2014). *Biomedyczne zastosowania termowizji*. Wrocław: Oficyna Wydawnicza Politechniki Wrocławskiej.

Pogrel, M. A., Erbez, G., Taylor, R. C., & Dodson, T. B. (1989). Liquid crystal thermography as a diagnostic aid and objective monitor for TMJ dysfunction and myogenic facial pain. *Journal of Craniomandibular Disorders*, *3*(2), 65–70. PMID:2606998

Polin, L., Corbett, T. H., Roberts, B. J., Lawson, A. J., Leopold, W. R., III, White, K., . . . Horwitz, J. P. (2011). Transplantable Syngeneic Rodent Tumors: Solid Tumors in Mice. In Tumor Models in Cancer Research (pp. 43-78). Humana Press.

Poljak-Blazi, M., Kolaric, D., Jaganjac, M., Zarkovic, K., Skala, K., & Zarkovic, N. (2009). Specific thermographic changes during Walker 256 carcinoma development: Differential infrared imaging of tumour, inflammation and haematoma. *Cancer Detection and Prevention*, *32*(5), 431–436. doi:10.1016/j.cdp.2009.01.002 PMID:19232842

Portela, A., Vasconcelos, M., Fernandes, M. H., Garcia, M., Silva, A., Gabriel, J., & Cavalheiro, J. et al. (2013). Highly focalised thermotherapy using a ferrimagnetic cement in the treatment of a melanoma mouse model by low temperature hyperthermia. *International Journal of Hyperthermia*, *29*(2), 121–132. doi:10.3109/02656736.2013.767478 PMID:23418916

Potente, M., Gerhardt, H., & Carmeliet, P. (2011). Basic and therapeutic aspects of angiogenesis. *Cell*, *146*(6), 873–887. doi:10.1016/j.cell.2011.08.039 PMID:21925313

Practice Guidelines Committee of the American Academy of Thermology. (2012a). *Guidelines for Breast Thermography*. Retrieved from http://www.aathermology.org/

Practice Guidelines Committee of the American Academy of Thermology. (2012b). *Guidelines for Neuromusculoskeletical Infrared Thermography Sympathetic Skin Response (SSR) Studies*. Retrieved from http://www.aathermology.org/

Priego Quesada, J. I., Carpes, F. P., Bini, R. R., Salvador Palmer, R., Pérez-Soriano, P., & Cibrián Ortiz de Anda, R. M. (2015). Relationship between skin temperature and muscle activation during incremental cycle exercise. *Journal of Thermal Biology*, *48*(0), 28–35. doi:10.1016/j.jtherbio.2014.12.005 PMID:25660627

Priego Quesada, J. I., Martínez, N., Salvador Palmer, R., Psikuta, A., Annaheim, S., Rossi, R. M., & Pérez-Soriano, P. et al. (2016). Effects of the cycling workload on core and local skin temperatures. *Experimental Thermal and Fluid Science*, *77*, 91–99. doi:10.1016/j.expthermflusci.2016.04.008

Purohit, R. (2009). Standards for thermal imaging in veterinary medicine.*Proceedings of the XIth European Congress of Thermology. Mannheim, Germany. Thermology International, 19*, 99.

Purohit, R. C., Bergfeld, W. A., McCoy, M. D., Thomson, W. M., & Sharman, R. S. (1977). Value of clinical thermography in veterinary medicine. *Auburn Veterinarian*, *33*(3), 104–108.

Purohit, R. C., & McCoy, M. D. (1980). Thermography in the diagnosis of inflammatory processes in the horse. *American Journal of Veterinary Research*, *41*(8), 1167–1174. PMID:7447110

Purvis, A. J., & Cable, N. T. (2000). The effects of phase control materials on hand skin temperature within gloves of soccer goalkeepers. *Ergonomics*, *43*(10), 1480–1488. doi:10.1080/001401300750003916 PMID:11083129

Purvis, A. J., & Tunstall, H. (2004). Effects of sock type on foot skin temperature and thermal demand during exercise. *Ergonomics*, *47*(15), 1657–1668. doi:10.1080/00140130412331290880 PMID:15545238

Pušnik, I., & Čuk, I. (2014). Thermal imaging of hands during simple gymnastics elements on the wooden bar with and without use of magnesium carbonate. *Science of Gymnastics Journal*, *6*(1), 67–72.

Raczkowski & Zagrobelny. (1990). *Technical and physiological aspects of whole body cooling*. Materials of IV Science and Training Conference of Polish Cryomedical Society.

Raffetto, J. D., & Khalil, R. A. (2008). Mechanisms of varicose vein formation: Valve dysfunction and wall dilation. *Phlebology*, *23*(2), 85–98. doi:10.1258/phleb.2007.007027 PMID:18453484

Ramdy, D. W. (1997). Prospective evaluation of fore limb flexion tests in practice: clinical response, radiographic correlation and predictive value for future lameness.*Proceedings of the Annual Convention American Association of Equine Practitioners*, *43*, 116-120.

Ramos e Côrte, A. C., & Hernandez, A. J. (2016). Termografía médica infravermelha aplicada à Medicina do Esporte. *Revista Brasileira de Medicina do Esporte*, *22*(4), 315–319. doi:10.1590/1517-869220162204160783

Ranson, S. (1933). The anatomy of the autonomic nervous system with special reference to the innervation of the skeletal muscles and blood vessels. *Annals of Internal Medicine*, *6*(8), 1013–1021. doi:10.7326/0003-4819-6-8-1013

Renault, G., Bonnin, P., Marchiol-Fournigault, C., Gregoire, J. M., Serriere, S., Richard, B., & Fradelizi, D. (2006). High-resolution ultrasound imaging of the mouse. *Journal de Radiologie*, *87*(12 Pt 2), 1937–1945. doi:10.1016/S0221-0363(06)74179-8 PMID:17211308

Richards, R. E., Allen, J., Burnett, S., Howell, K. J., & Smith, R. E. (2013). Evaluation of three thermal imagers for skin temperature measurement using a blackbody source and a spatial resolution test object. *Thermology International*, *23*, 17–23.

Rich, P. B., Dulabon, G. R., Douillet, C. D., Listwa, T. M., Robinson, W. P., Zarzaur, B. L., & Katz, L. M. et al. (2004). Infrared thermography: A rapid, portable, and accurate technique to detect experimental pneumothorax. *The Journal of Surgical Research*, *120*(2), 163–170. doi:10.1016/j.jss.2004.02.026 PMID:15234209

Ring & Ammer. (2000). The technique of infrared imaging in medicine. *Thermol. Intern.*, *10*(1), 7-14.

Ring & Ammer. (2000). The technique of infrared imaging in medicine. *Thermol Intern*, *10*, 7–14.

Ring & Ammer. (2012a). Infrared thermal imaging in medicine. *Physiological Measurement*, *33*(3), R33-46.

Ring & Ammer. (2012b). Thermal imaging in rheumatology - An overview. *Thermology International*, *22*(2), 68-69.

Ring, E. F. (1990). Quantitative thermal imaging. *Clin Phys Physiol Meas*, *11*(SA), 87-95.

Ring, E. F. J., & Ammer, K. (2000). The technique of infrared imaging in medicine. *Thermology International*, *10*(1), 7-14.

Ring, Jung, Kalicki, Zuber, Rustecka, & Vardasca. (2013). New Standards For Fever Screening With Thermal Imaging Systems. *Journal of Mechanics in Medicine and Biology*, *13*(2).

Ring. (1999). Thermal Symmetry of Human Skin Temperature. *Thermology International*, *9*(2), 53-55.

Ring. (2001). Provocation tests in thermal imaging. *Abs. Thermology Int.*, *11*, 2.

Ring, E. F. J. (2007). The historical development of temperature measurement in medicine. *Infrared Physics & Technology*, *49*(3), 297–301. doi:10.1016/j.infrared.2006.06.029

Ring, E. F. J. (2014). Pioneering progress in infrared imaging in medicine. *Quantitative InfraRed Thermography Journal*, *11*(1), 57–65. doi:10.1080/17686733.2014.892667

Ring, E. F. J., & Ammer, K. (2000). The technique of infrared imaging in medicine. *Thermol Int.*, *10*(1), 7–14.

Ring, E. F. J., & Ammer, K. (2012). Infrared thermal imaging in medicine. *Physiological Measurement*, *33*(3), R33–R46. doi:10.1088/0967-3334/33/3/R33 PMID:22370242

Ring, E. F. J., Ammer, K., Jung, A., Murawski, P., Wiecek, B., Zuber, J., & Jones, B. F. et al. (2003, December). Standardization of infrared imaging. *Conference Proceedings; ... Annual International Conference of the IEEE Engineering in Medicine and Biology Society. IEEE Engineering in Medicine and Biology Society. Conference*, *2*, 1183–1185. PMID:17271897

Ring, E. F. J., Hartmann, J., Ammer, K., Thomas, R., Land, D., & Hand, J. W. (2010). Infrared and Microwave Medical Thermometry. *Experimental Methods in the Physical Sciences*, *43*, 393–448. doi:10.1016/S1079-4042(09)04307-0

Ring, F. J. (1990). Quantitative thermal imaging. *Clinical Physics and Physiological Measurement*, *11*(4A), 87–97. doi:10.1088/0143-0815/11/4A/310 PMID:2286052

Ring, F., Jung, A., & Zuber, J. (2009). New opportunities for infrared thermography in medicine. *Acta Bio-Optika et Informatica Medica*, *15*, 28–30.

Ring, J. F., & Mercer, J. (2007). Thermal Imaging for Fever Screening. *The Magazine of the International Organization for Standardization*, *4*, 33–35.

Ritchie, S., Soulen, R. L., & Lapayowker, M. S. (1979). Thermographic diagnosis of deep venous thrombosis. *Radiology*, *131*(2), 341–344. doi:10.1148/131.2.341 PMID:441316

Rochcongar, P., & Schmitt, M. (1979). Thermographic study of muscular lesions in sport (author's transl). *Journal Belge de Medecine Physique et de Rehabilitation. Belgisch Tijdschrift voor Fysische Geneeskunde en Rehabilitatie*, *2*(4), 335–342. PMID:549939

Rodrigues, H. F., Mello, F. M., Branquinho, L. C., Zufelato, N., Silveira-Lacerda, E. P., & Bakuzis, A. F. (2013). Real-time infrared thermography detection of magnetic nanoparticle hyperthermia in a murine model under a non-uniform field configuration. *International Journal of Hyperthermia*, *29*(8), 752–767. doi:10.3109/02656736.2013.839056 PMID:24138472

Rok. (2012). *The use of thermovision in diagnostics and therapy* (Doctoral Thesis). Jagiellonian Univeristy, Kraków, Poland.

Ronikier. (2008). *Physiology of exercise in sports, physiotherapy and recreation*. Centralny Ośrodek Sportu, Warszawa.

Rosenberg & Marchese. (1963). Perforator vein localisation by heat emission detection. *Surgery*, *53*, 575–578. PMID:13974907

Rossdale, P. D., Hopes, R., Wingfield-Digby, N. J., & Offord, K. (1985). Epidemiological study of wastage among racehorses 1982 and 1983. *The Veterinary Record*, *116*(3), 66–69. doi:10.1136/vr.116.3.66 PMID:3976145

Ross, W., Ward, R., Leahy, R., & Day, J. (1982). Proportionality of Montreal Athletes. In J. Carter (Ed.), *Physical Structure of Olympic Athletes: Part 1. The Montreal Olympic Games Anthropological Project*. Basel: Karger. doi:10.1159/000406782

Rouard, A., & Clarys, J. (1995). Cocontraction in the elbow and shoulder muscles during rapid cyclic movements in an aquatic environment. *Journal of Electromyography and Kinesiology*, *5*(3), 177–183. doi:10.1016/1050-6411(95)00008-N PMID:20719649

Rowland, D. J., & Cherry, S. R. (2008, May). Small-animal preclinical nuclear medicine instrumentation and methodology. *Seminars in Nuclear Medicine*, *38*(3), 209–222. doi:10.1053/j.semnuclmed.2008.01.004 PMID:18396180

Rutherford, P., & Comerota, K. (2000). Venous severity scoring: An adjunct to venous outcome assessment. *Journal of Vascular Surgery*, *31*(6), 1307–1312. doi:10.1067/mva.2000.107094 PMID:10842165

Ruwe, P. A., Pink, M., Jobe, F. W., Perry, J., & Scovazzo, M. L. (1994). The Normal and the Painful Shoulders During the Breaststroke Electromyographic and Cinematographic Analysis of Twelve Muscles. *The American Journal of Sports Medicine*, *22*(6), 789–796. doi:10.1177/036354659402200610 PMID:7856803

Rybak, Kuliński, Misztela, & Podgórski. (1995). Zastosowanie Krioterapii W Leczeniu Następstw Blizn Kanału Kręgowego Baln.[In Polish]. *Pol*, *37*(3-4), 29–30.

Ryer, A., & Light, V. (1997). *Light measurement handbook*. Academic Press.

Rymaszewska, Biały, Zagrobelny, & Kiejna. (2000). The Influence Of Whole Body Cryotherapy On Mental Health. *Psychiatria Polska, 34*(4), 649 – 653.

Rymaszewska, R., Ramsey, D., & Chładzińska-Kiejna, S. (2008). Whole - body cryotherapy as adjunct treatment of depressive syndrome and anxiety disorders. *Archivum Immunologiae et Therapiae Experimentalis*, *56*(1), 63–68. doi:10.1007/s00005-008-0006-5 PMID:18250970

Sacharuk, V. Z., Lovatel, G. A., Ilha, J., Marcuzzo, S., Pinho, A. S. D., Xavier, L. L., & Achaval, M. et al. (2011). Thermographic evaluation of hind paw skin temperature and functional recovery of locomotion after sciatic nerve crush in rats. *Clinics (Sao Paulo)*, *66*(7), 1259–1266. doi:10.1590/S1807-59322011000700023 PMID:21876984

Sampedro, J., Piñonosa Cano, S., & Fernández-Cuevas, I. (2012). Thermography as a new assessment tool in basketball. Pilot study carried out with a professional player in the ACB. *Cuadernos de Psicología del Deporte*, *12*, 51–56. doi:10.4321/S1578-84232012000300012

Sanches, I. J. (2009). *Sobreposição de Imagens de Termografia e Ressonância Magnética: uma nova modalidade de imagem médica tridimensional*. Curitiba: Universidade Tecnológica Federal do Paraná, Engenharia Elétrica e Informática Industrial.

Sanchis-Sánchez, E., Salvador-Palmer, R., Codoñer-Franch, P., Martín, J., Vergara-Hernández, C., Blasco, J., & Cibrián, R. et al. (2014). Infrared thermography is useful for ruling out fractures in paediatric emergencies. *European Journal of Pediatrics*, 1–7. doi:10.1007/s00431-014-2425-0 PMID:25241828

Sanchis-Sánchez, E., Vergara-Hernández, C., Cibrián, R. M., Salvador, R., Sanchis, E., & Codoñer-Franch, P. (2014). Infrared thermal imaging in the diagnosis of musculoskeletal injuries: A systematic review and meta-analysis. *AJR. American Journal of Roentgenology*, *203*(4), 875–882. doi:10.2214/AJR.13.11716 PMID:25247955

Sands, W. A., McNeal, J. R., & Stone, M. (2011). Thermal imaging and gymnastics injuries: A means of screening and injury identification. *Science of Gymnastics Journal*, *3*(2), 5–12.

Saxena, A. K., & Willital, G. H. (2008). Infrared thermography: Experience from a decade of pediatric imaging. *European Journal of Pediatrics*, *167*(7), 757–764. doi:10.1007/s00431-007-0583-z PMID:17762940

Saxena, V., Marcu, L., & Karunasiri, G. (2008). A novel noninvasive all optical technique to monitor physiology of an exercising muscle. *Physics in Medicine and Biology*, *53*(21), 6211–6225. doi:10.1088/0031-9155/53/21/021 PMID:18854609

Sayre, K., Kelechi, T. J., & Neal, D. (2007). Sudden increase in skin temperature predicts venous ulcers: A case study. *Journal of Vascular Nursing*, *25*(3), 46–50. doi:10.1016/j.jvn.2007.06.002 PMID:17723909

Schmidt, K. L., Mäurer, R., & Rusch, D. (1979). Zur Wirkung örtlicher Wärme und Kälteanwendungen auf die Hauttemperatur am Kniegelenk. *Zeitschrift fur Rheumatologie*, *38*, 213–219. PMID:573031

Schroder & Anderson. (1995). *Kryo- und Thermotherapie. Grundlangen und praktische Anwendung*. New York: Gustaw Hischer Verlag.

Schulze-Rath, R., Hammer, G. P., & Blettner, M. (2008). Are pre-or postnatal diagnostic X-rays a risk factor for childhood cancer? A systematic review. *Radiation and Environmental Biophysics*, *47*(3), 301–312. doi:10.1007/s00411-008-0171-2 PMID:18528700

Schwartz, R. (2006). Guidelines for neuromusculoskeletal thermography. *Thermology International, 16*(1), 5-9.

Schwartz, R. G. (2006). Guidelines for Neuromusculoskeletal Thermography. Wheeling. *Thermol Int*, *16*(1), 5–9.

Scott, LaMorte, Gorin, & Menzoian. (1995). Risk factors for chronic venous insufficiency: A Dual case-control study. *J Vasc Surg., 22*(5), 622-628.

Seixas, A., Gonjo, T., Vardasca, R., Gabriel, J., & Fernandes, R. (2014). *A preliminary study on the relationship between energy expenditure and skin temperature in swimming*. Paper presented at the 12th International Conference on Quantitative InfraRed Thermography, Bordeaux. doi:10.21611/qirt.2014.097

Seixas, A., Silva, A., Vardasca, R., & Gabriel, J. (2012). The Effect of Whole-body Vibration in the Skin Temperature of Lower Extremities in Healthy Subjects. *Thermology International, 22*(3), 59-66.

Selfe, J., Alexander, J., Costello, J. T., May, K., Garratt, N., Atkins, S., & Richards, J. et al. (2014). The effect of three different (-135 degrees c) whole body cryotherapy exposure durations on elite rugby league players. *PLoS ONE, 9*(1), e86420. doi:10.1371/journal.pone.0086420 PMID:24489726

Shah, J. P., Danoff, J. V., Desai, M. J., Parikh, S., Nakamura, L. Y., Phillips, T. M., & Gerber, L. H. (2008). Biochemicals associated with pain and Inflammation are elevated in sites near to and remote from active myofascial trigger points. *Archives of Physical Medicine and Rehabilitation, 89*(1), 16–23. doi:10.1016/j.apmr.2007.10.018 PMID:18164325

Shejbal, D., Drvis, P., & Bedekovic, V. (2012). Thermography-measured effect of capsaicin, methylprednisolone and mitomycin on the survival of random skin flaps in rats. *Skin Research and Technology, 18*(2), 157–161. doi:10.1111/j.1600-0846.2011.00547.x PMID:21545651

Shojaei, F. (2012). Anti-angiogenesis therapy in cancer: Current challenges and future perspectives. *Cancer Letters, 320*(2), 130–137. doi:10.1016/j.canlet.2012.03.008 PMID:22425960

Shor & Pronin. (2006). Local signs of the reperfusion syndrome in obliterating atherosclerosis of the lower extremity arteries and their treatment. *Klin Khir, 1*, 34–37. PMID:16719070

Sieroń & Cieślar. (2003a). *The Application Of Cold In Medicine - Cryosurgery And Cryotherapy*. A-Medica Press Bielsko-Biala Poland. (in Polish)

Sieroń & Cieślar. (2003b). The theoretical basis for cooling treatment. The application of cold medicine - cryosurgery and cryotherapy. α-Medica Press.

Sieroń & Cieślar. (2007). Cryotherapy – cold treatment. α-Medica Press.

Sieroń, Cieślar, & Stanek. (2010). *Cryotherapy. Theoretical bases, biological effects, clinical applications*. α-Medica Press Bielsko Biała.

Sieroń, Stanek, & Cieślar. (Eds.). (2014). *Wellness, Spa, Anti-aging*. PZWL.

Sieroń, Pastuszka, Marniok, Wiśniowska, & Jagodziński, Ślusarczyk, … Stanek. (2004). Influence of low temperature on lymph formation and lymph flow velocity in mice. *Thermol. Int., 14*, 127–130.

Sieroń, Stanek, Cieślar, & Pasek. (2007). Cryorehabilitation - the role cryotherapy in modern rehabilitation. *Fizjoterapia, 15*(2), 3–8.

Sillero Quintana, M., Conde Pascual, E., Gómez Carmona, P. M., Fernández-Cuevas, I., & García-Pastor, T. (2012). Effect of yoga and swimming on body temperature of pregnant women. *Thermology International, 22*, 143-149.

Sillero Quintana, M., Gómez Carmona, P. M., García de la Concepción, M. Á., Fernández Cuevas, I., Piñonosa Cano, S., & Cordente, C. A. (2010). *Application of thermography as injury prevention method and monitoring of the injury recovery in Athletics*. Paper presented at the World Congress on Science in Athletics, Barcelona, Spain.

Sillero Quintana, M., Gómez Carmona, P. M., Noya Salces, J., Núñez, F. J., & Fernández Rodríguez, I. (2009). Comparation of infrared thermography with tensiomyography as injury prevention method in professional soccer players. *Journal of Sports Sciences*, S174.

Sillero-Quintana, M., Fernández-Jaén, T., Fernández-Cuevas, I., Gómez-Carmona, P. M., Arnaiz-Lastras, J., Pérez, M.-D., & Guillén, P. (2015). Infrared Thermography as a Support Tool for Screening and Early Diagnosis in Emergencies. *Journal of Medical Imaging and Health Informatics, 5*(6), 1223–1228. doi:10.1166/jmihi.2015.1511

Silva, C. T., Naveed, N., Bokhari, S., Baker, K. E., Staib, L. H., Ibrahim, S. M., & Goodman, T. R. et al. (2012). Early assessment of the efficacy of digital infrared thermal imaging in pediatric extremity trauma. *Emergency Radiology, 19*(3), 203–209. doi:10.1007/s10140-012-1027-2 PMID:22362422

Silverman, Tuncali, Adams, von Sonnenberg, Zou, Kacher, … Jolesz. (2000). MR imaging-guided percutaneous cryotherapy of liver tumors: Initial experience. *Radiology, 217*, 657-664.

Simmons, G. H., Wong, B. J., Holowatz, L. A., & Kenney, W. L. (2011). Changes in the control of skin blood flow with exercise training: Where do cutaneous vascular adaptations fit in? *Experimental Physiology, 96*(9), 822–828. doi:10.1113/expphysiol.2010.056176 PMID:21602295

Simon, E. L., Gaughan, E. M., Epp, T., & Spire, M. (2006). Influence of exercise on thermographically determined surface temperatures of thoracic and pelvic limbs in horses. *Journal of the American Veterinary Medical Association, 229*(12), 1940–1944. doi:10.2460/javma.229.12.1940 PMID:17173534

Simons, D. G. (1988). Myofascial pain syndromes: Where are we? Where are we going? *Archives of Physical Medicine and Rehabilitation, 69*(3 Pt 1), 207–212. PMID:3279935

Simons, D. G. (2004). Review of enigmatic MTP as a common cause of enigmatic musculoskeletal pain and dysfunction. *Journal of Electromyography and Kinesiology, 14*(1), 95–107. doi:10.1016/j.jelekin.2003.09.018 PMID:14759755

Simons, D. G., Travell, J. G., & Simons, L. S. (1999). *Travell & Simons' myofascial pain and dysfunction: the trigger point manual* (2nd ed.; Vol. 1). Baltimore, MD: Williams & Wilkins.

Singh, M., Murriel, C. L., & Johnson, L. (2012). Genetically engineered mouse models: Closing the gap between preclinical data and trial outcomes. *Cancer Research, 72*(11), 2695–2700. doi:10.1158/0008-5472.CAN-11-2786 PMID:22593194

Smith, B. L., Bandler, M. K., & Goodman, P. H. (1986). Dominant forearm hyperthermia: A study of fifteen athletes. *Thermology, 2*, 25–28.

Smriga, M., Murakami, H., Mori, M., & Torii, K. (2000). Use of thermal photography to explore the age-dependent effect of monosodium glutamate, NaCl and glucose on brown adipose tissue thermogenesis. *Physiology & Behavior, 71*(3), 403–407. doi:10.1016/S0031-9384(00)00350-4 PMID:11150573

Snekhalatha, U., Anburajan, M., Venkatraman, B., & Menaka, M. (2013). Evaluation of complete Freunds adjuvant-induced arthritis in a Wistar rat model. *Zeitschrift fur Rheumatologie, 72*(4), 375–382. doi:10.1007/s00393-012-1083-8 PMID:23208192

Song, C., Appleyard, V., Murray, K., Frank, T., Sibbett, W., Cuschieri, A., & Thompson, A. (2007). Thermographic assessment of tumor growth in mouse xenografts. *International Journal of Cancer, 121*(5), 1055–1058. doi:10.1002/ijc.22808 PMID:17487841

Soroko, M., & Davies - Morel, M.C.G. (2016). Equine Thermography in Practice, CABI, UK and US. doi:10.1079/9781780647876.0000

Soroko, M. (2011a). Analyses of superficial temperature distribution of lower part of the limbs in young racing horses. *Measurement. Automation and Monitoring, 57*(10), 1157–1160.

Soroko, M. (2011b). Thermographic diagnosis of sport horses' limbs. *Biomedical Engineering, 17*(2), 104–109.

Soroko, M., Dudek, K., Howell, K., Henklewski, R., & Jodkowska, E. (2014). Thermographic evaluation of racehorse performance. *Journal of Equine Veterinary Science, 34*(9), 1076–1083. doi:10.1016/j.jevs.2014.06.009

Soroko, M., Henklewski, R., Filipowski, H., & Jodkowska, E. (2013). The effectiveness of thermographic analysis in equine orthopedics. *Journal of Equine Veterinary Science*, *33*(9), 760–762. doi:10.1016/j.jevs.2012.11.009

Soroko, M., Henklewski, R., & Jodkowska, E. (2012a). Analiza wyników badań termograficznych, ultrasonograficznych i rentgenowskich w diagnozowaniu chorób ortopedycznych u koni wyścigowych[Comparison of thermographic, radiographic and ultrasonographic results in diagnosing racehorses orthopedic diseases]. *Medycyna Weterynaryjna*, *68*(11), 693–696.

Soroko, M., Jodkowska, E., & Dudek, K. (2015). Diagnoza termograficzna w monitorowaniu rocznego treningu koni wyścigowych[Thermography diagnosis in monitoring annual racehorses' training cycle]. *Medycyna Weterynaryjna*, *71*(01), 52–58.

Soroko, M., Jodkowska, E., & Zabłocka, M. (2012b). The use of thermography to evaluate back musculoskeletal responses of young racehorses to training. *Thermology International*, *22*(3), 152–156.

Spencer-Green, G. (1998). Outcomes in primary Raynaud phenomenon: A meta-analysis of the frequency, rates, and predictors of transition to secondary diseases. *Archives of Internal Medicine*, *158*(6), 595–600. doi:10.1001/archinte.158.6.595 PMID:9521223

Stanek, Cieslar, & Rosmus-Kucza. (2006). Influence of whole - body cryotherapy on blood morphology parameters in patients with ankylosing spondylitis and in healthy volunteers. *Acta Bio-Optica et Informatica Medica*, *12*(3), 207-210.

Stanek, Cholewka, & Cieslar, Rosmus-Kuczia, Drzazga, & Sieron. (2011). The assessment of the analgesic action of whole - body cryotherapy in patients with ankylosing spondylitis. *Fizjoterapia Polska*, *11*(1), 49–55.

Stanek, Cieslar, & Matyszkiewicz. (2005). Subjective estimation of therapeutic efficacy of whole - body cryotherapy in patients with ankylosing spondylitis. *Balneolologia Polska*, *47*(1-2), 24–32.

Stanek, Cieślar, & Matyszkiewicz. (2006). Changes in antioxidant status in patients with ankylosing spondylitis during cryotherapy. *European Journal of Clinical Investigation*, *36*(Suppl.1), 20.

Stanek, Cieslar, & Sieron. (2007). Therapeutic application of cryotherapy in clinical practice. *Balneologia Polska*, *49*(1), 37–45.

Stanek, Cieślar, & Sieroń. (2008). Application of cryotherapy in sport medcine. *Rehabilitacja w Praktyce*, *2*, 34–35.

Stanek, Cieslar, & Strzelczyk. (2010). Influence of cryogenic temperatures on inflammatory markers in patients with ankylosing spondylitis and healthy volunteers. *Polish Journal of Environmental Studies*, *19*(1), 167–175.

Stanek, Cieślar, Mrowiec, & Sieroń. (2006). Cryotherapy in clinical practice. *Rehabilitacja w Praktyce*, *1*, 27–31.

Stanek, Sieron, & Cieslar, Matyszkiewicz, & Rozmus-Kuczia. (2005). Influence of whole-body cryotherapy on parameters of spine mobility in patients with ankylosing spondylitis. *Ortopedia, Traumatologia, Rehabilitacja*, *5*(7), 549–554. PMID:17611448

Stanek, Wielkoszynski, & Cholewka. (2011). Influence of whole - body cryotherapy on some chosen non - enzymatic parameters of antioxidant status in patients with ankylosing spondylitis. *Acta Balneolgica*, *53*(4), 264–269.

Stannard, A. B., Brandenburg, J. P., Pitney, W. A., & Lukaszuk, J. M. (2011). Effects of wearing a cooling vest during the warm-up on 10-km run performance. *Journal of Strength and Conditioning Research*, *25*(7), 2018–2024. doi:10.1519/JSC.0b013e3181e07585 PMID:21448075

Stess, S., & Moss, G. (1986). Use of liquid crystal thermography in the evaluation of the diabetic foot. *Diabetes Care*, *9*(3), 267–272. doi:10.2337/diacare.9.3.267 PMID:3731992

Stromberg, B. (1972). Thermography of the superficial flexor tendon in race horses. *Acta Radiologica*, *319*(319 Suppl), 295–297. doi:10.1177/0284185172013S31954 PMID:4531198

Stromberg, B. (1974). The use of thermography in equine orthopedics. *Journal of the American Veterinary Radiology*, *15*(1), 94–97. doi:10.1111/j.1740-8261.1974.tb00676.x

Styczyński, Gasik, Krzemińska-Dąbrowska, & Pyskło. (2001). Ocena Przydatności Krioterapii U Chorych Na Bóle Krzyża Związane Z Dyskopatią I Zmianami Zwyrodnieniowymi Kręgosłupa Baln. *Pol.*, *43*(1-2), 50 – 55. (in Polish)

Sukovatykh & Kniazev. (2007). The mechanisms of critical impairments of microcirculation in patients with chronic ischemia of lower extremities. *Vestnik Khirurgii Imeni I. I. Grekova*, *166*(4), 20–24. PMID:17966649

Švestková & Pospíšilová. (1991). Risk Factors Of Chronic Venous Disease Inception. *Current Problems in Surgery*, *28*, 339–400.

Švestková & Pospíšilová. (2008). Risk Factors Of Chronic Venous Disease Inception. *Scripta Medica*, *81*(2), 117–128.

Swenson, S., Swärd, L., & Karlsson, J. (1996). Cryotherapy in sports medicine. *Scandinavian Journal of Medicine & Science in Sports*, *6*(4), 193–200. doi:10.1111/j.1600-0838.1996.tb00090.x PMID:8896090

Swerdlow, B., & Dieter, J. N. I. (1992). An evaluation of the sensitivity and specificity of medical thermography for the documentation of myofascial trigger points. *Pain*, *48*(2), 205–213. doi:10.1016/0304-3959(92)90060-O PMID:1589239

Tauchmannova, H., Gabrhel, J., & Cibak, M. (1993). Thermographic findings in different sports, their value in the prevention of soft tissue injuries. *Thermol Österr*, *3*, 91–95.

Tennvall, Andersso, & Bjellerup, Hjelmgren, & Oien. (2004). Treatment of venous leg ulcers can be better and cheaper. Annual costs calculation based on an inquiry study. *Lakartidningen*, *101*, 1506–1510, 1512–1513. PMID:15150953

Tepper, M., Shoval, A., Hoffer, O., Confino, H., Schmidt, M., Kelson, I., & Gannot, I. et al. (2013). Thermographic investigation of tumor size, and its correlation to tumor relative temperature, in mice with transplantable solid breast carcinoma. *Journal of Biomedical Optics*, *18*(11), 111410–111410. doi:10.1117/1.JBO.18.11.111410 PMID:23934014

Thomas, C., & Davies, J. (1989). Liquid crystal thermography and C reactive protein in the detection of deep venous thrombosis. *BMJ (Clinical Research Ed.)*, *299*(6705), 951–952. doi:10.1136/bmj.299.6705.951 PMID:2508949

Thomas, D., Siahamis, G., Marion, M., & Boyle, C. (1992). Computerised infrared thermography and isotopic bone scanning in tennis elbow. *Annals of the Rheumatic Diseases*, *51*(1), 103–107. doi:10.1136/ard.51.1.103 PMID:1540012

Thomas, R. A. (1999). *The thermography monitoring handbook*. Coxmoor Publ.

Torii, M., Yamasaki, M., & Sasaki, T. (1987). Skin surface temperatures during submaximal cycling observed by color thermography. *Annals of Physiological Anthropology*, *6*(1), 21–24. doi:10.2114/ahs1983.6.21 PMID:3675756

Torii, M., Yamasaki, M., Sasaki, T., & Nakayama, H. (1992). Fall in skin temperature of exercising man. *British Journal of Sports Medicine*, *26*(1), 29–32. doi:10.1136/bjsm.26.1.29 PMID:1600450

Torre, L. A., Bray, F., Siegel, R. L., Ferlay, J., Lortet-Tieulent, J., & Jemal, A. (2015). Global cancer statistics, 2012. *CA: a Cancer Journal for Clinicians*, *65*(2), 87–108. doi:10.3322/caac.21262 PMID:25651787

Traczyk. (2007). *Fizjologia człowieka w zarysie*. PZWL.

Tunley, B. V., & Henson, F. M. (2004). Reliability and repeatability of thermographic examination and the normal thermographic image of the thoracolumbar region in the horse. *Equine Veterinary Journal*, *36*(4), 306–312. doi:10.2746/0425164044890652 PMID:15163036

Turner, T. A. (1991). Thermography as an aid to the clinical lameness evaluation. *The Veterinary Clinics of North America. Equine Practice*, *7*(2), 311–338. PMID:1933566

Turner, T. A. (1998). The use of thermography in lameness evaluation.*Proceeding of the American Association of Equine Practitioners*, *44*, 224-226.

Turner, T. A. (2001). Diagnostic thermography. *The Veterinary Clinics of North America. Equine Practice*, *17*(1), 95–113. PMID:11488048

Turner, T. A. (2003). Back problems in horses.*49th Annual Convention of the American Association of Equine Practitioners*, New Orleans, LA.

Turner, T. A., Fessler, J. F., Lamp, M., Pearce, J. A., & Geddes, L. A. (1983). Thermographic evaluation of horses with podotrochlosis. *American Journal of Veterinary Research*, *44*(4), 535–539. PMID:6869948

Turner, T. A., Pansch, J., & Wilson, J. H. (2001). Thermographic assessment of racing Thoroughbreds.*Proceeding of the American Association of Equine Practitioners*, *47*, 344-346.

Turner, T. A., Rantanen, N. W., & Hauser, M. L. (1996). Alternate methods of soft tissue imaging.*1st Proceedings Dubai International Equine Symposium*, (pp. 165–176).

Turner, T. A., & Scroggins, R. D. (1989). Thermographic detection of gingering in horses. *Journal of Equine Veterinary Science*, *5*(1), 8–10. doi:10.1016/S0737-0806(85)80077-0

Turner, T. A., Waldsmith, J. K., & Wilson, J. H. (2004). How to assess saddle fit in horses. *Proceedings American Association of Equine Practice*, *50*, 196–201.

Tuszynski, J., & Dixon, J. (2002). *Biomedical applications for introductory physics*. New York: Wiley.

Uematsu, S. (1985). Symmetry of temperatures comparing one side of the other. *Thermology*, *1*, 4–7.

Usamentiaga, R., Venegas, P., Guerediaga, J., Vega, L., Molleda, J., & Bulnes, F. G. (2014). Infrared Thermography for Temperature Measurement and Non-Destructive Testing. *Sensors (Basel, Switzerland)*, *14*(7), 2305–2348. doi:10.3390/s140712305 PMID:25014096

Usuki, K., Kanekura, T., Aradono, K., & Kanzaki, T. (1998). Effects of nicotine on peripheral cutaneous blood flow and skin temperature. *Journal of Dermatological Science*, *16*(3), 173–181. doi:10.1016/S0923-1811(97)00049-2 PMID:9651814

Vaden, M. F., Purohit, R. C., McCoy, D., & Vaughan, J. T. (1980). Thermography: A technique for subclinical diagnosis of osteoarthritis. *American Journal of Veterinary Research*, *41*(8), 1175–1180. PMID:7447111

Vainer, B. G. (2005). FPA-based infrared thermography as applied to the study of cutaneous perspiration and stimulated vascular response in humans. *Physics in Medicine and Biology*, *50*(23), R63–R94. doi:10.1088/0031-9155/50/23/R01 PMID:16306642

Valvano, J.W., Allen, J.T., & Bowman, H.F. (1981). *The simultaneous measurement of thermal conductivity, thermal diffusivity, and perfusion in small volumes of tissue*. ASME 81- WA/HT-21.

Van Den Bosh, P. (2006). *Cycling: A year round plan*. Meyer & Meyer Sport.

Van den Oever, Hepp, Debbaut, & Simon. (1998). Socio-economic impact of chronic venous insufficiency. An underestimated public health problem. *International Angiology*, *17*, 161–167. PMID:9821029

Van Hoogmoed, L. M., & Snyder, J. R. (2002). Use of infrared thermography to detect injections and palmar digital neurectomy in horses. *Veterinary Journal (London, England)*, *164*(2), 129–141. doi:10.1053/tvjl.2002.0719 PMID:12359467

Van Hoogmoed, L. M., Snyder, J. R., Allen, A. K., & Waldsmith, J. D. (2000). Use of infrared thermography to detect performance - enhancing techniques in horses. *Equine Veterinary Education*, *12*(2), 102–107. doi:10.1111/j.2042-3292.2000.tb01772.x

Van Middendorp, J. J., Sanchez, G. M., & Burridge, A. L. (2010). The Edwin Smith papyrus: A clinical reappraisal of the oldest known document on spinal injuries. *European Spine Journal*, *19*(11), 1815–1823. doi:10.1007/s00586-010-1523-6 PMID:20697750

Vardasca, R. Â. R. (2012). *The effect of work related mechanical stress on the peripheral temperature of the hand.* Academic Press.

Vardasca, R., Ring, E. F. J., Plassmann, P., & Jones, C. D. (2012). Thermal symmetry of the upper and lower extremities in healthy subjects. *Thermology International, 22*(2), 53-60.

Vardasca, Ring, Plassmann, & Jones. (2012). Thermal symmetry of the upper and lower extermities in healthy subjects. *Thermology International, 22*(2), 53-60.

Vardasca, R. (2008). Symmetry of temperature distribution in the upper and the lower extremities. *Thermology International, 18*(4), 154.

Vardasca, R., Ring, E. F. J., Plassmann, P., & Jones, C. D. (2012). Thermal symmetry of the upper and lower extremities in healthy subjects. *Thermol Int*, *22*(3), 53–60.

Vardasca, R., & Simoes, R. (2013). Current Issues in Medical Thermography. In *Topics in Medical Image Processing and Computational Vision* (pp. 223–237). Springer Netherlands. doi:10.1007/978-94-007-0726-9_12

Vargas, J. V. C., Brioschi, M. L., Dias, F. G., Parolin, M. B., Mulinari-Brenner, F. A., Ordonez, J. C., & Colman, D. (2009). Normalized methodology for medical infrared imaging. *Infrared Physics & Technology*, *52*(1), 42–47. doi:10.1016/j.infrared.2008.11.003

Veghte, J. H., Adams, W. C., & Bernauer, E. M. (1979). Temperature changes during exercise measured by thermography. *Aviation, Space, and Environmental Medicine*, *50*(7), 708–713. PMID:486019

Verschooten, F., Desmet, P., & Verbeeck, J. (1997). Skin surface temperature measurements in horses by electronic thermometry. *Equine Practice*, *19*(4), 16–23.

Viskanta, R., & Toor, J. (1972). Radiant energy transfer in waters. *Water Resources Research*, *8*(3), 595–608. doi:10.1029/WR008i003p00595

Visscher, C. M., Lobbezoo, F., & Naeije, M. (2004). Comparison of algometry an palpation in the recognition of temporomandibular disorder pain complaints. *Journal of Orofacial Pain*, *18*(3), 214–219. PMID:15509000

von Schweinitz, D. G. (1999). Thermographic diagnosis in equine back pain. *The Veterinary Clinics of North America. Equine Practice*, *15*, 161–177. PMID:10218248

Wade, C. E., & Veghte, J. H. (1977). Thermographic evaluation of the relative heat loss by area in man after swimming. *Aviation, Space, and Environmental Medicine*, *48*(1), 16–18. PMID:831705

Walden, M., Hagglund, M., & Ekstrand, J. (2005). UEFA Champions League study: A prospective study of injuries in professional football during the 20012002 season. *British Journal of Sports Medicine*, *39*(8), 542–546. doi:10.1136/bjsm.2004.014571 PMID:16046340

Waldman, E.A., Luhm, K.R., Monteiro, S.A., Freitas, F.R. (2011). Surveillance of adverse effects following vaccination and safety of immunization programs. *Rev. Saude Publica., 45*(1), 173-84.

Waldsmith, J. K., & Oltman, J. I. (1994). Thermography: Subclinical inflammation, diagnosis, rehabilitation, and athletic evaluation. *Journal of Equine Veterinary Science*, *14*(1), 8–10. doi:10.1016/S0737-0806(07)80302-9

Wang, J.-G., & Toh, H. L. (2001, 2001). *Visualizing skin temperature before, during and after exercise for dynamic area telethermometry*. Paper presented at the Engineering in Medicine and Biology Society.

Ważny, Z. (1994). *Leksykon treningu sportowego*. Warszawa: AWF.

Weinstein, S. A., Weinstein, G., Weinstein, E. L., & Gelb, M. (1991). Facial thermography, basis, protocol, and clinical value. *Cranio*, *9*(3), 201–211. doi:10.1080/08869634.1991.11678368 PMID:1810666

Wendt, D., van Loon, L., & van Marken Lichtenbelt, W. (2007). Thermoregulation during Exercise in the heat. *Sports Medicine (Auckland, N.Z.)*, *37*(8), 669–682. doi:10.2165/00007256-200737080-00002 PMID:17645370

Westermann, S., Stanek, C., Schramel, J. P., Ion, A., & Buchner, H. H. (2013). The effect of airflow on thermographically determined temperature of the distal forelimb of the horse. *Equine Veterinary Journal*, *45*(5), 637–641. doi:10.1111/evj.12019 PMID:23294196

Wiącek, Rzymska-Klicha, Kaszuba, & Drobnik. (1999). The use of cryosurgical techniques in dermatology – own experiences. *Nowa. Klin.*, *6*(12), 1178–1184.

Wild, W., Schütte, S. R., Pau, H. W., Kramp, B., & Just, T. (2003). Infrared thermography as a non-invasive application for medical diagnostic. In *Proceedings XVII IMEKO World Congress* (pp. 22-27).

Wilkes, S., Stansby, G., Sims, A. J., Haining, S., & Allen, J. (2015). Peripheral arterial disease: Diagnostic challenges and how photoplethysmography may help. *The British Journal of General Practice*, *65*(635), 323–324. doi:10.3399/bjgp15X685489 PMID:26009528

Wilkinson, B., & Edwards, S. (1993). Leukocytes: Their role in the etiopathogenesis of skin damage in venous disease. *Journal of Vascular Surgery*, *17*(4), 669–675. doi:10.1016/0741-5214(93)90109-Y PMID:8464084

Williams, R. B., Harkins, L. S., Hammond, C. J., & Wood, J. L. (2001). Racehorses injuries, clinical problems and fatalities recorded on British racecourses from flat racing and National Hint racing during 1996, 1997 and 1998. *Equine Veterinary Journal*, *33*(5), 478–486. doi:10.2746/042516401776254808 PMID:11558743

Wiśniewski, S., & Wiśniewski, S. T. (2009). *Heat transfer* (6th ed.). Warszawa: WNT.

Woods, C., Hawkins, R., Hulse, M., & Hodson, A. (2003). The Football Association Medical Research Programme: an audit of injuries in professional football: an analysis of ankle sprains. *British Journal of Sports Medicine*, *37*(3), 233–238. doi:10.1136/bjsm.37.3.233 PMID:12782548

Wozniak, M.-K., Drewa, D., & Wozniak, O. (2001). Activity of chosen lisosome's enzymes in plasma of canoeists after whole - body cryotherapy. *Med Sport*, *17*, 322–327.

Xie, W., McCahon, P., Jakobsen, K., & Parish, C. (2004). Evaluation of the ability of digital infrared imaging to detect vascular changes in experimental animal tumours. *International Journal of Cancer*, *108*(5), 790–794. doi:10.1002/ijc.11618 PMID:14696108

Yamauchi, Nogami, & Miura. (1981). Various applications of extreme cryotherapy and strenuous exercise program - focusing on chronic rheumatoid arthritis. *Physiother Rehab*, *5*, 35–39.

Zagrobelny & Zimmer. (1999). The application of of cryogenic temperatures in medicine and physical sports therapy. *Med. Sport.*, *15*(94), 8–13.

Zagrobelny, Halawa, Jegierski, & Wawrowska. (1993). The influence of whole body cooling in cryogenic chamber on chosen haemodynamic markers and hormone concentration in serum of healthy people. *Physician Polish Weekly, 48*(14-15), 303-305.

Zagrobelny. (Ed.). (2003a). *Whole-body and local cryotherapy*. Urban & Partner.

Zagrobelny. (Ed.). (2003b). *Local and wholebody cryotherapy*. Urban & Partner.

Zaïdi, H., Taiar, R., Fohanno, S., & Polidori, G. (2007). The influence of swimming type on the skin-temperature maps of a competitive swimmer from infrared thermography. *Acta of Bioengineering and Biomechanics*, *9*(1), 47–51. PMID:17933104

Zatoń, M., Herbisz, R., & Herbisz, P. (2011). *Fizjologiczne podstawy treningu w kolarstwie górskim*. Wrocław: Wydawnictwo AWF Wrocław.

Zontak, A., Sideman, S., Verbitsky, O., & Beyar, R. (1998). Dynamic thermography: Analysis of hand temperature during exercise. *Annals of Biomedical Engineering*, *26*(6), 988–993. doi:10.1114/1.33 PMID:9846937

Żuber & Jung. (1997). *Thermographic methods in medical diagnostics*. Warszawa: Academic Press.

About the Contributors

Ricardo Vardasca holds a Ph.D. in Medical Informatics from University of South Wales (UK), currently he is a Postdoctoral fellow at INEGI and Faculty of Engineering of University of Porto, External Professor at University of Valencia (Spain) and General Secretary at the European Association of Thermology. He previously was a Postdoctoral fellow at University of Minho (Portugal), Invited Associated Professor at Polytechnic Institute of Leiria (Portugal) and Lecturer, Researcher and Consultant at the University of Glamorgan (actually University of South Wales, United Kingdom). He is associate member of the British Computer Society (Health Informatics group), honorary lifetime member of the Brazilian Association of Thermology, member of the Royal Photographic Society (Imaging Science group) and the Institute of Physics and Engineering in Medicine. He is at the editorial board of scientific journals: Thermology International, The Imaging Science Journal and International Journal of E-Health and Medical Communications. He acted as reviewer for many scientific journals and meetings scientific committees and was editor of 3 books, author of several book chapters, journal and conference proceeding articles, and presented more than 80 oral works at international meetings, serving in 25 as invited speaker. He has successfully supervised 7 MSc theses and co-supervised 1 PhD, actually is supervising 8 MSc students and co-supervising 5 PhD candidates Since January 2015 is member of the committee ISO/TC121/SC3-IEC62D/JWG8, Project Team 9 on Thermography. His main research interests are medical thermography, image processing and mobile computing.

Joaquim Gabriel received the degree in Mechanical Engineering from the Faculty of Engineering (UPorto, 1988), specialization of machine design; a post-graduation degree in Industrial Automation and Process Management; a Master in Industrial Computing, and a PhD in Industrial Electronics from the University of Minho. He was researcher fellow from JNICT (National Research Association), Portugal, 1989; and from the Japanese Ministry of Industry EU-STA at Kanagawa Science Park, Japan (1995-97) and invited researcher at Yokohama City University, Japan, 2002. Since 2003 he is with the Automation, Instrumentation and Control group of the Faculty of Engineering. His main interests are instrumentation, supervisory control and data acquisition - SCADA, industrial automation, medical devices, thermography. He is member of IEEE - Instrumentation and Measurement and of European Association of Thermology.

* * *

Ana Margarida Abrantes (PhD) Auxiliary Professor in Faculty of Medicine, University of Coimbra with 42 full papers published in international and national journals and 2 book chapters has been developing research work on biophysics, animal models of human diseases, Nuclear Oncology, radiobiology as well as new cancer therapies. She is researcher of CIMAGO- Centre of Investigation on Environment, Genetics and Oncobiology CNC.IBILI - Center for Neuroscience and Cell Biology and the Institute for Biomedical Imaging and Life Sciences Coimbra Health School, Polytechnic Institute of Coimbra, Portugal.

John Allen is Lead Clinical Scientist for Microvascular Diagnostics based in the Northern Medical Physics and Clinical Engineering Directorate at the Freeman Hospital, Newcastle upton Tyne, UK. He is the founder of the Newcastle measurement facility and leads service development and associated R&D. John is also an Honorary Clinical Senior Lecturer in the Faculty of Medical Sciences at Newcastle University. His PhD was awarded in 2002 on photoplethysmography and cardiovascular assessments. He has published and presented many papers on various clinical vascular optical measurements and has secured team awards at national level for medical technology and service innovations. He is also a Chartered Engineer and Scientist, a Fellow of the Royal Photographic Society (ASIS FRPS), and a member of the Editorial Board for the journal Physiological Measurement.

Kurt Ammer is the treasurer of the European Association of Thermology, the president of the Austrian Association of Thermology, the Editor in Chief of the Journal Thermology International, a Visiting Professor at Medical Imaging Research Unit, department of Computing, University of South Wales, U.K., and was the former the director of the Department of Physical Diagnosis, Ludwig Boltzmann Research Institute, Hanusch General Hospital, Viena (Austria).

Emiko S. Arita is a Professor of Postgraduate Course, Masters and PhD level at the Faculty of Dentistry, University of São Paulo. She acts as advisor to students of the Postgraduate Master's and Doctor's Examining Committee and participant in qualifying and defending theses. She is also a Visiting Professor and researcher of National University Corporation Okayama University, Department of Oral and Maxillofacial Radiology Okayama University Graduate School of Medicine, Dentistry and Pharmaceltical Sciences, Professor of Radiology of Specialization Course of Radiology. Actual Board, Commissions and Consulting, Scientific Council - São Paulo University, Faculty of Odontology. Specification: Council Member Actual Boards, Commissions and Consulting, Faculty of Dentistry, Department of Stomatology Specification: Co - Representative of Associate Professors at the Congregation Current Boards, Commissions and Consulting, Faculty of Dentistry, Department of Stomatology Specification: Representative of Associate Professors at the Department.

Usama I. Bajwa got both M.S. and Ph.D. degrees from CASE Islamabad, Pakistan in 2006 and 2013 respectively. He is presently serving as an Assistant Professor at Department of Computer Science, COMSATS Institute of Information Technology. After completing his M.S., he served as a visiting researcher at Medical Imaging Research Lab, University of South Wales, United Kingdom. He has authored/co-authored several research publications of international repute. His fields of interest are Medical Image Processing, Biometrics and Natural Language Processing.

Esther Ballester has a degree in Medicine (2005), and a PhD in Pediatrics (2015) from the University of Valencia, Spain. She is currently a pediatrician in the Pediatric Emergency Department of Doctor Peset University Hospital in Valencia and a clinical professor for the Department of Pediatrics, Ginecology and Obstetrics, University of Valencia. Her research interests include Pediatric Emergencies, Childhood Obesity and Physical Activity in children.

Filipa Barbosa has received a MSc in Bioengineering from Faculty of Engineering of University of Porto in 2014.

Jose María Blasco, PhD in Electronic Engineering and lecturer at the University of Valencia, has developed most of his work in the field of nuclear and medical physics applications, focusing on the development of instrumentation for radiation detection, hardware designs as well as the implementation of data processing approaches to optimize the exploitation of the available information of medical imaging and positioning systems.

Márcio Borgonovo-Santos received his degree in Physical Education in 2004, from the State University of Santa Catarina - UDESC. At the same time, attended the technical module of the Electronic Systems in 2006, at the Federal Institute of Santa Catarina - IFSC. He merges both areas, human and technological, in the Master of Sciences of Human Movement in 2009 at UDESC, specifically instrumentation in sports biomechanics. With the opportunity to do research in Europe, he comes from Brazil to Portugal since 2011, where he currently develops research activities at the Porto Biomechanics Laboratory - LABIOMEP, in the Faculty of Sports - FADE, of the University of Porto - UP. Participates in the doctoral program in Sports Sciences of UP as a Ph.D. candidate, which develops its project in Surf Biomechanics. This project has earned two awards with honorable mentions in business innovation contests, iUP25K and Pitch day of UPTEC in 2015.

Maria Filomena Botelho (MD, PhD) Full Professor in Faculty of Medicine, University of Coimbra, with 177 full papers published in international and national journals and 5 book chapters has been developing translational research work on Biophysics, animal models of human diseases, nuclear oncology Photodynamic therapy and Radiopharmacy. She is researcher of CIMAGO- Centre of Investigation on Environment, Genetics and Oncobiology CNC.IBILI - Center for Neuroscience and Cell Biology and the Institute for Biomedical Imaging and Life Sciences.

Marcos L. Brioschi is a Medical doctor since 1996, with specialty in General Surgery and Trauma, Forensic Sciencies and Thermology &Thermography at Faculty of Medicine at University of São Paulo (FMUSP), Currently he is a Research Professor at Faculty of Medicine at University of São Paulo (FMUSP). He also have been a Post-Doctoral in Medicine, Faculty of Medicine at University of São Paulo (FMUSP) and holds a Doctoral degree in Mechanical Engineering, Biothermodynamics, Federal University of Paraná (UFPR). He is the Coordinator and Professor of Postgraduate Course in Thermology and Thermography, Faculty of Medicine at University of São Paulo (FMUSP), President of the Brazilian Association of Thermology (ABRATERM), Director of the Brazilian Institute of Medical Thermology (IBTM), Actual Editor of the Pan American Journal of Medical Thermology (PAJMT) and of International Consensus and Guidelines of Medical Thermography (ICGMT). He is co-author of the book named "Dor Orofacial Crônica – diagnóstico por termografia infravermelha".

Armand Cholewka is an Associate Professor in Department of Medical Physics in University of Silesia, Katowice, Poland. He has been provided studies connected with thermal imaging in medicine and sports for last 15 years. His main academic interest focuses on medical physics and physical medicine mainly impact of extremely low temperatures (cryotherapy), application of extremely-low-frequency magnetic fields and low-energy lasers on human body He also perform functions: vice Director of Institute of Physics, the President of Silesian Branch of Polish Medical Physics Society and Main Board Member of Polish Medical Physics Society, the Dean of Youth University of Silesia and vice Director of Continuing Education Center.

Rosa Cibrián has both M.Sc. and Ph.D. degrees in Physics from the University of Valencia, Spain, in 1978 and 1987, respectively. She is currently professor of Biophysics in the Department of Physiology. She was head of that Department during three years and nowadays is Director of Master in Medical Physics. She has been involved in several projects related to image pattern analysis applied to Medicine and Sports. She has 4 research sexenis. She has co-authored over 110 publications at national and international journals, with high impact factor, book chapters, and more than 130 Congress communications. She has been the Director of 16 Doctoral Thesis, 3 of them with "extraordinary PhD award". She also has been Director of 14 Master thesis. She is member of different scientific associations and Member of the Organizing Committee of Scientific Congress.

Pilar Codoñer-Franch has a Ph.D. degree in Medicine (1987) from the University of Valencia, Spain. She is currently a full Professor at the Department of Pediatrics, Obstetrics and Gynecology, University of Valencia. His research interests include Childhood Obesity, Child Nutrition and Injuries in children. She is a Member of Spain Pediatric Association and President of Ethics Committee of Dr. Peset Hospital, Valencia (Spain).

Ana Domingues has received a MSc in Bioengineering from Faculty of Engineering of University of Porto in 2014.

Zofia Drzazga is a Professor of Medical Physics at University of Silesia in Katowice, a Head of Department of Medical Physics at Institute of Physics in Katowice and Silesian Center for Education and Interdisciplinary Research in Chorzow, Poland is coordinating the education in the field of medical physics in Silesia. She initiated and there was a chairwoman international symposium of medical physics in Poland (2001,2003,20009) She was awarded by of the Minister of Higher Education and Science 1988. Author and coauthor of more than 150 peer- reviewed articles published in journals and conference proceedings, 2 monographs, editor or co-editor of 6 books and 15 chapters in books. Research Interest Main fields of interest: Application of non-ionizing radiation in diagnostics and theraphy in vitro and in vivo . Her research interests include thermal imaging in medicine and sports, microcalorimetry measurements, fluorescence spectroscopy and microspectroscopy, CD spectroscopy of proteins, diffusion-weighted imaging (DWI), brain evoked potencials, functional magnetic resonance imaging (fMRI).

Ricardo Fernandes got his PhD in Sport Sciences from the Faculty of Sport - University of Porto (Portugal) in 2006. He has been teaching at the same institution (since 1995), researching at the Centre of Research, Education, Innovation and Intervention in Sport and part of on the Directive Board of the Porto Biomechanics Laboratory. He is interested in the biophysical characterization specially centred on the availability and use of energy in cyclic sports, particularly on the determination of the athlete's bioenergetical profile (understanding the kinetics of oxygen consumption and lactate production), and on the relationship of these physiological parameters with biomechanical variables. He also interested in planning and periodization, and training control and evaluation of athletes in cyclic sports. Most recently, he has been engaged in water polo game analysis, namely identifying the determinant factors that affect decisively the success of players and teams.

Ismael Fernández Cuevas has a research and professional background focused on the use of Infrared Thermography for injury prevention. He defended in 2012 his international PhD in Physical Activity and Sport Science in the Technical University of Madrid (Spain). He has published more than 15 research impact papers on the topic of Thermography and exercise, participated in more than 30 international congresses and 5 international R&D projects. He has been awarded 5 times for different works on this topic (including the award as the best PhD of the Technical University of Madrid). At the same time, Ismael is one of the cofounders of ThermoHuman, a company set up in 2008 and focused in the application of Infrared Thermography in humans in the sports and health sector, with experience in high performances teams and athletes from different sports (football, basketball, baseball, judo, etc.). In addition to that, he got in 2014 a MBA degree in International Business Administration by the Menéndez Pelayo International University (Spain)

Rui M. Gil da Costa is a veterinary pathologist working with animal models of cancer. He completed his PhD at the University of Porto with a thesis on the carcinogenic properties of bracken. HIs current research interests cover carcinogenesis and cancer prevention, as well as the development of new diagnostic methods and anti-neoplastic therapies.

Rolando J. González-Peña received his Master of Science degree in optics from the High Technology Institute of Havana in 1998 and his PhD in technical science from the High Technology Institute of Havana in 2001. His current research is focused on digital speckle interferometry and dynamic speckle laser. Currently, he is professor at the Physiology Department in the Faculty of Medicine and Odontology at the University of Valencia.

Denise S. Haddad is a Dentist since 2003, with specialty in temporomandibular disorder and orofacial pain., currently she is Post-Doctoral fellow in Dentistry, Faculty of Dentistry at University of São Paulo (FOUSP). She holds a Doctoral and a Master degrees in Dentistry, Faculty of Dentistry at University of São Paulo (FOUSP. She is Member of the Brazilian Association of Thermology (ABRATERM). She is actually at the Board of Technical Chamber of Temporomandibular Disorder and Orofacial Pain - Regional Council of Dentistry of São Paulo (CROSP). She is co-author of the book named "Dor Orofacial Crônica – diagnóstico por termografia infravermelha".

Andreas Hoffmann completed his DVM in Berlin at the Humboldt University in 1976 and continued his career in the fields of veterinary immunology, microbiology, vaccine control, generation of monoclonal antibodies and experimental allergy. From 2013 he changed to the unit of veterinary pharmacovigilance unit at the Paul-Ehrlich Institute in Langen (Germany). There he initiated several thermografic project´s following the 3R-concept in animal experiments and monitoring of vaccine side effects.

Carl Jones is a member of the Medical Imaging Research Unit at the University of South Wales and was involved in the development of a reference database of infrared images of normal subjects. The database was developed to assist clinicians in the diagnosis of various pathological conditions. The progress of this research has been published in refereed journals and has been presented to a variety of audiences at national and international conferences. He is currently involved in the continued research and development of the Mavis project. Mavis is a 3D imaging system developed for the non-contact measurement of chronic wounds. The device is also currently used for 3D measurement in the cosmetics industry. In September 2013, he was awarded with the Saxby Award for achievement in the field of three-dimensional imaging by the Royal Photographic Society.

Joanna Kajewska is a PhD student in Department of Medical Physics in University of Silesia, Katowice, Poland. University graduate in 2014 master's degree obtained from Medical Physics. On the PhD studies she is probing in thermal imaging on biological objects. Her purpose in researches is to find how infrared thermography could help in medical diagnosis.

Teresa Kasprzyk is a PhD student in Department of Medical Physics in University of Silesia, Katowice, Poland. University graduate in 2014 master's degree obtained from Medical Physics. On the PhD studies she is probing in thermal imaging on biological objects. Her purpose in researches is to find how infrared thermography could help in sport medicine.

Jose Martín has a B.S. degree in Physics (1997), a B.S. degree in Electronic Engineering (1999), a M.S. Degree in Electronic Engineering (2001) and a Ph.D. degree in Machine Learning (2004) from the University of Valencia, Spain. He is currently an Associate Professor at the Department of Electronic Engineering, University of Valencia. His research interests include Machine Learning and Computational Intelligence, with special emphasis in Reinforcement Learning and Quantum Machine Learning. He is a Member of the Medical Data Analysis Task Force (Data Mining Technical Committee, IEEE Computational Intelligence Society).

Paula A. Oliveira is an associated Professor in the area of Pharmacology and Animal Research. She graduated in Veterinary Medicine in 1996, obtained her PhD in Veterinary Sciences at University of Trás-os-Montes and Alto Douro in 2006 and her Habilitation in Pharmacology at University of Trás-os-Montes and Alto Douro in 2010. Presently, she teaches the courses of Pharmacology and Pharmacy, Pharmacology and Therapeutics, and Animal Research. She has supervised more 20 MSc and PhD students. Her main fields of research are animal models of cancer to evaluate new therapies.

Eduardo M. Pereira holds a Licenciatura (5-year degree) in Electronics and Telecommunications Engineering by Universidade de Aveiro (2004), a post-graduation in Computer Graphics and Virtual Environments by Universidade do Minho (2005), and achieved his Ph.D. under a collaboration between UT Austin-Texas University and Universidade do Porto in 2016. His research focuses on motion representations supported by relational-context features for the analysis of human activity in video frames captured from different camera-based devices. He has a large experience on the industry field where he has been exploring several topics from physical simulation environment, passing through 3D animation and game development, to analysis of human body gesture in space, until interactive technologies and natural user interfaces. He participated on the team that created the first 3D feature film in Portugal and Spain, at Dygrafilms. He was a co-founder, art-director and computer graphics developer of doubleMV, a game development company. He was the leader developer of the computer vision research and solutions at Edigma, trademark Displax. He also takes part on the development of an innovative capacitive multitouch patent platform, and related SDK. His last experience was at CoVii company, where he worked as a developer and consultor. He developed ViiMotion software/product that was on the top-ten finalist at ZON prize 2012, among other products.

Peter Plassmann is graduated in Electrical Engineering from the University and Fachhochschule of Hannover, Germany. He gained his PhD from the University of Glamorgan in 1992 for the development of an instrument for the non-contact three-dimensional measurement of human leg ulcers. While working as a Research Officer at the Wound Healing Research Unit, University Hospital of Wales, in Cardiff he developed this technology further to receive the RPS Williamson Award for Imaging Science Technology in 1993. Starting as a Research Fellow in 1994 at the University of South Wales he published over 30 papers on 3D and thermal imaging and was awarded the British Computer Society's Information Technology Medal in 1996. In 2007 he co-founded Photometrix Imaging Ltd. and is currently the company's managing director while simultaneously working as a Reader at the University of South Wales' School of Computing and Mathematical Sciences.

Jose I Priego-Quesada is a researcher in the Biophysics and Medical physics group (Physiology Department) and in the Research Group in Sport Biomechanics (Department of Physical Education and Sports) of the University of Valencia. Thermographer of level 1 by the Infrared Training Center. Previously, he worked for two years in the Biomechanics Institute of Valencia (IBV). His research topics of interest are the use of infrared thermography in sport assessment, cycling biomechanics, sport biomechanics and footwear assessment.

Francis Ring is head of Medical Imaging Research Unit and Professor at the department of Computing and Mathematical Sciences, Faculty of Computing, University of South Wales, U.K. Served in the Royal Air Force medical branch as a medical laboratory scientist, and then joined the Rheumatism Research Unit in Bath in 1959. He received a master's degree in 1975 in pharmacology and produced a thesis on the use of IR imaging to monitor the effect of drugs on the human body. He was awarded a Doctor of Science degree at Bath University in 1991 on account more than 250 papers on thermal imaging in medicine. He is Vice Chairman of The William Herschel Society in Bath and Academic Liaison Officer for The Royal Photographic Society, Imaging Science Group, in the UK.

Ana Rocha is master in Veterinary Medicine and PhD student in Veterinary Sciences. She has got experience in teaching. Her main areas of interest are oncology, angiogenesis and imaging. She is author/ co-author of 22 papers in ISI reputed journals, 28 abstracts in ISI journals, 6 papers in international journals with referee, 56 publications in proceedings books of international and national conferences, 17 oral communications and 50 posters in national and international meetings. She is also member of editorial board of three scientific journals and has collaborated as reviewer in several journals.

Rosario Salvador-Palmer graduated in Physics from the University of Valencia, Spain, in 1978 and received her PhD in Physics from the same university in 1987. She is currently professor of Biophysics and Medical Physic in the Department of Physiology, director of the Master's Degree in Physiology and Coordinator of the Doctoral Programme in Physiology of the University of Valencia. Her current research is focused on non-lesive medical image techniques as structured light and thermography and digital speckle procedures. She is member of different scientific associations and Member of the Organizing Committee of some Scientific Congresses.

Enrique Sanchis has a PhD in Physics from the University of Valencia Estudi General (UVEG) and Professor in the area of Electronic Technology at the University of Valencia. His basic research activity is focused on the field of Electronics for radiation detectors. He has participated in particle physics experiments at CERN, where he has developed contributions to the design of the trigger system and data acquisition detector. He is author of many international publications in international journals of high impact (Institute of Electrical and Electronic engineers). He has chaired the 13th IEEE Congress on Real Time (Nuclear and Plasma Sciences Society). In applied research he has carried out activities in technological innovation for industrial applications, having directed an Institutional Chair in the field of audio and videocommunications for inmotic applications. Besides this, he has promoted, directed and developed joint projects for applied research centers and hospital units in the field of health, particularly in medical applications and disability. He is author of industrial patents. He has directed numerous doctoral theses and is reviewer of international journals both in basic and applied research. His research has led to activities in transfer knowledge to society, particularly in the industrial sector and health. He is Full Professor at the UVEG (School of Engineering and Physics Faculty), where he teaches Communications Technology, Technology for Radiation Detectors and Electronics. He is author of educational publications. He has held various positions of university management. Among others, the leadership of the Department of Electronic Engineering and deputy director of the School of Engineering and membership in the Faculty of the University of Valencia. He participated in the 2010 elections to the Rector of the UVEG, as candidate for Vice Chancellor for Knowledge Transfer.

Enrique Sanchis-Sanchez has B.S. degree in Physical Therapy (2011), a M.S. degree in 2012 and a Ph.D. degree (Infrared Thermal Imaging, diagnositc test accuracy) in 2014 from the University of Valencia, Spain. He is currently an Associate Professor at the Faculty of Health Sciences, European University of Valencia. His research interests include Orthopedic Manual Therapy, Screening tests and neuromusculoeskeletal rehabilitation.

Adérito Seixas is graduated in Physiotherapy and specialized in neuromusculoskeletal rehabilitation. He received his MSc from University of Porto for a thesis focused on the assessment of sensorimotor skills of abled and disabled athletes. Currently, alongside his work as a full time Professor on a Physiotherapy Graduate course and Master Program at Universidade Fernando Pessoa, he is carrying out research for his PhD and his focus is on thermal imaging applications in rehabilitation and sports, and on the assessment of the sensorimotor system. He is a board member of the European Association of Thermology and member of the International Society of Biomechanics and the Portuguese Association of Physiotherapists.

Karolina Sieroń-Stołtny is an Associate professor at the Department and Clinical Department of Internal Diseases, Angiology and at the Physical Medicine Department at the Chair of Physiotherapy, of the Medical University of Silesia in Bytom. She is a specialist in internal diseases. Her main academic interest focuses on gastroenterology and physical medicine.

Manuel Sillero Quintana has a PhD. in Physical Activity and Sport Sciences and is lecturer at the Faculty of Physical Activity and Sport Sciences (INEF) at the Technical University of Madrid. His teaching includes "Athletics" at graduate level and "New technologies for researching in Physical Activity and Sport Sciences" and "Kinanthropometry" at postgraduate level. His research experience includes more than 24 research National and International projects on the areas of thermography applied to humans, visual perception, sports vision, kinantropometry and body composition, having published, 4 chapter books, more than 24 articles in JCR impact journals and more than 50 entries in congresses proceedings including several invited lectures in International congresses. He is current member of the executive board of the European Association of Thermology (EAT) and the International Society for the Advancement in Kinanthropometry (ISAK).

António Silva has begun his academic career in the Polytechnic of Porto, Mechanical Engineering and subsequently obtained a Master Degree in Mechanical Engineering - Automation from the Faculty of Engineering of the University of Porto. It is currently a researcher at FEUP and is awaiting to present and defend his PhD thesis, Detection and Characterization of Defects in Composite Materials Using Thermography. He is the author and co-author of several international publications in the field of instrumentation, control and monitoring of living things - eg, Olympic athletes, musical performers, and animals. In the last years has dedicate his research activities to Non-destructive Test techniques using thermography.

Maria Soroko gained her PhD in Agricultural Science with a specialisation in Animal Husbandry from the University of Environmental and Life Sciences of Wroclaw, Department of Horse Breeding and Equestrian Studies in 2013. Her Masters degree in Equine Science was completed in 2010 at the Institute of Biological, Environmental and Rural Sciences, Aberystwyth University, Wales, United Kingdom. Since 2008 the author has practiced thermography extensively in equine physiotherapy and in veterinary medicine, cooperating with veterinarians, horse breeders and trainers. She is also the owner and director of the company "Equine Massage - Maria Soroko", www.eqma.pl, which offers equine rehabilitation and thermography services, professional courses and workshops associated with horse rehabilitation and the application of thermography in veterinary and sports medicine. Maria conducts research on the application of thermography in sport and racing horses, authoring numerous original publications and overview papers. She is also a member of the European Association of Thermology. She has many years of experience in equine physiotherapy, achieving qualifications as an Equine Body Worker in sport massage and remedial therapy. Maria is also a riding instructor at the British Horse Society. Her skills and experience were achieved both in Europe and Australia.

Agata Stanek is an Associate Professor of the Medical University of Silesia, Poland. She is a specialist in internal diseases, angiology and physical medicine. Her main academic interest focuses on oxidative stress in patients with rheumatic diseases, impact of extremely low temperatures (cryotherapy and cryostimulation) on human body (prooxidant-antioxidant status, inflammatory status, lipid profile) and photodynamic therapy as well as clinical application of extremely-low-frequency and weak variable magnetic fields- magnetotherapy and magnetostimulation and low-energy lasers. She is also an expert in thermography imaging in medicine. She is a scientist highly respected not only in Poland but also abroad, with scientific achievements such as participating in academic publications. She is a member of many domestic and foreign scientific associations.

Index

V

W

www.ingramcontent.com/pod-product-compliance
Lightning Source LLC
LaVergne TN
LVHW080536300926
849162LV00007B/1615